Essentials of
Head and Neck Cancer

Essentials of
Head and Neck Cancer

Edited by

ALBERTO STAFFIERI
PAUL SEBASTIAN
MADAN KAPRE
BIPIN T. VARGHESE
REHAN KAZI

BYWORD BOOKS™

The mention of specific companies or of certain manufacturers' products does not imply that they are endorsed or recommended by the authors in preference to others of a similar nature that are not mentioned. The names of proprietary products are distinguished by initial capital letters.

Dosage, treatment schedule and methods are being constantly revised and new side-effects recognized. The reader is thus strongly urged to consult the printed instructions of drug companies before administering any of the drugs recommended in this book. It is possible that errors might have crept in despite our best efforts.

The publication of this book is supported by educational and research grants from the Cancer Aid and Research Foundation (CARF), Mumbai, India, and Head and Neck Cancer Research Service, United Kingdom.

First published 2012

10 9 8 7 6 5 4 3 2 1

ISBN 978-81-8193-071-2

Cover design: Netra Shyam
Typesetting: Jacob Thomas, Shailesh Misra

Published by
Byword Books Private Limited
GF-15, Virat Bhavan
Mukherjee Nagar Commercial Complex
Delhi 110009, India; Phone: 011-47038040
email: bywordbooks@gmail.com
website: www.bywordbooks.in

Printed in India by Manipal Technologies Ltd, Manipal, India

Contents

Foreword .... *vii*

Preface .... *ix*

Contributors .... *xi*

Abbreviations .... *xv*

1. Epidemiology, aetiology and natural history of head and neck cancer 1
   RAGHAV C. DWIVEDI, EDWARD CHISHOLM, NAMITA KANWAR, ANDRZEJ KOMOROWSKI, REHAN KAZI

2. Evaluation, management and outcomes of head and neck cancer 19
   RAGHAV C. DWIVEDI, NISHANT AGRAWAL, RAVI C. DWIVEDI, K.A. PATHAK, REHAN KAZI

3. Pathology of head and neck cancer 33
   JAYASREE K, THARA SOMANATHAN, BIPIN T. VARGHESE, PAUL SEBASTIAN

4. Radiology of head and neck malignancies 47
   K. RAMACHANDRAN, M. VENUGOPAL, V. JIJI, S.M. KOSHY, ANIL PRAHLADAN

5. Role of radiotherapy in head and neck cancer 57
   R. REJNISH KUMAR, CESSAL THOMMACHAN, K. RAMADAS, B. RAJAN

6. Role of chemotherapy in head and neck cancer 67
   CESSAL THOMMACHAN, K. RAMADAS, REJNISH KUMAR, B. RAJAN

7. Reconstruction in head and neck cancer 72
   SHAJI THOMAS, SUBRAMANIA IYER, SOWRABH KUMAR ARORA, BIPIN T. VARGHESE

8. Management of cervical metastases 93
   JOHANNES J. FAGAN

9. Cancer of the lip and oral cavity 103
   PAUL SEBASTIAN, ELIZABETH MATHEW IYPE, SAJITH BABU, BIPIN T. VARGHESE

10. Cancer of the oropharynx 114
    N. KANNAN, BIPIN T. VARGHESE, K. CHANDRAMOHAN, PAUL SEBASTIAN

11. Cancer of the larynx—early stage 123
    ALBERTO STAFFIERI, GINO MARIONI, BIPIN T. VARGHESE

12. Cancer of the larynx—advanced stage 136
    UMANATH NAYAK, REHAN KAZI

13. Cancer of the hypopharynx 143
UMANATH NAYAK, REHAN KAZI

14. Cancer of the nose and paranasal sinuses 150
RANJIT RAJAN, ALOK THAKAR, DAN FLISS, BIPIN T. VARGHESE

15. Cancer of the nasopharynx 167
CESSAL THOMMACHAN, REJNISH KUMAR, K. RAMADAS, B. RAJAN

16. Cancer of the thyroid and parathyroid glands 175
MADAN KAPRE

17. Cancer of the major salivary glands 185
MADAN KAPRE

18. Cancer of the skull base 193
C. RAYAPPA, K. KUMARESH

19. Cancer of the skin and ear 212
B.E. MOSTAFA, P. ARUN, BIPIN T. VARGHESE

20. Swallowing rehabilitation following head and neck cancer 225
KAPILA MANIKANTAN, RAGHAV C. DWIVEDI, REHAN KAZI

21. Speech and olfactory rehabilitation following head and neck cancer 237
PRASHANT PAWAR, SUHAIL SAYED, RAGHAV C. DWIVEDI, REHAN KAZI

22. Quality of life (QOL) outcomes in head and neck cancer 247
SUHAIL SAYED, RAGHAV C. DWIVEDI, ALOK PATHAK, REHAN KAZI

23. TNM classification of head and neck cancer 253
KAPILA MANIKANTAN, RAGHAV C. DWIVEDI, K.A. PATHAK, REHAN KAZI

24. Novel therapeutic approaches to head and neck cancer 256
KEVIN J. HARRINGTON

25. Post-treatment surveillance in head and neck cancer 267
KAPILA MANIKANTAN, RAGHAV C. DWIVEDI, REHAN KAZI

Index 275

Foreword

It is indeed a great pleasure and special honour for me to write this Foreword for *Essentials of Head and Neck Cancer* edited by Drs Staffieri, Sebastian, Kapre, Varghese and Kazi. Clearly, this is a gathering of senior head and neck surgeons who have undertaken an outstanding job of compiling multidisciplinary management of head and neck cancer. The theme of the book is to present the current advances and comprehensive management of head and neck cancer in the state–of-the-art fashion. The book includes several chapters on the principles of management of head and neck cancers including epidemiology, evaluation, pathology, radiology, multidisciplinary treatment, chemotherapy and reconstruction. There are several individual organ-site chapters discussing treatment approaches to different regions in the head and neck including thyroid tumours.

There are also many excellent chapters on swallowing, speech rehabilitation and quality of life. There is a dedicated chapter on novel therapeutic approaches and post-treatment surveillance. The compilation of these chapters represents a considerable thought process among the editors. Each chapter is written by well recognized head and neck surgeons with one or two senior authors. The book has been formatted very well with excellent tables, figures and colour combinations. It is easy to read and easy to digest. I have enjoyed reading several chapters and am quite confident this will be a handy book for head and neck trainees, practical clinicians and specialists. It will provide a road map for the treatment of head and neck cancer worldwide, especially Southeast Asia. The rich experience of Indian editors will be helpful for the Indian subcontinent to use this book as a decision-maker in patients with head and neck cancer presenting with early and advanced stages.

I would like to congratulate the editors and individual authors for accomplishing their goals of producing *Essentials of Head and Neck Cancer*. I think this book represents not only the essentials, but also the advances and state-of-the-art of management of head and neck cancer. I would strongly recommend this book as a handy reference source.

ASHOK R. SHAHA
Professor of Surgery
Jatin P. Shah Chair in Head and Neck Oncology
Memorial Sloan-Kettering Cancer Center
New York

Preface

Head and neck cancer is the fifth commonest cancer in the world. Although it is a rare cancer in the western world, it accounts for nearly one-third of all cancer cases in high-risk countries such as India, Pakistan, Bangladesh and Sri Lanka. It comprises a heterogeneous group of neoplasms arising in anatomically and physiologically diverse regions—the head and neck. These constitute the area from the dura to the pleura, and contain organs/structures essential for basic sensations such as vision, hearing, smell and taste. The area is traversed by virtually all the vital nerves, and vessels and tracts important for the survival of a human being. Head and neck tumours are anatomically and histopathologically diverse; approximately 35 different anatomical sites are present in the head and neck region and over 35 different types of tumours are known to occur in just one site (salivary glands).

Nowhere else in the human body is the effect of a disease process more readily apparent, more functionally and psychologically disturbing, and more aesthetically deforming than in the head and neck region. Moreover, the chances of distant metastases in head and neck cancer are very low compared with any other region, which makes the illness more protracted. In many cases, catastrophic loco-regional effects (e.g. bleeding and airway obstruction) serve as eventual life-takers. Aggressive loco-regional therapy is therefore warranted in all cases at least to circumvent these effects, if not to enhance survival. Each site has its own peculiar presentation; and anatomical, physiological and functional considerations. The natural history of the tumours is also different, which makes treating these cancers a challenging task. Therefore, optimal management of patients with head and neck cancer should be individualized and expert inputs are needed from various disciplines. Three decades ago, this led to the adoption of a multidisciplinary team approach to the management of patients with head and neck cancer, and is still the gold standard of practice.

Over the past few decades, our knowledge of the disease process, and epidemiological and aetiopathogenic factors has increased immensely owing to a better understanding of molecular, epigenetic and genetic interactions involved in the development, progression and metastatic spread of head and neck cancers. There has also been tremendous progress in diagnostic and imaging modalities, which help in early detection and accurate staging of the disease, leading to better outcomes. Remarkable progress has also been made in every treatment modality; surgery is now more refined, less radical and more functional as a result of incorporation of lasers and robotic operative techniques, and microvascular reconstructive techniques. Radiotherapy has become more target-specific and less destructive; addition of chemotherapeutic agents has improved outcomes. Incorporation of functional outcome and quality-of-life aspects have changed the face of rehabilitation for these patients resulting in their early integration in society, which was a far-fetched dream three decades ago.

This book brings together a broad, comprehensive and balanced view of current approaches to the multidisciplinary management and underlying biology of head and neck cancers. It also covers a wide range of exciting new findings in both the clinical and the basic sciences relevant to head and neck cancer. A generational equipoise has been aimed at by combining contributions from established leaders and upcoming stars. We hope that this book will provide the necessary grounding for residents, speech language therapists, otolaryngologists, head and neck surgeons, and oncologists.

REHAN KAZI
BIPIN T. VARGHESE

Contributors

NISHANT AGRAWAL
Department of Otolaryngology-Head & Neck Surgery, Johns Hopkins University School of Medicine, 601 N Caroline St, JHOC 6, Baltimore, MD 21287, USA; nagrawal@jhmi.edu

SOWRABH KUMAR ARORA
Head and Neck Services, Division of Surgical Oncology, Regional Cancer Centre, Thiruvananthapuram, Kerala, India; sowrabhinus@yahoo.com

P. ARUN
Department of Head and Neck Surgery, Tata Medical Centre Cancer Hospital, Rajarhat Newtown, Kolkata 700156, West Bengal, India; Fellow, National Institutes of Health (USA); arunpattu@gmail.com

SAJITH BABU T.P.
Department of Surgical Oncology, Malabar Cancer centre, Thalassery, Kannur, Kerala, India; drsajith@gmail.com

K. CHANDRAMOHAN
Division of Surgical Oncology, Regional Cancer Centre, Thiruvananthapuram, Kerala, India; drchandramohan@gmail.com

EDWARD CHISHOLM
Department of ENT, Musgrove Park Hospital, Taunton, Somerset, UK; edwardchisholm@doctors.org.uk

RAVI C. DWIVEDI
Department of Internal Medicine, MB Centre for Proteomics & Systems Biology, University of Manitoba, Winnipeg, MB, R3E 3P4, Canada; dwivedi@cc.umanitoba.ca

RAGHAV C. DWIVEDI
Department of Head and Neck Surgery, Head and Neck Unit, Royal Marsden Hospital, London, SW3 6JJ, UK; raghav_dwivedi@rediffmail.com

JOHANNES J. FAGAN
Division of Otolaryngology, Faculty of Health Sciences, University of Cape Town, H53 OMB, Groote Schuur Hospital, Observatory, Cape Town, 7925, South Africa; Johannes.fagan@uct.ac.za, fagan@iafrica.com

DAN FLISS
Department of Otolaryngology Head and Neck Surgery, Tel Aviv Sourasky Medical Center and the Faculty of Medicine, Tel Aviv University, 6 Weizmann St., Tel Aviv 64239, Israel; fliss@tasmc.health.gov.il; danf@tasmc.health.gov.il

K.J. HARRINGTON
Division of Experimental Biological Therapies, The Institute of Cancer Research, Targeted Therapy Laboratory, Chester Beatty Laboratories, 237 Fulham Road, London SW3 6JB, UK; kevin.harrington@icr.ac.uk

SUBRAMANIA IYER
Division of Reconstructive Surgery and Head and Neck Surgery, Amrita Institute OF Medical Sciences, Kochi, Kerala, India

ELIZABETH MATHEW IYPE
Division of Surgical Oncology, Regional Cancer Centre, Thiruvananthapuram, Kerala, India; elizabethrcc@gmail.com

V. JIJI
Division of Imageology, Regional Cancer Centre, Thiruvananthapuram, Kerala, India

JAYASREE K.
Division of Pathology, Regional Cancer Centre, Thiruvananthapuram, Kerala, India; jayasreeramdas@gmail.com

NAMITA KANWAR
Department of Internal Medicine, MB Centre for Proteomics & Systems Biology, University of Manitoba, Winnipeg, MB, R3E 3P4, Canada; kanwar@cc.umanitoba.ca

N. KANNAN
Department of Surgical Oncology, Army Hospital (R&R), New Delhi 110010, India; majkannan@gmail.com

MADAN KAPRE
Neeti Clinics, Nagpur, Madhya Pradesh, India; madankapre@gmail.com

REHAN KAZI
Institute of Head & Neck Studies & Education [InHanse], University Hospital Coventry & CTU, Warwick Medical School, Clifford Bridge Road, Coventry CV2 2DX, UK; Secretary-General: Cancer Aid & Research Foundation, India; rehan_kazi@yahoo.com

ANDRZEJ KOMOROWSKI
Servicio de Cirugia General, Hospital Virgen del Camino, 11540 Sanlúcar de Barrameda (CADIZ), Spain; alkomorowski@wp.pl

S.M. KOSHY
Division of Imageology, Regional Cancer Centre, Thiruvananthapuram 695011, Kerala, India

R. REJNISH KUMAR
Division of Radiation Oncology, Regional Cancer Centre, Thiruvananthapuram, Kerala, India; rejinish@yahoo.com

K. KUMARESH
Department of ENT-Head and Neck Surgery, Apollo Hospital, Bangalore, Karnataka, India

KAPILA MANIKANTAN
Department of ENT and Head & Neck Surgery, St Johns National Academy of Health, Sciences, Sarjapur Road, Bangalore 560034, Karnataka, India; kapila.manikantan@gmail.com

GINO MARIONI
Department of Medical and Surgical Specialties, Section of Otolaryngology, University of Padova, Via Giustiniani 2, 35100 Padova, Italy; gino.marioni@unipd.it

BADR E. MOSTAFA
Department of ENT-HNS, Ain-Shams Faculty of Medicine, 48 Ibn El Nafess treet, 11371-Nasr City, Cairo, Egypt;
bemostafa@yahoo.com, bemostafa@med.asu.edu.eg

UMANATH NAYAK
Cancer Institute, Apollo Health City, Jubilee Hills, Hyderabad 500033, India; drumanathnayak@gmail.com

K.A. PATHAK
Head and Neck Surgical Oncology, University of Manitoba, and Head & Neck Surgical Fellowship, Cancer Care Manitoba,
GF 440 A, 820 Sherbrook Street, Winnipeg R3A 1R9, Canada; kapathak@gmail.com

PRASHANT PAWAR
Department of Otolaryngology and Head & Neck Surgery, Grant Medical College and Sir J.J. Group of Hospitals, Byculla,
Mumbai, India; pawarvprashant@yahoo.co.in

ANIL PRAHLADAN
Division of Imageology, Regional Cancer Centre, Thiruvananthapuram 695011, Kerala, India; dr.anil2000@gmail.com

B. RAJAN
Department of Oncology, National Oncology Centre, Royal Hospital, Muscat

RANJIT RAJAN
Department of Otorhinolaryngology, Amala Institute of Medical Sciences, Thrissur 680555, Kerala, India;
ranjitrajan.ent@gmail.com

K. RAMACHANDRAN
Division of Imageology, Regional Cancer Centre, Thiruvananthapuram, Kerala, India; drkramachandran@hotmail.com

K. RAMADAS
Division of Head and Neck Oncology, Regional Cancer Centre, Thiruvananthapuram, Kerala, India; ramdasrcc@gmail.com

C. RAYAPPA
ENT-Head and Neck and Skull Base Surgeon, Apollo Speciality Hospital, Chennai, Tamil Nadu, India; drrayappa@yahoo.com

SUHAIL SAYED
Department of Otolaryngology and Head & Neck Surgery, Grant Medical College and Sir J.J. Group of Hospitals, Byculla,
Mumbai, India; drsuhailsayed@gmail.com

PAUL SEBASTIAN
Division of Surgical Oncology, Regional Cancer Centre, Thiruvananthapuram, Kerala, India; psebastian2091@gmail.com

THARA SOMANATHAN
Division of Pathology, Regional Cancer Centre, Thiruvananthapuram, Kerala, India; drtharas@gmail.com

ALBERTO STAFFIERI
Department of Medical and Surgical Specialties, Section of Otolaryngology, University of Padova, Via Giustiniani 2,
35100 Padova, Italy; alberto.staffieri@unipd.it

ALOK THAKAR
Department of Otolaryngology & Head Neck Surgery, All India Institute of Medical Sciences, New Delhi 110029, India;
drathakar@gmail.com

SHAJI THOMAS
Division of Surgical Oncology, Regional Cancer Centre, Thiruvananthapuram, Kerala, India; shajircc@gmail.com

K. CESSAL THOMMACHAN
Division of Head and Neck Oncology, Regional Cancer Centre, Thiruvananthapuram, Kerala, India; drcessalthomas@gmail.com

BIPIN T. VARGHESE
Head and Neck Services, Division of Surgical Oncology, Regional Cancer Centre, Thiruvananthapuram 695011, Kerala, India; bipinrcc@gmail.com

M. VENUGOPAL
Division of Imageology, Regional Cancer Centre, Thiruvananthapuram 695011, Kerala, India; drvenurcc@gmail.com

Abbreviations

3-D CRT	3-D conformal radiotherapy		EAC	external auditory canal
ACC	adenoid cystic carcinoma		EAM	external auditory meatus
ACS	American Cancer Society		EBV	Epstein–Barr virus
AJCC	American Joint Committee on Cancer		ECS	extracapsular spread
ALDH	aldehyde dehydrogenase		EGFR	epidermal growth factor receptor
ALT (flap)	anterolateral thigh (flap)		EMA	epithelial membrane antigen
APUD	amine precursor uptake and deamination		EMZBCL	extranodal marginal zone B cell lymphoma
ASCO	American Society of Clinical Oncology		END	elective neck dissection
ASR	age-standardized incidence rates		EORTC	European Organization for Research and Treatment of Cancer
ASTA	anterior branch of the superficial temporal artery		EUA	examination under anaesthesia
ATP	adenosine triphosphate		EWS/PNET	Ewing sarcoma/primitive neuroectodermal tumour
BCC	basal cell carcinoma		FA	Fanconi anaemia
bFGF	basic fibroblast growth factor		FACT-G	Functional Assessment of Cancer Therapy-General
BFI	Brief Fatigue Inventory			
BIPP	bismuth subnitrate iodoform paraffin paste		FDG	2-[18F] fluoro-2-deoxy-d-glucose
BOT	base of tongue		FEES	functional endoscopic evaluation of swallowing
BPI	Brief Pain Inventory			
CASTLE	carcinoma with thymus-like features		FNA	fine-needle aspiration
CDK	cyclin-dependent kinase		FNAB	fine-needle aspiration biopsy
CDKi	cyclin-dependent kinase inhibitor		FNAC	fine-needle aspiration cytology
CEA	carcino-embroyonic antigen		FOSS	functional outcome of the swallowing scale
CFR	craniofacial resection		GFR	growth factor receptor
CHEP	cricohyoidoepiglottopexy		GP	galeo-pericranial flap
CHP	cricohyoidopexy		GSPN	greater superficial petrosal nerve
CI	confidence interval		Gy	Gray
CNS	central nervous system		HBO	hyperbaric oxygen
CPA	cerebello pontine angle		HIV	human immunodeficiency virus
CRT	chemoradiation		HME	heat and moisture exchanger
CSF	cerebrospinal fluid		HNC	head and neck cancer
CT	computed tomography		HNSCC	head and neck squamous cell carcinoma
CTA	CT angiography		HPV	human papillomavirus
DCIA (flap)	deep circumflex iliac artery (flap)		HRQOL	health related QOL
DLBCL	diffuse large B cell lymphoma		IAP	inhibitor of apoptosis proteins
DLT	dose-limiting toxicity		ICA	internal carotid artery
DM	desmoplastic melanoma		IGRT	image-guided radiation therapy
DP	deltopectoral			

IJV	internal jugular vein
IMRT	intensity-modulated radiation therapy
ITF	infratemporal fossa
IVRS	interactive voice response system
KID	keratitis, ichthyosis and deafness
LET	linear energy transfer
LM	lentigo maligna
MAB	monoclonal antibody
MALT	mucoid-associated lymphoid tissue
MDADI	MD Anderson Dysphagia Inventory
MDT	multidisciplinary team
MEN	multiple endocrine neoplasia
MND	modified neck dissection
MNG	multinodular goitre
MOS	Medical Outcomes Study
MRA	MR angiography
MRI	magnetic resonance imaging
MRSA	methicillin-resistant *Staphylococcus aureus*
MTC	medullary thyroid carcinoma
NAIM	nasal airflow inducing manoeuvre
NCDB	National Cancer Data Base
NCI	National Cancer Institute
NG	nasogastric
NICE	National Institute for Clinical and Health Excellence
NIH	National Institute of Health
NPC	nasopharyngeal carcinoma
NPV	negative predictive value
NTL	near total laryngectomy
NTLER	near total laryngectomy with epiglottic reconstruction
OER	oxygen enhancement ratio
OPG	orthopantogram
OPL	open partial laryngectomy
OPSE	oropharyngeal swallowing efficiency
ORN	osteoradionecrosis
OSCC	oral squamous cell carcinoma
PDGF	platelet derived growth factor
PDT	photodynamic therapy
PE	pharyngoesophageal
PEG	percutaneous endoscopic gastrostomy
PES	pharyngo-oesophageal sphincter
PET	positron emission tomography
PET-CT	positron emission tomography-CT
PMD	potentially malignant disorder
PMMC	Pectoralis major myocutaneous
PND	prophylactic neck dissection
PNI	perineural invasion
PNS	paranasal sinus
PTEN	phosphatase and tensin homologue
QOL	quality of life
RBE	relative biological effectiveness
rCBF	regional cerebral blood flow
RND	radical neck dissection
RNS	reactive nitrogen species
ROS	reactive oxygen species
RT	radiotherapy
RTOG	Radiation Therapy Oncology Group
SAN	spinal accessory nerve
SCC	squamous cell carcinoma
SCL	supracricoid laryngectomy
SCM	sternocleidomastoid muscle
SEER	Surveillance Epidemiology and End Results
SES	socioeconomic status
SETTLE	spindle and epithelial thymus-like tumours
SIADH	syndrome of inappropriate antidiuretic hormone secretion
SIP	Sickness Impact Profile
SLC	secondary lymphoid organ chemokine
SND	selective neck dissection
SPECT	single photon emission computerized tomography
SPL	supracricoid partial laryngectomy
SRT	surgery followed by radiation
SUV	standardized uptake value
TANIS	Tumour and Node Integer Score
TBO	trial balloon occlusion
TE	tracheo-oesophageal
TEP	TE puncture
TFL-IC (flap)	tensor fascia lata–iliac crest (flap)
TG	thyroglobulin
TGF-α	transforming growth factor alpha
TGF-β	transforming growth factor beta
TK	tyrosine kinase
TKI	TK inhibitor
TNF-α	tumour necrosis factor alpha
TNM	tumour, node, metastasis (classification)
TRH	thyrotropin-releasing hormone
TSG	tumour suppressor gene
TSH	thyroid stimulating hormone
UADT	upper aerodigestive tract
UCLA	University of California, Los Angeles
UICC	Union International Contre le Cancer
USFDA	United States Food and Drug Administration
USG	ultrasonography
USGFNAC	ultrasound-guided fine-needle aspiration cytology
UWQOL	University of Washington QOL questionnaire
VEGF	vascular endothelial growth factor
VPL	vertical partial laryngectomy
VRQOL	voice-related QOL
WHO	World Health Organization
XIAP	X-linked IAP
XIn	spinal accessory nerve

Epidemiology, aetiology and natural history of head and neck cancer

RAGHAV C. DWIVEDI, EDWARD CHISHOLM, NAMITA KANWAR,
ANDRZEJ KOMOROWSKI, REHAN KAZI

Head and neck cancer (HNC) is a deadly disease known to exist ever since the origins of the human race. The oldest proof of HNC comes from a fossilized human mandibular fragment, probably dating back to the middle Pleistocene epoch of the Cenozoic era (>500,000 years ago). The fossil shows an extensive, irregular lesion extending onto the lingual and labial surfaces of the jaw in the region of the mandibular symphysis[1] and is regarded to be the oldest known instance of a tumour in a human species.

The oldest written documentation of HNC dates back to 1600–1550 BC, with Ebers Papyrus containing a description of treating an 'eating ulcer on the gums'.[2] However, this document is believed to contain descriptions originating from as early as 3000–2500 BC.[2] According to Ebers Papyrus, the ancient Egyptians appear to have treated oral cavity cancer with a mixture of cinnamon, gum, honey and oil.[2] Hippocrates (460 BC) was the first to use the term 'carcinoma'.[3] In ancient Rome, Aurelius Cornelius Celsus (AD 30) treated cancer of the face and lip by excision. Galen (AD 200) advocated the humoral theory of disease and postulated that cancer was a systemic disease and therefore had to be treated systemically.[3] Medical knowledge stagnated in the following centuries because of religious concerns about anatomical dissections and surgical operations.[4] During the Renaissance (AD ≈1500–1760) the influence of Galen's doctrine slowly declined and scientists, notably Andreas Vesalius, used anatomical studies to broaden their medical knowledge.[3] Before the introduction of tobacco in the late 16th century, oral cancer was seldom mentioned in medical writings.[5] Obviously, this changed in subsequent years. In 1650, Richard Wiseman[6] gave the first

detailed report on the treatment of oral cancer, and in 1664 Marchetti[7] described the first glossectomy for cancer. The 18th century witnessed the emergence of the first theories about the pathogenesis of cancer and the opening of the first cancer hospital in Rheims, France.[3] Awareness of the importance of nodal metastasis appeared in the medical literature around 1790.[8] The 19th century brought many breakthroughs in diagnostic tools, anaesthetic techniques, surgical therapy and understanding of pathological mechanisms.[4] By 1860, scientists had studied the dynamics of lymphatic spread and defined five different phases as the crucial events in metastatic spread, viz. liberation, transportation, deposition, establishment, and growth of malignant cells.[8] Rudalph Virchow (1821–1902) initiated the histological approach to tumours and his concept of cellular pathology finally made it possible to overturn the concept of humoral pathology.[9] In the late 19th century, Thiersch[10] and Waldeyer[11,12] proved that cancer originated from the epithelial surface and invaded the stroma. The surgeons Carl Ruge, Johan Veit and Friedrich von Esmarch regarded surgical biopsies as an essential tool for diagnosis.[13,14] Although the acceptance of histological examination of biopsies was slow, by the end of 19th and the beginning of the 20th century histological evaluation of tumours became standard practice.[15]

By the second half of 19th century advances in antisepsis, anaesthesia and airway management opened new possibilities for surgical treatment of HNC.[4] A major breakthrough was the introduction of general anaesthesia by Horace Wells (1815–1848), William Thomas Green Morton (1819–1868) and John Collins Warren (1778–1856). On 16 October 1846,

Dr Warren removed a cervical tumour from a patient with ether anaesthesia, administered by Morton.[4] This successful procedure, witnessed by a number of important colleagues, established a place for general anaesthesia in surgery, and opened the door to performing major surgical procedures of all types, including those on the head and neck.[4] The first total laryngectomy in cancer patients was performed by Billroth on 31 December 1873. Five years later, in 1878, he was again the first to perform a hemilaryngectomy. Vertical and horizontal laryngectomies had to await the developments of the 20th century.[4]

The 20th century witnessed further advances in medicine and surgery. The first half of the century was interrupted by two world wars which spawned the specialty of reconstructive or plastic surgery, but by mid-century, the availability of blood transfusion, antibiotics and modern closed-system anaesthesia permitted the concepts of earlier surgeons to be developed by their modern counterparts into safe, effective and reproducible operations.[4] A major development in the 20th century was the discovery of non-surgical methods of treatment, viz. irradiation, and later, chemotherapy. These provided alternative methods of treatment, as well as layers of additional, or adjuvant, treatment—'multimodality therapy'. Thus the surgeon was relieved of the burden of having the only effective means of treating cancer.[4] With the development of modern technologies, the second half of 20th century and first few years of the 21st century witnessed an exponential growth in the understanding, diagnosis and treatment of HNCs, which, it is hoped continues at even a faster pace.

Epidemiology

HNC is a heterogeneous group of neoplasms with diverse natural history arising in one anatomical region. It is a broad term, which encompasses tumours arising from the mucosa of the upper aerodigestive tract (UADT), including the paranasal sinus, nasal cavity, oral cavity, pharynx and larynx. It also includes tumours arising from salivary glands, thyroid and parathyroid, bony tumours, and those arising from the skin and soft tissues of this anatomical region. Consequently, tumours arising at different sub-sites within the head and neck region have their own unique sets of epidemiological, pathological and treatment considerations. By far the most common histological type of HNC is squamous cell carcinoma (SCC), which constitutes >90% of all HNCs, and occurs commonly in the oral cavity, oropharynx, larynx and hypopharynx.[16,17] Other less common histological variants of this region are lymphoma, adenocarcinoma, adenoid cystic carcinoma, melanoma and basal cell carcinioma, which collectively account for <10% of all HNCs.

HNC is the fifth commonest cancer worldwide,[18] with an extensively variable incidence of 0.5–43.1 per 100,000 (Fig. 1) and represents approximately 6% of the entire global cancer

burden.[19] According to a recent estimate, >784,880 new cases and >387,100 cancer deaths are reported each year throughout the world[18] (Table 1). Although HNCs are categorized under the 'rare cancers' in the developed world, with <4% of all newly diagnosed cancer cases, they represent the commonest form of cancers in certain high-risk areas (e.g. Sri Lanka, India, Bangladesh and Pakistan), and may contribute to as high as 25%–37.5% of all new cancer cases.[18] Nearly two-thirds of these HNC cases come from less developed or developing countries (Fig. 2).[18] Excluding thyroid cancers and looking specifically at the commonest HNC variant, viz. SCC of the head and neck (HNSCC) alone, then HNC ranks sixth among all cancers with >640,000 new cancer cases and >350,000 cancer deaths per year globally (Table 1).[18] Among all the forms of HNSCC, oral cancer alone is the most common cancer and is responsible for >274,000 new cases and >127,000

Table 1. Global incidence of and mortality due to various cancers (data from reference 18)

Rank	Site	No. of cancer cases	No. of cancer deaths
1.	Lung	1,352,132	1,178,918
2.	Breast	1,151,298	410,712
3.	Colon and rectum	1,023,152	528,978
4.	Stomach	933,937	700,349
5.	Head and neck (all sub-sites included)	784,882	387,115
6.	Prostate	679,023	221,002
7.	Liver	626,162	598,321
8.	Cervix uteri	493,243	273,505
9.	Oesophagus	462,117	385,892
10.	Bladder	356,557	145,009
11.	Non-Hodgkin lymphoma	300,571	171,820
12.	Leukaemia	300,522	222,506
13.	Oral cavity[a]	274,289	127,459
14.	Pancreas	232,306	227,023
15.	Kidney, etc.	208,480	101,895
16.	Ovary	204,499	124,860
17.	Corpus uteri	198,783	50,327
18.	Brain (including nervous system)	189,485	141,650
19.	Melanoma (cutaneous)	160,177	40,781
20.	Larynx[b]	159,241	89,956
21.	Thyroid[c]	141,013	35,375
22.	Pharynx (other)[d]	130,296	83,993
23.	Multiple myeloma	85,704	62,535
24.	Nasopharynx[e]	80,043	50,332

[a] Overall individual ranking 12   [b] Overall individual ranking 19
[c] Overall individual ranking 20   [d] Overall individual ranking 21
[e] Overall individual ranking 23

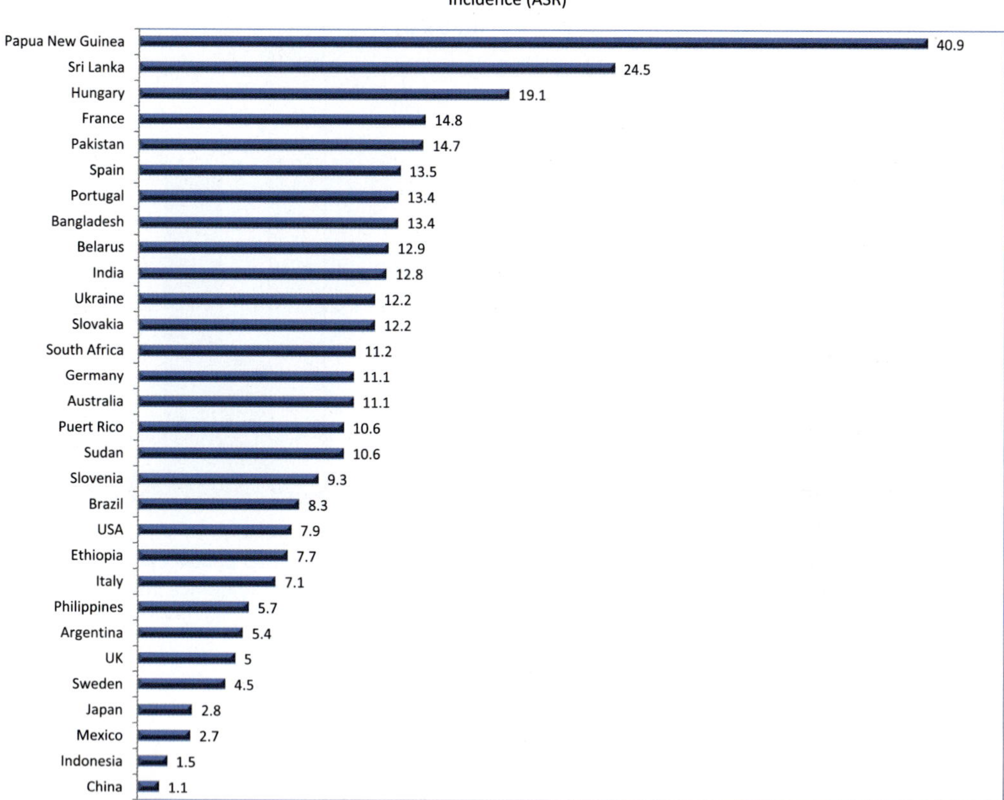

Fig. 1a. Worldwide age-standardized incidence rates (ASR) per 100,000 cases of oral cancers among men (adapted from reference 18)

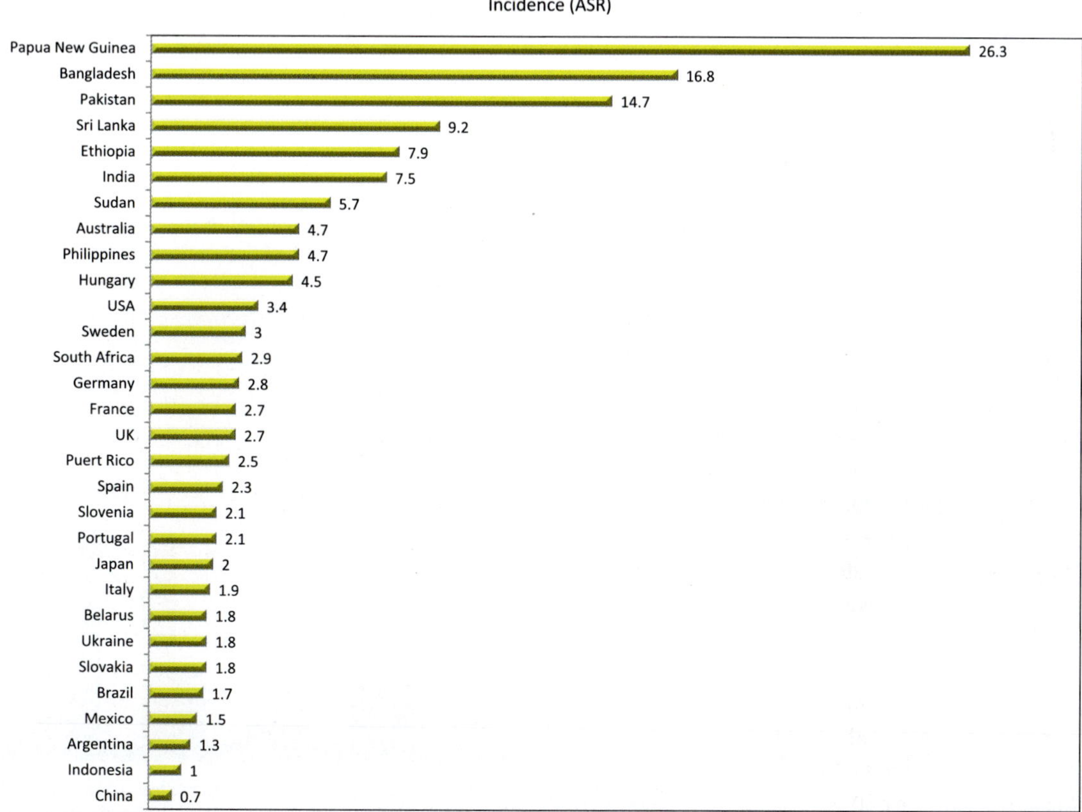

Fig. 1b. Worldwide age-standardized incidence rates (ASR) per 100,000 cases of oral cancers among women (adapted from reference 18)

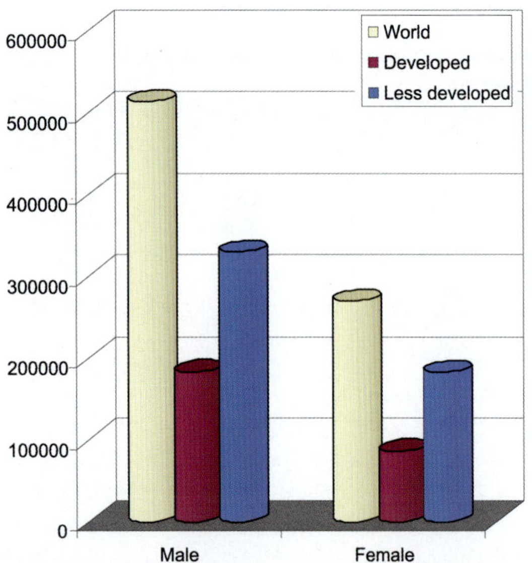

Fig. 2a. Incidence of HNC in patients in developed and less developed countries (data from reference 18)

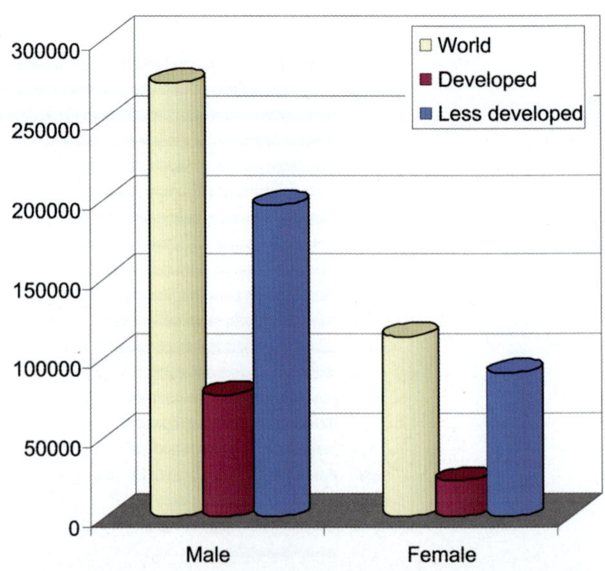

Fig. 2b. Mortality of HNC patients in developed and less developed countries (adapted from reference 18)

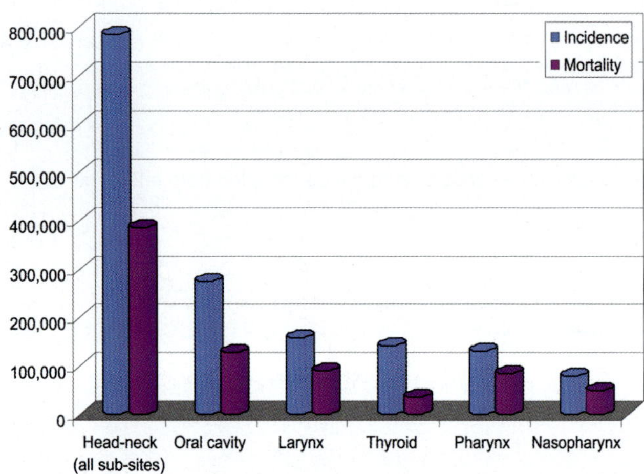

Fig. 3. Global incidence and mortality of HNC (adapted from reference 18)

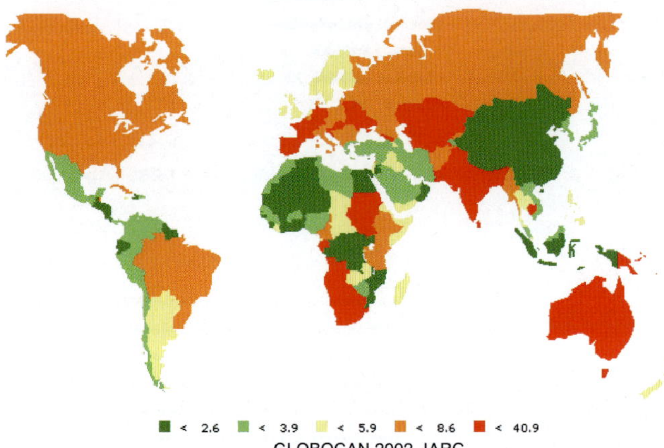

Fig. 4. Global distribution of age-standardized incidence rates (ASR) per 100,000 cases of oral cancers among men (adapted from reference 18)

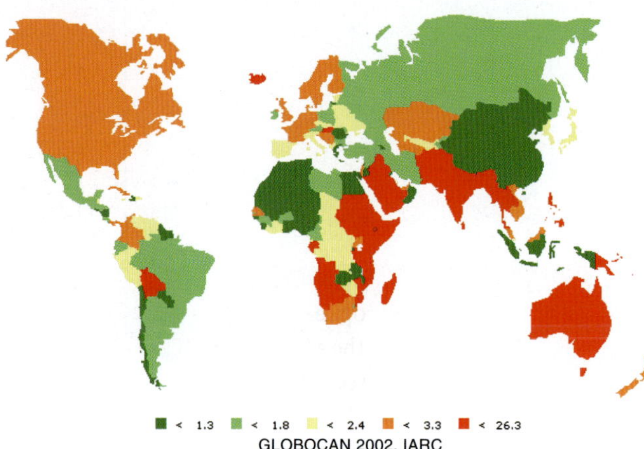

Fig. 5. Global distribution of age-standardized incidence rates (ASR) per 100,000 cases of oral cancers among women (adapted from reference 18)

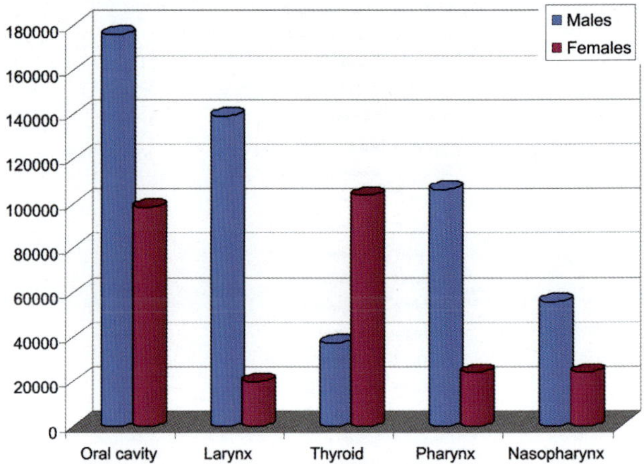

Fig. 6. Incidence of different HNCs, depending on sub-sites (adapted from reference 18)

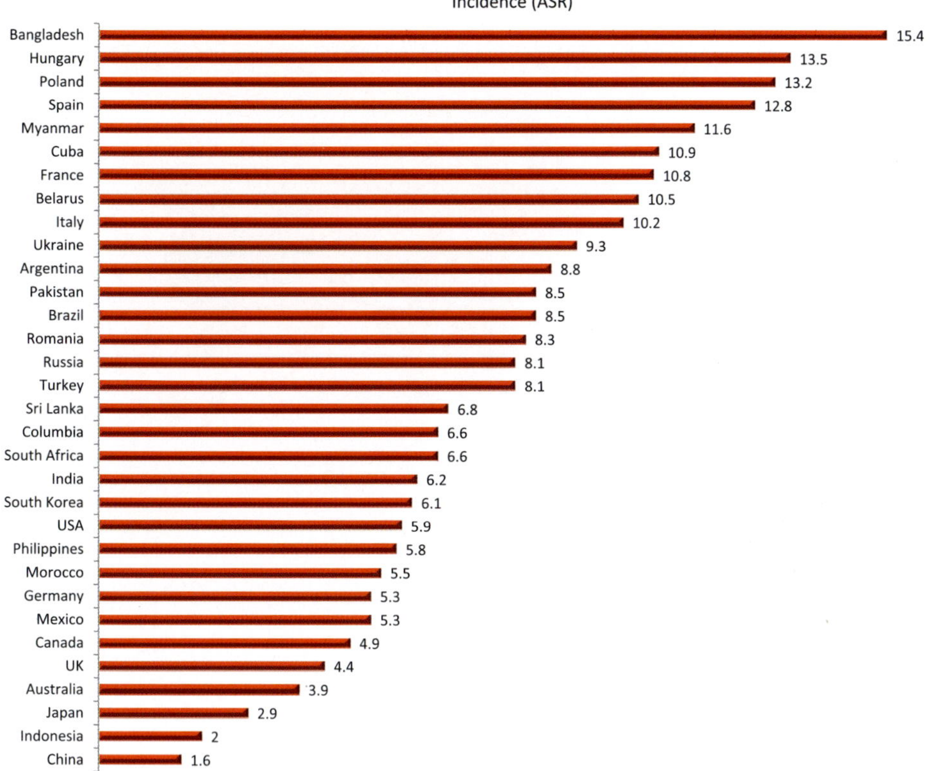

Fig. 7. Worldwide geographical variation in age-standardized incidence rates (ASR) per 100,000 cases of laryngeal cancers among men (adapted from reference 18)

cancer deaths worldwide; it ranks twelfth among all cancers. Laryngeal cancer is the second most common HNC, and is responsible for >159,000 new cases and about 90,000 cancer deaths each year worldwide (Fig. 3, Table 1).[18]

The wide geographical variation in the incidence and mortality of oral cancer around the world (Figs 4 and 5)[18,20] may be secondary to environmental, industrial, ethnic and social influences. The incidence and mortality of HNSCC also show immense variation between different sub-sites and gender; the male:female ratio varies between 2:1 and 15:1, depending on the anatomical sub-site and geographical area (Fig. 6). The highest incidence worldwide was reported in Somme, France, where men showed an average rate of 43.1 new cases per 100,000; the women, on the other hand, had a significantly lower incidence rate of 4.7 cases per 100,000.[21] The highest worldwide incidence of HNSCC in women was seen in Bangalore, India, with an average rate of 11.2 cases per 100,000.[21] The lowest worldwide incidence in men was reported in Quito, Ecuador, with an average of 2.4 new cases per 100,000. Although women in Ecuador had similar incidence rates during this time period, with 1.8 new cases per 100,000, the lowest worldwide incidence in women was reported in Kangwha County, Korea, with an average rate of 0.05 per 100,000.[21]

The incidence rates of oral cancer vary between 0.7 and 40.9 per 100,000 population (Fig. 1).[18] Some of the areas reporting the highest incidence in men are Melanesia (Papua New Guinea), southeast Asia (Sri Lanka, Bangladesh, India, Pakistan), western Europe (France, Germany), eastern Europe (Hungary, Slovakia, Slovenia), parts of Latin America and the Caribbean (Brazil, Puerto Rico), and southern Europe (Spain, Portugal) (Figs 1a and 4). Similar trends of oral cancers are also reflected in women in these areas (Figs 1b and 5).[18]

Laryngeal cancers are more prevalent in men as compared with women (Fig. 6).[18] Global incidence rates for laryngeal cancers are higher in southeast Asia (Bangladesh, Myanmar, Pakistan, Sri Lanka, India), eastern Europe (Hungary, Poland, Ukraine, Russia, Belarus), southern Europe (Spain, France, Italy), Cuba, South America (Argentina, Brazil) and western Asia (Turkey) (Figs 7 and 8).[18]

Thyroid cancers are more commonly seen in women than in men (Fig. 6) throughout the world; however, the reported incidence rates are higher in the USA, Canada and western Europe, with pockets of high incidence in Belarus and France (Fig. 9).[18]

Like oral and laryngeal cancers, pharyngeal cancers (excluding those of the nasopharynx) are also more common in men (Fig. 6).[18,20] Some of the areas reported with the highest incidence of pharyngeal cancers are eastern Europe (Hungary, Romania, Poland, Ukraine, Russia), western Europe (France, Germany), southeast Asia (India, Myanmar, Sri Lanka, Pakistan) and southern Europe (Spain, Portugal) (Fig. 10).[18]

A higher incidence of nasopharyngeal carcinoma (NPC) is reported in southeast Asia (Singapore, Malaysia, Vietnam,

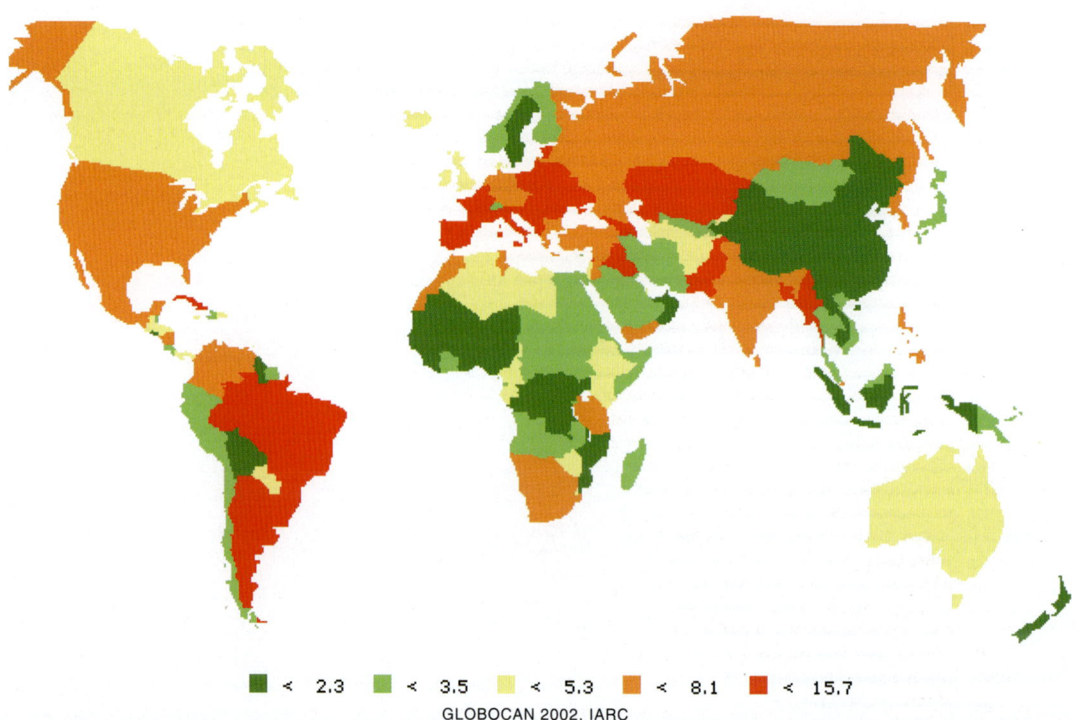

Fig. 8. Worldwide distribution of age-standardized incidence rates (ASR) per 100,000 cases of laryngeal cancers among men (adapted from reference 18)

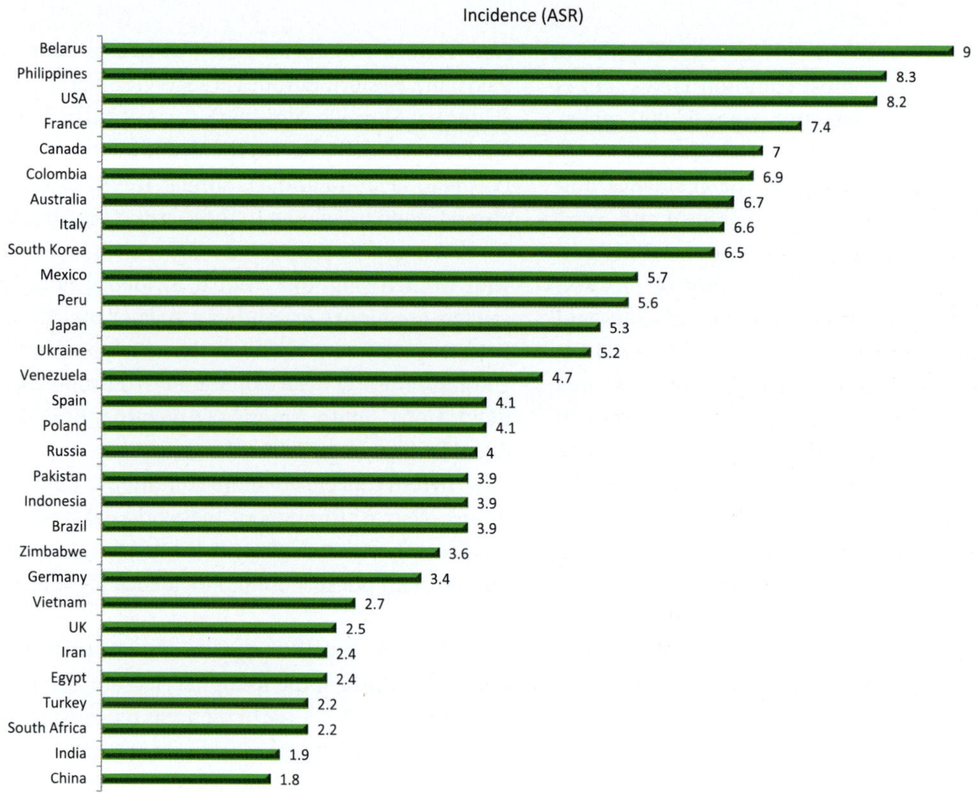

Fig. 9. Worldwide geographical variation in age-standardized incidence rates (ASR) per 100,000 cases of thyroid cancer among women (adapted from reference 18)

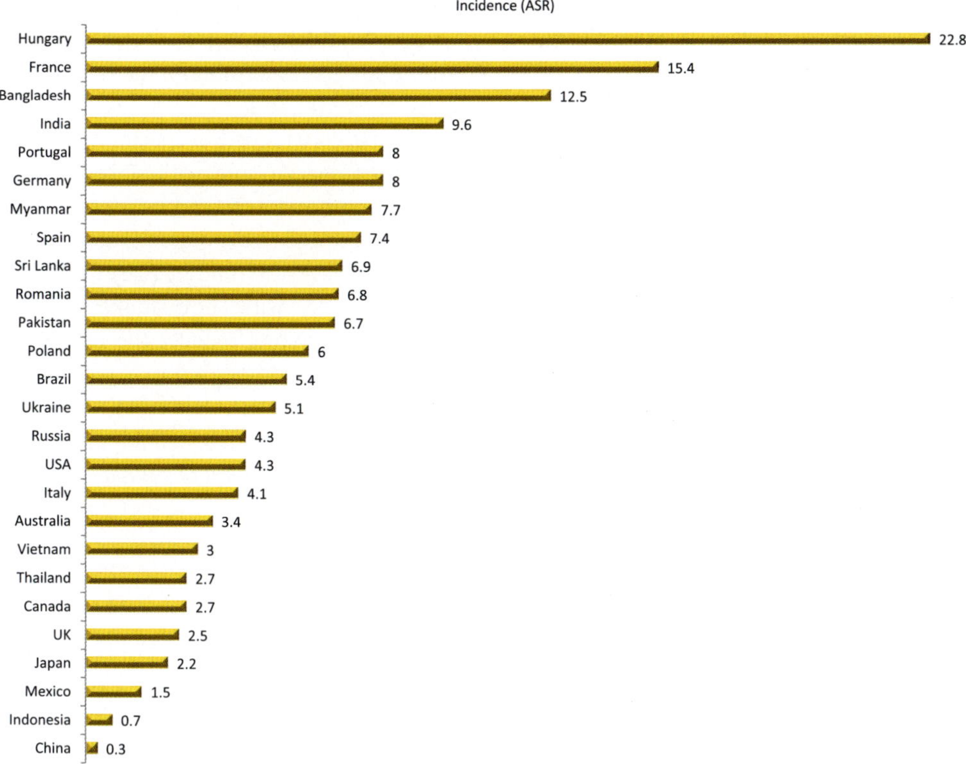

Fig. 10. Worldwide geographical variation in age-standardized incidence rates (ASR) per 100,000 cases of pharyngeal cancer (excluding nasopharynx) among men (adapted from reference 18)

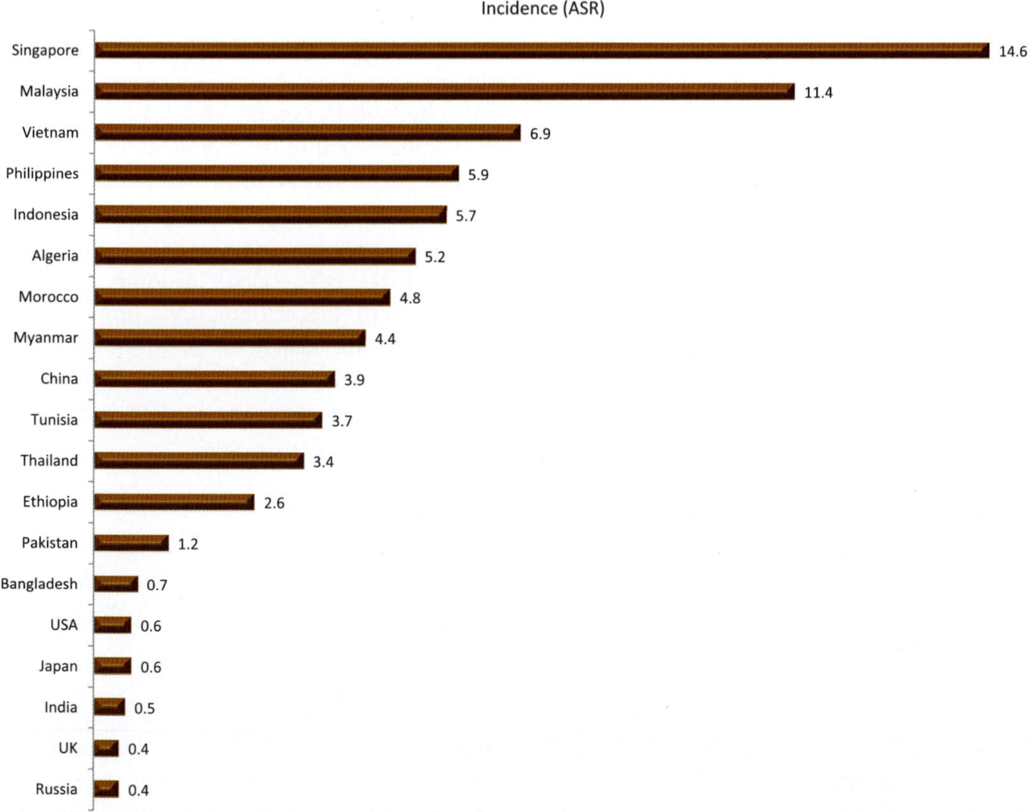

Fig. 11. Worldwide geographical variation in age-standardized incidence rates (ASR) per 100,000 cases of nasopharyngeal cancer among men (adapted from reference 18)

the Philippines, Indonesia) and China, with areas of high incidence in northern Africa, especially Algeria, Morocco and Tunisia (Fig. 11).[18]

Aetiology

HNC, like any other cancer, is multi-factorial in origin. Most HNCs result from a combination of genetic predisposition and environmental factors, such as exposure to carcinogens, often due to lifestyle habits (Table 2). Lifestyle habits play a significant role, as 8 of 10 HNC cases are known to arise from them, which potentially can be avoided. Although these habits are widespread, their preponderance varies according to the geographical region, and social and cultural beliefs. According to recent worldwide estimates, one billion men and 250 million women smoke cigarettes, 600–1200 million people chew betel quid, and two billion consume alcohol. An unbalanced diet is a common factor among people in developed and developing countries.[22] Tobacco and alcohol consumption alone are implicated in 75% of all HNSCC cases, and the effect is synergistic rather than simply additive.[23–25]

Tobacco

Tobacco is the single most important aetiological factor in HNCs, as well as in cancers in general. Tobacco consumption has now reached the proportion of a global epidemic.[22] Tobacco companies are producing cigarettes at the rate of 5.5 trillion a year, i.e. nearly 1000 cigarettes for every man, woman and child on the planet.[26] Worldwide, 20%–30% of all oral cancers can be directly attributed to tobacco usage (smoking/chewing).[22] Tobacco contains more than 19 known carcinogens (collectively known as tar) and more than 4000 chemicals, most of which have been identified as toxic, tumorogenic and carcinogenic.[27,28] Burning of tobacco releases methylchloranthrene, benzopyrine, benzanthracene and other polycyclic aromatic hydrocarbons, which reach the cellular surface of the epithelium in the smoke or by dissolution in saliva. Arylhydrocarbon hydroxylation breakdown of these carcinogens produces secondary carcinogenic epoxides that bind to DNA and RNA molecules, damaging them and initiating cancer formation.[29] N-nitroso compounds, well-known carcinogens in tobacco smoke, play a major role in the malignant transformation of UADT mucous membranes.[30]

Tobacco users have a high frequency of p53 mutation,[31] which is a key feature of all cancers. The developmental process of the carcinoma depends on many possible determinants that are both pro- and anti-cancer, such as the type of tobacco used, the length and intensity of carcinogen exposure, type of vehicle used, response of the epithelium (production of mucous and ciliary paralysis), genetically determined arylhydrocarbon hydroxylase inducibility, and the intake of fresh fruits (containing naturally occurring antioxidants that are cancer-protective) and other dietary factors.[32]

Regional differences in the form and method of tobacco consumption are responsible for the varied prevalence of HNC. The use of *bidi* (a crude form of cigarette with approximately 0.2 g of tobacco wrapped in specific tree leaf), tobacco quid, and *khaini* (tobacco quid with slaked lime) is prevalent in India and southeast Asia, and it is responsible for the higher prevalence of HNC in the region (Figs 4, 5 and 8).[18,20]

Smokers have a six-fold increase in the risk of developing HNC compared with non-smokers.[33] Quitting tobacco and stopping smoking reduces the risk of cancers and pre-malignant lesions, although it may take 10–20 years or more for a former smoker's risk to reduce to that of a non-smoker.[34,35] Second-hand smoke (passive smoking) and smokeless tobacco are also established causes of HNC, especially of the larynx and pharynx.[36]

Betel quid and areca nut

Approximately 600–1200 million people are estimated to chew betel quid in India and southeast Asia (prevalence of 80%–90% in some areas and among some rural ethnic groups).[37,38] Betel quid, or *paan*, generally consists of areca nut, slaked lime, catechu and often tobacco wrapped in a betel leaf. Use of paan masala (dry mixture of areca nut, catechu and flavouring agents) and *gutka* (a similar mixture with tobacco) is widespread in India, and they are the main culprits in this mammoth rate of HNC, especially oral and oropharyngeal cancers[29,39] (Figs 4, 5 and 10). *Paan masala* and *gutka* contain over 2000 chemicals, many of which are proven carcinogens.[40] Carcinogenic nitrosamines derived from the areca nut, the primary ingredient in betel quid, are formed in the saliva of chewers. Areca nut is known to induce oral preneoplastic lesions with a high propensity to progress to cancer.

Besides having a direct irritating effect on the mucosa, chewing betel quid causes genomic instability.[41] It also interferes with the cell-mediated immunity, which might play a role in the malignant transformation of the oral and oropharyngeal mucous membranes.[42] Betel quid chewing is associated with a five- to six-fold increase in the risk of developing oral cavity cancers.[43,44]

Alcohol

Alcohol is a well established risk factor for the development of HNC as well as other cancers. It alone is responsible for as many as 19% of all oral cancers worldwide. Nearly 2 billion adults consume alcoholic beverages regularly, with an average daily consumption of 13 g ethanol (equivalent of about one drink).[22,45] Alcohol drinking results in exposure to acetaldehyde, derived from the beverage itself and formed endogenously. Acetaldehyde is a genotoxic compound that is detoxified by aldehyde dehydrogenase (ALDH). The ALDH2*2

Table 2. Aetiological factors for head and neck cancers

Agent		Sub-site predisposition
Tobacco		Oral cavity, oropharynx, larynx, hypopharynx, cervical oesophagus, nose and paranasal sinus
Betel quid and areca nut		Oral cavity, oropharynx, larynx, hypopharynx, cervical oesophagus
Alcohol		Oral cavity, oropharynx, hypopharynx, larynx, cervical oesophagus
Viruses		
	Human papillomavirus	Oropharynx (especially tonsil), oral cavity and larynx
	Human immunodeficiency virus	Oral cavity, oropharynx, larynx, hypopharynx
	Epstein–Barr virus	Nasopharyngeal cancer
Dietary factors		Oral cavity, oropharynx, larynx, hypopharynx, cervical oesophagus
Familial and genetic factors		Oral cavity, oropharynx, larynx, hypopharynx, cervical oesophagus
Immunosuppression		Oral cavity, oropharynx, larynx, hypopharynx, cervical oesophagus
Occupation		
	Wood workers	Nasal cavity, paranasal sinuses, nasopharynx
	Formaldehyde exposure	Paranasal sinuses, nasal cavity, larynx
	Rubber manufacturing	Larynx, cervical oesophagus
	Alcohol manufacturing	Nasal cavity, larynx, oral cavity, pharynx
	Leather workers	Nasal cavity, paranasal sinus
	Nickel refiners	Nasal cavity and paranasal sinus
	Chromium compounds	Nasal cavity and paranasal sinus
	Asbestos	Larynx, pharynx
	Sulphar mustard	Larynx
	Radium-dial painters	Paranasal sinus (because of radiation-induced affects)
	Textile workers	Larynx, pharynx, oral cavity
	Paint and printing	Paranasal sinus, larynx, oral cavity, pharynx
	Metal workers*	Larynx, oropharynx, oral cavity
	Sulphuric acid*	Larynx
	Plastics*	Larynx, oral cavity, pharynx
	Car mechanics*	Larynx, oral cavity
	Pesticides*	Larynx
	Cement and concrete*	Larynx
	Coal and stone dust*	Larynx
	Naphthalene*	Larynx
Radiation		
	Radioiodine including iodine-131	Thyroid cancers (especially in paediatric population), sarcomas, non-Hodgkin lymphoma and laryngeal cancers
	Radium-226, radium-228 and decay products	Paranasal sinus, mastoid process (radium-226 only)
	X-radiation or gamma-radiation	Salivary glands, cervical oesophagus, basal cell carcinoma
Others		
	Chronic irritation, diabetes mellitus, candidiasis, syphilis, marijuana, atmospheric pollution	Oral cavity, oropharynx, larynx, hypopharynx

* Weak association/ insufficient data

variant allele, which encodes an inactive enzyme, is prevalent (up to 30%) in east Asian populations. Heterozygous carriers, who have approximately 10% enzyme activity, accumulate acetaldehyde and have higher relative risk of alcohol-related HNC compared with individuals with the common alleles.[46]

The chronic consumption of alcohol is estimated to increase the risk of UADT cancer by 2–3 times.[23,47] Alcohol affects oncogenes at initiation and promotion stages of carcinogenesis, impairs the cell's ability to repair its DNA, and causes overexpression of certain oncogenes responsible for the formation of the cancer.

Alcohol, when consumed, has a synergistic carcinogenic effect with tobacco, the risk of developing HNSCC being 20–120 times that of a teetotaller and non-smoker.[23,24] The nitrocarbon carcinogens in tobacco are relatively insoluble in normal saliva but are soluble in alcohol, because of which they are more readily absorbed into the surface epithelium.[27] Alcohol also dehydrates cell walls and hence enhances the ability of tobacco carcinogens to permeate the local tissues; additionally, it retards the body's natural defence mechanisms and depletes antioxidants, which have a protective role in cancers.[47] Some alcoholic beverages contain chemical impurities, such as N-nitrosodiethylamine and polycyclic aromatic hydrocarbons, which are well known carcinogens.[48,49] Similar to smoking, the incidence and severity of HNC is directly affected by the quantity, quality and duration of alcohol consumed.[50,51]

Viruses

Human papillomavirus

The role of human papillomavirus (HPV) as an aetiological factor in HNSCCs has been established over two decades. HPV, especially the mucosal high-risk types HPV-16 and HPV-18, have been directly implicated in the causation of oropharyngeal cancers (25%–30%) and oral cancers (3%). Over 90% of the HPV-positive oral cancers are HPV-16 positive, and the rate of positivity is even greater (95%) in oropharyngeal cancers.[52] HPV infection is now regarded as an independent risk factor for HNC, especially for oropharyngeal cancers.[53] This finding is further supported by identification of HPV in cervical nodes of patients presenting with an occult primary, confirming that they come from the oropharynx.[54]

Two oncogenic proteins of HPV-16—E6 and E7—can target two critical areas of the Rb and p53 tumour suppressor pathways and subsequently cause genomic instability through the deregulation of important cellular processes, including DNA repair, cell cycle control and apoptosis.[55]

HPV infection is particularly prevalent in young, sexually active males who are non-smokers, and may be responsible for the changing trends of HNCs (especially of oropharyngeal cancers) towards younger, non-smoking populations in the developed world.[24,56] As risk factors for HPV infection include having a large number of sexual partners and the first intercourse at a younger age, changing sexual practices in our society may increase the effect of HPV infection on the development of HNC and pre-malignant lesions, especially in younger adults.[57] Oral sex practices have been associated recently with the increased risk of developing oropharyngeal cancers, especially tonsillar carcinomas.[58] It has been shown that HPV infection is synergistic with smoking and chronic alcohol consumption in the causation of UADT SCCs.[59]

Human immunodeficiency virus

Human immunodeficiency virus (HIV) probably accelerates the development of HNSCC in high-risk patients. A study showed that HIV infection was present in approximately 5% of all HNC patients and that the disease was relatively more advanced at the time of presentation than in non-HIV HNC patients.[27]

Epstein–Barr virus

Epstein–Barr virus (EBV) has been shown to have a strong association with the development of NPC.[60] The presence of EBV DNA in the UADT mucosa varies extensively across different areas of the world, with a high prevalence in the southeast Asian population, especially in Singapore, Malaysia, Philippines, Indonesia and China (Fig. 11), where NPC is one of the commonest cancers.[18]

Dietary factors

Dietary deficiencies have repeatedly been associated with the development of HNC and other cancers in general. About 10%–15% of oral and oropharyngeal cancers can be directly attributed to dietary deficiencies or imbalances.[22,29] Increased risk has been reported from the high intake of high-calorie foods, such as starchy foods, certain meats, especially processed meats, charcoal-grilled meat, pork and eggs.[61,62] Ingestion of salted meat has also been shown to be a risk factor in oral cavity and pharyngeal carcinomas.[63]

Reactive oxygen species (ROS) and reactive nitrogen species (RNS) can function both as initiators and promoters in carcinogenesis, whereas antioxidants provide protection against the cellular and molecular damage caused by ROS and RNS.[64] Fruits and vegetables have naturally occurring antioxidants; similarly vitamins A and C, which are also antioxidants, protect cells from the development of cancers.[65] It has been shown that dietary deficiencies, particularly of vitamins A (and related carotenoids), C and E, and iron, folate, selenium and trace elements have been linked to an increased risk of HNC.[66–68]

Familial and genetic factors

Cigarette smoking cannot be the sole aetiological factor, as only a small percentage of smokers develop HNC. This indicates that tobacco-associated susceptibility to HNSCC is influenced by host factors as well.[69] Several studies have suggested that the risk for developing HNSCC is inherited, as individuals with a first degree family member with cancer have a 2- to 14-fold increase in HNSCC.[70,71]

Accumulation of p53 in tumour cell nuclei predicts a significantly increased risk of death, independent of tumour grade, stage and lymph node status.[72] Some other genetic factors associated with increased risk of HNC include abnormal inducibility of cytochrome P450[73-76] and mutagen sensitivity,[77] which reflect a defect in DNA repair. Patients with xeroderma pigmentosum, Fanconi anaemia, ataxia telangiectasia, Li-Fraumani syndrome and hereditary non-polyposis colorectal cancers are known to have an increased risk of developing HNSCC.[78]

Immunosuppression

An increased incidence of HNC has been documented in chronic immunodeficiency states.[79-82] Oral SCC has been reported in younger persons undergoing immunosuppression regimes following organ transplantation.[83]

Occupation

Epidemiological evidence exists for an association between workers exposed to wood dust, leather dust,[84] formaldehyde, and inorganic acid mist, and an increased risk of developing different HNCs[85] (Table 2).

Radiation

Long-term radiation exposure is known to cause HNC, especially thyroid cancers, because of the radioiodines, particularly iodine-131, during childhood and adolescence. This was reported after the Chernobyl disaster.[86,87] Prolonged exposure to radium-228 is known to cause paranasal sinus carcinomas, whereas radium-226 exposure may lead to the development of mastoid process carcinoma.[86]

Other factors

Chronic irritants, poor dental hygiene (polymicrobial supra-gingival dental plaque),[88] candidiasis,[89] diabetes,[90] syphilis[91] and marijuana smoking[92] have also been identified as predisposing factors in UADT carcinoma.

Pathogenesis and natural history

HNC may result from an uncontrolled cell growth in susceptible patients resulting from a disruption of normal mechanisms that regulate cellular proliferation, differentiation and cell death, or apoptosis. Recent developments in molecular medicine have elucidated a plethora of genetic events leading to inactivation of tumour suppressor genes or activation of proto-oncogenes, or both, which govern the development of HNSCC.[19] Molecular techniques have further identified genetic and epigenetic alterations (Fig. 12a) in pre-malignant and invasive lesions, which has made it possible to delineate a classical hypothetical progression model for HNSCC.[93-95] It is now known that HNSCC follows a definite histological evolution, running from normal tissue to hyperplastic changes, to dysplasia, to carcinoma *in situ*, and finally to the development of an invasive carcinoma (Fig. 12b). A similar pattern of sequential progression of a frank SCC is also well known. The majority of HNCs progress in a relatively orderly and predictable fashion from a small primary to a larger lesion, to lymph node metastasis and distant metastasis. Several factors/characteristics influence the natural history of HNSCC, which can be broadly studied under three subheadings: Primary lesion, lymphatic spread and distant spread.

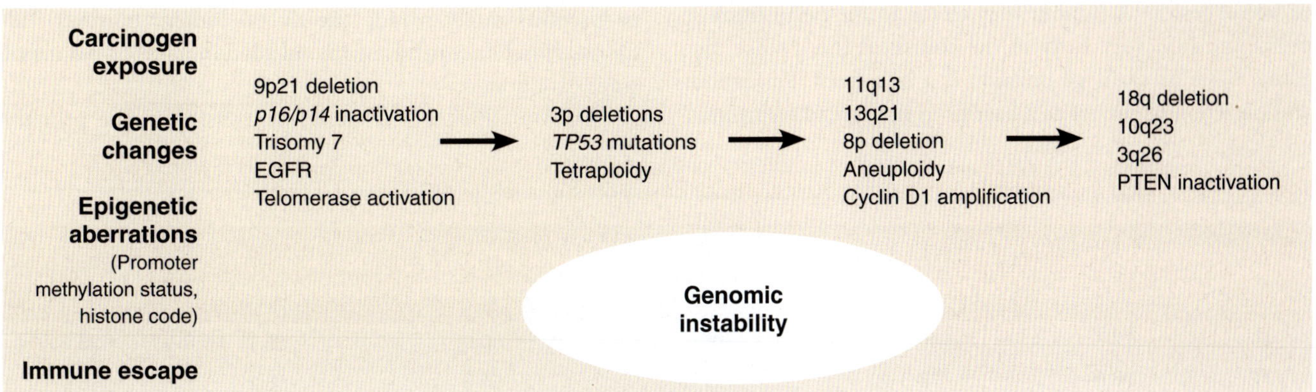

Fig. 12a. Genetic and epi-genetic events in head and neck carcinogenesis
EGFR epidermal growth factor receptor   PTEN phosphatase and tensin homologue

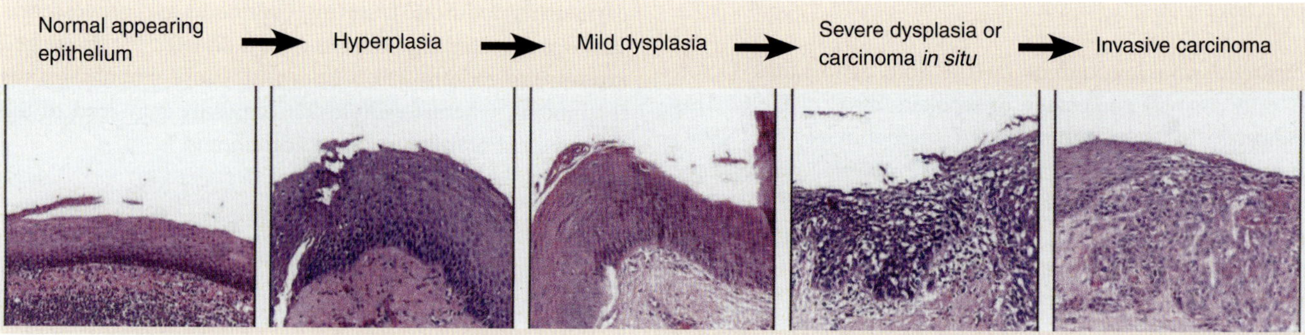

Fig. 12b. Parallel phenotypical progression and histological evolution of HNC shown in haematoxylin and eosin (adapted with permission from references 19, 93 and 94)

Primary lesion

The size of the primary lesion and the disease spread are directly related. The dictum, 'the larger the tumour the worse the prognosis', is generally valid. In fact, it forms one of the three components of the classical TNM (tumour, node, metastasis) system of cancer staging. This is particularly true for oral cavity cancer, laryngeal cancers, and nose and paranasal sinus cancers. However, carcinomas arising in the floor of the mouth may have a larger surface component but show only superficial invasion of the lamina propria. Such tumours are less likely to disseminate to regional lymph nodes and tend to have a better prognosis than deeply invasive ones. On the other hand, nasopharyngeal, hypopharyngeal, oropharyngeal and supraglottic laryngeal cancers, although small, may demonstrate a propensity of early lymphovascular invasion, because of the rich lymphovascular system in these areas, resulting in early and more marked nodal involvement and distant metastasis compared with other sub-sites (Table 3).

Most HNCs begin as a surface lesion of the UADT and each anatomical sub-site within the head and neck region has its own particular pattern of spread. Although these cancers originate from the mucosal surface, muscular invasion is commonly seen and a tumour may spread along muscle or facial planes for a considerable distance from the palpable or visible lesion. A tumour may attach to the periostium or perichondrium very early in the course of the disease, but actual bone or cartilage invasion is a late event. Periostium and perichondrium act as a barrier to the spread of primary disease, and these structures are generally spared until the tumour has explored easier avenues of growth, either by themselves (by activation of host osteoclasts by local tumour-derived products) or along neural pathways. This pattern of local spread is seen in oral cavity, oropharyngeal and laryngeal cancers.

Perineural invasion is an important pathway of tumour spread and is more common than previously thought. It is regarded as an ominous sign that correlates with an increased incidence of local recurrence, regional lymph node metastasis and decreased survival.[102] It is a histological sign of the biological aggressiveness of the tumour and is independent of the size of the primary lesion.[102] No site or histology is immune to it; SCC and its variants and minor salivary gland tumours, especially adenoid cystic carcinoma, may show this pattern, the latter more so. Also, local recurrence increases the likelihood of perinural involvement and the tumours may track along a nerve to the base of the skull. Patients with perinural invasion will often develop minor neurological symptoms and if nerve palsies are noted, they are most often secondary to compression or entrapment rather than the actual nerve invasion.

Invasion of the parapharyngeal space allows tumours to spread superiorly or inferiorly from the base of the skull to the hyoid bone. Tumours arising from ducts of minor salivary glands or major salivary glands (submandibular, sublingual or parotid) rarely invade the ductal lumen; however, the nasolacrimal duct is frequently invaded in nasal or paranasal sinus carcinomas.

Tumour thickness or depth of invasion of the primary

Table 3. Neck node metastasis (%) in head and neck cancer based on sub-sites and T-stage of the disease

T-stage	Nasopharynx (Wang et al.[96])	Pyriform fossa (De Zinis et al.[97])	Postcricoid region (Farrington et al.[98])	Base of Tongue (Session et al.[99])	Tonsil (Hannisdal et al.[100])	Supraglottic Larynx (Sheahan[101])
T1	77.7	50.0	06.0	50.0	68.1	25.0
T2	76.8	72.0	17.0	54.6	58.2	70.0
T3	78.0	89.0	38.0	65.0	67.1	80.0
T4	70.6	81.0	50.0	71.0	67.6	80.0

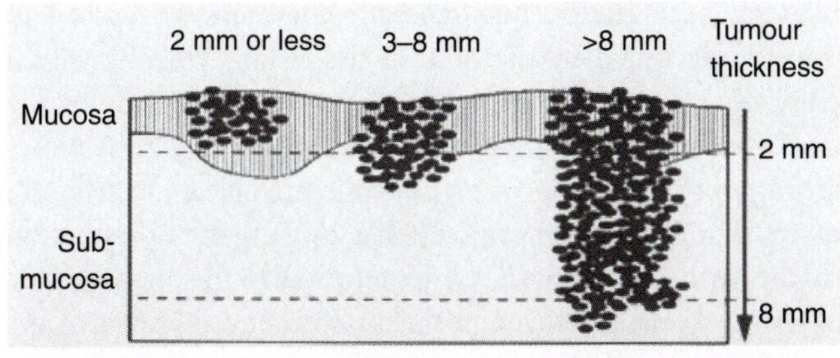

Tumour thickness	Risk of occult nodal metastasis	Overall incidence of nodal metastasis	Treatment failure	Patients died of disease
2 mm or less	7%	13%	2%	3%
3–8 mm	26%	46%	45%	17%
8 mm or more	41%	65%	45%	35%

Fig. 13 and Table 4. Risk of nodal metastases, treatment failure and death in relation to thickness of primary SCCs of the tongue and floor of the mouth (adapted with permission from reference 104)

tumour is one of the most important indicators of the aggressive nature of the disease. This is particularly true in cases of oral cavity cancers, where it has been linked directly with the occurrence of nodal involvement, treatment failure and poor survival[103] (Fig. 13 and Table 4).

Local spread of HNC also depends on differentiation (grade) of tumour, pattern of tumour invasion, and inflammatory response to the tumour. Poorly differentiated tumours, in general, tend to have a more rapid doubling time and metastasize earlier than more differentiated types. It is noted that the tumours composed of large cohesive masses of cells are less likely to metastasize than those that invade in a non-cohesive pattern of single and small aggregates of cells. All HNCs are known to produce an immunological response and, in general, the greater the immunological response to the tumour, the better the prognosis.

Lymphatic spread

The status of regional lymph nodes is one of the most important parameters that determines prognosis in patients with HNC. The presence of even a single positive node decreases survival by as much as 50%.[105,106] The risk of lymph node metastasis may be predicted by the differentiation of the tumour (the more poorly differentiated, the greater the risk), by the size and the depth of invasion of the primary tumour, and by the availability of the capillary lymphatics, as explained above. Also, the risk of lymphatic spread increases with recurrence of the tumour.

No histological type is excluded from the lymphatic spread; mere access of capillary lymphatics determines the opportunity for lymphatic spread. Minor salivary gland tumours and sarcomas, for example, assume the risk of

lymphatic metastasis similar to SCC for each anatomical site. For instance, a minor salivary gland tumour or sarcoma arising in the nasopharynx would have a relatively high risk for lymphatic metastasis, whereas should the same tumour arise from the maxillary antrum, it would have a relatively low risk.

Embryonically, the lymphatic system arises by budding from the venous system, which explains the close anatomical relationship of these two drainage systems. The blood capillaries have narrow endothelial junctions and do not normally resorb larger molecules and cells. However, lymphatic capillaries have relatively open endothelial junctions that permit the larger molecules and cells to be absorbed/pass, explaining why tumour cells enter the lymphatic system more readily than the vascular system. The lymphatic system of the head and neck region consists of lymphatic capillaries, lymphatic trunks and lymph nodes; a detailed understanding of which holds the key to the successful management of HNCs.

The epithelium, bone and cartilage are devoid of capillary lymphatics; a few occur in the periosteum and perichondrium, but they are abundant in the submucosa and the dermis. Because of the absence of lymphatics in the epithelium, a tumour must penetrate the lamina propria before lymphatic invasion can occur. In the superficial layer, the diameter of the lymphatic capillaries is usually narrower than it is in the deeper layers. The richness of capillary network in any given head and neck site may be predicted by the relative incidence of lymph node metastases. The nasopharynx, pyriform sinus (hypopharynx), supraglottic larynx and oropharynx have the most profuse network of capillary lymphatics, which is reflected clinically by the presence of neck nodes at the time of initial presentation (Table 3). The paranasal sinus, middle ear and vocal cords have few or no capillary lymphatics, which is in agreement with their low rate of lymph node metastasis when the tumour is confined to these sites. The capillary lymphatic system, particularly in the larynx and trachea, tends to atrophy with age.

The capillary lymphatics converge to form lymphatic trunks that have semilunar valves, which direct lymph flow to a lymph node. However, the dermal lymphatic vessels are devoid of valves, and once the cancer invades this system, flow is unpredictable and erratic, with skin nodules surfacing at remote distances from the original area of skin invasion. The lymphatic trunks eventually empty into a large vein, usually near the junction of the internal jugular vein and the axillary vein, the so-called venous angle. However, the lymphatic vessels, particularly those of the thyroid, may occasionally empty directly into the internal jugular vein or subclavian vein well above the venous angle. Lymphaticovenous connections exist between lymphatic trunks and veins or within the lymph node. The lymphaticovenous connections between the vessels are probably of little importance until a lymphatic trunk is obstructed. The lymphatic trunks function as lymph transportation channels and the direction of lymphatic flow for each anatomical site is predictable, although aberrant pathways may occur. The intercalated nodes (inconsistent 1–2 mm nodes) may occur anywhere along the course of a lymph vessel between its origin and its entrance to a large lymph node, and may uncommonly account for the odd recurrences.

Obstruction of a lymph channel has the effect of re-routing the lymphatic flow. Complete obstruction by surgical transection will cause major changes in the expected pathway of lymph node metastasis. Radiation therapy causes partial obstruction, the degree of obstruction being dose-dependent. Lymph nodes that are replaced by a tumour may cause partial or complete obstruction, especially when the mass becomes large enough to compress or invade the afferent lymphatic trunks. Approximately 300 lymph nodes are located above the clavicle, i.e. nearly one-third of the total lymph nodes in the body.[106] The arrangement of these nodes within the head and neck region is archetypal, and each group receives drainage (either directly or indirectly) from specific areas; they drain into a deep cervical group (terminal group for the head and neck region) before finally draining into the lymphatic duct (right)/thoracic duct (left) or jugulosubclavian junction via the jugular trunk (Fig. 14).

Lymph node involvement in HNC usually follows an orderly progression but, rarely, skip metastasis may be seen.[108,109] Well lateralized lesions spread to ipsilateral neck nodes. Lesions on or near the midline and lateralized tongue and nasopharyngeal lesions may spread to contralateral or bilateral neck nodes, but generally they tend to spread to the side occupied by the bulk of the lesion. Patients with a clinically positive lymph node in the ipsilateral side of the neck are at risk of contralateral disease, especially if the nodes are large or if multiple lymph nodes are involved. Obstruction of the lymphatic pathways caused by surgery or radiation therapy will also shunt the lymphatic flow to the opposite side of the neck, mainly through the anastomotic channels of the submaxillary and submental areas.

Distant spread

Development of distant metastasis results from vascular invasion by tumour cells and involves clonal selection of cells that are able to overcome mechanical and immunological barriers. It is an ominous sign indicating an aggressive behaviour of the disease, adversely affecting patient survival.[110] The incidence of distant metastasis from HNC varies according to the source of the data. The reported incidence rates from clinical studies fluctuate between 7% and 23%,[110] whereas in autopsy findings they can range between 30% and 50%.[111]

Almost half of all distant metastases are detected clinically within 9 months of treatment, 80% within 2 years, 90% within 3 years and 99% within 5 years. Their presence is a poor prognostic factor, as 90% of the patients are dead within 2 years of detection of the first metastasis.

The lung is the most common site of a distant metastasis (50%–75% cases), whereas bone, liver, brain, skin and soft tissue metastases account for 10%–44%, 4%–34%, 3%–13%,

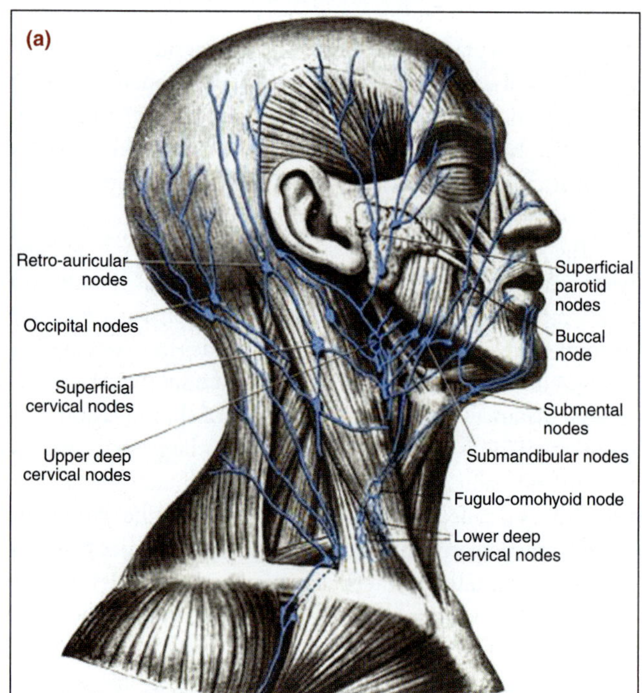

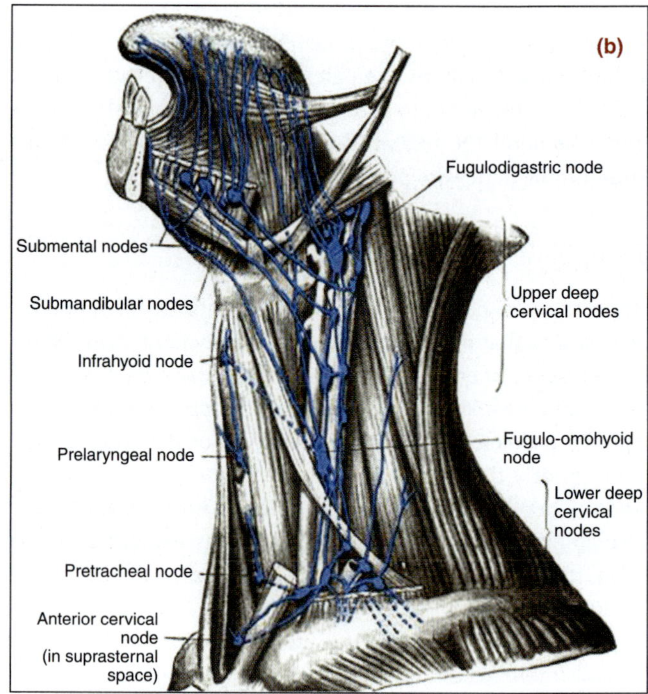

Fig. 14a. Superficial lymph nodes and lymph vessels of the head and neck region. **(b).** Deep cervical chain/groups of lymph nodes (after removal of the left sternocleidomastoid muscle and left hemimandible) (adapted with permission from reference 107)

3%–31% and 2%–9%, respectively.[110,112–114] The probability of developing distant metastasis is related to the site, nodal stage, tumour stage and overall stage of the cancer.[110,112,114] Tumours of the hypopharynx, supraglottic larynx, nasopharynx and oropharynx are more likely to disseminate than those of the oral cavity, paranasal sinuses and the glottis larynx.

The incidence of distant metastasis is strongly related to the initial control of the cancer, especially in the neck. Distant metastasis in the absence of nodal metastasis is very rare in head and neck SCC.[110] Untreated occult disease in the neck may shed tumour cells in the lymphaticovenous system and produce distant metastasis while the lymph node is growing slowly to a size that can be detected. It is seen that patients with advanced nodal disease have a high incidence of distant metastasis, particularly in the presence of jugular vein invasion or extensive soft tissue disease in the neck.[110] The rate of distant metastasis increases up to 27.6% for N3 disease as against 9.2% for N2 disease.[110]

Overall, the clinical stage and treatment modality adopted also have an effect on distant metastasis. Reported rates of distant metastasis for stages I, II, III and IV HNSCC are 1%, 14%, 15% and 20%, respectively.[110] Development of distant metastases are typically preceded by locoregional recurrence; however, 10%–20% patients develop them even if the disease is deemed to be locoregionally controlled.[111]

Multiple primaries

Five per cent to 36% of patients with HNC either have or will develop additional primary malignancies during their lifetime.[115] These can be classified according to their temporal sequence as synchronous (diagnosed at the same time or within 6 months of the diagnosis of the primary lesion) or metachronous (those developing over 6 months after the index tumour) carcinomas. Most of these are found in the head and neck region, in the lungs or in the oesophagus.

About two-thirds of these reported second primaries occur within the head and neck region at the rate of approximately 2% per patient-year of follow-up.[116] The frequent development of second/third or multiple primary tumours may well be explained by the 'field cancerization theory' proposed by Slaughter *et al.*[117] in 1953, which was later supported by other researchers.[118,119] This theory proposes that tumours develop in a multifocal fashion within a field of tissue chronically exposed and sensitized to carcinogens. Development of multiple primaries is classically seen in the oral cavity, oropharyngeal and hypopharyngeal cancers.

For multiple primaries occurring outside the head and neck region, pharyngeal primary HNSCC is most closely linked with subsequent development of oesophageal carcinoma (digestive axis). However, a careful search should also be made in whole of the UADT, including the respiratory axis.[120] It is important to recognize this phenomenon because the discovery of a second primary tumour may alter the initial therapeutic approach to the index tumour. It represents a more aggressive, life-threatening neoplasm and a compromised previously successful treatment. Continued exposure to carcinogens (especially tobacco and alcohol) after treatment has been associated with an increased risk of developing multiple primary tumours within the head and neck region and the UADT.[121,122]

References

1. Brothwell D. The evidence of neoplasms. In: Brothwell D, Sandison AT (eds). *Diseases in antiquity: A survey of diseases, injuries and surgery of early populations.* Springfield, IL: Charles C. Thomas; 1967:320–40.
2. Butterfield WC. Tumor treatment 3000 BC. *Surgery* 1966;**60**:476–9.
3. Kardinal CG. An outline of the history of cancer. Part I. *Mo Med* 1977;**74**:662–6.
4. Folz BJ, Silver CE, Rinaldo A, *et al.* An outline of the history of head and neck oncology. *Oral Oncol* 2008;**44**:2–9.
5. Nelson WR. In search of the first head and neck surgeon. *Am J Surg* 1987;**154**:342–6.
6. Martin H. Richard Wiseman on cancer. *Cancer* 1951;**4**:907–12.
7. Marchetti P. *Observationum medico-chirurgicarum rariorum sylloge.* Amstelodami: Ex officina Petri le Grand; 1665.
8. Onuigbo WI. Historical data on the dynamics of lymphatic metastasis. *Oncology* 1972;**26**:505–14.
9. Nezelof C. European roots of pathology. *Pathol Res Pract* 1994;**190**:103–14.
10. Thiersch C. *Der Epithelialkrebs, namentlich der Haut.* Leipzig: Engelmann; 1865.
11. Waldeyer W. Die Entwicklung der Carcinome. *Arch Pathol Anat* 1867;**41**:470–522.
12. Waldeyer W. Die Entwicklung der Carcinome. *Arch Pathol Anat* 1872;**55**:67–158.
13. Ruge C, Veit J. 1870. Quoted by Nezelof C1.
14. von Esmarch F; 1889. Quoted by Nezelof C1.
15. Dhom G. Zur Geschichte der mikroskopischen Krebsdiagnose. *Pathologe* 1992;**13**:308–13.
16. Forastiere A, Koch W, Trotti A, *et al.* Head and neck cancer. *N Engl J Med* 2001;**345**:1890–900.
17. Mendenhall WM, Riggs CE Jr, Cassisi NJ. Treatment of head and neck cancers. In: DeVita VT Jr, Hellman S, Rosenberg SA (eds). *Cancer: Principles and practice of oncology.* Philadelphia; Pa: Lippincott Williams and Wilkins; 2005:662–732.
18. Bray FF, Pisani P, Parkin DM. GLOBOCAN 2002: Cancer Incidence, Mortality and Prevalence Worldwide. IARC Cancer Base No. 5. version 2.0. Lyon: IARC Press; 2004. http://www-dep.iarc.fr/
19. Argiris A, Karamouzis MV, Raben D, *et al.* Head and neck cancer. *The Lancet* 2008;**371**:1695–709.
20. Dwivedi RC, Rhys-Evans PH, Patel SG. Tumors of the oropharynx. In: Montgomery PQ, Rhys-Evans PH, Gullane PJ (eds). *Principles and practice in head-neck surgery and oncology.* New York: Informa Healthcare; 2009:192–232.
21. Parkin DM, Whelan SL, Farlay J, *et al.* Cancer incidence in five continents. Lyon: IARC Scientific Publications; 2002.
22. Petti S. Lifestyle risk factors for oral cancer. *Oral Oncol* 2009;**45**:340–50.
23. Pelucchi C, Gallus S, Garavello W, *et al.* Cancer risk associated with alcohol and tobacco use: Focus on upper aero-digestive tract and liver. *Alcohol Res Health* 2006;**29**:193–98.

24. Laronde DM, Hislop TG, Elwood JM, *et al.* Oral cancer: Just the facts. *J Can Dent Assoc* 2008;**74**:269–72.

25. Vineis P, Alavanja M, Buffler P, *et al.* Tobacco and cancer: Recent epidemiological evidence. *J Natl Cancer Inst* 2004;**96**:99–106.

26. Mackay J, Eriksen M. *The tobacco atlas.* Geneva: WHO; 2002.

27. Singh B, Balwally AN, Shaha AR, *et al.* Upper aerodigestive tract squamous cell carcinoma—The human immunodeficiency virus connection. *Arch Otolaryngol Head Neck Surg* 1996;**122**:639–43.

28. Hoffmann D, Hoffmann I. Chemistry and toxicology. In: US Department of Health and Human Services. *Cigars, smoking and tobacco control.* Monograph: National Institutes of Health, National Cancer Institute; 1998:55–104.

29. Kapil U, Singh P. Nutritional risk factors in oral carcinoma. *Pak J Nutr* 2004;**3**:366–70.

30. Patel BP, Rawal UM, Shah PM, *et al.* Study of tobacco habits and alterations in enzymatic antioxidant system in oral cancer. *Oncology* 2005;**68**:511–19.

31. Lazarus P, Stern J, Zwiebel N, *et al.* Relationship between p53 mutation incidence in oral cavity squamous cell carcinomas and patient tobacco use. *Carcinogenesis* 1996;**17**:733–9.

32. Riboli E, Kaaks R, Esteve J. Nutrition and laryngeal cancer. *Cancer Causes Control* 1996;**7**:147–56.

33. LaVecchia C, Tavani A, Franceschi S, *et al.* Epidemiology and prevention of oral cancer. *Oral Oncology* 1997;**33**:302–12.

34. Mayne S, Morse D, Winn D. Cancers of the oral cavity and pharynx. In: Schottenfeld D, Fraumeni J Jr (eds). *Cancer epidemiology and prevention.* New York: Oxford University Press; 2006:647–96.

35. Cawson RA, Langdon JD, Eveson JW. *Surgical pathology of the mouth and jaws.* Oxford: Wright; 1996:204–8.

36. Lee YC, Boffetta P, Sturgis EM, *et al.* Involuntary smoking and head and neck cancer risk: Pooled analysis in the international head and neck cancer epidemiology consortium. *Cancer Epidemiol Biomarkers Prev* 2008;**17**:1974–81.

37. Secretan B, Straif K, Baan R, *et al.* WHO International Agency for Research on Cancer Monograph Working Group. A review of human carcinogens—Part E: Tobacco, areca nut, alcohol, coal smoke, and salted fish. *Lancet Oncol* 2009;**10**:1033–4.

38. Gupta PC, Ray CS. Epidemiology of betel quid usage. *Ann Acad Med Singapore* 2004;**33** (Suppl):31S–36S.

39. Bedi R. Betel-quid and tobacco chewing among the United Kingdom's Bangladeshi community. *Br J Cancer Suppl* 1996;**74**:73–7.

40. Chaturvedi P, Chaturvedi U, Sanyal B. Prevalence of tobacco consumption in school children in rural India—an epidemic of tobaccogenic cancers looming ahead in the third world. *J Cancer Educ* 2002;**17**:6.

41. Zienolddiny S, Aguelon AM, Mironov N, *et al.* Genomic instability in oral squamous cell carcinoma: Relationship to betel-quid chewing. *Oral Oncology* 2004;**40**:298–303.

42. Chang MC, Chiang CP, Lin CL, *et al.* Cell-mediated immunity and head and neck cancer: With special emphasis on betel quid chewing habit. *Oral Oncology* 2005;**41**:757–75.

43. Balaram P, Sridhar H, Rajkumar T, *et al.* Oral cancer in southern India: The influence of smoking, drinking, paan-chewing and oral hygiene. *Int J Cancer* 2002;**98**:440–45.

44. Dikshit RP, Kanhere S. Tobacco habits and risk of lung, oropharyngeal and oral cavity cancer: A population-based case–control study in Bhopal, India. *Int J Epidemiol* 2000;**29**:609–14.

45. Baan R, Straif K, Grosse Y, *et al.* WHO International Agency for Research on Cancer Monograph Working Group. Carcinogenicity of alcoholic beverages. *Lancet Oncol* 2007;**8**:292–3.

46. Yokoyama A, Omori T. Genetic polymorphisms of alcohol and aldehyde dehydrogenases and risk for esophageal and head and neck cancers. *Alcohol* 2005;**35**:175–85.

47. Seitz HK, Becker P. Alcohol metabolism and cancer risk. *Alcohol Res Health* 2007;**30**:38–41, 44–7.

48. Klienjans JC, Monnen EJ, Dallinga JW. Polycyclic Aromatic hydrocarbons in whiskey. *The Lancet* 1996;**348**:1731.

49. Rogers MA, Vaughan TL, Davis S, *et al.* Consumption of nitrate, nitrite and nitrosodimethylamine and the risk of upper aerodigestive tract cancer. *Cancer Epidemiol Biomarkers Prev* 1995;**4**:29–36.

50. Rodriguez T, Altieri A, Chatenoud L, *et al.* Risk factors for oral and pharyngeal cancer in young adults. *Oral Oncology* 2004;**40**:207–13.

51. De Stefani E, Boffetta P, Oreggia F, *et al.* Smoking patterns and cancer of the oral cavity and pharynx: A case–control study in Uruguay. *Oral Oncology* 1998;**34**:340–6.

52. Kreimer AR, Clifford GM, Boyle P, *et al.* Human papillomavirus types in head and neck squamous cell carcinomas worldwide: A systematic review. *Cancer Epidemiol Biomarkers Prev* 2005;**14**:467–75.

53. Rose Ragin CC, Taioli E. Second primary head and neck tumor risk in patients with cervical cancer—SEER data analysis. *Head Neck* 2008;**30**:58–66.

54. Begum S, Gillison ML, Ansari-Lari MA, *et al.* Detection of human papillomavirus in cervical lymph nodes: A highly effective strategy for localizing site of tumor origin. *Clin Cancer Res* 2003;**9**:6469–75.

55. Dahlstrom KR, Little JA, Zafereo ME, *et al.* Squamous cell carcinoma of the head and neck in never smoker-never drinkers: A descriptive epidemiologic study. *Head Neck* 2008;**30**:75–84.

56. Shiboski CH, Schmidt BL, Jordan RC. Tongue and tonsil carcinoma—Increasing trends in the US population ages 20–44 years. *Cancer* 2005;**103**:1843–9.

57. D'Souza G, Kreimer AR, Viscidi R, *et al.* Case–control study of human papillomavirus and oropharyngeal cancer. *N Engl J Med* 2007;**356**:1944–56.

58. Johns Hopkins Medical Institutions (2007, May 10). Oral sex increases risk of throat cancer. ScienceDaily. Retrieved March 13, 2010, from http://www.sciencedaily.com /releases/2007/05/070509210142.htm

59. Smith EM, Ritchie JM, Summersgill KF, *et al.* Human papillomavirus in oral exfoliated cells and risk of head and neck cancer. *J Natl Cancer Inst* 2004;**96**:449–55.

60. Bouvard V, Baan R, Straif K, *et al.* WHO International Agency for Research on Cancer Monograph Working Group. A review of human carcinogens—Part B: Biological agents. *Lancet Oncol* 2009;**10**:321–2.

61. Gupta PC, Hebert JR, Bhonsle RB, *et al.* Influence of dietary factors on oral precancerous lesions in a population-based case–control study in Kerala, India. *Cancer* 1999;**85**:1885–93.

62. Franceschi S, Bidoli E, Baron AE, *et al.* Nutrition and cancer of the oral cavity and pharynx in north-east Italy. *Int J Cancer* 1991;**47**:20–5.

63. Destefani E, Oreggia F, Ronco A, *et al.* Salted meat consumption as a risk factor for cancer of the oral cavity and pharynx—A case–control study from Uruguay. *Cancer Epidemiol Biomarkers Prev* 1994;**3**:381–5.

64. Rasheed MH, Beevi SS, Geetha A. Enhanced lipid peroxidation and nitric oxide products with deranged antioxidant status in patients with head and neck squamous cell carcinoma. *Oral Oncology* 2007;**43**:333–8.

65. World Cancer Research Fund International and American Institute for Cancer Research. Mouth, pharynx, and larynx. Food, nutrition, physical activity and the prevention of cancer: A global perspective. Washington, DC: AICR, 2007:245–49.

66. Key T, Schatzkin A, Willett WC, *et al.* Diet, nutrition and the prevention of cancer. *Public Health Nutrition* 2004;**7**:187–200.

67. Bosetti C, Gallus S, Trichopoulou A, *et al.* Influence of the mediterranean diet on the risk of cancers of the upper aerodigestive tract. *Cancer Epidemiol Biomarkers Prev* 2003;**12**:1091–4.

68. Pelucchi C, Talamini R, Negri E, *et al.* Folate intake and risk of oral and pharyngeal cancer. *Ann Oncol* 2003;**14**:1677–81.

69. Llewellyn CD, Johnson NW, Warnakulasuriya KA. Risk factors for squamous cell carcinoma of the oral cavity in young people—A comprehensive literature review. *Oral Oncology* 2001;**37**:401–18.

70. Ho T, Wei QY, Sturgis EM. Epidemiology of carcinogen metabolism genes and risk of squamous cell carcinoma of the head and neck. *Head Neck* 2007;**29**:682–99.

71. Lynch HT, Fusaro RM, Lynch J. Hereditary cancer in adults. *Cancer Detect Prev* 1995;**19**:219–33.

72. Caminero MJ, Nunez F, Suarez C, *et al.* Detection of p53 protein in oropharyngeal carcinoma—Prognostic implications. *Arch Otolaryngol Head Neck Surg* 1996;**122**:769–72.

73. Scully C, Field JK, Tanzawa H. Genetic aberrations in oral or head and neck squamous cell carcinoma (SCCHN): 1. Carcinogen metabolism, DNA repair and cell cycle control. *Oral Oncology* 2000;**36**:256–63.

74. Katoh T, Kaneko S, Kohshi K, *et al.* Genetic polymorphisms of tobacco- and alcohol-related metabolizing enzymes and oral cavity cancer. *Int J Cancer* 1999;**83**:606–9.

75. Sato M, Sato T, Izumo T, *et al.* Genetic polymorphism of drug-metabolizing enzymes and susceptibility to oral cancer. *Carcinogenesis* 1999;**20**:1927–31.

76. Tanimoto K, Hayashi S, Yoshiga K, *et al.* Polymorphisms of the CYP1A1 and GSTM1 gene involved in oral squamous cell carcinoma in association with a cigarette dose. *Oral Oncology* 1999;**35**:191–6.

77. Brennan JA, Boyle JO, Koch WM, *et al.* Association between cigarette-smoking and mutation of the P53 gene in squamous-cell carcinoma of the head and neck. *N Engl J Med* 1995;**332**:712–17.

78. Foulkes WD, Brunet JS, Sieh W, *et al.* Familial risks of squamous cell carcinoma of the head and neck: Retrospective case–control study. *BMJ* 1996;**313**:716–21.

79. Quon H, Hershock D, Feldman M, *et al.* Cancer of the head and neck. In: Abeloff M, Armitage J, Niederhuber J, Kastan M, McKenna W (eds). *Clinical oncology.* Orlando: Churchill Livingstone (Elsevier); 2004:1499–500.

80. Bhatia S, Louie AD, Bhatia R, *et al.* Solid cancers after bone marrow transplantation. *J Clin Oncol* 2001;**19**:464–71.

81. Curtis RE, Rowlings PA, Deeg HJ, *et al.* Solid cancers after bone marrow transplantation. *N Engl J Med* 1997;**336**:897–904.

82. Streilein JW. Immunogenetic factors in skin-cancer. *N Engl J Med* 1991;**325**:884–7.

83. Varga E, Tyldesley WR. Carcinoma arising in cyclosporine-induced gingival hyperplasia. *Br Dent J* 1991;**171**:26–7.

84. Straif K, Benbrahim-Tallaa L, Baan R, *et al.* WHO International Agency for Research on Cancer Monograph Working Group. A review of human carcinogens—part C: Metals, arsenic, dusts, and fibres. *Lancet Oncol* 2009;**10**:453–4.

85. Baan R, Grosse Y, Straif K, *et al.* WHO International Agency for Research on Cancer Monograph Working Group. A review of human carcinogens—Part F: Chemical agents and related occupations. *Lancet Oncol* 2009;**10**:1143–4.

86. El Ghissassi F, Baan R, Straif K, *et al.* WHO International Agency for Research on Cancer Monograph Working Group. A review of human carcinogens—part D: Radiation. *Lancet Oncol* 2009;**10**:751–2.

87. Cardis E, Howe G, Ron E, *et al.* Cancer consequences of the chernobyl accident: 20 years on. *J Radiol Prot* 2006;**26**:127–40.

88. Bloching M, Reich W, Schubert J, *et al.* The influence of oral hygiene on salivary quality in the ames test, as a marker for genotoxic effects. *Oral Oncology* 2007;**43**:933–9.

89. Rautemaa R, Hietanen J, Niissalo S, *et al.* Oral and oesophageal squamous cell carcinoma: A complication or component of autoimmune polyendocrinopathy-candidiasis-ectodermal dystrophy (APECED, APS-I). *Oral Oncology* 2007;**43**:607–13.

90. Goutzanis L, Vairaktaris E, Yapijakis C, *et al.* Diabetes may increase risk for oral cancer through the insulin receptor substrate-1 and focal adhesion kinase pathway. *Oral Oncology* 2007;**43**:165–73.

91. Hashibe M, Ford DE, Zhang ZF. Marijuana s/moking and head and neck cancer. *J Clin Pharmacol* 2002;**42**:103S–107S.

92. Lingen M, Sturgis EM, Kies MS. Squamous cell carcinoma of the head and neck in non-smokers: Clinical and biologic characteristics and implications for management. *Curr Opin Oncol* 2001;**13**:176–82.

93. Califano J, van der Riet P, Westra W, *et al.* Genetic progression model for head and neck cancer: Implications for field cancerization. *Cancer Res* 1996;**56**:2488–92.

94. Perez-Ordonez B, Beauchemin M, Jordan RC. Molecular biology of squamous cell carcinoma of the head and neck. *J Clin Pathol* 2006;**59**:445–53.

95. Ha PK, Califano JA. Promoter methylation and inactivation of tumour-suppressor genes in oral squamous-cell carcinoma. *Lancet Oncol* 2006;**7**:77–82.

96. Wang X, Li L, Hu C, *et al.* Patterns of level II node metastasis in nasopharyngeal carcinoma. *Radiother Oncol* 2008;**89**:28–32.

97. De Zinis LO, Cavalleri M, Casirati C, *et al.* Surgical treatment of neck lymph nodes in squamous cell carcinoma of the pyriform sinus. *Acta Otorhinolaryngol Ital* 2001;**21**:341–9.

98. Farrington WT, Weighill JS, Jones PH. Post-cricoid carcinoma (a ten-year retrospective study). *J Laryngol Otol* 1986;**100**:79–84.

99. Sessions DG, Lenox J, Spector GJ, *et al.* Analysis of treatment results for base of tongue cancer. *Laryngoscope* 2003;**113**:1252–61.

100. Hannisdal K, Boysen M, Evensen JF. Different prognostic indices in 310 patients with tonsillar carcinomas. *Head Neck* 2003;**25**:123–31.

101. Sheahan P, Ganly I, Rhys-Evans PH, *et al.* Tumors of the larynx. In: Montgomery PQ, Rhys-Evans PH, Gullane PJ (eds). *Principles and practice in head-neck surgery and oncology.* New York: Informa Healthcare; 2009:257–90.

102. Soo KC, Carter RL, O'Brien CJ, *et al.* Prognostic implications of perineural spread in squamous carcinomas of the head and neck. *Laryngoscope* 1986;**96**:1145–8.

103. Shah JP, Gil Z. Current concepts in management of oral cancer—surgery. *Oral Oncol* 2009;**45**:394–401.

104. Spiro RH, Huvos AG, Wong GY, *et al.* Predictive value of tumor thickness in squamous carcinoma confined to the tongue and floor of the mouth. *Am J Surg* 1986;**152**:345–50.

105. Shah JP, Andersen PE. Evolving role of modifications in neck dissection for oral squamous carcinoma. *Br J Oral Maxillofac Surg* 1995;**33**:3–8.

106. Audet N, Beasley NJ, MacMillan C, *et al.* Lymphatic vessel density, nodal metastases, and prognosis in patients with head and neck cancer. *Arch Otolaryngol Head Neck Surg* 2005;**131**:1065–70.

107. Giabella G. Cardiovascular. In: Williams PL, Bannister LH, Berry M, *et al.* (eds). *Gray's anatomy.* 38th ed. New York: Churchill Livingstone; 1995:1611–12.

108. Shah JP. Patterns of cervical lymph node metastasis from squamous carcinomas of the upper aerodigestive tract. *Am J Surg* 1990;**160**:405–9.

109. Stoeckli SJ. Sentinel node biopsy for oral and oropharyngeal squamous cell carcinoma of the head and neck. *Laryngoscope* 2007;**117**:1539–51.

110. Dwivedi RC, Kazi R, Agrawal N, *et al.* Comprehensive review of small bowel metastasis from head and neck squamous cell carcinoma. *Oral Oncol* 2010;**46**:330–5.

111. Zbären P, Lehmann W. Frequency and sites of distant metastases

in head and neck squamous cell carcinoma. An analysis of 101 cases at autopsy. *Arch Otolaryngol Head Neck Surg* 1987;**113**: 762–4.

112. Leon X, Quer M, Orus C, *et al*. Distant metastases in head and neck cancer patients who achieved loco-regional control. *Head Neck* 2000;**22**:680–6.

113. de Bree R, Deurloo EE, Snow GB, *et al*. Screening for distant metastases in patients with head and neck cancer. *Laryngoscope* 2000;**110**:397–401.

114. Ferlito A, Shaha AR, Silver CE, *et al*. Incidence and sites of distant metastases from head and neck cancer. *ORL J Otorhinolaryngol Relat Spec* 2001;**63**:202–7.

115. Vaamonde P, Martin C, Del Rio M, *et al*. Second primary malignancies in patients with cancer of the head and neck. *Otolaryngology-Head and Neck Surgery* 2003;**129**:65–70.

116. Bhattacharyya N, Nayak VK. Survival outcomes for second primary head and neck cancer: A matched analysis. *Otolaryngology-Head and Neck Surgery* 2005;**132**:63–8.

117. Slaughter DP, Southwick HW, Smejkal LW. Field cancerization in oral stratified squamous epithelium: Clinical implications of multicentric origin. *Cancer* 1953;**6**:963–8.

118. Braakhuis BJ, Tabor MP, Kummer JA, *et al*. A genetic explanation of Slaughter's concept of field cancerization: Evidence and clinical implications. *Cancer Res* 2003;**63**:1727–30.

119. Braakhuis BJ, Tabor MP, Leemans CR, *et al*. Second primary tumors and field cancerization in oral and oropharyngeal cancer: Molecular techniques provide new insights and definitions. *Head Neck* 2002;**24**:198–206.

120. Leon X, Quer M, Diez S, *et al*. Second neoplasm in patients with head and neck cancer. *Head Neck* 1999;**21**:204–10.

121. Do KA, Johnson MM, Doherty DA, *et al*. Second primary tumors in patients with upper aerodigestive tract cancers: Joint effects of smoking and alcohol (United States). *Cancer Causes Control* 2003;**14**:131–8.

122. Khuri FR, Kim ES, Lee JJ, *et al*. The impact of smoking status, disease stage, and index tumor site on second primary tumor incidence and tumor recurrence in the head and neck retinoid chemoprevention trial. *Cancer Epidemiol Biomarkers Prev* 2001;**10**:823–9.

2

Evaluation, management and outcomes of head and neck cancer

RAGHAV C. DWIVEDI, NISHANT AGRAWAL, RAVI C. DWIVEDI,
K.A. PATHAK, REHAN KAZI

EVALUATION

Owing to the complex anatomy and delicate physiology of the region, head and neck cancer (HNC) and its treatment often adversely affect patients in many ways, requiring a variety of medical and allied medical specialties to work in close coordination to abate disease and restore function. Therefore, evaluation of an HNC patient essentially involves a multidisciplinary team (MDT) approach[1,2] (Table 1). A comprehensive evaluation in a MDT setting ensures that the patient has been assessed thoroughly to optimize survival, functional outcomes and quality of life (QOL). A brief schema of patient evaluation is provided in Table 2.

History-taking

History is often the most important key in the management of HNC. A careful history can generate a complete differential diagnosis in the majority of patients, ensuring that all diagnostic possibilities have been considered before establishing a definitive diagnosis. HNCs are a diverse group of cancers, which affect different anatomical sub-sites that perform complex physiological functions; these results in varied clinical presentations and a diverse symptomatology.

Presenting symptoms often relate to pathology and signal a possible site of the disease. For instance, hoarseness indicates probable laryngeal involvement. Furthermore, the presence of risk factors, including smoking and alcohol intake, increases the likelihood of a malignant process. Other common symptoms of cancer in this region include oral ulceration, bleeding, otalgia, hearing loss/unilateral otitis media, nasal obstruction, sore throat, dysphagia, odynophagia, breathing difficulty and cervical lymphadenopathy.

Apart from diagnosis, the history provides estimates of

Table 1. Specialties involved in the management of HNCs

Components of a multidisciplinary team
• Head and neck surgeon
• Radiologist
• Pathologist
• Radiation oncologist
• Medical oncologist
• Plastic and reconstructive surgeon
• Dental oncologist/ prosthodontist
• Speech and swallowing therapist
• Clinical nurse specialist
• Dietician
• Clinical social worker

Table 2. A schema of evaluation of an HNC patient

Evaluation of an HNC patient
• History-taking
• Physical examination
• Metastatic work-up
• Medical evaluation
• Nutritional assessment
• Psychosocial assessment
• Investigations
—Radiological evaluation
—Pathological evaluation
—Endoscopic evaluation under anaesthesia

prognosis and aids in treatment selection. The duration, type, severity, progression of symptoms and degree of functional impairment are good indicators of the extent and severity of the disease process. The presence of symptoms, such as jaundice, bone pain and haemoptysis, indicate systemic spread of the disease, and indicate a poor prognosis. The presence of co-morbid medical conditions should be evaluated as these may considerably affect a patient's prognosis, treatment planning and outcome.

Physical examination

The importance of a proper physical examination cannot be overstated and a clinician should be able to evaluate the physical integrity of the head and neck region in detail. All symptoms and physical findings must be correlated with the patient's clinical presentation. The common dictum of inspection, palpation and auscultation (if necessary) should be strictly followed. A careful inspection and palpation of the surfaces and cavities of the head and neck region should be able to localize and characterize the pathological changes causing the patient's symptoms.

The clinician should pay special attention to abnormalities in the texture and colour of the mucosal linings of the upper aerodigestive tract (UADT). The earliest surface lesions may show only erythema and a slightly elevated, smooth or minimally roughened or ulcerated mucosa, which always deserve consideration for biopsy. The extent of involvement is often misleading on inspection, therefore digital/bimanual palpation of the suspicious area must be undertaken in all patients, especially with oral cavity and oropharyngeal lesions.

In patients presenting with isolated neck node enlargement, a thorough search should be conducted in the corresponding areas drained by that particular group of lymph nodes to locate the primary lesion. A thorough search is generally productive, although, in 5%–10% patients the primary lesion remains undectable (unknown primary carcinoma).

Examination of the neck must be carried out systematically and each level must be carefully palpated to detect lymph node enlargement or deep invasion of the tumour (Fig. 1 and Table 3).[3] The dictum of site, size, shape, number, consistency should always be followed. The deep cervical chain of nodes is particularly difficult to assess correctly, especially if the patient has a thick neck or if there is muscle spasm. At best, clinical examination of the neck has a 30% inaccuracy rate[4] with 10%–30% false-negative and/or false-positive rates.[5]

Nodal metastases from squamous cell carcinomas (SCCs) are typically hard and irregular and, when small, are generally mobile. As they enlarge, those in the deep cervical chain (levels II, III and IV) initially become attached to the structures in the carotid sheath and the overlying sternomastoid muscle with

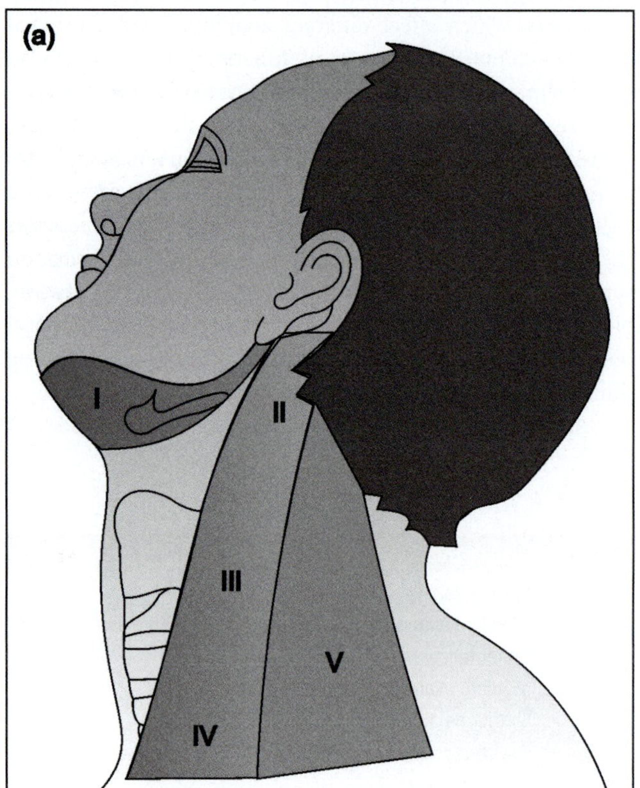

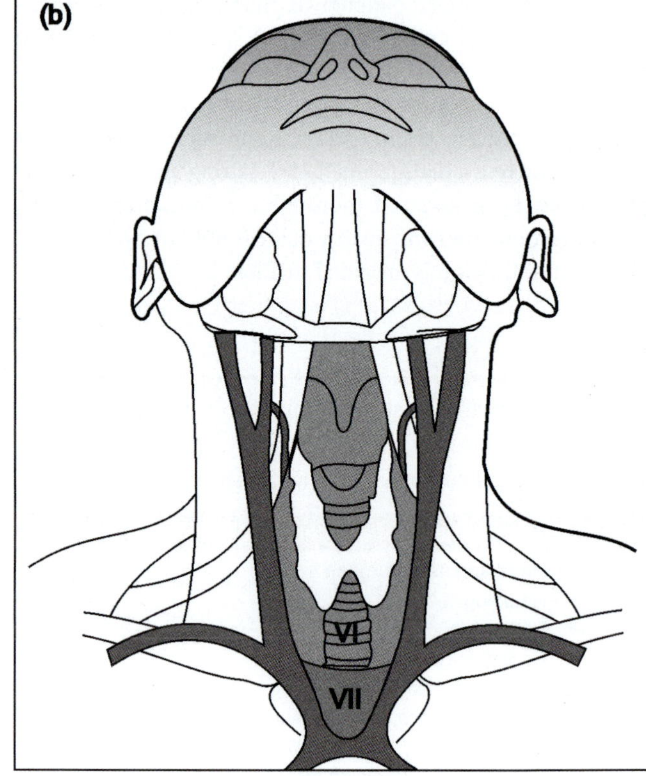

Fig. 1. Lymph node groups in the head and neck region with boundaries. (a) lateral view; (b) anterior view (adapted with permission from reference 3).

Table 3. Description of neck node levels in the head and neck region with clinical and surgical landmarks (adapted with permission from reference 3)

Nodal level	Clinical landmarks	Surgical landmarks
Level I	Submental and submandibular triangle	*Superiorly* Lower border of the body of the mandible *Inferiorly* Hyoid bone *Anteriorly* Midline of the neck *Posteriorly* Posterior belly of the diagastric muscle
Level II	Upper jugular lymph nodes	*Superiorly* Base of skull *Inferiorly* Hyoid bone *Anteriorly* Posterior belly of the diagastric muscle *Posteriorly* Posterior border of the sternocleidomastoid muscle
Level III	Middle jugular lymph nodes	*Superiorly* Hyoid bone *Inferiorly* Cricoid cartilage *Anteriorly* Lateral limit of the sternohyoid muscle *Posteriorly* Posterior border of the sternocleidomastoid muscle
Level IV	Lower jugular lymph nodes	*Superiorly* Cricoid cartilage *Inferiorly* The Clavicle *Anteriorly* Lateral limit of the sternohyoid muscle *Posteriorly* Posterior border of the sternocleidomastoid muscle
Level V	Posterior triangle lymph nodes	*Superiorly* Base of skull *Inferiorly* The Clavicle *Anteriorly* Posterior border of the sternohyoid muscle *Posteriorly* Anterior border of the trapezius muscle
Level VI	Lymph nodes in the anterior compartment of the neck	*Superiorly* Hyoid bone *Inferiorly* Suprasternal notch *Medially* Imaginary midline *Laterally* Medial border of the carotid sheath
Level VII	Superior mediastinal lymph nodes	Suprasternal notch

restriction of vertical mobility, but later become attached to the deeper structures in the prevertebral region with absolute fixation. Cystic degeneration or necrosis in a metastatic jugulodigastric node may cause rapid enlargement and may initially be confused for a branchial cyst, with potential delay in accurate diagnosis. Lymphomatous nodes have a firm and rubbery consistency and are generally larger and multiple with matting of adjacent nodes.

Examination of the head and neck region is deemed incomplete without a sensory–motor examination. A complete sensory and motor examination of the head and neck region should always be done, particularly mobility of the tongue as well as fixation. A hypoglossal nerve paralysis causes wasting of the ipsilateral tongue with deviation to the affected side on protrusion, but in the early stages only fasciculations may be apparent. Palatal movement may be impaired by the tumour mass but a palsy of the vagus nerve near the skull base will also cause weakness, often leading to vocal cord palsy in addition. An impaired sensation over the anterior chin distribution of the mental nerve and the lateral part of the tongue is an ominous sign, indicating invasion of the inferior alveolar nerve or the lingual nerve in the infratemporal fossa.

Fibreoptic endoscopes are usually available in most of the clinics and should be used routinely. Fibreoptic examination under a local anaesthetic has greatly enhanced the ease of examination of the pharynx and larynx, particularly in assessing the lower extent of the tumour and mobility of structures at or below the level of the hyoid. It is also valuable for estimating invasion of the nasopharynx. Indirect laryngoscopy with a mirror is no longer deemed sufficient for optimum assessment, but should always be performed if the facilities of fibreoptic endoscopy are not routinely available.

Metastatic work-up

Although HNC is generally considered a local or locoregional disease, because of the propensity of regional lymph node involvement, the possibility of distant spread should not be overlooked. Patients with advanced disease (large primary tumours, bulky/multiple/bilateral neck nodes, lower deep-cervical lymph node involvement), recurrent disease, second primary tumours, or with tumours of high-risk areas (supraglottic larynx, hypopharynx and oropharynx) are especially prone to early nodal and distant spread of the disease, mandating a thorough metastatic work-up.[6] As the majority of distant metastasis from HNC involve the lungs, a minimum of one screening chest radiograph (or preferably a CT scan) should always be performed, to avoid futile extensive treatments.[7,8]

At centres having the facility of a CT scan, neck imaging should always be undertaken and the screening field should preferably be extended to include the head, chest and upper abdomen to screen the lungs, skull and liver and to rule out pulmonary, bone or liver metastasis. Rarely, a bone scan may be required if there is suspicion of a bony metastasis. However, it is not performed routinely, as in the absence of obvious lung metastasis, the chances of bone metastasis are extremely low in HNC.[6]

Medical evaluation

A general medical evaluation of patients is important to identify and assess any associated co-morbid condition that may affect selection of the treatment modality, outcomes and prognosis of a patient. Also, evaluation of a patient's performance status should be followed from pre-treatment phase through recovery, as it is a good predictor of post-treatment medical complications and prognosis.

Nutritional assessment

The majority of HNC patients present with malnutrition and nutritional deficiencies because of the disease process and/or poor dietary intake secondary to dysphagia and odynophagia. Also, most of the HNC patients are tobacco and alcohol abusers, which further aggravate nutritional depletion. Malnutrition is known to decrease wound healing, compromise immunological functions and increase susceptibility to infections, all of which may affect outcome and prognosis. All patients should receive nutritional support, irrespective of the modality and course of treatment.

Psychosocial assessment

The dysfunction and disfigurement of structures of the head and neck, which arises from HNC and its treatment, have a great psychological impact on patients and may lead to social isolation. These patients also have problems with self-esteem secondary to changes in self-image,[9] which may further pose a challenge to treating clinicians. Therefore, pre-treatment assessment should focus on coping skills, family support, personality disorders, psychiatric illness and substance abuse. Patients should be encouraged to meet with former patients, speech therapists and support groups, as this helps them understand post-treatment changes, provides a firm evidence of survival and reduces uncertainty.

MANAGEMENT

Investigations

Accurate evaluation of local disease and regional metastasis is critical in planning the management of HNC patients. In general, physical examination of the head and neck region, augmented by radiological evaluation, forms the basis of the TNM classification and staging system.

Radiological investigations

Although endoscopy is the ideal investigation for mapping the superficial extent of the lesion, the critical role of imaging is to define the deeper extent of the disease and the relationship of the tumour to various structures that are key determinants of the surgical approach and potential resectability.

Computed tomography (CT) and magnetic resonance imaging (MRI)

CT scan and/or MRI are usually the first line of investigations in patients clinically suspected of having a cancer of the head and neck. CT delineates muscle from fat and gives an excellent image of bone. The tumour can be identified by its effects on the fat planes, which become important landmarks throughout the head and neck region. MRI uses a magnetic field (unlike CT which utilizes ionizing radiation) that provides better soft tissue delineation than CT but takes a much longer time to perform. These imaging techniques are extensively used in the head and neck region. However, a detailed description of these techniques and their advantages and disadvantages are beyond the scope of this chapter.

The extent of the primary tumour and its relation to adjacent soft tissue structures is better determined by MRI than CT because the density of the soft tissue is often identical to that of tumour on a CT. MRI is particularly useful for small tongue base tumours to determine the extent of soft tissue invasion.[10] The interface between tumour and paranasal sinuses can frequently be visualized on CT but it is more consistently delineated on MRI. MRI is also very useful in defining intracranial extension of skull-base and paranasal sinus tumours and to rule out dural or brain involvement compared with a CT scan. The main disadvantages of MRI include longer imaging time and motion artifacts during normal physiological processes, such as breathing and deglutition.

CT scan is the gold standard for investigating any bony invasion.[10] CT is also highly accurate for evaluating the neck to assess the presence, site, size and invasive potential of cervical lymphadenopathy and, in particular, its relation to important structures, such as the carotid artery and internal jugular vein. After radiotherapy to the neck, these examinations are less dependable in accurately assessing the disease, especially in the carotid sheath region, because of post-radiotherapy fibrosis, which sometimes may be mistaken for the tumour itself.

CT scan is extremely useful in assessing clinically N0 necks, particularly in obese patients, those with a thick neck, or where there is a spasm. It helps in identifying possible nodes in the jugular chain, or in the spinal accessory chain deep to the sternomastoid (Fig. 14 of Chapter 1). CT is also sensitive in evaluating retropharyngeal nodes (nodes of rouviere) and parapharyngeal nodes, which are clinically undetectable. A rounded (non-oval), low attenuation lymph node with a definable rim and a dark central portion represents carcinomatous replacement of a lymph node and mandates further investigation, irrespective of the size of the node. The calculated sensitivity of CT and MRI for detecting lymph node metastases ranges from 36% to 94%, whereas the specificity ranges from 50% to 98%.[11]

Positron emission tomography (PET) and PET-CT

Malignant tumour cells are known to be metabolically more active than the cells within normal surrounding tissue. This metabolic hyperactivity is represented by increased tracer (a glucose analogue tagged with a positron-emitting isotope of fluorine: 2-[18F] fluoro-2-deoxy-d-glucose [FDG]) uptake on PET in the area of the tumour cells, allowing for the use of FDG-PET imaging in the detection of HNCs.[12] Underlying infection, inflammation and normal lymphoid tissue may lead to false-positive PET scan results, because of increased tracer uptake in these conditions.[13,14]

The sensitivity of FDG-PET in detecting cervical lymph node metastases of HNCs varies between 67% and 96%, whereas the specificity ranges between 82% and 100%.[15,16] FDG-PET is also more accurate in detecting primary tumours in general, as well as in patients with unknown primary carcinoma.[17] Although PET imaging does not provide anatomical definition, the combination of FDG-PET and CT has been reported to be more accurate than either alone in the detection and anatomical localization of HNCs, and thus may affect patient care and final outcome.[18,19] PET has also been shown to be of value in detecting recurrent SCC of the head and neck (HNSCC).[20] Potential clinical applications of FDG-PET are summarized in Table 4.

Plain X-ray films

Plain X-ray radiographs have a limited role in the imaging of

Table 4. Potential applications of FDG-PET in HNC

Applications of FDG-PET in HNC
• To detect occult metastatic nodal disease, which is not amenable to detection by clinical examination or any other imaging modality
• To assess occult distant metastatic disease
• To detect second primary carcinomas
• In pre-treatment staging; diagnosis may be upstaged in up to 20% of patients, requiring gross alteration in treatment regimen, especially from M0 to M1
• To detect unknown primary carcinoma
• To detect recurrent disease
• For treatment monitoring
• For proper intensity modulated radiotherapy (IMRT) planning
• As a prognostic marker in HNSCC

tumours involving the head and neck region. They provide minimal information about soft tissues because the densities of the various components of similar soft tissues are nearly equal. However, plain X-rays of the chest are still used in routine examinations to rule out metastatic carcinoma, synchronous bronchial primary tumours, and any coexisting acute or chronic pulmonary disease. A special form of plain X-ray, the orthopantomogram, may be necessary in cases of oral and oropharyngeal cancers for assessing mandibular invasion should a mandibulatomy be planned, or to visualize the dentition before commencing radiotherapy.

Ultrasound examination

Ultrasound examination is also of limited use in the head and neck region. However, it is used extensively in lesions of the thyroid and parathyroid gland, because of their easy accessibility by the ultrasound probes. Ultrasound is also used occasionally in the evaluation of tumours of the salivary glands, especially submandibular and parotid glands. Ultrasound examination of the neck to detect metastatic nodal disease is more sensitive than palpation and has a specificity of approximately 75%. The specificity is improved to >90% with the use of ultrasound-guided aspiration cytology, compared with CT and MRI scans (approximately 80%).[21] This technique is highly dependable in experienced hands and has proven to be an excellent method of neck node evaluation.

Fine-needle aspiration cytology (FNAC) and fine-needle aspiration biopsy (FNAB)

Any suspicious swelling or node within the head and neck region should have FNAC at the initial consultation, which should allow rapid differentiation between a cancerous and non-cancerous tumour. Aspiration of cystic fluid from a necrotic metastatic node may give a false-negative result and should be repeated to sample the solid portion or wall of the tumour, if necessary under ultrasound guidance. It requires the skills of a well-trained cytopathologist to demonstrate the excellent diagnostic accuracy of these examination techniques. If the findings of FNAC or FNAB do not correlate with the clinical picture of the patient, the clinician should pursue further diagnostic evaluation until he or she is confident of the findings. In cases of lymphoma, FNAC is usually inconclusive, mandating FNAB or an open biopsy.

Examination under anaesthesia (EUA) and biopsy

A biopsy may be taken under local anaesthesia in the clinic when appropriate, especially when there could be unacceptable risks with a general anaesthetic, as in the case of the elderly or infirm patients. However, in all other patients a full examination of the UADT using pan-endoscopy

Table 5. Rationale for examination under anaesthesia (EUA) in HNC patients

Reasons for performing EUA in HNC patients
• To biopsy the lesion
• To search for possible synchronous lesions
• To assess fixation of the primary lesion
• For bimanual palpation, particularly lesions of the tongue base
• To assess the extent of involvement
• For evaluation of the neck and to perform FNAC, if necessary
• For evaluation of the airway and to carry out a tracheostomy, if necessary
• For dental extraction before treatment, if required
• For bone marrow aspiration in case of lymphoma
• For PEG (percutaneous endoscopic gastrostomy) insertion if nutritional support is required

(bronchoscopy, oesophagoscopy and laryngoscopy) under general anaesthesia should be performed as a matter of routine (Table 5).

Classification of HNC

The standardization of cancer classification provides universal definitions to ensure uniform collection and reporting of cancer-related information in cancer registries. Without standard definitions for reporting of tumours and cancer patients, confusion arises in cancer statistics, including those for reporting the results and evaluation of treatments.

It is for this reason that a TNM classification was proposed in 1944[22] and later incorporated in 1953 by the Union Internationale Contre le Cancer (UICC) into a formal classification system for cancer. The TNM system came into clinical use in the United States of America in 1959 when the American Joint Committee on Cancer (AJCC) adopted it in staging and end-result reporting of cancer.[23] During the past five decades, the AJCC has worked to develop TNM definitions and stage classifications for all anatomical sites and sub-sites, revise definitions and classifications from results of clinical studies, and educate physicians and other healthcare professionals about the TNM classification system.[24] The latest version of the TNM system (7th edition) became effective in 2010.[25] The main objectives of TNM classification include: (i) Aiding the clinicians in planning treatment; (ii) giving an indication of prognosis; (iii) assisting in the evaluation of end results; (iv) facilitating the exchange of information between treatment centres; and (v) assisting in the continuing investigation of cancer.

Gross morphological classification

Morphological classification attempts to establish standard measures of the physical extent of the cancer across different anatomical sites. Owing to the variability in clinical presentation,

Table 6. T-stage classification of HNCs, depending on the anatomical sub-site (adapted with permission from reference 26)

Oral cavity, including lip

Tx	Primary tumour cannot be assessed
T0	No evidence of primary tumour
Tis	Carcinoma *in situ*
T1	≤2 cm
T2	>2–4 cm
T3	>4 cm
T4a	Oral cavity: Through cortical bone, deep/extrinsic muscles of tongue, maxillary sinus, skin Lip: Through cortical bone, inferior alveolar nerve, floor of mouth, skin
T4b	Masticator space, pterygoid plates, skull base, internal carotid artery

Larynx

Supraglottis

T1	One sub-site, normal mobility
T2	Mucosa of more than one adjacent sub-site of supraglottis, or glottis, or adjacent region outside the supraglottis, without fixation
T3	Cord fixation or invasion of postcricoid area, pre-epiglottic tissue, paraglottic space, thyroid cartilage erosion
T4a	Through thyroid cartilage, trachea, soft tissue of neck, deep/extrinsic muscles of tongue, strap muscles, thyroid, oesophagus
T4b	Prevertebral space, mediastinal structures, carotid artery

Glottis

T1	Limited to vocal cord/s, normal mobility a: One cord b: Both cords
T2	Supraglottis, subglottis, impaired cord mobility
T3	Cord fixation, paraglottic space, thyroid cartilage erosion
T4a	Through thyroid cartilage, trachea, soft tissue of neck, deep/extrinsic muscles of tongue, strap muscles, thyroid, oesophagus
T4b	Prevertebral space, mediastinal structures, carotid artery

Subglottis

T1	Limited to subglottis
T2	Extends to vocal cord/s with normal/impaired mobility
T3	Cord fixation
T4a	Through thyroid cartilage, trachea, soft tissue of neck, deep/extrinsic muscles of tongue, strap muscles, thyroid, oesophagus
T4b	Prevertebral space, mediastinal structures, carotid artery

Pharynx

Nasopharynx

T1	Nasopharynx
T2	Soft tissue a: Oropharynx/nasal cavity without parapharyngeal extension b: Tumour with parapharyngeal extension
T3	Bony structures, paranasal sinuses
T4	Intracranial extension, cranial nerves, infratemporal fossa, hypopharynx, orbit, masticator space

Oropharynx

T1	≤2 cm
T2	>2–4 cm
T3	>4 cm
T4a	Larynx, deep/extrinsic muscles of tongue, medial pterigyoid, hard palate, mandible
T4b	Lateral pterygoid muscle, pterygoid plates, lateral nasopharynx, skull base, carotid artery

Hypopharynx

T1	≤2 cm or limited to one sub-site
T2	>2–4 cm or invasion of more than one sub-site
T3	>4 cm or with fixation of hemilarynx
T4a	Thyroid/cricoid cartilage, hyoid bone, thyroid gland, oesophagus, or central compartment soft tissue
T4b	Prevertebral fascia, encases carotid artery, or involves mediastinal structures

Thyroid

Papillary, follicular and medullary carcinoma

T1	≤2 cm, intrathyroidal
T2	>2–4 cm, intrathyroidal
T3	>4 cm or minimal extension
T4a	Subcutaneous, larynx, trachea, oesophagus, recurrent laryngeal nerve
T4b	Prevertebral fascia, mediastinal vessels, carotid artery

Anaplastic/undifferentiated carcinoma

T4a	Tumour limited to thyroid
T4b	Tumour beyond thyroid capsule

tumours from all sites are classified in general terms, according to the anatomical extent of the primary tumour (T), regional nodal involvement (N), and presence of distant metastatic disease (M)—the TNM classification system.

T categories

The general criteria for categorizing tumours of the head and neck region are surface spread and size of the tumour. The T classification for cancers involving the varying sub-sites is different, but the basic principle remains the same (Table 6).

N categories

The general criteria for the classification of regional lymph node spread are based on size, number, distribution and level of involvement (Table 7). Size is one of the most important criteria in nodal classification, but it may be difficult to determine it clinically. A superficial node that is >0.5 cm in diameter is usually palpable, whereas a deeper node must reach 1 cm in diameter before if becomes palpable.

The level of lymph node involvement is generally discussed in terms of stations (echelon), which refers to a regular stopping place in a stage of progression. The first echelon is the cluster

Table 7. N-stage classification of HNCs, depending on the anatomical sub-site (adapted with permission from reference 26)

N-stage for all sub-sites except thyroid and nasopharynx

N1	Ipsilateral single ≤3 cm
N2	a: Ipsilateral single >3–6 cm
	b: Ipsilateral multiple ≤6 cm
	c: Bilateral, contralateral ≤6 cm
N3	>6 cm

N-stage for thyroid

N1a	Level VI nodes
N1b	Other regional node/s

N-stage for nasopharynx

N1	Unilateral node/s ≤6 cm, above supraclavicular fossa
N2	Bilateral node/s ≤6 cm, above supraclavicular fossa
N3	a: >6 cm
	b: In supraclavicular fossa

of lymph nodes receiving direct drainage of a specific site or organ. The second echelon refers to nodes that commonly receive lymphatic drainage from other lymph nodes, rather than directly from the site or organ. The level of lymph node involvement has been shown to be of prognostic importance; however, it is not included in the N classification.

M categories

Metastasis is classified as either present or absent, i.e. as M1 or M0. When the metastatic work-up has not been completed and the probability of metastasis is low, the designation MX should be used.

Microscopic morphological classification

The cancers can also be classified on the basis of the degree of differentiation of tumours into the following grades: GX, grade cannot be assessed; G1, well differentiated; G2, moderately differentiated; G3, poorly differentiated; and G4, undifferentiated.

Staging of HNC

Staging must not be confused as the classification of cancer; it is in fact a separate entity and involves grouping of tumours with similar crude survival rates. For each cancer, the individual T, N, and M category ratings, if combined in tandem, will form different expressions. Because there are five categories of T, four categories of N and two categories of M, a total of 40 different combinations of TNM expressions are possible, which are grouped as I, II, III and IV (Table 8).

Table 8. Stage grouping of various HNCs (adapted with permission from reference 26)

All sites except thyroid and nasopharynx

Stage 0	Tis	N0	M0
Stage I	T1	N0	M0
Stage II	T2	N0	M0
Stage III	T1, T2	N1	M0
	T3	N0, N1	M0
Stage IVa	T1, T2, T3	N2	M0
	T4a	N0, N1, N2	M0
Stage IVb	Any T	N3	M0
	T4b	Any N	M0
Stage IVc	Any T	Any N	M1

Thyroid

Papillary or follicular, under age of 45 years

Stage I	Any T	Any N	M0
Stage II	Any T	Any N	M1

Papillary or folloicular, above 45 years of and medullary carcinoma

Stage I	T1	N0	M0
Stage II	T2	N0	M0
Stage III	T3	N0	M0
	T1, T2, T3	N1a	M0
Stage IVa	T1, T2, T3	N1b	M0
	T4a	N0, N1	M0
Stage IVb	T4b	Any N	M0
Stage IVc	Any T	Any N	M1

Anaplastic/undifferentiated

Stage IVa	T4a	Any N	M0
Stage IVb	T4b	Any N	M0
Stage IVc	Any T	Any N	M1

Nasopharynx

Stage 0	Tis	N0	M0
Stage I	T1	N0	M0
Stage IIa	T2a	N0	M0
Stage IIb	T1	N1	M0
	T2a	N1	M0
	T2b	N0, N1	M0
Stage III	T1	N2	M0
	T2a, T2b	N2	M0
	T3	N0, N1, N2	M0
Stage IVa	T4	N0, N1, N2	M0
Stage IVb	Any T	N3	M0
Stage IVc	Any T	Any N	M1

Treatment

General principles

The aims of the treatment of HNCs are cure, organ preservation, attenuation of the morbidities associated with therapy, and improvement in QOL.[2] For patients who achieve cure, second primary cancers pose a significant risk; therefore, prevention of second malignancies are the goals of therapy in the treatment of patients with HNCs.[27]

Table 9. Factors determining the choice of the initial treatment of HNCs

Tumour factors
• Site of the tumour
• Sub-site of the tumour
• Size of the tumour
• Stage of the tumour
• Grade of the tumour
• Status of the neck nodes
• Depth of tumour invasion
• Proximity to bone, cartilage, nerves and great vessels
• Previous treatment

Patient factors
• Age of the patient
• Lifestyle of the patient (smoking or drinking)
• Occupation
• General medical condition
• Performance status of the patient
• Socioeconomic considerations
• Previous treatment

Clinician factors
• Surgery
• Radiotherapy
• Chemotherapy
• Nursing and rehabilitation
• Support services
• Dental and prosthetic rehabilitation

In general, the choice of treatment for a patient depends on a number of tumour factors, patient factors and clinician factors (Table 9). Tumour factors influencing selection of treatment modality depend on the variables that affect the natural history of the disease. The most notable factors are site, size and depth of invasion of the primary tumour. Where cure rates for surgery and radiotherapy are similar, the choice is usually that which causes the least functional disability.[28] Deeply ulcerative lesions are best treated with initial surgery followed by postoperative radiation therapy, as the results of salvage surgery in this setting are poor.

It is well established that the single most important prognostic factor in HNC is the nodal status of the disease at the time of initial presentation.[29,30] The presence of nodal metastases in the neck at presentation reduces the prognosis by about 50%.[31,32] Although radical radiotherapy may be effective in N0 and early N1 nodal disease, optimum treatment for N+ disease usually involves a combination of primary surgery (including neck dissection) with postoperative radiotherapy in high-risk patients.[33]

Curative treatment of HNC depends on the stage of the disease. In general, early stage (stage I or II) disease can be cured by either surgery or radiotherapy alone. Curative intent for advanced stage is either by surgery followed by adjuvant radiotherapy with possible chemotherapy, depending on the final pathological characteristics, or concurrent chemoradiotherapy with possible salvage surgery. Primary chemotherapy and newer forms of biological therapy or immunotherapy are still in the evolving phase and do not appear to give consistent results. Hence, they are reserved for the adjuvant or palliative setting.

Surgery

Surgery is a time-tested standard treatment for HNC but is frequently limited by the anatomical extent of the tumour and desire to achieve organ preservation.[34] Advances in microsurgical free tissue transfer for reconstruction of surgical defects have made major reconstructive procedures commonplace at many centres, and have facilitated the reconstruction of locally advanced tumours. By use of modern surgical techniques, improved functional outcomes are often possible for patients who need extensive surgical resections, even in the setting of salvage surgery after failure of chemoradiotherapy.[34] Although HNCs do not have uniform general unresectability criteria, most surgeons accept invasion of the carotid artery, base of skull or pre-vertebral musculature as unresectable.[34] The several advantages in adopting a surgical management of HNC are summarized in the Table 10.

Neck dissection is routinely carried out when surgery is the primary modality of HNC treatment and provides the basis of accurate disease staging. The disease is often upstaged in apparently clinically negative necks by histological identification of micrometastasis, which may affect adjuvant treatment decisions.[35] However, after treatment with primary chemoradiotherapy, neck dissection in usually recommended when residual disease is suspected, on the basis of physical examination, anatomical imaging or metabolic imaging; whereas its role remains controversial in the setting of complete response.[36,37]

Table 10. Advantages of surgical management of HNCs

Advantages of surgery
• Exact pathological staging of the disease is obtained by virtue of direct examination of the primary tumour and the regional lymph nodes. It often upstages the disease and thereby provides guide to adjuvant treatment decisions.
• Shorter treatment time
• Limited amount of tissue is exposed to treatment.
• Provides good functional preservation by avoiding risk of immediate and late radiation sequelae, especially for smaller tumours.
• Radiation therapy can be reserved for recurrent or subsequent tumours, which are known to occur in >50% of the cases.
• Microsurgical treatment with the use of endoscopic laser, robotic techniques and high resolution optics saves costs and provides good functional results.

Table 11. Advantages of radiotherapy in the management of HNCs

Advantages of radiotherapy
• Avoidance of a major surgery
• No immediate threat to life (avoidance of operative or postoperative mortality)
• Avoidance of scars and cosmetic defects
• Preservation of organ function (is still debated as anatomical preservation does not essentially mean functional preservation)
• Nearly equal outcomes with surgery for early disease.

Radiotherapy

Radiotherapy is most effective in eradicating microscopic disease that is less amenable to surgery (Table 11).[38] It is an integral part of primary or adjuvant treatment for HNC. Radiotherapy alone can control disease in early-stage glottic, base of tongue, and tonsillar cancers.[34] Newer radiotherapy techniques, such as altered fractionation (hyperfractionation and accelerated fractionation), intensity-modulated radiotherapy and 3-D conformal radiotherapy (3-D CRT) have dramatically changed management approaches for some of the HNCs, most notably laryngeal and oropharyngeal cancers. A detailed description of various radiotherapy techniques is beyond the scope of this chapter.

Chemotherapy

The role of chemotherapy has evolved from palliative care to a central component of curative programmes for locally advanced HNC,[39] although it is still in its early stages. The platinum-based compound, cisplatin, is regarded as a standard agent in combination with radiation or with other agents.[34] Neo-adjuvant chemotherapy (given prior to radiotherapy or surgery) is known to improve local control and may allow greater organ preservation, but it does not affect overall survival.[38] However, concurrent chemotherapy does show an 8% absolute survival benefit compared with radiotherapy alone.[40] Chemotherapy along with radiotherapy may have improved organ preservation and survival, but this remains under investigation.[38]

Newer agents

Novel agents, such as epidermal growth factor receptor inhibitors, angiogenesis inhibitors, single-selective or multi-selective tyrosine kinase inhibitors, monoclonal antibodies and nucleic acid-directed approaches for the management of HNC are also being explored currently.[34,41] The combination of these novel agents with chemotherapy and radiotherapy is also under investigation and may offer some breakthrough in the management of HNC in the near future.

Treatment of early stage HNC

Early-stage disease (stages I and II) is generally best treated by single modality, either radiotherapy or surgery, with equivalent results.[42] The estimated cure rates for HNC treated with curative intent, either with surgery or radiotherapy, are high for early HNC; for stage I they reach up to 90%, whereas for stage 2 disease they are around 70%.[34] Treatment approaches differ according to the site of the primary tumour. Surgery or radiotherapy can be used for early-stage oral cavity cancer, but surgery is usually preferred to avoid the late toxic effect of radiation.[43] Elective ipsilateral functional neck dissection remains a standard practice in patients with a high-risk of occult nodal metastasis.[44] Radiotherapy, as well as open or endoscopic surgery, are acceptable options for treating early-stage laryngeal cancers.[45–47] Radiotherapy is generally preferred over surgery for early-stage oropharyngeal and hypopharyngeal cancers, because of comparable survival rates, lower morbidity, and better functional results associated with the former.[48,49]

Treatment of advanced-stage HNC

For locally advanced lesions (stages III and IV), combined therapy with surgery (if deemed resectable) followed by postoperative radiotherapy or chemo-radiotherapy is generally accepted as giving the best chance of cure.[42,50] In general, oral cavity primaries are usually treated with surgery, as the cosmetic and functional results are regarded as satisfactory and patients might be spared aggressive chemo-radiotherapy, which can sometimes leave an anatomically intact but dysfunctional organ. However, locally advanced oropharyngeal cancers are usually treated by chemo-radiotherapy with good efficacy and functional results.[51] Patients with locally advanced laryngeal and hypopharyngeal cancers should be considered for organ preservation as an option.[34] In patients with unresectable, locally advanced HNC, chemo-radiotherapy is standard,[52] unless the addition of chemotherapy is contraindicated because of poor performance status or co-morbid illness.

Follow up and rehabilitation

Follow up and rehabilitation of patients who have had treatment for HNC is often a prolonged process. Apart from a great deal of patience, successful rehabilitation requires close cooperation between the members of the MDT. Regular post-treatment follow up provides an opportunity for patients and clinicians to achieve the goals of the treatment and to provide surveillance for recurrent or new disease. The time-scale of post-treatment follow up for HNC patients is crucial, as recurrence of the disease and/or emergence of multiple primaries (because of field cancerization) is extremely common. All patients should be examined by a clinician on a monthly basis for the first post-treatment year, every 2 months in the second year, every 3 months in the third year, and every 6 months thereafter.[53] A baseline follow-up CT or MRI imagining taken between 3 and 6 months after completion of therapy is essential. Persistent or recurrent tissue asymmetry or increased tissue enhancement should arouse suspicion for residual or recurrent disease, mandating further investigations. In case of no apparent clinical correlation, an additional PET or PET-CT may be useful. It is even more difficult to detect persistent or recurrent disease in patients who have undergone a flap reconstruction for the post-excision defect. A high index of suspicion is required in these cases and in presence of persistent or progressive tissue changes, a biopsy should always be performed as a rule.

OUTCOMES

Survival

Despite advancements in the therapeutic modalities, the long-term survival rates of most HNCs have not improved, the exact reasons for which are still under investigation. HNCs are notorious for local and locoregional recurrence, as evident by the fact that over half of the cases recur in the period of 2 years following the treatment. Although we have been successful in achieving good local and locoregional control of HNC, more patients are now known to develop distant metastasis that may result from failure to achieve disease control, which accounts for the poor survival rates of patients with HNC.

Nearly two-thirds of patients with HNC present with advanced stage (stages III or IV).[34,54] Survival rates of HNC

depend considerably on the stage of the disease at the time of initial presentation. In general, better survival rates are reported for patients presenting with early-stage disease (stage I and II) compared with those presenting with an advanced disease (stages III and IV) (Fig. 2), irrespective of the treatment modality.[56]

The site of the primary lesion also affects the survival rates in HNC. The reported 5-year survival rates are poor for cancers arising in the hypopharynx, supraglottic larynx and base of tongue, compared with the oral tongue and glottic cancers. The cancers arising in the former are clinically silent, and these sites have rich lymphatics, which collectively are responsible for late presentation and early disease spread. On the other hand, tumours that have better 5-year survival rates are those that arise in sites that are highly visible to the patient, do not involve vital structures early in the disease process, compromise function early in the course of the disease, and arise in areas relatively devoid of lymphatics.

A marked difference (10%–20%) is observed in 5-year survival rates between poor and affluent patients, even in developed countries. This may be linked to a delay in diagnosis, more advanced stage of the disease at the initial presentation, poor general health, poor access to optimal healthcare, and lower compliance with treatment in poor people (Fig. 3).[38,57] Similar trends of deprivation effect are reflected across the globe, with higher mortality rates in less developed countries compared with the developed nations (Fig. 4).[58]

Functional outcomes and QOL

The impact of a diagnosis of HNC on the patient and the consequences of its treatment cross multiple domains that have a clear and direct influence on the patient's post-treatment well-

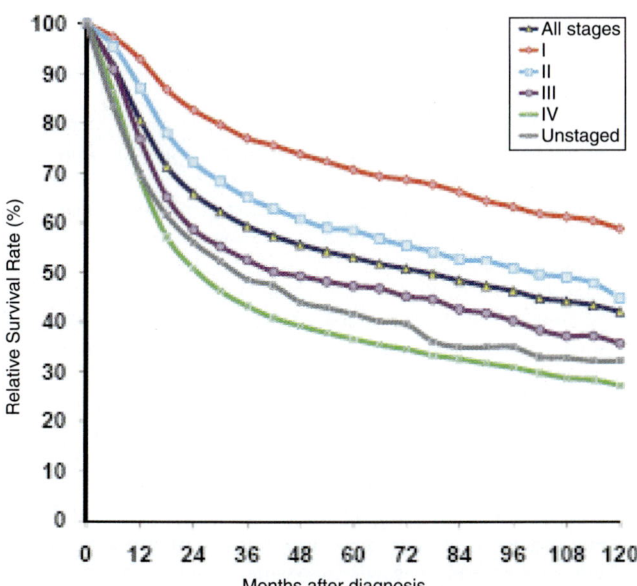

Fig. 2. Relative survival rates (%) of tongue cancer, depending on the stage of the disease (adapted from reference 55)

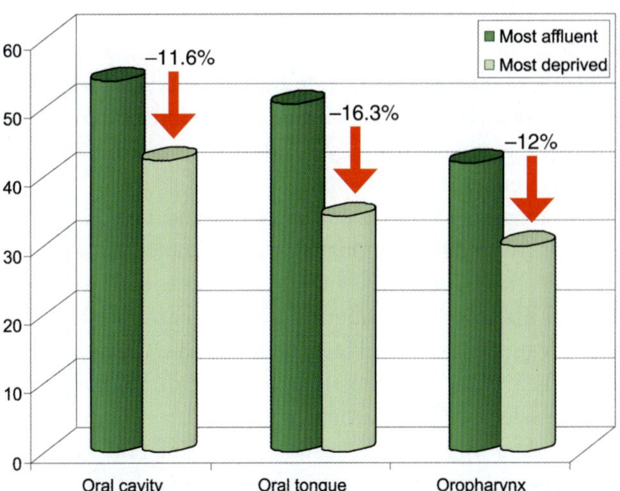

Fig. 3. Comparison of 5-year survival (%) difference between the most affluent and most deprived HNC patients in England and Wales (adapted from reference 57)

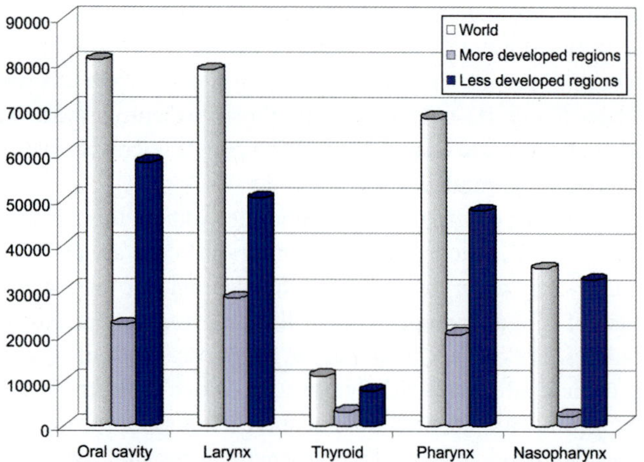

Fig. 4a. Mortality from HNCs in males in developed and less developed countries (adapted from reference 58)

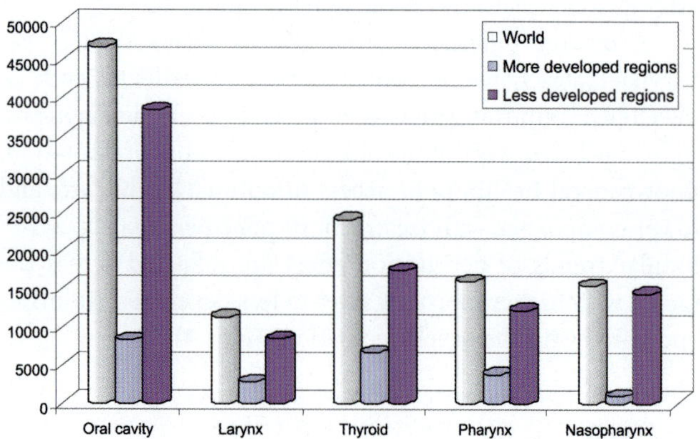

Fig. 4b. Mortality of HNCs in females in developed and less developed countries (adapted from reference 58)

being, functional outcomes, and QOL.[59] Besides the functional impairments (speech/voice, swallow and respiration/breathing), HNC patients are often rendered vulnerable to psychosocial problems, because social interactions and emotional expression depends, to a great extent, upon the structural and functional integrity of the head and neck region.[60] Therefore, accomplishing optimal functional integrity is of vital importance in the management of HNC patients.

Evaluation of functional outcomes and QOL may help to improve treatment modalities, to promote restoration of patients' daily functions, and to accelerate their return to normal life. Also, estimation of the influence of HNCs and their treatment on important functions and QOL can serve as a means by which the most appropriate treatment approach can be selected for a particular patient. To restore optimal functions, a thorough understanding of different aspects of QOL and treatment variables is a must. It may help clinicians to improve assessment and management of patients, identify specific impediments at an early stage during the follow up, and direct specific interventions to patients who are at increased

risk and with poor outcomes.[61,62] Also, early access of patients to detailed information about their disease can make them better adjusted to an imminent medical condition.[63,64] Finally, and most importantly, post-treatment functional outcomes and QOL should be a decisive factor in choosing between different therapies having nearly equal locoregional control and survival rates.[65]

References

1. Peters LJ. Changes in radiotherapeutic management of head and neck cancer: A 30-year perspective. *Int J Radiat Oncol Biol Phys* 2007;**69**:S8–S11.
2. Yao M, Epstein JB, Modi BJ, *et al.* Current surgical treatment of squamous cell carcinoma of the head and neck. *Oral Oncol* 2007; **43**:213–23.
3. Ganly I, Tay HN, Patel SG, *et al.* Management of the neck. In: Montgomery PQ, Rhys-Evans PH, Gullane PJ (eds). *Principles and practice in head-neck surgery and oncology.* New York: Informa Healthcare; 2009:291–315.
4. Shoaib T, Soutar DS, MacDonald DG, *et al.* The accuracy of head and neck carcinoma sentinel lymph node biopsy in the clinically N0 neck. *Cancer* 2001;**91**:2077–83.
5. Ali S, Tiwari RM, Snow GB. False-Positive and False-Negative Neck Nodes. *Head and Neck Surgery* 1985;**8**:78–82.
6. Brouwer J, de Bree R, Hoekstra OS, *et al.* Screening for distant metastases in patients with head and neck cancer: Is chest computed tomography sufficient? *Laryngoscope* 2005;**115**:1813–7.
7. Senft A, de Bree R, Hoekstra OS, *et al.* Screening for distant metastases in head and neck cancer patients by chest CT or whole body FDG-PET: A prospective multicenter trial. *Radiother Oncol* 2008;**87**:221–9.
8. Dwivedi RC, Kazi R, Agrawal N, *et al.* Comprehensive review of small bowel metastasis from head and neck squamous cell carcinoma. *Oral Oncol* 2010 Feb 25.
9. Gamba A, Romano M, Grosso IM, *et al.* Psychosocial adjustment of patients surgically treated for head and neck cancer. *Head Neck* 1992;**14**:218–23.
10. Weber AL, Romo L, Hashmi S. Malignant tumors of the oral cavity and oropharynx: Clinical, pathologic, and radiologic evaluation. *Neuroimaging Clin N Am* 2003;**13**:443–64.
11. Lin DT, Cohen SM, Coppit GL, *et al.* Squamous cell carcinoma of the oropharynx and hypopharynx. *Otolaryngol Clin North Am* 2005;**38**:59–74.
12. Braams JW, Pruim J, Kole AC, *et al.* Detection of unknown primary head and neck tumors by positron emission tomography. *Int J Oral Maxillofac Surg* 1997;**26**:112–15.
13. Kim MR, Roh JL, Kim JS, *et al.* Utility of F-18-fluorodeoxyglucose positron emission tomography in the preoperative staging of squamous cell carcinoma of the oropharynx. *Eur J Surg Oncol* 2007; **33**:633–8.
14. Paulus P, Sambon A, Vivegnis D, *et al.* FDG-PET for the assessment of primary head and neck tumors: Clinical, computed tomography, and histopathological correlation in 38 patients. *Laryngoscope* 1998; **108**:1578–83.
15. Ng SH, Yen TC, Chang JT, *et al.* Prospective study of [F-18] fluorodeoxyglucose positron emission tomography and computed tomography and magnetic resonance imaging in oral cavity squamous cell carcinoma with palpably negative neck. *J Clin Oncol* 2006;**24**:4371–6.
16. Ng SH, Yen TC, Liao CT, *al.* F-18-FDG-PET and CT/MRI in oral

cavity squamous cell carcinoma: A prospective study of 124 patients with histologic correlation. *J Nucl Med* 2005;**46**:1136–43.

17. Rusthoven KE, Raben D, Ballonoff A, *et al.* Effect of radiation techniques in treatment of oropharynx cancer. *Laryngoscope* 2008;**118**:635–9.

18. Branstetter BF 4th, Blodgett TM, Zimmer LA, *et al.* Head and neck malignancy: Is PET/CT more accurate than PET or CT alone? *Radiology* 2005;**235**:580–6.

19. Schoder H, Yeung HWD, Gonen M, *et al.* Head and neck cancer: Clinical usefulness and accuracy of PET/CT image fusion. *Radiology* 2004;**231**:65–72.

20. Wong RJ, Lin DT, Schoder H, *et al.* Diagnostic and prognostic value of [F-18] fluorodeoxyglucose positron emission tomography for recurrent head and neck squamous cell carcinoma. *J Clin Oncol* 2002;**20**:4199–208.

21. Castelijns JA, van den Brekel MW. Imaging of lymphadenopathy in the neck. *Eur Radiol* 2002;**12**:727–38.

22. Denoix PF. Tumor, Node and Metastasis (TNM). *Bull Inst Nat Hyg (Paris)* 1944;**1**:1–69.

23. American Joint Committee on Cancer. *Manual for Staging of Cancer.* 4th ed. Philadelphia: JB Lippincott; 1992.

24. Patel SG, Shah JP. TNM staging of cancers of the head and neck: Striving for uniformity among diversity. *CA Cancer J Clin* 2005;**55**:242–58.

25. Edge SB, Byrd DR, Compton CC (eds). *AJCC Cancer Staging Manual.* 7th ed. New York, NY: Springer; 2010.

26. van der Schroeff MP, Baatenburg de Jong RJ. Staging and prognosis in head and neck cancer. *Oral Oncol* 2009;**45**:356–60.

27. Vokes EE, Weichselbaum RR, Lippman SM. Head and neck-cancer—reply. *N Engl J Med* 1993;**328**:1784.

28. Fu KK, Pajak TF, Trotti A, *et al.* A Radiation Therapy Oncology Group (RTOG) phase III randomized study to compare hyperfractionation and two variants of accelerated fractionation to standard fractionation radiotherapy for head and neck squamous cell carcinomas: First report of RTOG 9003. *Int J Radiat Oncol Biol Phys* 2000;**48**:7–16.

29. Layland MK, Sessions DG, Lenox J. The influence of lymph node metastasis in the treatment of squamous cell carcinoma of the oral cavity, oropharynx, larynx, and hypopharynx: N0 versus N+. *Laryngoscope* 2005;**115**:629–39.

30. Leemans CR, Tiwari R, Nauta JJP, *et al.* Regional lymph-node involvement and its significance in the development of distant metastases in head and neck-carcinoma. *Cancer* 1993;**71**:452–6.

31. Audet N, Beasley NJ, MacMillan C, *et al.* Lymphatic vessel density, nodal metastases, and prognosis in patients with head and neck cancer. *Arch Otolaryngol Head Neck Surg* 2005;**131**:1065–70.

32. Shah JP, Andersen PE. Evolving role of modifications in neck dissection for oral squamous carcinoma. *Br J Oral Maxillofac Surg* 1995;**33**:3–8.

33. Leemans CR, Tiwari R, Vanderwaal I, *et al.* The efficacy of comprehensive neck dissection with or without postoperative radiotherapy in nodal metastases of squamous-cell carcinoma of the upper respiratory and digestive tracts. *Laryngoscope* 1990;**100**:1194–8.

34. Argiris A, Karamouzis MV, Raben D, *et al.* Head and neck cancer. *The Lancet* 2008;**371**:1695–709.

35. Greenberg JS, El Naggar AK, Mo V, *et al.* Disparity in pathologic and clinical lymph node staging in oral tongue carcinoma. Implication for therapeutic decision making. *Cancer* 2003;**98**:508–15.

36. Pfi ster DG, Laurie SA, Weinstein GS, *et al.* American Society of Clinical Oncology clinical practice guideline for the use of larynx-preservation strategies in the treatment of laryngeal cancer. *J Clin Oncol* 2006;**24**:3693–704.

37. Argiris A, Stenson KM, Brockstein BE, *et al.* Neck dissection in the combined-modality therapy of patients with locoregionally advanced head and neck cancer. *Head Neck* 2004;**26**:447–55.

38. Balfour A, Rhys-Evans PH, Patel SG. Head and neck malignancy: An overview. In: Montgomery PQ, Rhys-Evans PH, Gullane PJ (eds). *Principles and practice in head-neck surgery and oncology.* New York: Informa Healthcare; 2009:1–13.

39. Cohen EE, Lingen MW, Vokes EE. The expanding role of systemic therapy in head and neck cancer. *J Clin Oncol* 2004;**22**:1743–52.

40. Pignon JP, Bourhis J, Domenge C, *et al.* Chemotherapy added to locoregional treatment for head and neck squamous-cell carcinoma: Three meta-analyses of updated individual data. MACH-NC Collaborative Group. Meta-Analysis of Chemotherapy on Head and Neck Cancer. *The Lancet* 2000;**355**:949–55.

41. Karamouzis MV, Grandis JR, Argiris A. Therapies directed against epidermal growth factor receptor in aerodigestive carcinomas. *JAMA* 2007;**298**:70–82.

42. Parsons JT, Mendenhall WM, Stringer SP, *et al.* Squamous cell carcinoma of the oropharynx—Surgery, radiation therapy, or both. *Cancer* 2002;**94**:2967–80.

43. Shah JP. Surgical approaches to the oral cavity primary and neck. *Int J Radiat Oncol Biol Phys* 2007;**69** (Suppl 2):S15–S18.

44. Duvvuri U, Simental AA Jr, D'Angelo G, *et al.* Elective neck dissection and survival in patients with squamous cell carcinoma of the oral cavity and oropharynx. *Laryngoscope* 2004;**114**:2228–34.

45. Mendenhall WM, Werning JW, Hinerman RW, *et al.* Management of T1-T2 glottic carcinomas. *Cancer* 2004;**100**:1786–92.

46. Dey P, Arnold D, Wight R, *et al.* Radiotherapy versus open surgery versus endolaryngeal surgery (with or without laser) for early laryngeal squamous cell cancer. *Cochrane Database Syst Rev* 2002;**2**:CD002027.

47. Jones AS, Fish B, Fenton JE, *et al.* The treatment of early laryngeal cancers (T1-T2 N0): Surgery or irradiation? *Head Neck* 2004;**26**:127–35.

48. Nakamura K, Shioyama Y, Kawashima M, *et al.* Multi-institutional analysis of early squamous cell carcinoma of the hypopharynx treated with radical radiotherapy. *Int J Radiat Oncol Biol Phys* 2006;**65**:1045–50.

49. Mendenhall WM, Morris CG, Amdur RJ, *et al.* Definative radiotherapy for tonsillar squamous cell carcinoma. *Am J Clin Oncol* 2006;**29**:290–7.

50. Poulsen M, Porceddu SV, Kingsley PA, *et al.* Locally advanced tonsillar squamous cell carcinoma: Treatment approach revisited. *Laryngoscope* 2007;**117**:45–50.

51. Allal AS, Nicoucar K, Mach N, *et al.* Quality of life in patients with oropharynx carcinomas: Assessment after accelerated radiotherapy with or without chemotherapy versus radical surgery and postoperative radiotherapy. *Head Neck* 2003;**25**:833–9.

52. Adelstein DJ, Li Y, Adams GL, *et al.* An intergroup phase III comparison of standard radiation therapy and two schedules of concurrent chemoradiotherapy in patients with unresectable squamous cell head and neck cancer. *J Clin Oncol* 2003;**21**:92–8.

53. Dwivedi RC, Rhys-Evans PH, Patel SG. Tumors of the oropharynx. In: Montgomery PQ, Rhys-Evans PH, Gullane PJ (eds). *Principles and practice in head-neck surgery and oncology.* New York: Informa Healthcare; 2009:192–232.

54. Ries LAG, Melbert D, Krapcho M, *et al.* (eds). *SEER Cancer Statistics Review,* 1975–2004, National Cancer Institute. Bethesda, MD, http://seer.cancer.gov/csr/1975_2004/, based on November 2006 SEER data submission, posted to the SEER Web site, 2007.

55. Piccirillo J, Costas I, Reichman M. Cancers of the head and neck. In: Ries LA, Young JL, Keel GE, Eisner MP, Lin YD, Horner MJ (eds). *SEER survival monograph: Cancer survival among adults.* U.S. SEER Program, 1988–2001, Patient and tumor characteristics. NIH

Pub. No. 07-6215. Bethesda (MD): National Cancer Institute, SEER Program; 2007:7–22.

56. Shah JP, Gil Z. Current concepts in management of oral cancer—surgery. *Oral Oncol* 2009;**45**:394–401.

57. Coleman MP, Babb P, Damiecki P. Cancer Survival Trends in England and Wales, 1971–1995: Deprivation and NHS Region (Studies in medical and Population Subjects, No. 61). London: The Stationary Office, 1999.

58. Ferlay J, Bray F, Pisani P, *et al.* GLOBOCAN 2002: Cancer Incidence, Mortality and Prevalence Worldwide IARC CancerBase No. 5, version 2.0, IARCPress, Lyon, 2004. http://www-dep.iarc.fr/

59. Kazi R, De Cordova J, Kanagalingam J, *et al.* Quality of life following total laryngectomy: Assessment using the UW-QOL scale. *ORL J Otorhinolaryngol Relat Spec* 2007;**69**:100–6.

60. Sayed SI, Elmiyeh B, Rhys-Evans P, *et al.* Quality of life and outcomes research in head and neck cancer: A review of the state of the discipline and likely future directions. *Cancer Treat Rev* 2009;**35**:397–402.

61. Gil Z, Abergel A, Spektor S, *et al.* Quality of life following surgery for anterior skull base tumors. *Arch Otolaryngol Head Neck Surg* 2003;**129**:1303–9.

62. Fitzpatrick R, Fletcher A, Gore S, *et al.* Quality of life measures in healthcare, I: Applications and issues in assessment. *BMJ* 1992;**305**:1074–7.

63. Gil Z, Fliss DM. Contemporary management of head and neck cancers. *Isr Med Assoc J* 2009;**11**:296–300.

64. Portenoy RK. Quality of life issues in patients with head and neck cancer. In: Harrison LB (ed). *Head and Neck Cancer*. New York, NY: Plenum Press; 1995:218–31.

65. Boscolo-Rizzo P, Stellin M, Fuson R, *et al.* Long-term quality of life after treatment for locally advanced oropharyngeal carcinoma: Surgery and postoperative radiotherapy versus concurrent chemoradiation. *Oral Oncol* 2009;**45**:953–7.

3

Pathology of head and neck cancer

JAYASREE K., THARA SOMANATHAN, BIPIN T. VARGHESE, PAUL SEBASTIAN

The head and neck constitute a region in which the different structures have a variety of functions, such as respiration, phonation, vision, alimentation, metabolism, and support of the musculoskeletal system.

Tumours of this region include epithelial and mesenchymal tumours. The former arise from the mucosal lining, and seromucinous and endocrine glands. Mesenchymal tumours arise from the soft tissue, bone, cartilage, neural/neuroectodermal tissue and haemolymphoid cells in the oral cavity, oropharynx, nasal cavity, paranasal sinuses, nasopharynx, hypopharynx, larynx, trachea and ear.

Epithelial tumours

Epithelial tumours include squamous lesions that originate from the squamous epithelial lining, and glandular lesions that arise from the seromucinous glands.

Squamous papillomas

The papilloma is a common, benign tumour, which arises from the squamous epithelium. It is often mistaken clinically for other benign lesions, such as fibroma in the oral cavity.[1] It is an exophytic, well circumscribed growth with small finger-like projections giving it a cauliflower-like appearance. It is often pedunculated; sometimes sessile. Intraorally it is found in the tongue, lips, buccal mucosa, gingiva and palate. Most squamous papillomas are a few millimetres in diameter, but larger lesions may also be seen.

Microscopically, the papilloma shows many long, thin, finger-like projections above the surface mucosa. The

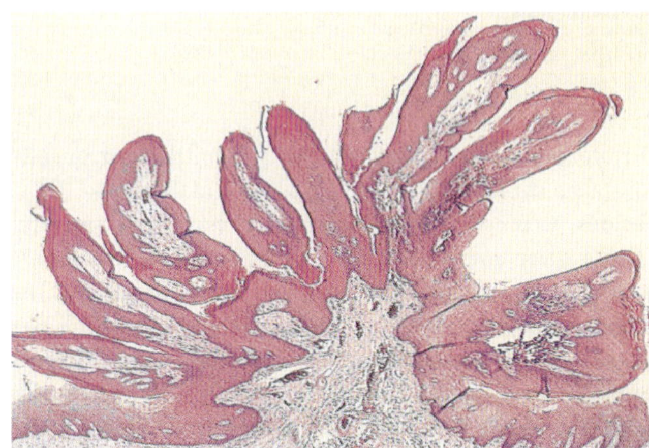

Fig. 1. Squamous papilloma

projections have a thin fibrovascular core surrounded by squamous epithelium (Fig. 1).

Laryngeal papillomas are the most common benign epithelial tumour of the larynx, and are caused by human papillomavirus (HPV) infection.[2] They often occur in multiples and can recur. Juvenile papillomas are characterized by extensive growth and rapid recurrence. Adult papillomas usually do not have a dramatic clinical course.

Papilloma of the sinonasal tract

These are also called Schneiderian papilloma, transitional cell papilloma and cylindrical cell papilloma. Papillomas of the sinonasal tract tend to recur. Invasive squamous cell carcinomas (SCCs) may co-exist with these lesions or may, rarely, arise from them.[2]

Papillary squamous hyperplasia

Nodular or papillary lesions frequently seen in the palate and lateral border of the tongue[1] arise commonly in response to injury from ill fitting dentures or bad teeth. Lesions may also be seen in xerostomia or in people with a high, arched palate. The lesions may be florid in immunosuppressed individuals. Microscopically, papillomatous hyperplasia of the epithelium with parakeratinization or orthokeratanization is evident.

Focal epithelial hyperplasia

The labial and buccal mucosa and the tongue, usually in children, adolescents and young adults, are the most common sites for multiple oral papillomas. They are induced by infection with HPV 13 and 32. Lesions are seen as multiple, soft, rounded or flat sessile swellings, pink or white in colour, and 2–10 mm in diameter. Microscopic examination reveals a lesion with a sharply demarcated zone of acanthosis with koilocytes, and the characteristic 'mitosoid bodies' (nuclei with coarse, clumped heterochromatin resembling a mitotic figure). This lesion has no malignant potential and it resolves spontaneously.

Keratoacanthoma

Keratoacanthoma is a benign epithelial lesion that is frequently mistaken clinically and histologically for malignancy.[2] These lesions occur on the exposed skin, cheeks, nose and lips. They appear umbilicated or crateriform with a central core or plug, 1.0–1.5 cm in diameter, and are often painful. The lesion begins as a small nodule that develops to its full size within 4–6 weeks, remains the same and then undergoes spontaneous regression over several months. Microscopically, the lesion is cup-shaped or crateriform, and filled with keratin and a dense inflammatory infiltrate in the underlying stroma. The deep margin of the tumour may occasionally show islands of epithelium appearing to be invading. It is often difficult to distinguish this area from a SCC.

Epithelial premalignant lesions

A precursor or premalignant lesion is an altered epithelium with an increased likelihood of progression to carcinoma.[2] The altered epithelium shows various cytological and architectural changes termed 'dysplasia', 'squamous intraepithelial neoplasia' or 'squamous intraepithelial lesions'. Clinically, these precursor lesions may appear as a leukoplakia (white patch), erythroplakia (red patch) or as mixed white and red lesions. Leukoplakias have a lower risk of malignant transformation than the mixed lesions. Pure erythroplakias have the highest risk of malignant transformation.

Microscopically, the precursor lesions are usually

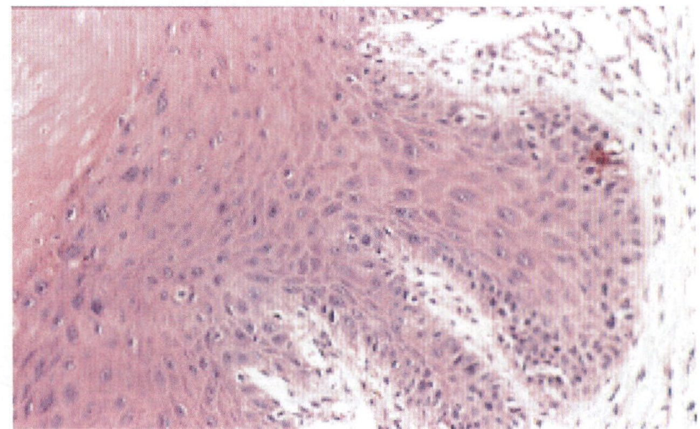

Fig. 2. Leukoplakia with mild dysplasia

thickened, although some may be atrophic. They show hyperkeratosis and/or parakeratosis, hyperplasia (acanthosis and/or basal cell hyperplasia) and dysplasia. The dysplasias are graded as mild, moderate or severe, depending on the severity of cytological atypia and thickness of the epithelium involved (Fig. 2).[2]

Carcinoma *in situ*

These are lesions in which malignant transformation has occurred within the epithelium, but invasion into the underlying stroma is not present. Some of the precursor lesions persist as such, some regress and some progress to SCCs. The histopathological degree of severity of these lesions can be a predictive factor.

Oral submucous fibrosis

Oral submucous fibrosis is a precancerous condition strongly associated with chewing areca nuts. Precancerous conditions are generalized clinical states associated with a significantly increased risk for SCC.[2] Clinically, the patients have a burning sensation in the mouth and intolerance to spicy food. Vesicle formation, ulceration and stomatitis can be seen. In advanced cases, there is difficulty in opening the mouth and swallowing. There is a juxta-epithelial inflammatory reaction followed by a fibroelastic change of the lamina propria with epithelial atrophy leading to stiffness of the oral mucosa. Fibrous bands and mucosal pallor are seen.

Histologically, epithelial atrophy with severe hyalinization and homogenization of the collagen bundles in the underlying connective tissue is evident. Twenty-five per cent of the cases may show varying degrees of epithelial dysplasia and some of them develop SCC (Fig. 3).[3]

Invasive SCC

This is an invasive epithelial neoplasm with varying degrees of squamous differentiation, occurring predominantly in alcohol

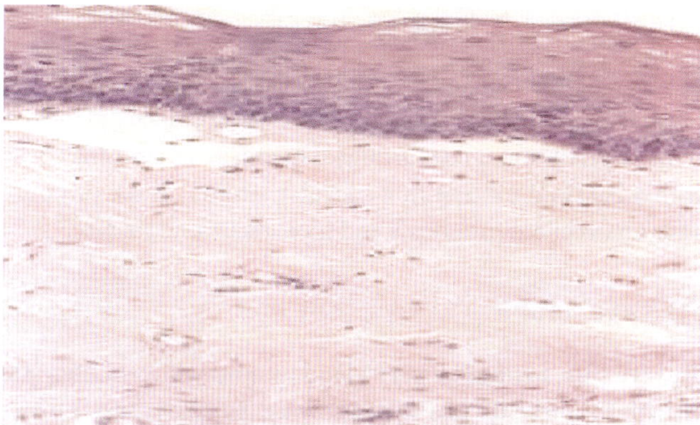

Fig. 3. Submucous fibrosis

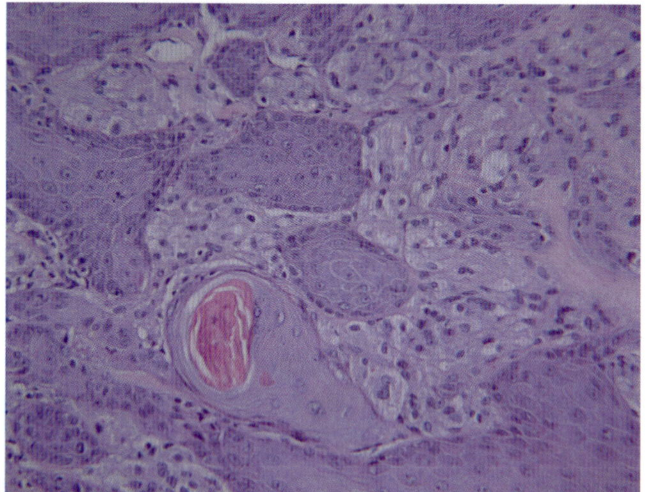

Fig. 4. Squamous cell carcinoma

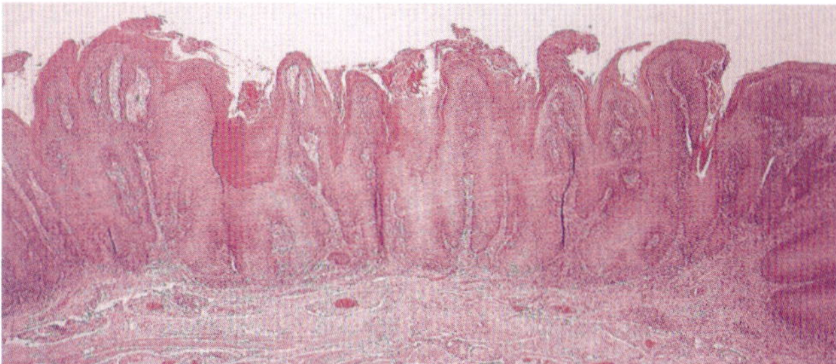

Fig. 5. Verrucous carcinoma

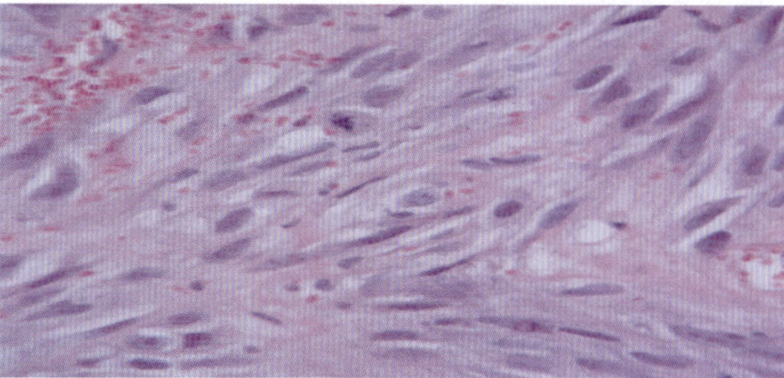

Fig. 6. Spindle cell variant of squamous cell carcinoma

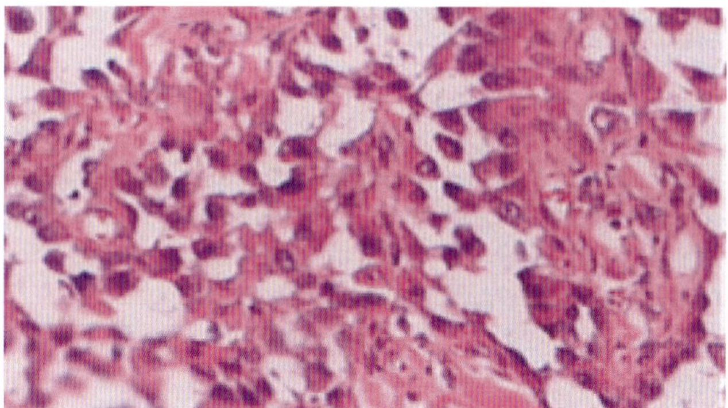

Fig. 7. Acantholytic sqamous cell carcinoma

and tobacco using adults. Recent studies suggest that the HPV may be responsible for some oral and oropharyngeal SCCs.[2]

Squamous differentiation, seen as keratinization with keratin pearl formation and invasive growth, are features of SCC (Fig. 4). These tumours are graded as: well, moderate or poorly differentiated. Well differentiated SCC resembles the normal squamous epithelium with abundant keratinization. Moderately differentiated SCC shows more nuclear atypia and mitotic activity and less keratinization. Poorly differentiated SCC shows immature cells with minimal keratinization.

Variants of SCC

Verrucous carcinoma

It is an exophytic, warty, slow-growing variant of SCC. It erodes the underlying stroma, rather than invading it. The pushing advancing margin of the tumour is bulbous and broad. The tumour cells are well differentiated and often lack the criteria of malignancy (Fig. 5). One-fifth of these tumours may have a co-existing SCC and such tumours have a greater risk of recurrence and metastasis.

Spindle cell carcinoma

Seen more commonly in the oropharynx, larynx and hypopharynx, these tumours are usually polypoid masses. Some develop after radiation exposure.[4]

Histopathologically they resemble a sarcoma (Fig. 6). Special procedures to demonstrate epithelial differentiation, such as immunohistochemistry, have to be used to differentiate them from a sarcoma or a melanoma.

Acantholytic SCC

This is a variant of SCC with acantholysis of the tumour cells, which produces a pseudoglandular appearance (Fig. 7).

Basaloid SCC

Common in the oropharynx, basaloid SCC is an aggressive variant of SCC with basaloid and squamous components. It has a poor prognosis.

Glandular lesions

Glandular lesions in the head and neck region arise from the major and minor salivary glands and from the mucous glands.

Tumours of the salivary glands

Pleomorphic adenoma

Pleomorphic adenoma, or mixed tumour, is a benign tumour with epithelial and myo-epithelial elements in a mucoid, myxoid or chondroid matrix. These tumours are the most common type of salivary gland tumours, 80% of which arise in the parotid gland. They are slow growing, painless masses. The epithelial cells may be cuboidal, squamous, basaloid, spindly, plasmacytoid, or clear cells in sheets or duct-like structures. The myoepithelial cells may be plasmacytoid or spindly, seen in sheets or in a reticular pattern. The matrix is mucoid, myxoid, chondroid or hyalinised. These tumours recur and can undergo malignant transformation.[2]

Myoepithelioma

Myoepithelioma is a benign salivary gland tumour composed predominantly of myoepithelial cells that may be plasmacytoid, spindly, epithelioid or clear, and which are seen in sheets, cords or nests. Forty per cent of these tumours occur in the parotid. They are well circumscribed and slow growing. They may recur or undergo malignant transformation.[2]

Basal cell adenoma

Basal cell adenoma is a rare benign neoplasm composed of basaloid cells. They occur most commonly in the parotid gland. Basal cell adenomas are solitary and well defined. Microscopically, the basaloid cells are seen in solid, trabecular, tubular and membranous patterns. These tumours usually do not recur. Malignant transformation is a rare possibility.[2]

Warthin tumour

These are benign salivary gland tumours that are almost always seen in the parotid gland and the periparotid lymph nodes. Microscopically, they show glandular, cystic and papillary structures lined by inner columnar oncocytic cells and outer small basal cells. The intervening stroma shows lymphoid tissue. These tumours have a low recurrence rate and malignant change is rare.[2]

Oncocytoma

This is a benign salivary gland tumour comprising of oncocytic cells, and is seen chiefly in the parotid gland. Local recurrence is rare.[2]

Canalicular adenoma

This is a benign salivary gland neoplasm with a predilection for the upper lip; it rarely involves the major salivary glands. It is made of columnar cells arranged in thin anastomosing cords with a basaloid pattern in a vascular stroma. These tumours have an excellent prognosis and local recurrence is rare.[2]

Cystadenoma

This is a rare, benign salivary gland tumour with a multicystic growth.[2] It presents as a slow-growing, painless mass, mostly in the minor salivary glands, lips and buccal mucosa.

Acinic cell carcinoma

Acinic cell carcinoma is a malignant epithelial tumour of the salivary glands; 80% of them occur in the parotid.[2] They are slow growing malignant epithelial neoplasms with the tumour cells showing serous acinar cell differentiation with cytoplasmic zymogen granules. These tumours have a recurrence rate of 35%. Multiple recurrences and metastasis to cervical lymph nodes indicate a poor prognosis. Distant metastasis can also occur.

Mucoepidermoid carcinoma

Mucoepidermoid carcinoma is the most common malignancy of the salivary gland in adults and children.[2] Fifty-three per cent of these tumours are seen in the major salivary glands, mostly in the parotid. Microscopically, these tumours are composed of squamoid cells, mucous cells, and intermediate types of cells in varying proportions (Fig. 8). They can spread to the regional lymph nodes and can have widespread distant metastasis to lung, liver, bone and brain. Most patients have a good prognosis.

Adenoid cystic carcinoma

These tumours, comprising approximately 10% of all

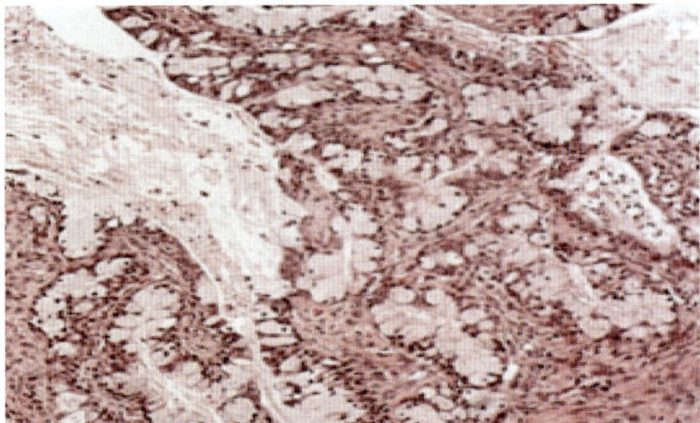

Fig. 8. Mucoepidermoid carcinoma

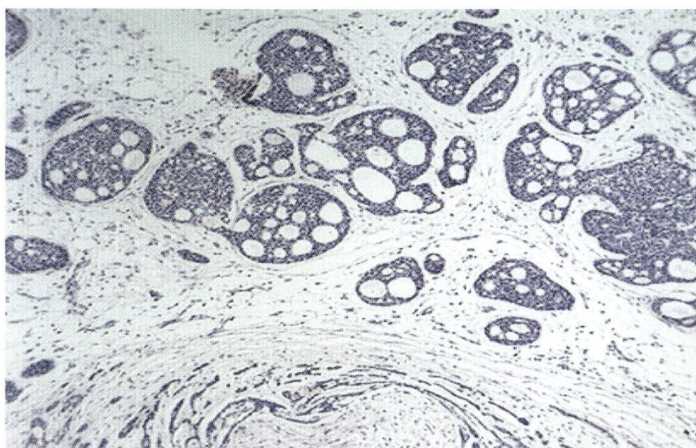

Fig. 9. Adenoid cystic carcinoma

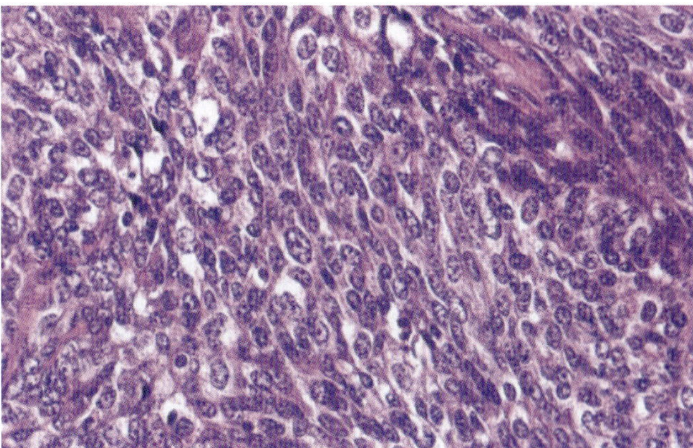

Fig. 10. Myoepithelial carcinoma

epithelial salivary gland tumours, commonly involve the parotid, submandibular and minor salivary glands.[2] They are slow growing. Pain caused by perineural tumour infiltration is frequently present.

These tumours consist of epithelial and myoepithelial cells in tubular, cribriform and solid patterns. Hyaline or basophilic mucoid material fills the lumina (Fig. 9). Tumours with >30% solid areas have a more aggressive course. The local recurrence rate ranges from 16% to 85%. Eighty per cent to 95% of patients die of the disease in 10–15 years. The lung, bone, brain and liver are common sites of distant metastases.

Polymorphous lowgrade adenocarcinoma

Sixty per cent of these tumours occur in the palate.[2] Major salivary glands are seldom involved. These tumours have an infiltrative growth in many patterns: Lobular, papillary, trabecular, cystic, cribriform, etc. The tumour cells are small to medium with cytological uniformity. These tumours have a good prognosis.

Epithelial–myoepithelial carcinoma

These are malignant tumours seen mostly in the major salivary glands, notably in the parotid.[2] They are composed of inner epithelial and outer myoepithelial cells lining duct-like spaces. These tumours recur in approximately 40% of cases; metastases are seen in 14%.

Salivary duct carcinoma

This is a rapidly growing tumour, most commonly involving the parotid. It is an aggressive tumour resembling duct carcinoma of the breast. Most patients develop local recurrences and distant metastasis.[2]

Myoepithelial carcinoma

This is a locally destructive tumour seen mostly in the parotid

gland, composed of cells showing myoepithelial differentiation in a myxoid or hyaline stroma (Fig. 10). The tumours may develop in a pre-existing pleomorphic adenoma or benign myoepithelioma, or they may arise *de novo*. Myoepithelial carcinomas are locally aggressive.

Carcinoma ex-pleomorphic adenoma

Carcinoma arising in a pleomorphic adenoma is most frequently seen in the parotid gland.[2] Patients give a history of a long standing mass with a recent rapid increase in size, or of that of a previously excised pleomorphic adenoma at the same site. The malignant component is a poorly differentiated adenocarcinoma or an undifferentiated carcinoma. These tumours may be non-invasive, minimally invasive (<1.5 mm extracapsular invasion) or invasive (>1.5 mm extracapsular invasion). Patients with non-invasive or minimally invasive carcinoma have an excellent prognosis, whereas those with invasive carcinoma have a bad outcome.

Neuroendocrine tumours

They are a group of tumours that may be benign to highly malignant with histological, immunohistochemical and ultra-structural evidence of neuroendocrine differentiation. The following types of neuroendocrine carcinoma are seen: Typical carcinoid or well differentiated (grade I), atypical carcinoid or moderately differentiated (grade II), small cell or poorly differentiated (grade III), combined small cell carcinoma and non-small cell (squamous or adenocarcinomas) carcinoma and paragangliomas.

The atypical carcinoids are aggressive tumours. Metastasis to cervical lymph nodes, skin and soft tissues, lung, liver and bone can occur. Small cell neuroendocrine carcinoma is also an aggressive tumour with a propensity for early regional and distant metastasis.

Neuroendocrine tumours are rare in the nasal cavity, paranasal sinuses and nasopharynx. Typical and atypical carcinoids of the nasal cavity and paranasal sinuses are rare.

Neuroendocrine tumours occur infrequently in the larynx where atypical carcinoids are more common.

Sinonasal undifferentiated carcinoma

This is a rare, highly aggressive carcinoma involving the nasal cavity, maxillary antrum and ethmoid sinus, and presents with locally extensive disease.[2] Microscopically, it is composed of cells in sheets, nests and trabeculae, with a high rate of mitosis and prominent necrosis. These tumours have a poor prognosis. Metastasis can occur in regional lymph nodes and distant sites, such as the liver, lung and bone.

Nasopharyngeal carcinoma

Nasopharyngeal carcinoma arises in the nasopharyngeal mucosa and shows evidence of squamous differentiation.[2] It includes SCC, non-keratinizing carcinoma (differentiated and undifferentiated) and basaloid SCC. Epstein–Barr virus is thought to play a role in the genesis of these tumours. Cervical lymph node metastasis occurs frequently.

Neuroectodermal tumours

Ewing sarcoma/primitive neuroectodermal tumour (EWS/PNET)

These are high-grade small, round cell tumours with neuroectodermal differentiation. Sinonasal EWS/PNET is rare, occurring mostly in children and young adults, commonly in the maxillary sinus and nasal fossa.[2] The tumour comprises of small, round cells with high mitotic activity and necrosis. These tumours have a better prognosis in the head and neck. Metastasis is usually to the lungs and bone.

Olfactory neuroblastoma

This is a malignant neuroectodermal tumour seen most frequently in the upper nasal cavity in the region of the cribriform plate; it is thought to arise from the olfactory membrane.[2] Microscopically, the tumour cells are round in a neurofibrillary matrix, which are tangles of neuronal cell processes. Homer Wright type of pseudorosettes and Flexner-Wintersteiner type of true rosettes can be seen. Fifteen per cent to 70% of patients have local recurrence, 10%–25% have cervical lymph node metastasis and 10%–60% have distant metastases.

Melanotic neuroectodermal tumour of infancy

This is a rare tumour in infants, involving the maxilla, mandible and skull; it appears as rapidly growing pigmented masses.[2] Histologically, these tumours show a dual population of cells—small neuroblastic cells and large melanin containing epithelial cells in a dense fibrous stroma. Local recurrence may occur if not excised completely. Some tumours metastasize to lymph nodes, liver, bone, adrenal gland, or soft tissue.

Mucosal malignant melanoma

This is a malignant tumour arising from mucosal melanocytes.[2] They are typically evident in the nasal cavity, and less so in the paranasal sinuses and other sites. Microscopically, these tumours show spindly, epithelioid or plasmacytoid cells with pleomorphic nulcei containing prominent nucleoli. The cytoplasm may contain melanin pigment. Local recurrence is common. Regional lymph node involvement is seen in 10%–20% of cases and distant metastasis in approximately 10% of cases.

Nasal glioma

These are heterotypic glial tissue, which present as a mass in and around the nose.[2] Most of these cases are seen at birth and/or by the age of 2 years. In 60% of the cases the mass is extranasal, on or near the nasal bridge. The mass is intranasal in 30% of cases and presents as a nasal obstruction or deformity. Heterotopic glial tissue may be seen in the paranasal sinuses, nasopharynx, tongue, palate, pharynx, tonsil and orbit.

Glial tissue with astrocytes is observed microscopically. Neurones are rare or absent. Incomplete excision may lead to recurrence.

Nasophyaryngeal angiofibroma

This is a benign mesenchymal tumour seen in the nasopharynx of boys, adolescents and young men.[2] Patients present with nasal obstruction, epistaxis, sinusitis, tinnitus, diplopia, facial deformity or anosmia. Histologically, the tumour shows proliferating vascular spaces, which lack the muscle layer in a fibrous stroma. These tumours are locally aggressive and may recur.

Germ cell tumours

Germ cell tumours with features similar to those in the gonads are rarely seen in the sinonasal tract.

Immature teratomas

Rarely seen in the sinonasal tract and nasopharynx, these tumours consist of immature tissue elements: neuroepithelial tissue and tissues derived from the three embryonic germ layers. They are present in infancy and childhood.

Mature teratoma

These are benign germ cell tumours occurring in the sinonasal region. Six per cent of all teratomas are seen in the head and neck. Most cases are seen in neonates and infants. Microscopically, these tumours show skin with or without appendage, fat, muscle, cartilage, bone, glial tissue, various types of epithelia, etc. Complete excision is curative.

Sinonasal teratocarcinosarcoma

This is a malignant tumour with features of teratoma and carcinosarcoma.[2] Benign and malignant epithelial, mesenchymal and neural elements are seen. These tumours are rare and occur in adults. They are usually located in the ethmoid sinus and maxillary antrum.

Microscopically different types of tissues derived from the germ layers, in varying degrees of maturation, are seen along with carcinomas and sarcomatous elements. Nests of fetal appearing squamous cells are commonly seen. Neuroblastoma-like areas may also be evident. These tumours are locally aggressive and can metastasize to regional lymph nodes and distant sites.

Odontogenic tumours

- Ameloblastoma
- Calcifying epithelial odontogenic tumours
- Ameloblastic odontoma
- Complex odontoma
- Myxoma (fibromyoma)
- Adenomatoid odontogenic tumours

Ameloblastoma

Ameloblastoma is the most common of the odontogenic tumours. It comprises 1% of all tumours in the jaw bones.[5] Young adults are mostly affected. Women predominate, with a female to male ratio of 4:3. Eighty per cent of lesions occur in

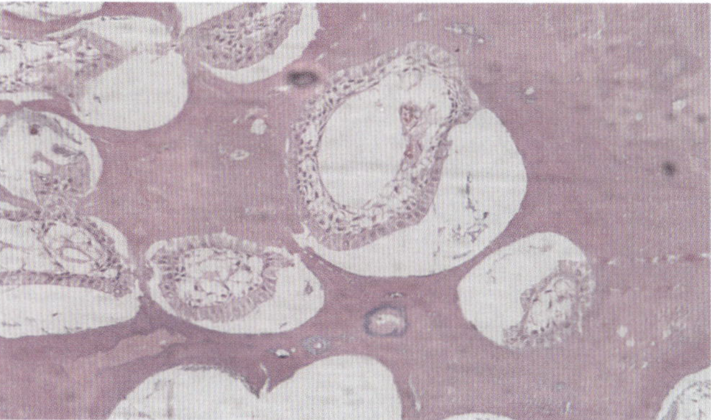

Fig. 11. Ameloblastoma: Epithelial cells in palisading pattern with stellate reticulum at the centre H and E; magnification 250x

the mandible. They are painless, slow growing tumours seen mostly in the molar-angle region. Radiologically, they show a coarsely trabeculated appearance of a multilobular cystic cavity giving a honeycomb or soap bubble appearance.

The histology reveals proliferation of epithelial cells with varying amounts of fibrous tissue. Epithelial cells are arranged in a palisading pattern at the periphery with central loose tissue, suggesting a stellate reticulum (Fig. 11). A cellular variant resembling spindle cell sarcoma is seen rarely. Some tumours show extensive squamous metaplasia, suggestive of a diagnosis of SCC. Ameloblastomas are locally aggressive tumours. It is suggested that the cystic variant of ameloblastoma has a better prognosis.[5]

Ameloblastic carcinoma

- *Metastasizing ameloblastoma:* This is an ameloblastoma that metastasizes in spite of a benign histological appearance. Metastatic deposits are seen in the lungs in most of the cases.
- *Ameloblastic carcinoma* (primary type): These are ameloblastoma with cytological atypia.
- *Ameloblastic carcinoma* (secondary type)—Intraosseous: This arises in a pre-existing benign ameloblastoma.

Calcifying epithelial odontogenic tumours (Pindborg tumours)

Pindborg tumour may be a variant of ameloblastoma. It occurs in adults. The radiograph shows a well defined defect that may be calcified. Epithelial cells predominate with tiny spherules of calcific foci in between. It is common to find eosinophilic amorphous material that stains like amyloid.

Adenomatoid odontogenic tumour (ameloblastic adenomatoid tumour)

This is a cystic neoplasm that responds to conservative surgical removal and has little tendency to recur. Most of the tumours occur in the maxilla. It produces a cyst-like zone on radiological examination, which may display calcific material in a stippled pattern. The cyst often contains an unerupted tooth and resembles a dentigerous cyst. Histologically, the tumours show tubular or duct-like structure with a central space surrounded by cuboidal to columnar cells. A thin hyaline-like lining is present. Small calcified spherules or larger mineralized masses may be found. The prognosis is excellent.

Ameloblastic fibroma (soft mixed odontoma)

This is a rare lesion affecting young males, especially boys who are usually <10 years old. The lesion may be found incidentally on plain radiographs, producing a well circumscribed radiolucent zone. Grossly, the tissue is a soft fibrous mass. Proliferation of mesenchymal and epithelial elements characterizes these tumours, which are benign. Fibrosarcoma rarely develops from stroma.

Myxoma (fibromyxoma)

Myxomas of bone always occur in the jaw bones. Hence, it is thought that they have an odontogenic origin, which is supported by their resemblance to the mesenchymal portion of the tooth germ.

Most of the patients are young adults. Grossly, the tumour is soft and semi-translucent. Loose stellate cells predominate in a myxoid stroma. Some of the tumours have bizarre nuclei or a cellular stroma.

Myxomas of the jaw may recur, but do not metastasize. Fibrosarcomas, chondrosarcomas and osteosarcomas of the jaw can have myxoid features, which may simulate myxoma and must therefore be differentiated carefully from it.

Bone tumours of the jaws and skull

Osteoid producing tumours

Osteoma of skull

This is a rare, single, unilateral lesion with a pedicle, occurring in the region of the tympanosquamous or tympanomastoid suture line. It is rarely seen in the mastoids, temporal bone, internal auditory canal, glenoid fossa, eustachian tube and styloid process.

Osteoma also involves paranasal sinuses. A few of these dense 'ivory' osteomas contain softer zones of fibro-osseous dysplasia. Skeletal osteomas of various bones, particularly involving those of the skull and jaw, are associated with intestinal polyps, fibromatous and other lesions of connective tissue and epidermal cysts in gardner syndrome.

Some of the solid odontomas may be osteomas because formed elements of tooth structure cannot be absolutely identified. Dentin can become ossified. These lesions of the head may produce symptoms through deformity or proptosis, or they may be incidental finding on radiographs.

Osteoid osteoma in the jaw bones are extremely rare. Lesions, such as fibrous dysplasia, have areas simulating osteoid osteoma. Hence, painless osteoid osteoma should be viewed with caution. The pain experienced in osteoid osteoma is said to be caused by high levels of prostaglandins.

Osteoblastoma, on the other hand, are reported in jaw bones, especially the mandible.[6] Radiologically, most of them are benign, but 10% can show a malignant appearance. Hence, distinction from osteosarcoma is difficult.

Histologically both types of tumour are similar in

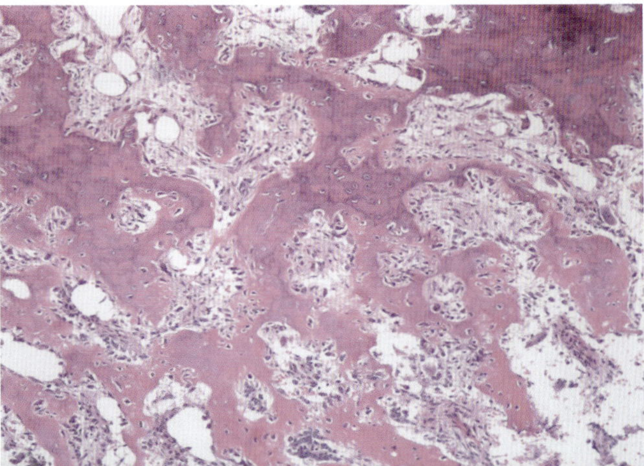

Fig. 12. Osteoblastoma: Woven bone with fibrovascular stroma. H and E; magnification 250x

appearance, with a nidus in the centre surrounded by sclerotic bone. The nidus is composed of woven (immature) bone, rimmed by osteoblasts and loose fibrovascular stroma. Osteoid osteoma is small (<1 cm) and osteoblastoma is usually >2 cm (Fig. 12).

Osteosarcoma

The average age of patients with osteosarcoma of jaw bones is significantly greater than that of patients with tumours in conventional sites; they occur in the second to fourth decades of life.[7,8] The maxilla and mandible are almost equally affected. Approximately 50% of the osteosarcoma of the jaws show chondroblastic differentiation (Fig. 13). Osteoid production is usually minimal and difficult to recognize. Cellular anaplasias are minimal and most of them are graded as intermediate. Chondroid differentiation in a lesion of the jaw should be viewed with suspicion because it is never found in benign conditions, except in callus, in these bones.

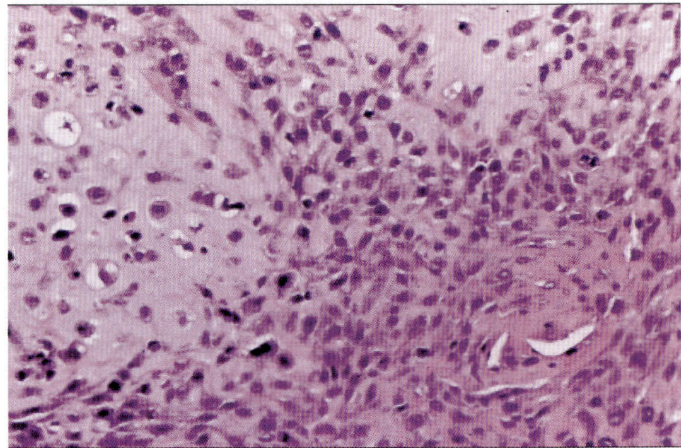

Fig. 13. Chondroblastic osteosarcoma: High-grade cartilage with peripheral spindling of cells and tumour osteoid. H and E; magnification 250x

Osteosarcoma of the jaw usually has a good prognosis with radical surgery; the 5-year survival rate is 80%. Haematogenous spread is unusual in these cases. Patients who die do so from uncontrolled local disease.

Patients with osteosarcoma of the skull have an extremely poor prognosis. Patients with secondary osteosarcoma of the skull have a poor prognosis, whereas those with primary osteosarcoma do much better.

Chondroid tumours

Cartilage tumours in the head and neck region are rare because skull bones are formed by intramembranous ossification.[15] However, uncommon examples can be seen. Osteochondromas and enchondromas are not described in skull and jaw bones. But rarely, chondroma of the meninges can occur. The temporal bone is a common site for chondroblastoma.[14] Chondromyxoid fibromas are rare in skull and jaw bones.

Chondrosarcomas usually involve the nasal bones. Most of the lesions described in the maxilla seem to arise in the nasal bones. Chondrosarcomas of maxilla, mandible and hyoid bone can occur rarely. Usually, malignant cartilage tumours of jaw bones are chondroblastic osteosarcoma. Chondrosarcomas are described in the base of skull region.[12]

Clear cell chondrosarcoma is a rare tumour found in the nasal bones. Skull and jaw bones are preferred sites for mesenchymal chondrosarcomas.[13] Jaw bones, especially the mandible, is a common site. Mesenchymal chondrosarcoma is also described in the meninges.[10]

Chordoma

Chordomas are seen in the base of skull.[11] Chondroid chordomas mostly occur at this site. It is difficult to differentiate between chondroid chordoma from chondrosarcoma (Fig. 15).

Fibrous dysplasia

This is a benign intramedullary proliferation of woven bone admixed with fibrous tissue, affecting children and adults. Skull and facial bones are affected in 10%–20% of cases. The temporal bone, internal auditory canal and lateral semicircular canal and its ossicles may be involved.

Microscopy of chondrosarcomas

Chondrosarcoma is a hyaline cartilage tumour and is usually of low grades, i.e. grades 1 and 2. Increase in cellularity, double or multiple nuclei and myxoid changes are worrisome histological features. Permeation sign is the diagnostic feature that defines a hyaline cartilage tumour as malignant, i.e. permeation of tumour in between pre-existing bony spicules.

The cells in clear-cell chondrosarcomas have a clear cytoplasm and areas of osteoid and bone formation can be seen. Foci of calcification are also noted.

Mesenchymal chondrosarcoma, on the other hand, is a small round cell tumour with vascular channels in between that form a haemangiopericytomatous pattern. Islands of cartilage cells are seen amidst the round cells. Round cells have scanty cytoplasm and hyperchromatic nuclei (Fig. 14). An important differential diagnosis in a small biopsy is Ewing sarcoma and other small round cell tumours, such as rhabdomyosarcoma, lymphoma, etc.

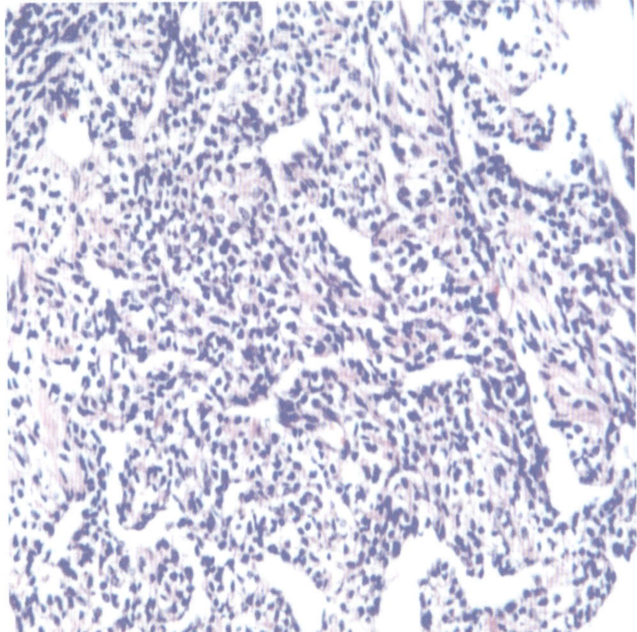

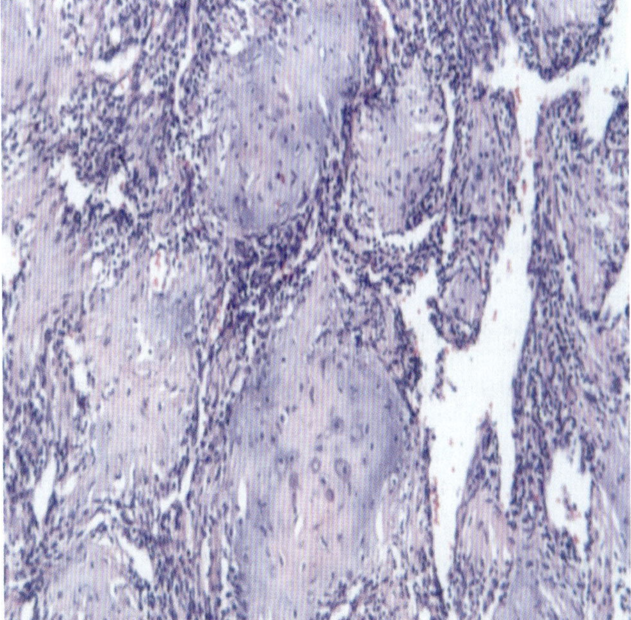

Fig. 14. Mesenchymal chondrosarcoma: Small round cells, haemangiopericytomatous pattern of vessels and chondroid islands.

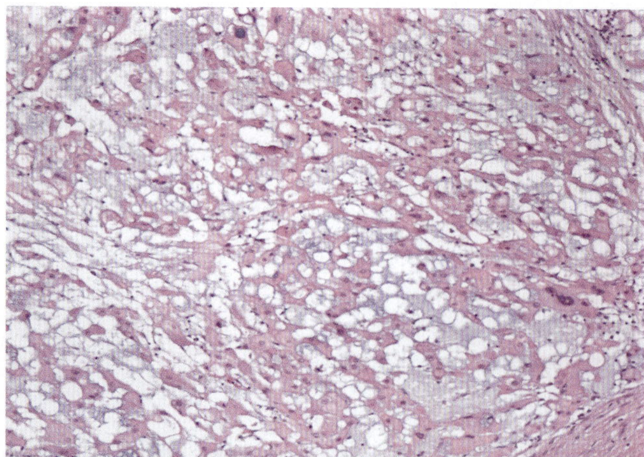

Fig. 15. Chords of cells floating in mucoid background. H and E; magnification 250x

Cytogenetics: A peculiar Robertsonian translocation der $(13;21)(q10;q10)$ is described in mesenchymal chondrosarcomas.

Metastatic tumours in the head and neck

Metastasis to lymph nodes

The lymph nodes in the neck are a common site for metastasis from tumours in the head and neck and from other sites. The most common type of metastatic carcinoma of the head and neck is SCC. Metastatic adenocarcinomas in cervical nodes may be from the thyroid, salivary gland, prostate, stomach, breast, lung, etc. Metastatic neuroendocrine tumours are usually from the lung or thyroid.

Metastasis to craniofacial bones and sinuses

The mandible and skull are two common sites of bony metastasis in the head and neck, the others being the maxillary sinuses and orbit.[20] The frequent primary sites are kidney, lung, breast, thyroid and prostate. Metastasis to the nasopharynx, larynx, hypophyarynx and trachea are extremely rare.

Paraganglioma

Paragangliomas in the head and neck are found at the bifurcation of the common carotid artery in the middle ear, temporal bone, along the vagus nerve, and rarely in the orbit, nasal cavity, paranasal sinuses, nasopharynx, larynx and thyroid.

Carotid body paraganglioma

These are neuroendocrine neoplasms derived from the carotid body paraganglia. They usually occur in adults. Microscopically they are made up of chief cells and sustentacular cells arranged in an organoid of 'Zellballen' pattern. Paragangliomas are considered to be malignant only in the presence of regional lymph node or distant metastasis.

Jugulotympanic paragangliomas

They arise form paraganglia near the jugular bulb or in the middle ear. They are slow growing tumours.

Vagal paraganglioma

They arise from the paraganglia within or adjacent to the vagus nerve. They are more common in women. Seven per cent of vagal paragangliomas are malignant.

Laryngeal paraganglioma

They are derived from the superior or inferior paraganglia of the larynx. They are more common in women, and occur mostly in the supraglottic larynx. Approximately 2% are malignant.

Tumours of the ear

Most of the tumours in the external ear arise from the skin and the ceruminous glands.

Squamous cell carcinoma (SCC)

SCC arises from the skin covering the pinna and external auditory canal; they are prevalent mostly in the pinna. The lesions in the pinna are identified earlier and have an aggressive course with local recurrence. Lesions in the auditory canal have a worse prognosis because of the delay in diagnosis and infiltration into deep structures.

Tumours from the ceruminous glands

These are rare tumours which can be benign or malignant.

Adenoma of the ceruminous glands

These are benign tumours comprising of apocrine glands.

Chondroid syringoma

A benign tumour similar to pleomorphic adenoma.

Syringocystadenoma papilliferum

This is a benign adnexal tumour, which is seen usually in children or young adults and which occurs on the face or scalp, and sometimes in the auditory canal.

Cylindroma

This is a benign adnexal tumour that may be seen in the pinna or external canal. Malignant tumours of the ceruminous glands may be adenocarcinoma, adenoid cystic carcinoma, or mucoepidermoid carcinoma.

Embryonal rhabdomyosarcoma

This is a premature malignant tumour with skeletal muscle differentiation. Most of the tumours occur in the middle ear, extending into the external auditory canal as a polyp.

Extostosis

These are common, broad-based lesions, often bilateral and deep in the ear canal.

Angiolymphoid hyperplasia with eosinophilia

These benign vascular neoplasms, occurring in the third to fifth decades of life, are seen more commonly in women. These lesions appear as a long standing nodule and are sometimes painful or pruritic; they occur frequently on the forehead, scalp, ear and periauricular area. They can bleed easily. Histologically they have vascular and inflammatory components, predominantly eosinophils and lymphoid follicles. They may recur locally, but have no metastatic potential.

Tumours of the middle ear

Adenoma of the middle ear is a benign glandular tumour with neuroendocrine differentiation and mucin secretion. It arises from the lining epithelium of the middle ear. It can recur locally.

Schneiderian papilloma and inverted papilloma

Histologically these tumours are similar to those seen in the sinonasal region.

Papillary adenocarcinoma of the middle ear

This aggressive papillary tumour may be found in any part of the middle ear. It is thought to arise from the endolymphatic sac. The tumour is often seen filling the middle ear and the bone is often invaded. Microscopically, they show complex papillae lined by a single layer of low cuboidal to columnar cells. Some of these cases are associated with Von Hippel Lindau disease.

Acoustic neuroma

Vestibular schwannoma is the most common benign neoplasm of the temporal bone. Patients often present with unilateral hearing loss, headache, vertigo and tinnitus. They are benign nerve sheath tumours showing cellular Antoni A areas with verocay bodies and fewer cellular Antoni B areas.

Endolymphatic sac tumour

This is a rare neoplasm in adults. It is slow growing, but with extensive bone infiltration. It is often associated with Von Hippel Lindau disease. It is a papillary adenocarcinoma of endolymphatic sac origin. It is not known to metastatize.

Langerhans cell histocytosis

This is a rare neoplastic proliferation of Langerhans cells, and occurs mostly in children. Unifocal disease usually involves the bone, mostly the skull bone, followed by the femur, pelvic bones and ribs. Sometimes it may be confined to a lymph node, lung or skin. In multifocal unisystem disease many sites in one organ, usually bones, are affected. In multifocal multisystem disease, bones, skin, liver, lymph nodes, spleen and bone marrow may be involved.

The diagnosis is made by identifying the Langerhans cell with a grooved coffee bean-shaped nuclei admixed with eosinophils, lymphocytes, plasma cells, and neutrophils. The prognosis is good in patients with limited disease.

Tumours of the thyroid

Tumours of the thyroid are classifed as[21] differentiated tumours which include papillary and follicular carcinomas, undifferentiated or anaplastic carcinoma, medullary carcinoma, squamous cell carcinoma, microepidermal carcinoma, sclerosing mucoepidermoid carcinoma, mucinous carcinoma, mixed medullary and follicular carcinoma with thymus-like differentiation, mixed medullary and spindle cell carcinoma with thymus-like differentiation and other tumours which include teratoma, malignant lymphoma, sarcoma, paraganglioma, solitary fibrous histiocytosis, Langerhan cell histiocytosis and secondary tumours.

Papillary carcinoma

This is a malignant epithelial tumour showing evidence of follicular cell differentiation and with distinctive nuclear features. Grossly, tumours appear as well encapsulated with irregular borders. The cut surface is whitish. Microscopically, cells are arranged in a papillary pattern. Cells are cuboidal

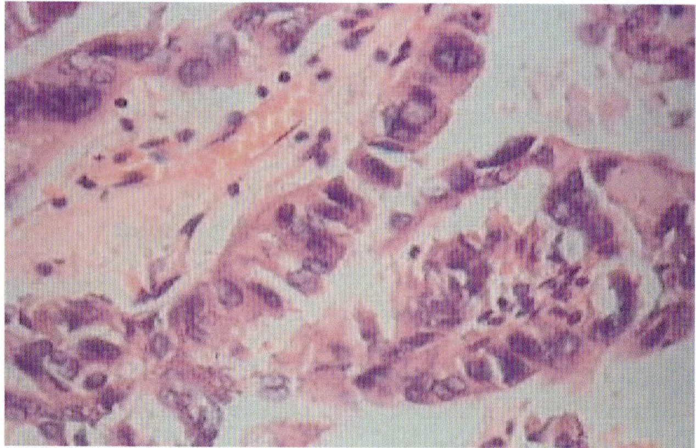

Fig. 16. Papillary carcinoma: Papillae lined by cells with pale cytoplasm, vesicular ground-glass nuclei with nuclear overlapping and grooves. H and E; magnification 400x

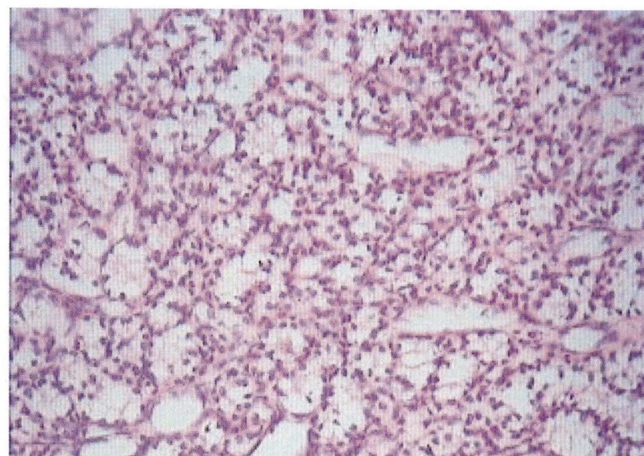

Fig. 17. Follicular adenoma: Cells in follicular pattern. H and E; magnification 100x

with pale/clear cytoplasm and nuclei show typical clearing or a ground-glass appearance. Nuclear grooves, overlapping of nuclei, and nuclear pseudo inclusion are common features (Fig. 16). Squamous metaplasia is another feature. Psammoma bodies are rounded and concentrically laminated calcifications and are seen in association with tumour cells.

Variants

- Follicular variant—tumour cells arranged in follicular pattern
- Macrofollicular variant—rarest form; confused with adenomas because most are encapsulated
- Tall cell variant—cells are tall columnar; height of cells twice the width of cell
- Columnar cell variant—cells are columnar and stratification is evident;[17] hyperchromasia of nuclei and prominent nucleolus; typical nuclear features of papillary carcinoma lacking
- Diffuse sclerosing variant—grossly diffuse enlargement of thyroid; histological evidence of extensive sclerosis of stroma; abundant psammoma bodies and squamous metaplasia present
- Warthin-like variant—resembles Warthin tumour of salivary gland
- Papillary microcarcinoma—tumour size <1 cm
- Oncocytic variant—cells with abundant eosinophilic cytoplasm
- Clear cell variant—cells with clear cytoplasm
- Encapsulated variant—well-encapsulated tumour with absence of capsule infiltration
- Solid variant—tumour cells in sheets without specific pattern.

Poor prognostic types include—tall cell, columnar cell, diffuse sclerosing and solid variants.

Follicular neoplasm

- Follicular adenoma (Fig. 17)
- Follicular carcinoma: Malignant epithelial tumour with follicular cell differentiation and lacking the diagnostic nuclear features of papillary carcinoma. Cells are arranged in follicles, solid or trabecular pattern. Capsular and/or vascular invasion of tumour cells is present.
  - Minimally invasive—tumour cells invade the capsule and/or vessel, but not beyond the capsule.
  - Widely invasive—tumour cells infiltrate widely outside the capsule to adjacent thyroid tissue and/or blood vessels.
- Hurthle cell carcinoma-tumour cells have abundant eosinophilic cytoplasm and are considered as a variant of follicular carcinoma.

Medullary thyroid carcinoma (MTC)

MTC is a malignant tumour of the thyroid gland showing C-cell differentiation. Twenty-five per cent of medullary carcinomas are hereditary (MEN type 2A and 2B, and familial MTC) with an autosomal dominant mode of inheritance.[16] Rest of the MTCs are sporadic.

The characteristic histological features are sheets, nests or trabeculae of polygonal, round or spindle cells in lobules or organoid pattern. Tumour cells have round or oval regular nuclei with coarse powdery/stippled chromatin. Cytoplasm is granular eosinophilic with ill-defined margins (Fig. 18).

Poorly differentiated carcinoma (insular carcinoma)

These tumours are intermediate between differentiated (follicular and papillary carcinomas) and undifferentiated (anaplastic) carcinomas.[18] Histopathologically three different patterns are recognized: insular, trabecular and solid. Infiltrative

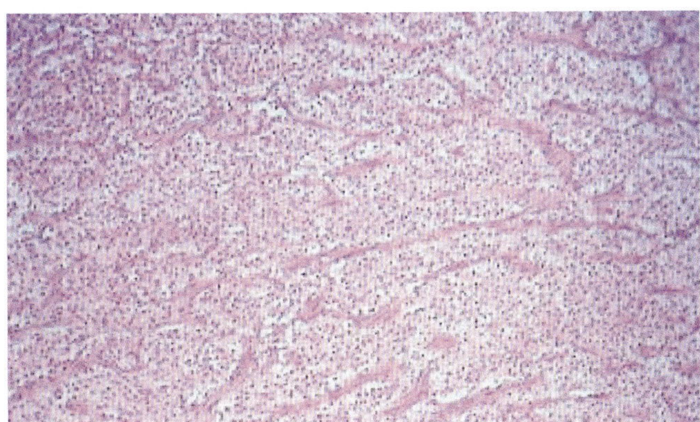

Fig. 18. Medullary carcinoma: Small cells in nests with scanty cytoplasm, vesicular nuclei with fine powdery chromatin. H and E; magnification 100x

patterns of growth, necrosis and vascular invasion are seen commonly. Cells are small and uniform with hyperchomatic nuclei. Mitotic figures are widespread (Fig. 19).

Undifferentiated (anaplastic) carcinoma

These are highly malignant tumours composed of undifferentiated cells that exhibit immunohistochemical and ultrastructural features of epithelial differentiation. The tumours are large, fleshy with areas of haemorrhage and necrosis; most show invasion to surrounding soft tissue (Table 1).

Histologically, the tumours are widely invasive with a mixture of spindle cells, pleomorphic giant cells and epithelial cells. Sometimes, cells have squamoid features. Frequent mitotic figures are seen. Extensive necrosis and vascular invasion are common findings. Osteoclast-like giant cells may be seen.[9] Exclusively spindle cell tumours are often confused with sarcomas (Fig. 20).

Primary squamous cell carcinomas

These are rare aggressive tumours in the thyroid.[19]

Table 1. Immunohistochemistry

Papillary carcinoma	High molecular weight CK19, RET, thyroglobulin, TTF-1 – positive Synaptopysin and chromogranin – negative
Follicular carcinoma	Low molecular weight CK, thyroglobulin, TTF-1 – positive
Medullary carcinoma	Calcitonin, synaptophysin, chromogranin – positive. TTF-1 may be positive CK19, thyroglobulin – negative

TTF–1 thyroid transcription factor 1   CK cytokeratin

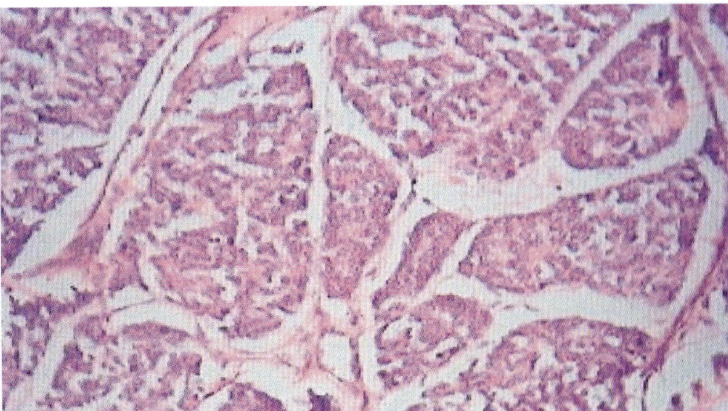

Fig. 19. Insular carcinoma: Small tumour cells in insular pattern. H and E; magnification 250x

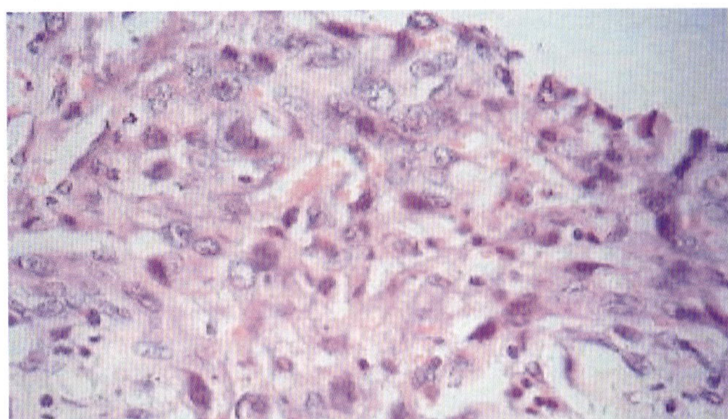

Fig. 20. Anaplastic carcinoma: Pleomorphic malignant cells with hyperchromatic nuclei. H and E; magnification 400x

Malignant lymphoma

Most cases of extranodal malignant lymphoma of the thyroid are associated with chronic lymphocytic thyroiditis or Hashimoto thyroiditis. The lymphomas of the thyroid include EMZBCL (extranodal marginal zone B cell lymphoma) and DLBCL (diffuse large B cell lymphoma). Follicular lymphomas are rare.

Sarcomas of the thyroid

The thyroid is reported to have angiosarcoma, leiomyosarcoma, malignant peripheral nerve sheath tumour, etc. These lesions should be differentiated from anaplastic carcinoma by using appropriate immunohistochemical markers.

Paraganglioma

This is an intrathyroidal neuroendocrine tumour of paraganglionic origin. These tumours are extremely rare in the thyroid.

Secondary tumours

Metastases to thyroid are seen in up to 25% of disseminated malignancies. The most common primary sites are the kidney, lung, uterus and skin (melanomas). Hodgkin lymphoma of the thyroid is usually a direct extension from a lymph node or thymic mass.

References

1. Cawson RA, Binnie WH, Speight PM, *et al. Lucas pathology of tumours of the oral tissues.* 5th ed. Churchill Livingstone; 1998.
2. World Health Organization Classification of tumours. In: Barnes L, Eveson JW, Riechart P, Sidransky D (eds). *Pathology and Genetics, Head and Neck Tumours.* Lyon: IARC Press; 2005.
3. Franco EL, Rohan TE (eds). *Cancer precursors epidemiology, detection and prevention.* New York: Springer-Verlag; 2002.
4. Sternberg SS (ed). *Diagnostic surgical pathology.* 3rd ed. Lippincott William and Wilkins; 1999.
5. Unni KK, Inwards CY. Odontogenic and related tumors. *Dahlins Bone Tumours – General aspects and Data on 10,165 cases.* 6th ed. Lippincott William and Wilkins; 2009: 381–91.
6. Lucas DR, Unni KK, Mcleod RA, *et al.* Osteoblastoma: Clinicopathologic study of 306 cases. *Hum Pathol* 1994;**25**:117–34.
7. Nora FE, Unni KK, Pritchard DJ, *et al.* Osteosarcoma of extragnathic craniofacial bones. *Mayo Clinic Proc* 1983;**58**:286–72.
8. Clark JL, Unni KK, Dahlin DC, *et al.* Osteosarcoma of the jaw. *Cancer* 1983;**51**:2311–16.
9. Gaffey MJ, Lack EE, Christ ML, *et al.* Anaplastic thyroid carcinoma with osteoclast like giant cells—a clinicopathologic, immunohistochemical and ultrastructural study. *Am J Surg Pathol* 1991;**15**:160–8.
10. Scheithauer BW, J Rubinstein LJ. Meningeal mesenchymal chondrosarcoma: Report of 8 cases with review of the Literature. *Cancer* 1978;**42**:2744–52.
11. Hoch BL, Nielsen GP, Liebsch NJ, *et al.* Base of skull chordomas in children and adolescents: A clinicopathologic study of 73 cases. *Am J Surg Pathol* 2006;**30**:811–18.
12. Rosenberg AE, Nielsen GP, Keel SB, *et al.* Chondrosarcoma of the base of the skull: A clinicopathologic study of 200 cases with emphasis on its distinction from chondroma. *Am J Surg Pathol* 1999;**23**:1370–8.
13. Vencio EF, Reeve CM, Unni KK, *et al.* Mesenchymal chondrosarcoma of the jaw bones: Clinicopathologic study of 19 cases. *Cancer* 1998;**82**:2350–5.
14. Feely M, Keohan C. Chondroblastoma of the Skull. *J Neurol Neurosurg Psychiatry* 1984;**47**:1348–50.
15. Chaudhry A, Robinovitch M, Mitchell D, *et al.* Chondrogenic tumours of the jaws. *Am J Surgery* 2009;**102**:403–11.
16. Kaserer K, Scheuba C, Neuhold N, *et al.* Sporadic versus familial medullary thyroid microcarcinomas: A histopathologic study of 50 consecutive patients. *Am J Surg Pathol* 2001;**25**:1245–51.
17. Gaertiner EM, Davidson M, Wenig BM. The columnar cell variant of thyroid papillary carcinoma: Case report and discussion of an unusually aggressive thyroid papillary carcinoma. *Am J Surg Pathol* 1995;**19**:940–7.
18. Carcangin ML, Zampi G, Rosai J. Poorly differentiated ('Insular') thyroid carcinoma. A reinterpretation of Langhans' 'wuchernde struma'. *Am J Surg Pathol* 1984;**8**:655–68.
19. Lam KY, Lo C-Y, Liu M-C. Primary squamous cell carcinoma of the thyroid gland: An entity with aggressive clinical behaviour and distinctive cytokeratin expression profile. *Histopathology* 2001;**39**:279–86.
20. Shrikhande SS (ed). Biopsy interpretation. Guidelines to selected areas in oncopathology. Bombay: Professional Education Department, Tata Memorial Hospital, Tata Memorial Centre.
21. DeLellis RA, Williams ED. Tumours of the thyroid and parathyroid. WHO classification of tumours—pathology and genetics. In: DeLellis RA, Lloyd RV, Heitz PU, *et al. Tumours of endocrine organs.* Lyon: IARC Press; 2004: 50.

4

Radiology of head and neck malignancies

K. RAMACHANDRAN, M. VENUGOPAL, V. JIJI, S.M. KOSHY, ANIL PRAHLADAN

The role of imaging in head and neck malignancies, by and large, is indicated in defining local spread of disease and staging of a diagnosed lesion. This is especially so, taking into account the inherent inability of all current modalities in characterizing a pure mucosal disease. Computed tomography (CT) is currently the most commonly used imaging modality due to its ability to adequately assess bone involvement and nodal status, so much so that it has almost obviated the role of conventional radiography. In recent times, magnetic resonance imaging (MRI) has emerged as an equally competent, if not superior, examination with its exquisite soft tissue resolution and lack of ionizing radiation. However, long imaging times and exclusivity, including cost, have not made it popular. In experienced hands, ultrasound still has a role in assessment of neck nodes and imaging of thyroid tumours. This chapter aims to provide an overview of imaging findings in various head and neck malignancies.

Malignant lesions of the oral cavity

Malignant lesions account for approximately 7% of oral cavity lesions. Squamous cell carcinoma (SCC) accounts for approximately 90% of these.[1] Other less common malignancies include the following:

- Minor salivary gland tumours
  —Adenoid cystic carcinoma
  —Adenocarcinoma
  —Mucoepidermoid carcinoma
- Lymphoma
  —Hodgkin
  —Non-Hodgkin
- Sarcoma
  —Liposarcoma
  —Rhabdomyosarcoma
  —Fibrosarcoma
  —Angiosarcoma
  —Leiomyo sarcoma
- Neoplasms of the mandible
  —Osteogenic sarcoma
  —Ewing sarcoma
  —Chondrosarcoma
  —Metastasis

CT and MRI help mainly in detecting the extent of the involvement of these tumours in deeper tissues and invasion of adjacent structures (including neurovascular bundles), bone and lymph nodes. Imaging also can aid in staging the primary malignancies on the basis of the tumour, node, metastasis (TNM) system.

Squamous cell carcinoma (SCC)

As the squamous epithelium of the oral cavity is derived from the ectodermal elements, it is more prone to being affected by less aggressive lesions than those of the oropharynx, which is of endodermal origin.[2] SCC occurs more commonly between the ages of 50 and 70 years, predominantly in men who have a history of prolonged tobacco and alcohol abuse.[3,4] Even though it can arise from any mucosal surface, SCC has a predilection for the floor of the mouth, ventrolateral tongue and the soft palate complex.[5] These lesions carry a potential for neurovascular involvement. Vascular invasion is often also associated with an increased likelihood of cervical nodal metastases.[6] Perineural invasion permits tumour extension beyond the expected tumour margins.[7] Neurovascular invasion indicates aggressive behaviour and greater metastatic potential.[8,9]

As 30%–65% of patients with SCC of the oral cavity have a positive nodal status at the time of initial presentation,[10–13] cervical lymph node chains should also be included in the imaging of the primary tumour.[14] This can be accomplished by either CT or MRI modalities. Modern generation CT seems to be more precise with its ability to demonstrate extranodal tumour spread and central necrosis accurately, compared with MR techniques.[15,16]

On CT scan, SCC has a density similar to that of muscle and shows moderate enhancement with contrast, whereas on MRI the signal intensity is similar to muscle on T_1, and an inhomogeneously increased signal on T_2-weighted images are noticed with some degree of enhancement on administering gadolinium.[17,18]

When evaluating SCC of the floor of the mouth the following three points should be noted: (i) The presence and extent of mandibular involvement; (ii) the degree of submucosal extension; and (iii) the status of regional lymph nodes.[19] Contrast-enhanced CT is the preferred modality for detecting cortical bone invasion[20] and lymph node metastasis, and MRI is ideal in evaluating bone marrow involvement and perineural tumour spread.[21–23] In the absence of a tumour, the marrow in T_1-weighted images is displayed as high signal intensity, which in the presence of a tumour is seen as low signal intensity. Inflammatory enlargement of the submandibular and sublingual glands with duct dilatation can be seen because of obstruction of the ostium by tumour infiltration. The tumour spreads to the submental, submandibular and internal jugular nodes (levels I and II) in lesions of the floor of the mouth.

SCC of the oral tongue occurs mostly on its ventrolateral surface. The lesions may extend along the extrinsic muscles to their attachment, viz. hyoid bone, mandible, styloid process, etc. They can involve the floor of the mouth (Fig. 1), tonsils, mandible and pharyngeal walls by submucosal extension. Superiorly, they can extend to the soft palate via the palatoglossus muscle and nasopharynx via the veli palatini muscles.[17] Assessing the extent of the tumour across the midline with involvement of contralateral lingual neurovascular bundle is important in its surgical planning. These tumours also drain to bilateral submandibular and internal jugular nodes (levels I and II).

Buccal mucosa SCCs commonly originate along the lateral walls and lateral submucosal extension along the buccinator muscle to the pterygomandibular raphe with erosion of the underlying bone which is the most common method of spread.

Lower gingival lesions may erode the mandible and spread by perineural or intramedullary extension.

Primary SCC of the hard palate is rare and usually

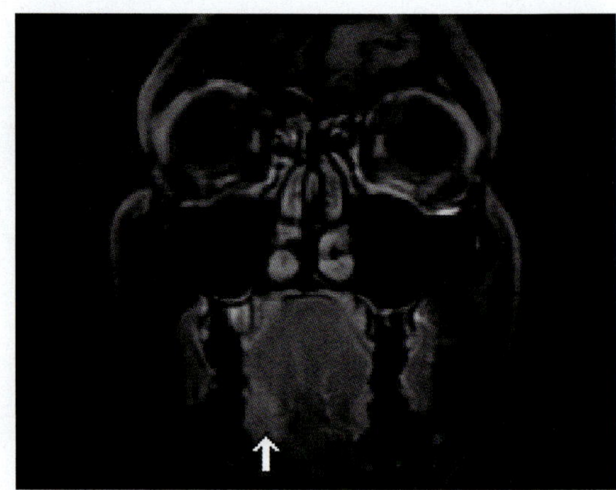

Fig. 1. Post-contrast coronal T_1-weighted image showing a mass in the right lateral border of the tongue in a patient with SCC

represents an extension from the gingival SCC. These lesions may erode the floor of the nasal cavity or maxillary sinus, or involve the soft palate. Perineural spread can occur along the lesser and greater palatine nerves back to the pterygopalatine fossa to involve the maxillary division of the trigeminal nerve.[19] This spread is best imaged by MRI in the coronal plane.

Retromolar trigone SCC may extend deep to the maxillary tuberosity to involve the buccal space fat posterolateral to the maxillary antrum. It may also extend anteriorly along the orbicularis oris and buccinator muscles, and posteriorly to the superior pharyngeal constrictor muscle. Cavernous sinus spread through the maxillary and mandibular nerves[19] can occur when the lesion extends to the pterygopalatine fossa and masticator space. Mandibular ramus spread must be assessed in imaging of this area (Fig. 2).

Lymphoma

Hodgkin and non-Hodgkin lymphomas can occur in the head and neck region. Lymph node enlargement is the commonest presenting symptom. Hodgkin lymphoma tends to be nodal whereas non-Hodgkin lymphoma frequently involves extranodal sites.[24,25] Affected lymph nodes may vary in size. They have a homogeneous texture and may manifest as peripheral rim enhancement. Central necrosis occurs only after treatment.[24] Lymph nodes involved by Hodgkin/non-Hodgkin lymphomas are usually not distinguishable from metastasis by CT and MRI.

Adenoid cystic carcinoma

Adenoid cystic carcinoma (ACC) accounts for only 5% of major salivary gland neoplasms, whereas it comprises >25% of minor salivary gland malignancies. Three histological subtypes are identifiable: tubular, cribriform and solid. The degree of cellularity increases from the tubular to the solid form.[26] ACC is characterized by slow, relentless growth and a tendency towards extensive local invasion and perineural extension

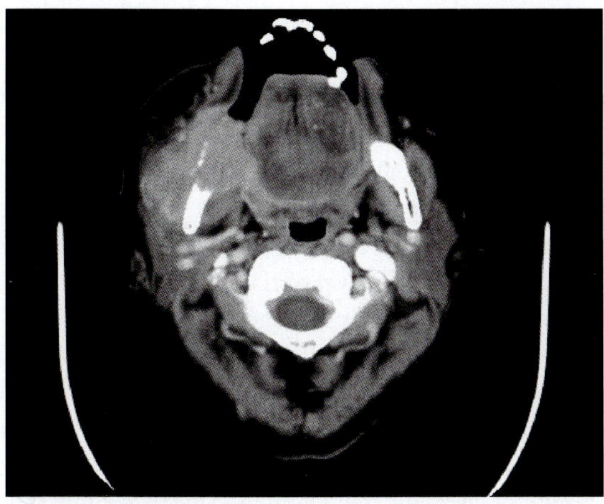

Fig. 2. Post-contrast axial CT showing destruction of mandible in SCC of retromolar trigone

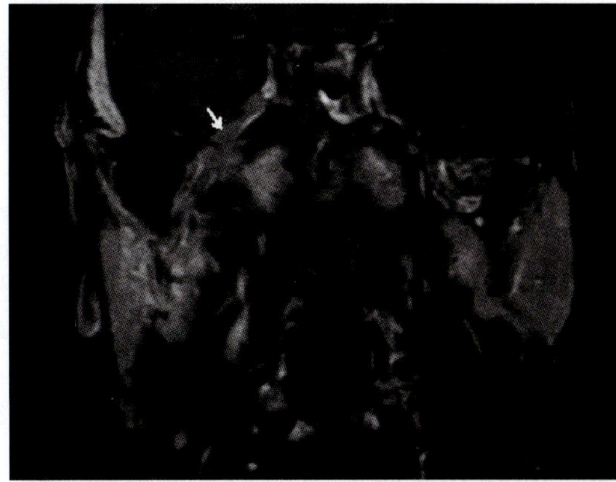

Fig. 3. Post-contrast coronal T_1-image showing perineural tumour extension along the right mandibular nerve in adenocarcinoma of the salivary gland

(Fig. 3). On CT and MRI, ACC cannot be distinguished from other malignancies on the basis of density or signal intensity. A perineural tumour on CT is seen as an enlargement of skull base foramina and fissures; rarely, a diffusely enlarged nerve can also be seen. MRI may demonstrate increased thickness of nerve and diffuse or marginal enhancement.

Mucoepidermoid carcinoma

This arises from a glandular ductal epithelium. Nearly 30% of these arise from the minor salivary glands located in the buccal mucosa and palate. These tumours are classified into low-, intermediate- and high-grade lesions. Low-grade lesions have a benign imaging appearance with fairly well delineated, smooth margins. Cystic areas may be present and calcifications are rarely seen within. High-grade lesions are poorly circumscribed with indistinct infiltrating margins and demonstrate low-to-intermediate signal intensities on T_1- and T_2-weighted sequences.[27]

Liposarcoma

These are rare in the head and neck region and originate from lipoblasts. On CT, liposarcomas are inhomogeneous, having fat and soft-tissue elements. The density of the fat is greater than that of subcutaneous fat. On MRI they appear as fatty lesions but demonstrate signal intensities lower than that of subcutaneous fat on T_1.

Rhabdomyosarcoma

These are rare mesenchymal tumours of which approximately 36% occur in the head and neck region.[28] Oral rhabdomyosarcomas are more commonly seen in males in the first two decades of life.[29] They are seen as muscle density masses on CT and MRI; in T_2-weighted images they have higher signal intensity. They have a tendency to infiltrate

the surrounding structures and exhibit a variable amount of enhancement.

Miscellaneous malignancies

Apart from the above-mentioned common malignancies, various less common malignancies such as adenocarcinomas, fibrosarcomas, angiosarcomas, myosarcomas and leiomyosarcomas can also occur in the oral cavity. Contiguous lesions from the jaws, such as Ewing sarcomas, chondrosarcomas, osteosarcomas and metastasis, as well as lesions of the neural structures such as malignant schwannomas of the inferior alveolar nerves, can also extend into the oral cavity.

Nasopharynx, larynx and hypopharynx

Cancer of the nasopharynx

Often, a tumour arises in the fossa of Rosenmuller. The early stage of the cancer may show only subtle changes, such as obliteration of fat stripe between levator veli palatini and tensor veli palatini muscles, or otomastoiditis, or enlarged retropharyngeal node (node of Rouviere).

In advanced disease, CT and MRI are useful in assessing the extent of the disease. In CT, the mass is isodense with no significant enhancement. But in MRI, the mass is dark on T_1 imaging and slightly bright with enhancement on T_2 imaging. CT depicts bone destruction beautifully whereas MRI delineates bone marrow infiltration.

The purpose of imaging
1. Accurate tumour staging
2. Definition of tumour margins for radiation oncologist
3. Evaluate the response to chemotherapy/radiotherapy (RT).

Laterally, the tumour can spread to the parapharyngeal space through the sinus of Morgagni and enter the masticator space. In this case the mandibular nerve can be involved. The mandibular nerve acts as a cable through which the tumour can reach the gasserian ganglion in the Meckel cave through the foramen ovale and from there through the preganglionic segment of the nerve V to the pons.

The involved mandibular nerve is seen thickened between the lateral and medial pterygoid muscles and shows enhancement on contrast administration, better delineated in contrast-enhanced T_1-weighted image in the coronal plane, with fat suppression in MRI.

Posterolateral spread is to the retrostyloid parapharyngeal space where cranial nerves IX–XII can get involved.

Posterior spread can also be seen to the retropharyngeal space and from there to the prevertebral space. Infiltration of the prevertebral muscles is seen in T_2-weighted image as bright signals in the muscle, which may also be due to oedema. Sometimes, vertebral body destruction and spinal canal invasion may be seen.

Superiorly, the tumour can erode the skull base and extend intracranially. Intracranial extension may occur through the following routes:

- Foramen ovale—perineural/direct
- Foramen lacerum—along the internal carotid artery, reaching the cavernous sinus where cranial nerves III, IV and VI can be involved
- Direct destruction of the skull base at the attachment of the levator and tensor veli palatini muscles
- Direct invasion of the sphenoid sinus
- Through the foramen rotundum/superior orbital fissure
- Through the jugular foramen/foramen magnum into the posterior fossa. (In the posterior fossa, infiltration is demonstrated as dural thickening in contrast-enhanced coronal MRI.)

While assessing the response to chemotherapy/RT, one has to differentiate between residual/recurrent tissue and scar tissue. It is not difficult to differentiate mature scar tissue in MRI, as it appears dark in T_2 without enhancement. The immature scar, on the other hand, is bright in T_2, and enhancement is similar to that of tumours. It is better to have a baseline MRI 3–4 months post-treatment so that any changes from the baseline during the follow up can be detected immediately. A positron emission tomography (PET) scan using 18 FDG (fluorodeoxyglucose) and thallium 201, and a MR spectroscopy can help in distinguishing the tumour from scar tissue.

Cancer of the larynx

Imaging for mucosal tumours is not a substitute for direct visualization. Imaging is indicated when considering whether voice sparing surgery is possible. The treatment depends on the origin and extent of the tumour.

For supraglottic tumours, resection is done through the ventricle. Hence, if the tumour is crossing the ventricle, supraglottic laryngectomy cannot be considered. The important role of imaging is to rule out submucosal spread through the ventricle.

In axial sections, determining the level of the ventricle is a little difficult. The paraglottic space at the false vocal cord level consists of fat and at the true vocal cord level it is muscle. Tumour extension at the level of the true vocal cord needs to be ruled out for supraglottic laryngectomy.

Cartilage invasion is assessed by imaging. Although it can be assessed only by imaging, this is not always possible. Cartilage invasion is considered a contraindication for vertical hemilaryngectomy and supraglottic laryngectomy. The only reliable sign of cartilage involvement is extralaryngeal spread of the tumour. In CT, cartilage invasion may be implied by erosion or sclerosis. However, irregular ossifications of cartilages may cause erroneous interpretations. Often, arytenoid cartilages can be found sclerosed.

It is difficult to assess the non-ossified cartilage in CT, in which case MRI is more beneficial. If the T_1-weighted image is bright, the cartilage is non-infiltrated. If it is T_1 dark and T_2 dark, then it is ossified. If it is T_1 dark and T_2 intermediate or bright, then tumour infiltration may be considered. Extension to the pre-epiglottic space and involvement of the epiglottic cartilage are not contraindications for supraglottic laryngectomy.

For a true vocal cord tumour, the surgical options are resection, endoscopic laser resection, RT and vertical hemilaryngectomy. Surgery is contraindicated when there is an extension to the cricoid cartilage, deep invasion at the anterior commissure, involvement of more than one-third of the contralateral cord, and extension across the ventricle to the false vocal cord.

For subglottic tumours the only option is total laryngectomy. For submucosal laryngeal tumours, imaging is used not only to show the extent of the tumour but also to help identify the type of the tumour. It can be a chondroma or chondrosarcoma arising from the laryngeal cartilages, haemangioma or paraganglioma.

In post-treatment imaging, if an attempt is made to reconstruct the cord using a small slip taken from the strap muscle, it can lead to soft tissue density that cannot be readily distinguished from the tumour.

In RT, swelling of soft tissue and stranding of paraglottic fat represent local inflammation and oedema. Recurrent tumour presents as a small enhancing area. PET may play an important role in post-treatment management.

Cancer of the hypopharynx

The tumour can involve the pyriform sinus, posterior wall of the hypopharynx and post-cricoid region. The apex of the pyriform sinus corresponds to the level of the true vocal cord. The anterior pyriform sinus mucosa abuts the posterior paraglottic space. The post-cricoid region is part of the anterior wall of the lower hypopharynx.

Superficial lesions are best observed by direct clinical examination; CT and MRI help to assess submucosal spread. Hypopharyngeal tumours can extend easily to the larynx. Infiltration of prevertebral muscles is a contraindication for surgery. This can be better depicted in MRI as bright signals in the muscle in T_2-weighted images.

Sinonasal neoplasms

The sinonasal tract can harbour a variety of neoplasms derived from various tissue types. They can be classified broadly into those arising from epithelial and those arising from mesenchymal elements.

In comparison to inflammatory pathology, neoplasms are rare. Although carcinomas are by far the most common, they nevertheless constitute only 3% of all head and neck malignancies.[30,31] However, in spite of this, carcinomas are clinically significant with a grave prognosis. This is because they remain clinically silent until an advanced stage. With advances in imaging technology, superior tumour mapping and staging are now possible, permitting more realistic treatment planning for a cure, as against palliation.[32]

Challenges in imaging

A major imaging problem in sinonasal malignancies is differentiating the viable tumour from adjacent inflammation.[33,34] In this regard, MRI is superior to contrast-enhanced CT. On T_2W the cellular sinonasal tumour is less hyperintense than the inflammatory pathology. Benign or low-grade minor salivary gland tumours, schwannomas, inverted papillomas and rare haemangiomatous lesions show an intensely high T_2 signal, thus making mapping of these tumours inaccurate.

Bone destruction adjacent to the tumour allows for a more definite imaging diagnosis of neoplasms.[35–37] The size of the tumour matters as small tumours have no adjacent bone erosion, making diagnosis difficult. SCCs, metastases, and some sarcomas and lymphomas are associated with aggressive bone destruction. By comparison, mucocoeles, polyps, inverted papillomas and lesions, such as minor salivary gland tumours, schwannomas, olfactory neuroblastomas, most lymphomas and sarcomas tend to remodel rather than aggressively destroy bone. Bone sclerosis is also rare, with the neoplastic process being more in favour of infective/inflammatory pathology.

The size of the tumour is another important factor in determining imaging sensitivity. Small tumours often have MR characteristics that are indistinguishable from adjacent inflammatory pathology.

Contrast-enhanced CT and MRI in specifically indicated

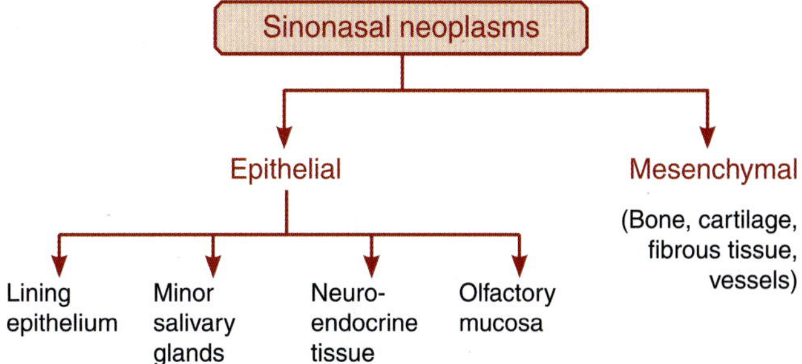

Fig. 4. Sinonasal neoplasms

cases remains the mainstay of diagnostic imaging in sinonasal malignancies. Although it is tempting to offer a pathological diagnosis on imaging features alone, very few cases show imaging findings to be pathognomonic. The role of imaging is primarily in accurate tumour mapping with special emphasis on involvement of critical anatomical sites that will influence treatment planning, rather than to offer a final pathological diagnosis.

Papillomas[38–41]

These constitute only 0.5%–5% of all sinonasal tumours. It is important to differentiate these from simple cysts or polyps because of the possibility of malignant degeneration.

1. *Fungiform papillomas* (50%)
   — Nearly always arise from nasal septum
   — Usually solitary (75%) and unilateral (96%)
   — Are not considered premalignant.
2. *Inverted papillomas* (47%)
   — Characteristically arise from the lateral nasal mall and may extend into sinuses, especially the maxillary sinus. Rarely, isolated sinus involvement has also been reported.
   — Carcinoma may develop (5%–25%) concurrently or subsequently, most commonly the SCCs.
   — Verrucous carcinoma, mucoepidermoid carcinoma and adenocarcinoma have also been reported.
   — Can have calcification within
   — Aggressive bone destruction along the margin of an inverted papilloma should be considered suspicious for malignant degeneration.
3. *Oncocytic papilloma* (3%)
   These are radiologically similar to inverted papillomas.

Imaging findings can range from a small nasal polypoidal mass to an expansile nasal mass with bone remodelling and extension to sinuses. CT and MRI are non-specific.

Carcinomas (Fig. 5)[42–44]

SCCs most commonly arise from the maxillary sinus; 25%–

60% arise from the maxillary antrum, 25%–35% from the nasal cavity, 10% from the ethmoids, and 1% from the frontal and sphenoid bones. Secondary extension to the maxillary sinus is most common (80%). The primary imaging feature is bone destruction even with only a small demonstrable mass.

Ten per cent of carcinomas are glandular in origin; adenoid cystic carcinomas and mucoepidermoid carcinomas, as well as intestinal-type adenocarcinomas, arise from the minor salivary glands.

T staging

T1 Limited to antral mucosal; no bone destruction
T2 Bone destruction but no extension beyond
T3 Extension to orbit, ethmoids or skin
T4 Extension to nasopharynx, sphenoid, cribriform plate or pterygopalatine fossa. Conventional radiographs show sinus opacification; 70%–90% show bone destruction. Contrast-enhanced CT and MRI better delineate the exent of the tumour, bone destruction and soft tissue component.

Adenoid cystic carcinomas (Fig. 6)[45–47]

These arise most commonly in the palate and extend into the nasal cavities and paranasal space. Among salivary neoplasms, the most common are adenoid cystic carcinomas (35%), followed by pleomorphic adenoma, mucoepidermoid carcinoma and lastly malignant plemorphic adenoma.

Adenoid cystic carcinomas have the following features:
- Perineural tumour invasion is characteristic.
- Skip lesions within nerves can occur.
- Locoregional recurrence is common.

Olfactory neuroblastomas (Figs 7, 8)[48–51]

These are uncommon tumours that arise from the neural crest cells in the roof of the nasal cavities. They are considered here because of their unique site of origin and route of spread.

Olfactory neuroblastomas have the following features:
- Bimodal peak; second and sixth decades of life
- Relatively slow growing for a malignant tumour
- Expand and remodel bone rather than frank destruction
- Can have calcification within
- Extend into ipsilateral maxillary and ethmoid sinuses (rarely into sphenoid)
- Intracranial extension through dura in the region of the cribriform plate.

Lymphomas[52–57]

- Mostly non-Hodgkin lymphoma
- Second most common sinonasal malignancy after SCCs; 10% are extranodal involving tonsils, sinonasal tract and thyroid
- Most commonly involve nasal cavity and maxillary sinuses; rarely ethmoid sinuses
- Mostly remodel, occasionally destroy bone
- Bulky soft tissue mass with moderate enhancement.

Imaging in thyroid malignancies

Thyroid malignancies are not uncommon and occur in both sexes and across all age groups. In recent decades, an increase in the incidence of these tumours has been attributed to low-dose radiation given as part of the treatment for head and neck cancers. The prognosis of these tumours, if detected sufficiently early and if amenable to surgical resection, is generally good. An exception is anaplastic carcinomas, which usually presents as advanced disease with survival measured in months.

Thyroid malignancies can arise from both follicular and parafollicular C cells. The major histopathological classification includes papillary, follicular, medullary and anaplastic carcinomas—in decreasing order of incidence and increasing order of mortality.

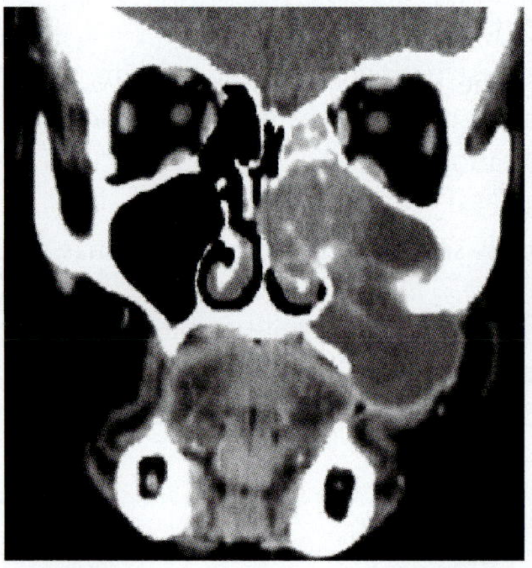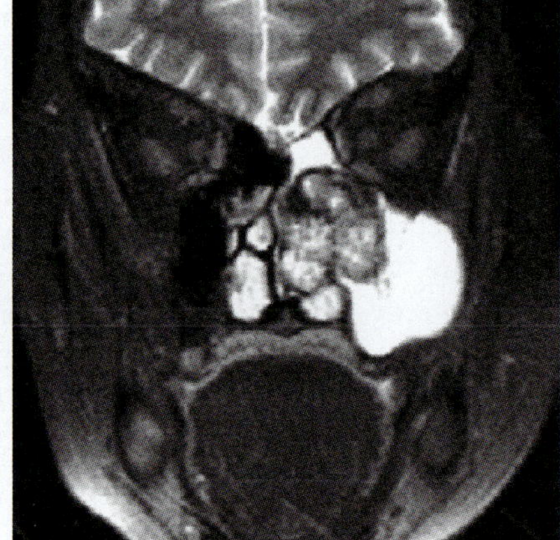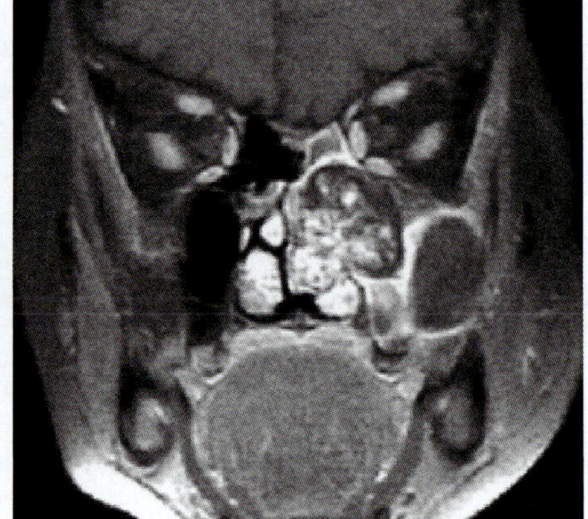

Fig. 5. Maxillary sinus carcinoma—Cor CT, Cor T$_2$ and post-Gd coronal MRI showing maxillary mass with co-existent inflammatory pathology; best differentiated on T$_2$W MRI

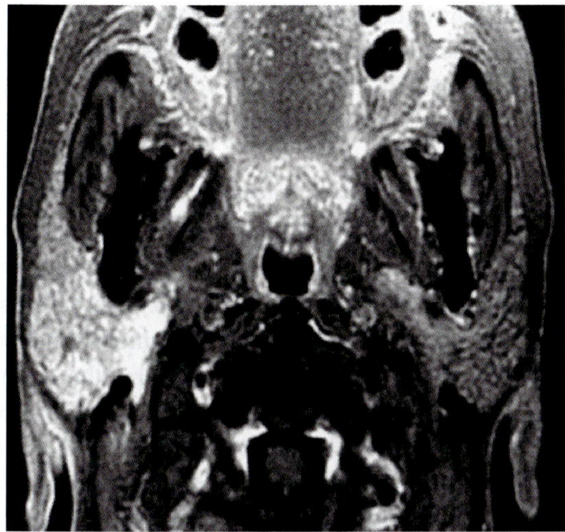
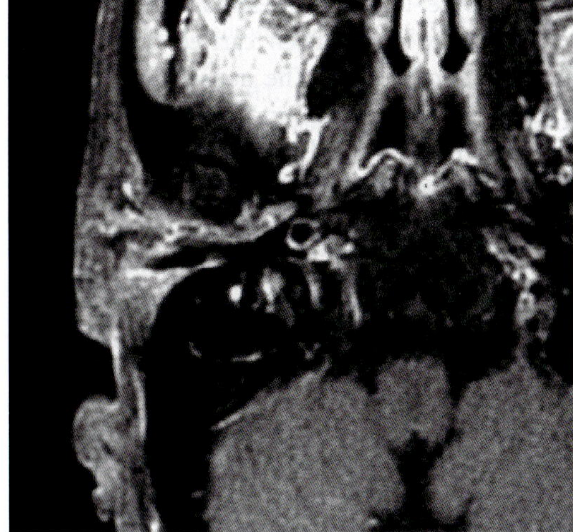

Fig. 6. Adenoid cystic carcinoma parotid gland with perineural invasion along cranial nerve VII

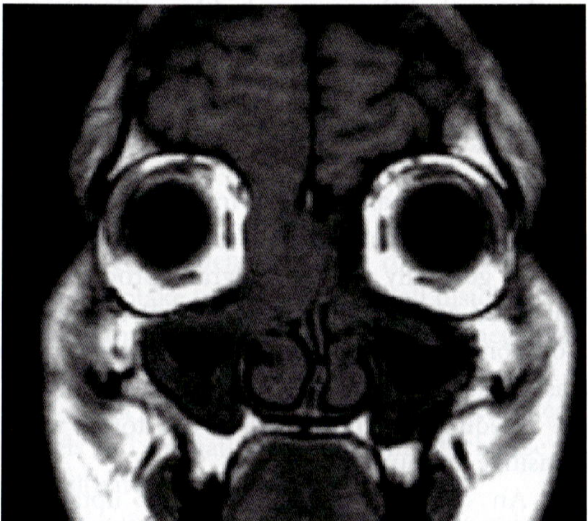
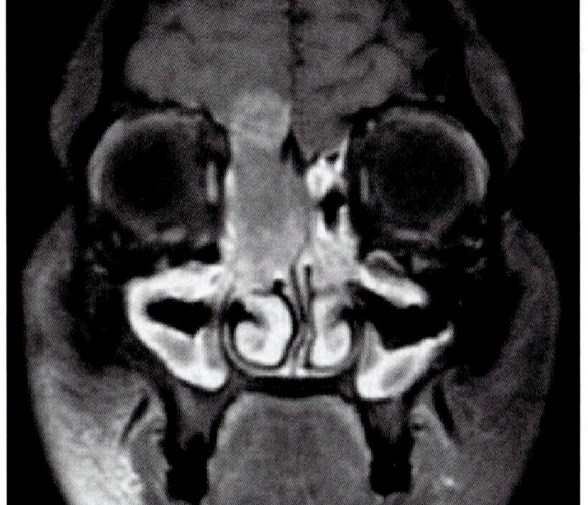

Fig. 7. Olfactory neuroblastoma—T_1W MRI plain

Fig. 8. Olfatory neuroblastoma—T_1 post-contrast

The diagnosis of primary thyroid carcinomas is mainly by histological, clinical and biochemical parameters. The role of imaging is limited chiefly to assessment of findings relating to a thyroid neoplasm, as features characteristic of a histological subtype are not evident with the currently available imaging modalities. Most features detected on imaging, such as calcifications, cystic areas and haemorrhage, show considerable overlap in both benign and malignant lesions. The main aims of cross-sectional imaging (ultrasound, CT and MRI) are to assess the following features:

- Adjacent structure infiltration (airway, vessels, soft tissue)
- Retrosternal extension
- Cervical nodal metastases
- Distant metastases (including bone)
- Guide for fine-needle aspiration (FNA) cytology/biopsy.

Nuclear scintigraphy, on the other hand, provides functional information, with the major aim being differentiation between 'hot' and 'cold' nodules, the latter being associated with a greater incidence (nearly four times) of malignancy.

Presently, morphological detail of the thyroid is assessed with technetium (^{99m}Tc) pertechnetate, iodine (I) 123 and I-131. I-131 is also used for determining 24-hour thyroid iodine uptake and for evaluation and treatment of thyroid cancers that concentrate iodine.

^{18}Fluorodeoxyglucose-(FDG) PET has recently emerged as a promising modality in imaging of metastatic thyroid tumours that do not concentrate radioiodine.

Salient features of the commonly used cross-sectional imaging modalities are described below.

Ultrasound (with linear high-frequency [7.5 MHz] probe)

- Safe (absence of ionizing radiation)
- Easily accessible, inexpensive and non-invasive
- Highly sensitive for differentiating cystic and solid lesions
- Real-time guidance for guided procedures
- Examiner-dependant
- Less sensitive for adjacent structure infiltration and lymphadenopathy.

33. Lloyd G, Lund V, Phelps PD, *et al*. Magnetic resonance imaging in the evaluation of nose and paranasal sinus disease. *Br J Radiol* 1987;**60**:957–68.

34. Som P, Shapiro M, Biller H, *et al*. Sinonasal tumors and inflammatory tissues: Differentiation with MR imaging. *Radiology* 1988;**167**:803–8.

35. Dubois P, Schultz J, Perrin R, *et al*. Tomography in expansile lesions of the nasal and paranasal sinuses. *Radiology* 1977;**125**:149–58.

36. Som P, Shugar J. The significance of bone expansion associated with the diagnosis of malignant tumors of the paranasal sinuses. *Radiology* 1980;**136**:97–100.

37. Som P, Shugar J. When to question the diagnosis of anaplastic carcinoma. *Mt Sinai J Med* 1981;**48**:230–5.

38. Barnes L, Verbin R, Gnepp D. Diseases of the nose, paranasal sinuses and nasopharynx. In: Barnes L (ed). *Surgical pathology of the head and neck*. Vol. 1. New York: Marcel Dekker; 1985:403–51.

39. Hyams V. Papillomas of the nasal cavity and paranasal sinuses: A clinicopathologic study of 315 cases. *Ann Otol Rhinol Laryngol* 1971;**80**:192–206.

40. Lasser A, Rothfeld P, Shapiro R. Epithelial papilloma and squamous cell carcinoma of the nasal cavity and paranasal sinuses: A clinicopathologic study. *Cancer* 1976;**38**:2503–10.

41. Vrabec D. The inverted schneiderian papilloma: A clinical and pathological study. *Laryngoscope* 1975;**85**:186–220.

42. Slootweg P, Richardson M. Squamous cell carcinoma of the upper aerodigestive system. In: Gnepp D (ed). *Diagnostic surgical pathology of the head and neck*. Philadelphia: WB Saunders; 2001:19–78.

43. Barton R. Nickel carcinogenesis of the respiratory tract. *J Otolaryngol* 1977;**6**:412–22.

44. Perzin K, Lefkowitch J, Hui R. Bilateral nasal squamous carcinoma arising in papillomatosis: Report of a case developing after chemotherapy for leukemia. *Cancer* 1981;**48**:2375–82.

45. Klintenberg C, Olofsson J, Hellquist H, *et al*. Adenocarcinoma of the ethmoid sinuses: A review of 38 cases with special reference to wood dust exposure. *Cancer* 1984;**31**:482–8.

46. Spiro R, Koss L, Hajdu S, *et al*. Tumors of minor salivary origin: A clinicopathologic study of 492 cases. *Cancer* 1973;**31**:117–29.

47. Yamamoto Y, Saka T, Makimoto K, *et al*. Histological changes during progression of adenoid cystic carcinoma. *J Laryngol Otol* 1992;**106**:1016–20.

48. Kadish S, Goodman M, Wine C. Olfactory neuroblastoma: A clinical nalysis of 17 cases. *Cancer* 1976;**37**:1571–6.

49. Miyamoto R, Gleich L, Biddinger P, *et al*. Esthesioneuroblastoma and sinonasal undifferentiated carcinoma: Impact of histological grading and clinical staging on survival and prognosis. *Laryngoscope* 2000;**110**:1262–5.

50. Som P, Lawson W, Biller H, *et al*. Ethmoid sinus disease: CT evaluation in 400 cases. Part III: Cranio-facial resection. *Radiology* 1986;**159**:605–9.

51. Morita A, Ebersold M, Olsen K. Esthesioneuroblastoma: Prognosis and management. *Neurosurgery* 1993;**32**:706–15.

52. McGurk M, Goepel J, Hancock B. Extranodal lymphoma of head and neck: A review of 49 consecutive cases. *Clin Radiol* 1985;**36**:455–8.

53. Fellbaum C, Hansmann M, Lennert K. Malignant lymphomas of the nasal and paranasal sinuses. *Virch Arch A Pathol Anat Histopathol* 1989;**414**:399–405.

54. Cleary K, Batsakis J. Sinonasal lymphomas. *Ann Otol Rhinol Laryngol* 1994;**103**:911–14.

55. Quraishi M, Bessell E, Clark D, *et al*. Non-Hodgkin's lymphoma of the sinonasal tract. *Laryngoscope* 2000;**110**:1489–92.

56. Rodriguez J, Romaguera J, Manning J, *et al*. Nasal-type T/NK lymphomas: A clinicopathologic study of 13 cases. *Leuk Lymphoma* 2000;**39**:139–44.

57. Cuadra-Garcia I, Proulx G, Wu C, *et al*. Sinonasal lymphoma: A clinicopathologic analysis of 58 cases from the Massachusetts General Hospital. *Am J Surg Pathol* 1999;**23**:1356–69.

58. Chen KTK, Rosai J. Follicular variant of thyroid papillary carcinoma. A clinicopathologic study of 6 cases. *Am J Surg Pathol* 1977;**1**:123–30.

59. Rosai J, Zampi G, Carcangiu ML. Papillary carcinoma of the thyroid. A discussion of its several morphologic expressions, with particular emphasis on the follicular variant. *Am J Surg Pathol* 1983;**7**:809–17.

60. Carcangiu ML, Zampi G, Pupi A, *et al*. Papillary carcinoma of the thyroid. A clinicopathologic study of 244 cases treated at the University of Florence, Italy. *Cancer* 1985;**55**:805–28.

61. Vickery AL. Thyroid papillary carcinoma. Pathological and philosophical controversies. *Am J Surg Pathol* 1983;**7**:797–807.

62. Hay ID. Papillary thyroid carcinoma. *Endocrinol Metab Clin North Am* 1990;**19**:545–76.

63. Hawk WA, Hazard JB. The many appearances of papillary carcinoma of the thyroid. *Cleve Clin Q* 1976;**43**:207–16.

64. Som PM, Brandwein M, Lidov M, *et al*. The varied appearance of papillary carcinoma cervical nodal disease: CT and MR findings. *AJNR* 1994;**15**:1129–38.

65. Franssila KO, Ackerman LV, Brown CL, *et al*. Follicular carcinoma. *Semin Diagn Pathol* 1985;**2**:101–2.

66. Roediger WEW. The oxyphil and C cells of the human thyroid gland. *Cancer* 1975;**36**:1758–70.

67. Bondeson L, Bondeson AG, Ljungberg O, *et al*. Oxyphil tumors of the thyroid. Follow-up of 42 surgical cases. *Ann Surg* 1981;**194**:677–80.

68. Gorman B, Charboneau JW, James EM, *et al*. Medullary thyroid carcinoma: Role of high-resolution US. *Radiology* 1987;**162**:147–50.

69. Melvin KEW, Miller HH, Tashjian AH. Early diagnosis of medullary carcinoma of the thyroid by means of calcitonin assay. *N Engl J Med* 1971;**285**:1115–20.

70. Steiner AL, Goodman AD, Powers SR. Study of a kindred with pheochromocytoma, medullary thyroid carcinoma, hyperparathyroidism, and Cushing's disease: Multiple endocrine neoplasia type 2. *Medicine* 1968;**47**:371–409.

71. Wolfe HJ, DeLellis RA. Familial medullary thyroid carcinomaand C-cell hyperplasia. *Clin Endocrinol Metab* 1981;**10**:351–65.

72. Kakudo K, Carney JA, Sizemore GW. Medullary carcinoma of thyroid: Biologic behavior of the sporadic and familial neoplasm. *Cancer* 1985;**55**:2818–21.

73. Busnardo B, Girelli ME, Simioni N, *et al*. Non-parallel patterns of calcitonin and carcinoembryonic antigen levels in the follow-up of medullary thyroid carcinoma. *Cancer* 1984;**53**:278–85.

74. Dörr U, Würstlin S, Frank-Raue K, *et al*. Somatostatin receptor scintigraphy and magnetic resonance imaging in recurrent medullary thyroid carcinoma: A comparative study. *Horm Metab Res Suppl* 1993;**27**:48–55.

75. Lebouthillier G, Morais J, Picard M, *et al*. Tc-99m sestamibi and other agents in the detection of metastatic medullary carcinoma of the thyroid. *Clin Nucl Med* 1993;**18**:657–61.

76. Krenning EP, Kwekkeboom DJ, Bakker WH, *et al*. Somatostatin receptor scintigraphy with [111-In-DTPA-D-phe]- and [I-123-tyr]-octreotide: The Rotterdam experience with more than 1,000 patients. *Eur J Nucl Med* 1993;**20**:716–31.

77. Dorr U, Sautter-Bihl ML, Heiner B. The contribution of somatostatin receptor scintigraphy to the diagnosis of recurrent medullary carcinoma of the thyroid. *Semin Oncol* 1994;**21**:42–5.

78. Takashima S, Morimoto S, Ikezoe J, *et al*. CT evaluation of anaplastic thyroid carcinoma. *AJR* 1990;**154**:1079–85.

79. Ohnishi T, Noguchi S, Murakami N, *et al*. MR imaging in patients with primary thyroid lymphoma. *Am J Neuroradiol* 1992;**13**:1196–8.

80. Haugen BR, Nawaz S, Cohn A, *et al*. Secondary malignancy of the thyroid gland: A case report and review of the literature. *Thyroid* 1994;**4**:297–300.

81. Czech JM, Lichtor TR, Carney JA, *et al*. Neoplasms metastatic to the thyroid gland. *Surg Gynecol Obstet* 1982;**155**:503–5.

5

Role of radiotherapy in head and neck cancer

R. REJNISH KUMAR, CESSAL THOMMACHAN, K. RAMADAS, B. RAJAN

Radiotherapy or radiation therapy (RT) is the treatment of diseases using ionizing radiation. Ionizing radiation is used for both therapeutic and diagnostic purposes. For therapy, high-energy radiation in megavoltage range is preferred whereas for diagnosis kilovoltage energy is used.

Principles of radiotherapy (RT)

RT is based on the basic principle that rapidly proliferating cells are more sensitive to ionizing radiation compared with normal cell. This differential cell kill is used for the treatment of tumours.

Radiobiology

When ionizing radiation passes through the tissue of a patient it affects the biology of both normal and tumour tissues. This radiation causes both direct and indirect effects on biological targets. The DNA of a cell may be directly affected by the secondary electrons generated as ionizing radiation interacts with tissue. The radiation may also have an indirect effect due to the formation of free radicals; these free radicals in turn cause most of the chemical damage to the DNA. In addition, there are a number of other cellular functions that are disrupted by radiation-induced damage. This damage is modified by oxygen concentration, temperature and other intracellular components.

The goal of RT is to sterilize tumour and to preserve adjacent normal tissue. Ionizing radiation deposits energy that injures or destroys cells by damaging their genetic material, making it impossible for these cells to continue to grow.[1]

- Lethal dose for normal and abnormal tissues is about the same.
- Normal tissues have greater ability to repair sublethal damage between doses of radiation than neoplastic cells.
- The effects produced depend on factors such as oxygen enhancement ratio (OER), linear energy transfer (LET), and relative biological effectiveness (RBE).
- OER is the ratio of doses of radiation required to produce a given amount of damage without and with oxygen.
- RBE is the ratio of dose of 250 kV X-rays to that of test radiation required to produce equal amount of biological effect.
- LET is the energy transferred by the radiation per unit length of track.
- Response of cells to radiation depends upon several factors such as radiation quality, dose rate, dose fractionation, oxygen tension, cell stage, presence of chemical protectors and sensitizers, and recovery and repair process. The presence of oxygen is among the best known sensitizers of radiation damage. High LET radiations such as neutrons and protons cause more radiation damage as compared to low LET radiations such as X-rays or gamma rays. Cells in S-phase are generally more radio-resistant as compared to cells in G2 and M phases.

Physical concepts in radiation oncology

Ionizing radiation used to treat cancers is divided into electromagnetic radiation and particle radiation. Electromagnetic radiation is the predominant therapeutic modality for RT. Energey levels of electromagnetic radiations are directly proportional to the frequency of radiation. Higher frequency electromagnetic radiations such as X-rays and gamma rays that are used for radiation therapy can have energy levels in the order of megavolts. Particle radiations include electrons, neutrons and protons.

Gamma rays have a higher frequency than X-rays. They differ in the ways they are produced. X-rays are produced by man-made devices by introducing a target material along the pathway of fast-moving electrons. Gamma rays are emitted from a radioactive isotope as part of the process of naturally occurring radioactive decay. Particle radiation involves the use of fast-moving subatomic particles to treat localized cancers. Most particles (neutrons, protons, etc.) deposit more energy while passing through tissues, thus causing more damage to the cells they hit. Recent advances in RT research include the use of radio-labelled antibodies to deliver doses of radiation directly to the cancer site (radioimmunotherapy). Tumour-specific antibodies against tumour antigens labelled with radioactive isotopes (radiolabelling) are injected into the body, which actively seek out the cancer cells and destroy them by the cytotoxic action of the radiation. This approach can minimize the risk of radiation damage to healthy cells.

Methods of delivery of RT

Based on the method of delivery, RT is classified into teletherapy, brachytherapy and internal therapy.

External beam RT (Teletherapy)

External RT is normally given as a series of short daily treatments, usually from Monday through Friday, in the radiotherapy department using teletherapy machine telecobalt/linear accelerator). While taking treatment, the patient will be alone in the treatment room. However he will be closely monitored through a closed circuit camera (Fig. 1). The patient can have normal social life and there will not be any radiation emitted from the patient.

Radiation given using machines kept at a distance away

from the patient. Based on the energy this is subdivided into:

- *Superficial therapy*
  Superficial voltage machine generate X-rays 30–125 kV. This is used to treat superficial tumours such as skin cancer.

- *Orthovoltage therapy (kilovoltage)*
  Orthovoltage machines produce medium energy X-rays in the range of 200–300 kV. Primarily used to treat superficially situated tumours. In this situation skin dose is high and cannot be used to treat deep-seated tumours.

- *Megavoltage therapy*
  Megavoltage machines such as telecobalt and linear accelerators generate radiations having energy above one megavoltage. These machines are used to treat deeply situated tumours delivering lesser dose to the overlying skin.

Telecobalt teletherapy (Co⁶⁰)

In telecobalt machine, radioactive isotope (Co^{60}) which emits gamma rays having an average energy of 1.25 MeV.

Linear accelerator

These are the most commonly used RT machines. This does not contain a continuously emitting radioactive isotope. In this machine electrons are generated, accelerated and made to strike a target to produce high voltage X-rays. The advantage of this machine is that both X-rays and electrons can be utilized for treatment. Electrons are commonly used to treat superficial tumours without damaging underlying critical structures.

Brachytherapy

The term brachytherapy was first proposed by Dr G. Forsell in 1931. It is derived from the greek word 'brachio', meaning short and refers to treatment with a radioisotope at a short distance <5 cm from a tumour. Interest in brachytherapy remained low due to the radiation exposure to operating staff. The introduction, in the early 1960s, of megavoltage linear accelerators capable of producing improved teletherapy dose distributions further slowed the use of brachytherapy. The development of safe after-loading technique especially the high dose rate remote after-loading methods has given renewed interest in this field. The advantage of brachytherapy is that it is a highly localized form of treatment causing minimal and excellent tumour control. Short treatment time is another advantage of this technique. The disadvantage is that it can be used only in selected cases especially in early stage disease at accessible site. It requires anaesthesia and excellent expertise. This is an invasive procedure.

Brachytherapy may be used either alone or in combination

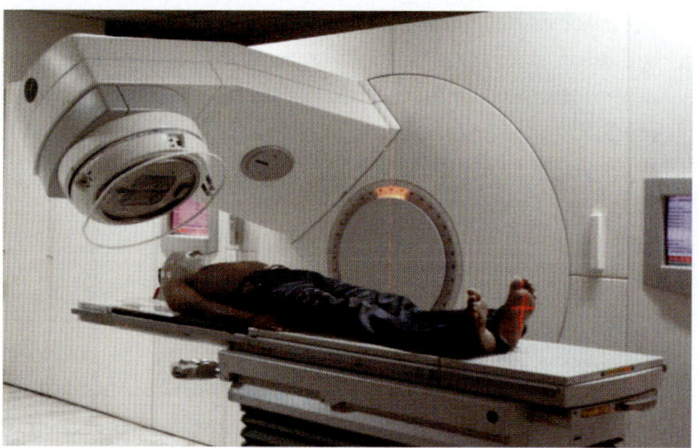

Fig. 1. Teletherapy

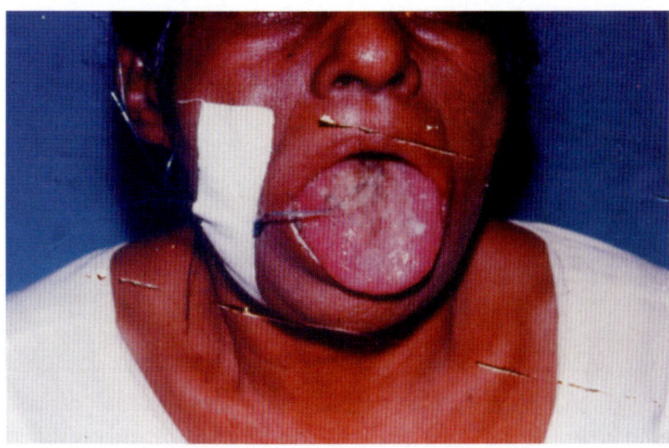

Fig. 2. Brachytherapy

with external beam radiation and/or surgery. The radioactive sources used for bachytherapy come in the form of small seeds, needles or wires. The dose of radiation and length of time prescribed will depend on the tumour size, location, and sensitivity to radiation. Generally a dose of 65 Gy over 6–7 days is given when it is used as the sole treatment.

Depending upon the loading, brachytherapy is classified into preload (Fig. 2) and afterload techniques. In preload technique radioactive isotope is directly handled by the staff and all staff members involved in the procedure get radiation whereas in afterload technique first metal or plastic tubes are inserted into the tumour and these tubes are later loaded with radioactive source. This can be done manually or with the help of machine (remote afterloading techniques). In remote after loading technique the radiation hazard is almost nil.

High-dose rate (HDR) brachytherapy

This is an outpatient form of radiation treatment that has become very popular in recent years. A small machine containing a HDR radioactive isotope is used for this. The source is transferred into the tubes kept within the tumour using a catheters attached to the machine. All the source movements are controlled with the help of computer.

Internal therapy

Radioisotope is either injected or taken as a drink to treat tumours. For example: radioactive iodine (I^{131}) in the treatment of thyroid cancer. Phosphorus-32 in the treatment of polycythemia vera.

Fractionation in RT

Fractionation is a term used to describe the manner in which daily dose of radiation is given.[2] Fractionation of the total dose of radiation helps in minimizing normal tissue reaction. The clinical effects of fractionated RT are influenced by the ability to repair sublethal damage, reoxygenation of tumour during the course of radiation, repopulation of tumour and normal tissues between fractions and redistribution of cells into a more sensitive phase in cell cycle treatment—the 4 R's of radiobiology.

Conventional fractionation

Conventional fractionation is the application of daily doses of 180–200 cGy and 5 fractions per week to a total dose of 40–70 Gy depending upon the type of tumour.

Hyperfractionation

Two or more fractions per day of reduced dose (115–120 cGy) with overall treatment time similar to that of conventional fractionation. Hyperfractionation helps in increasing the total dose without increasing the late reactions.

Accelerated fractionation

Accelerated fractionation is a means of decreasing the overall duration of treatment in an effort to reduce the repopulation of tumour cells in rapidly proliferating cancers. Repopulation (tumour–cell regeneration) occurs during treatment when the overall duration of treatment is increased. Shortening of overall treatment time can increase the tumour control in selected situation.

Accelerated hyperfractionation

Delivering two or more fractions per day of normal dose per fraction helps in reducing the overall treatment time without increasing the risk of late complication.

Concomitant-boost technique

A variant of accelerated fractionation is the concomitant boost technique. With this technique, treatment is delivered once daily for the first 3.5 weeks and then twice daily during the final 2–2.5 weeks, when tumour cells can begin to repopulate more rapidly.

Hypofractionation

Here <4 fractions per week with higher dose per fraction than conventional are planned. In selected situations this is found to be useful especially in the treatment of melanomas.

Split course therapy

Radiation is given in small courses with a rest period in between.

Side-effects of radiation in HNC patients

Radiotherapy side-effects are classified into acute and late.

Acute reaction

Acute reaction occurs during and immediately after treatment up to 6 weeks. Acute effects are related to dose per treatment, total dose, volume of tissue irradiated and the site. These reactions are limited to the area irradiated and not seen outside the treatment volume. This is mainly due to the inflammation of the tissues during treatment. Symptoms include xerostomia, pain in the mouth and throat, skin reactions and falling of hair within the treatment volume may occur. The mucous membrane within the irradiated area gets inflamed leading to patchy ulceration. Salivary secretion decreases during RT and it become thicker and forms a coating over the tongue. This causes change in the pH of the saliva, which can lead to changes in the bacteria flora. There will be alteration of taste during RT.

These acute reactions are self-limiting and subside usually in 2–3 weeks following completion of RT. There can be superadded bacterial and fungal infections. This is managed by antibiotic, antifungal and analgesics. During RT patients are advised to take high calorie non-spicy bland food. Frequent use of soda bicarbonate and saline mouthwash is advisable. They should not use very hot and very cold food during treatment. During treatment, patients should avoid application of creams and oils and rubbing of the skin with rough clothes.

Late reaction

This is the dose-limiting toxicity and usually occurs months or years after treatment. This depends upon the dose per fraction, total dose and volume of tissue irradiated. This includes dryness of mouth, intolerance to spicy food, hair loss and oedema of the skin with in the irradiated area. Necrosis, fistula formation, non-healing ulceration and osteonecrosis are rare. However, modern RT delivery is very precise and accurate and damage to critical structures are extremely rare.

Advantages of RT

- No tissue or functional loss
- Good cosmetic outcome compared to surgery control of subclinical disease in the regional nodes is possible without added morbidity
- Can simultaneously treat multiple primaries
- Better surgical salvage of RT failures than salvage of surgical failures.
- Rare treatment-related mortality

Disadvantages of RT

- Undesirable acute side-effects such as painful mucositis, loss of taste, dryness of mouth
- Potential late complications of soft tissues and bone
- Protracted treatment course
- Requires good infrastructures
- Rare possibility of development of second malignancy

Management of HNC

Head and neck cancer (HNC) is a locoregional disease and majority of these patients die because of uncontrolled locoregional disease. Distant metastasis is extremely rare in these tumours. Therefore, local forms of treatment like surgery and RT either alone or in combination plays an important role in the management of these cancers. Chemotherapy is used in recurrent or residual diseases for palliation of symptoms. In curative settings it is used along with surgery and/or RT.

The choice of treatment depends on factors such as cell type or degree of differentiation, site and extent of the primary lesions, gross characteristics of the tumour (exophytic, superficial vs endophytic, infiltrative), involvement of bone and muscle, metastatic nodal status, likelihood of complete surgical resection, possibility of preservation of speech or swallowing mechanisms, physical condition, social status and occupation of the patient, experience and skill of both the surgeon and the radiotherapist, infrastructure cooperation and wishes of the patient.

Baseline investigations

- Height, weight, performance status and nutritional status.
- Complete diagrammatic and descriptive documentation including measurements of the extent of primary and regional disease.
- ENT evaluation of the head and neck region including endoscopic evaluation.
- Routine blood tests such as TC, DC, BUN, serum creatinine and blood sugar estimation.
- Chest X-ray, orthopantomogram, and X-rays of the affected site.
- High resolution CT/MRI of the primary site and the neck—optional.
- Nodes not palpable and found only on CT or MRI scans: Size with imaging must be 1.0 cm in its minimal axial diameter/contain necrotic regions regardless of size.
- Biopsy from the primary site. If no primary is detected, FNAC from the regional node.
- Baseline quality-of-life (QOL) assessment (before the start of protocol treatment) and pregnancy test for women of child-bearing potential is also advocated.

Principles of radiotherapy in HNC

The use of RT in the management of squamous cell carcinoma (SCC) of the head and neck is based on the following principles.[3]

- SCC is generally radioresponsive and in early stage highly radiocurable.
- The more differentiated the tumour the less rapid the radiation response and resolution and the higher the radiation dose required.
- Exophytic and well oxygenated tumours are more radioresponsive than deeply ulcerative and infiltrative hypoxic tumours.
- SCC, when limited to the mucosa is highly radio-curable.
- Bone and muscle involvement by carcinoma adversely alters radioresponsiveness and subsequently decrease radiocurability.
- The early small metastases can be controlled with RT alone. Advanced cervical metastatic lymph nodes are better treated with combined surgery and radiation.

Indications of radiation

- T1–T2 lesions as single modality
- T3–T4 locally-advanced lesions.

Combined surgery and RT or combination of chemo-RT.

Combined surgery and RT

RT can be given before or after surgery. Each sequence has theoretical advantages and disadvantages. However, the results from randomized studies favour post-operative RT.[4,5] In practice, most surgeons also prefer to operate in an unirradiated field where frozen section control of resection margin can be obtained. In certain clinical settings, however, planned pre-operative RT may be favoured. These include situations where cancer is not resectable at presentation or when a free osteomyocutaneous graft is to be used for mandibular soft tissue reconstruction. In the latter situation avoidance of irradiating the graft and delivery of a lower dose to the mandibular stump than would be necessary in post-operative setting both facilitate integration of the vascular graft.

Indications for post-operative RT

- Positive resected margins
- Locally-advanced primary regardless of margin
- Multiple involved nodes
- Extracapsular extension
- Perineural spread
- Vascular and lymphatic emboli

Timing of radiation

The general guideline is to commence RT when tissues are well healed. RT should be started as early as possible after proper wound healing preferably within 6 weeks. The longer the interval before the commencement of radiation, the greater is the opportunity for presumed clonogens to proliferate. A delay of more than 6 weeks can adversely affect the outcome.[6]

Combined chemotherapy and RT treatment

Chemotherapy is generally used along with radiation in organ-conservation settings, especially in locally advanced tumours to avoid surgery. Chemotherapy can be combined with RT in various ways.[7]

Neoadjuvant /Anterior/Induction chemotherapy

Chemotherapy is given before local treatment such as RT and surgery. This has a survival benefit of 2%.

Concurrent or concomitant chemotherapy

Chemotherapy is given along with radiation. This has a survival benefit of 8%.

Adjuvant chemotherapy

Chemotherapy is given after local form of treatment such as RT or surgery. This has a survival benefit of 1%.

Dose of radiotherapy

The radiation dosage is determined by:
- Tumour site
- Size of the lesion
- Volume to be irradiated (target volume)
- No of fractions of treatment
- Various techniques of delivery of radiotherapy
- Tolerance of various structures
- Associated medical conditions like diabetes, collagen disorders, etc.

In general, a dose of 50–55 Gy in 25–30 fractions over 5–6 weeks is considered, adequate for sterilization of microscopic or occult diseases. A dose of 66–70 Gy over 7 weeks is required for control of gross tumour. The initial dose is usually 50 Gy to the primary lesion and the regional nodes using a wide field technique followed by boost dose up to 66–70 Gy using smaller volume covering gross disease. Spinal cord is shielded after 45 Gy.

Table 1. Survival rates in oral cancer

Relative survival rates in 11,375 cases			
Site	**Stage**	**No. of cases**	**5-year survival rate**
Lip	I–II	7125	95
	III–IV	288	78
Oral tongue	I–II	787	67
	III–IV	866	20
Floor of mouth	I–II	324	68
	III–IV	1669	41
Gingiva	I–II	70	55
	III–IV	822	44
Buccal mucosa	I–II	58	78
	III–IV	256	40

Newer radiation delivery techniques

New radiation delivery techniques offer powerful potential to diminish the severity of radiation toxicities. In conventional radiotherapy because of close proximity of head and neck tumours to critical organs such as spinal cord, eyes, optic chiasma, etc. quite often, delivery of maximal dose to tumour is not feasible. Advances in computer technology and engineering have facilitated delivery higher dose to the tumour sparing critical organs.

- *3D conformal radiotherapy:* In this the treatment volume confirms to the shape of the tumour using 3D planning technique, minimizing the dose to normal structures.
- *Intensity modulated radiotherapy (IMRT):* IMRT refers to a specific technique of linear accelerator based radiotherapy by which radiation beams are modulated in such a manner as to produce highly conformal dose distribution within the tumour while reducing the dose to normal structures

Drugs used to minimize the side-effects of RT

- *Amifostine:* Amifostine formely known as WR-2721 protects cell damage by scavenging free radicals. A dose of amifostine 200 mg/m^2 is given as rapid infusion 30 minutes before each fraction of radiation. This can minimize the side-effects of radiotherapy.
- *Pilocapine:* This drug is used against dryness of mouth to increase the salivary flow.
- *Erythropoietin:* 10,000 units given as subcutaneous injection 3 times a week is used to correct anaemia before RT.

Colony-stimulating factor (CSF): G-CSF and GM-CSF are used to diminish myelosuppression associated with chemo-RT. These agents also provide mucosal protection in patients treated with chemo-RT.

Palliative radiotherapy

Locally-advanced head and neck can benefit from palliative radiation to control localized symptoms including respiratory compromise, bleeding, discharge from exophytic lesions, functional difficulties in speech and swallowing, cranial nerve involvement and avoid fungation of lymph nodes. These patients are treated with short course of RT, unlike more protracted course in a curative setting.

Dental care and radiation

Dental care by a dental surgeon and oral surgeon plays a vital part in the treatment of HNCs. The teeth and the soft tissues should be well examined and any tooth which cannot be restored due to periodontitis or dental caries should be extracted before radiation and radiation should not be started without adequate healing of the sockets. Post-radiation extraction is possible, if the tooth lies away from the high-dose volume and extraction should be under a prolonged antibiotic coverage beginning ahead of extraction. Care should be taken to suture the extraction site to avoid infection and consequent osteradionecrosis.

Role of radiation in HNC

In almost all cancer hospitals across India as well as the South-East Asian countries, HNCs account for 30%–40% of all the cancers registered in the clinics. Of these 60% are advanced stage disease (stage III and IV) and locoregional failures account for the predominant recurrence pattern and mortality accounts from uncontrolled locoregional disease. RT has been the standard non-surgical treatment in this regard.

Radiation may be given as:
- *Radical treatment:* as external beam treatment or brachytherapy.
- *Palliative:* mostly external beam.
- *Adjuvant to surgery:* sometimes as chemo-RT also in high-risk cases.

The newer strategies of radiation led to a 10%–15% improvement in locoregional control, i.e. hyperfractionation, accelerated fractionation, etc. Nonetheless the most effective radiation regimens have resulted in local control rates of 50%–70% and disease-free survival of 30%–50%. Since HNCs can be aggressive it is important to adequately treat the gross as well as the microscopic disease. At the same time, many of the normal tissues in this region such as the salivary glands, larynx, constrictor muscles, etc. are sensitive to radiation and can result in long-term sequelae. This places the radiation oncologist in the difficult situation of attempting to provide high doses of radiation to tumour and target volumes and minimal doses of radiation to normal tissues. New technologies and increasing familiarity and experience with these technologies have allowed the practice of RT to increase the distance between tumour dose and normal tissue dose, which in turn improves the ratio of cancer cure to treatment morbidity. HNCs may be divided into, according to sites as: oral cavity (buccal mucosa, lips, upper and lower gingiva, the hard palate and the intra-oral tongue) oropharynx, larynx, hypopharynx and salivary gland tumours and the nasopharynx. The commonest histology are the SCCs which account for 90% of the HNCs and then the adenocarcinomas, the adenoid cystic carcinomas, muco-epidermoid carcinomas, lymphomas, melanomas, solitary plasmacytomas, etc.

Oral cavity

Though a number of subsites have been clubbed under a single site, they are actually a heterogeneous group of disease which behave differently. The buccal mucosa cancers in early stage disease T1 and T2 stages, can be managed either with surgery or radical radiation. The radical radiation treatment would include either external beam radiation or brachytherapy delivering 70 Gy in 35 fractions over 7 weeks which would treat the primary tumour and the first-station nodes. When being treated with brachytherapy, a dose equivalent of this may be given as high-dose rate, iridium implantation (most commonly used isotope). Brachytherapy is the most conformal type of radiation that can ever be given by radiation as there is a rapid fall off of dose and there is minimal or practically no dose received by adjacent structures when properly delivered. Depending on the volume of implantation, single plane, double plane or volume implants have been used to cover the tumour with a margin of 1 cm.[8]

T3 and T4 tumours of the buccal mucosa may be treated with combined modality treatment with surgery and post-operative radiation (as many clinical trials have shown that pre-operative radiation is inferior to postoperative radiation). In a few cases when medically inoperable they may be ideal candidates for chemoradiation. Even cases of T4a disease with minimal bone and skin infiltration maybe treated with concurrent chemoradiation. Buccal mucosal cancers which are mainly superficial tumours are a few groups of tumours which can be effectively treated with an ordinary cobalt60 machine without any sophisticated features. The dose for radical treatment is the same as previous, but in post-operative cases the dose is 60 Gy in 30 fractions over 6 weeks. However, in case the margins are positive or if there is extracapsular invasion of the lymph nodes in the post-operative pathology report the dose to these sites is boosted to 66 Gy in 33 fractions. These are the two absolute indications for post-operative chemoradiation.

In the oral tongue surgery is the treatment of choice for T1 and T2 disease and brachytherapy is an equally effective tool in properly selected cases. The main disadvantage with brachytherapy is that the neck nodes are not addressed and so proper selection of patients is extremely important with at least an ultrasonological assessment of the neck to call it negative. If the neck nodes are negative a radical dose of brachytherapy carries the same results as compared to surgery. As for T3 and T4 diseases of the tongue, surgery followed by post-operative radiation/chemoradiation is the treatment of choice. Radiation alone is being reserved for inoperable cases.[9–11]

Same is the case for early, i.e. T1 and T2 lesions of the lip which can be effectively treated with brachytherapy with excellent cosmesis. T3 and T4 disease may require combined modality treatment. The doses of RT are the same in all sites for radical and post-operative treatment except in certain regions where critical structures prevent full doses to be delivered.

In T1 and T2 lesions of the upper and lower gingiva external beam radiation given with a radical intent has 5-year survival rates of 80%–90%. The important aspect to be noted in buccal mucosa and gingival cancers are that the lymph node areas to be covered in the radiation portal are the involved nodes and one station of nodes ahead whereas in tongue lesions, except in early lesions all the nodes in the neck are at risk and have to be covered in the radiation portal. In T3 and T4 disease of the gingiva, surgery and post-operative radiation is the treatment of choice.

The lesions on the hard palate if superficial and without bone destruction are treated best with brachytherapy using HDR mould technique—T1 and most of the T2 lesions. However, T3 onwards chemoradiation is the treatment of choice. But if bone is involved, surgery with post-operative radiation is the treatment of choice.

Oropharynx

Oropharyngeal lesions include the lesions involving base tongue, vallecula and the tonsils. Since these regions are well networked by lymphatics, most of them present with advanced disease, with lymph nodal metastasis, with an overall metastatic rate of 45%. The nodal metastatic rate increases as the T status increases with T1 lesions having 10%, T2 having 30% and T3 and T4 lesions having 65%–70% nodal metastasis, respectively. The chance of distant metastasis in these group of lesions are 6.7% most of which appeared within the first 2 years, the lung being the commonest site.[12]

T1 and T2 disease of the base tongue and valleculae may be treated either with surgery, brachytherapy or external beam radiation. Combining external beam radiation and finally boosting the same with brachytherapy is also an acceptable option in bulky disease with poorly differentiated histology. With this the uninvolved nodes may be given a prophylactic dose of radiation. However, with the advent of newer technologies such as intensity-modulated radiation therapy (IMRT), image-guided radiation therapy (IGRT), etc., there is a trend to increase the dose with external beam radiation itself, since the normal structures can be avoided with safe doses and good tolerance. Brachytherapy being an invasive procedure requires anaesthesia and more expertise and may not be easily available in most centres. Surgery and postoperative radiation as in other sites may be the treatment options for T3 and T4 disease of the base tongue and valleculae. But, due to the morbidity due to surgery and organ preservation possible with chemoradiation and with newer drugs like monoclonal antibodies showing excellent responses, chemoradiation has come to stay in the treatment of advanced oropharyngeal lesions with moderate improvement in results but more importantly without causing too much morbidity. In advanced diseases even without any involved nodes, it is customary to treat the levels 3, 4 and 5 regions to a prophylactic dose. T3 and T4 disease of the base tongue and vallecula continues to have a bad prognosis in spite of all the newly available advances.[13,14]

For T1 and T2 lesions of the Tonsil, external beam radiation has excellent results and the radiation portal would include the primary and the ipsilateral level 2 nodes with a wedge pair technique that can be effectually delivered even on a regular cobalt machine. However, sophisticated treatment techniques like IMRT may be the preferred method now.[15,16] T3 and T4 tumours of the tonsil carry a better prognosis with chemoradiation rather than the corresponding stages in other sites in the same region. In advanced stages, treatment would include the primary tumour with the involved nodes and prophylactic radiation to the supraclavicular region. However as in other sites neck dissection may be done for residual nodes as per institutional policy. Since the role of surgery is not discussed in this chapter, I will not be highlighting the role of surgery in these cases.[17]

Larynx

Laryngeal cancers are probably the most exciting and rewarding tumours for the radiation oncologists to treat. The tumours of the larynx include the lesions of the supraglottis, glottic larynx and infraglottis. Purely infra-glottic cancers are extremely rare and are mostly infra-glottic extensions from the subsites. Of the 3 sites said above, supraglottic regions are highly vascular and the true glottis is almost devoid of any lymphatics. The lesions in these areas tend to remain compartmentalized, though there is no anatomic barrier. The nodal status at presentation for supraglottic tumours are 55% at diagnosis with 16% being bilateral. For T1 larynx the nodal metastasis is almost 0% and for T2 larynx it is almost 1.7%.[18] In all the stages the treatment intent is to cure and so the treatment modality should be carefully chosen. In T1 and T2 vocal cord cancers though a variety of surgical techniques have been described, radical radiation remains to be the standard of care throughout, with cure rates of 90%–95%. Since the chance of lymph nodal metastasis is very low the treatment volume does not include a prophylactic dose of radiation to the nodes and the morbidity with radiation is also very low. T3 disease, i.e. with fixed cord lesions, they may be divided into favourable disease (those with lesions confined to one side, good airway, etc.) and the unfavourable group (extensive bilateral disease with compromised airway, etc.). The favourable group may be offered radical chemoradiation with close follow-up and maybe recommended total laryngectomy even without biopsy proof, purely on clinical grounds, since there is a 5% chance of chondronecrosis if warranted. Advanced disease with thyroid, cricoid, and arytenoid cartilage involvement, compromised airway, etc. require primary surgery as the treatment of choice and should have post-operative radiation treatment.[19-21]

Early supraglottic lesions and moderately advanced lesions (T2 N0 and T3 N0) may be treated with external beam radiation to a radical dose with coverage of the primary and level 2, 3 and 4 nodal areas in the primary treatment portal. The alternative is to have conservative laryngectomies with total laryngectomy being reserved for treatment failures. The status of the neck usually determines the mode of treatment. The advent of chemoradiation has roped in a number of cases into the chemoradiation arm from surgery, though this modality carries with it higher morbidity. But, this has gained more acceptances considering the fact of organ preservation. Overall T1 and T2 lesions have a local control rate of 100% to 80% respectively and T3 and T4 lesions the local control comes down to 64% and 36%, respectively with radiation alone. No special mention is made on infra-glottic tumours since these tumours are extremely rare as a single site disease.[22-24]

Hypopharynx

This site is divided into the *pyriform fossa*, lateral pharyngeal wall and the postcricoid region. They are a group of highly networked region by the regional lymphatics. Due to this reason most of them present in advanced stages with extensive nodes. Even T1 and T2 lesions usually have a 30%–50% chance of regional lymph nodes and the value goes up to 60%–80% with T3 and T4 diseases. The mid-cervical and the upper deep cervical nodes are the most commonly involved nodes and also the retropharyngeal nodes are at high-risk of involvement. Hence, when planning radiation care must be taken to cover these groups of nodes at least to prophylactic doses when taken for radical treatment.[25-27]

T1 and T2 tumours of the pyriform fossa though uncommon can be treated with radical radiation with cure rates of 60%–70%. However, a few T3 diseases may also be treated with chemoradiation in a selected group. With nodal disease >3 cm, and advanced T stage, surgery plus post-operative radiation is the treatment of choice. In those patients who have curable primary tumours but with rather bulky nodal disease chemoradiation, followed by neck dissection has been used for preservation of function. There have been a few series in which neck dissection followed by radical radiation has also been tried with similar results for early T-stage and advanced N-stage. However this has never become the standard practice due to lack of phase 3 data. The best results with radiation alone have been obtained in small lesions limited to one or two walls, less bulky and those diseases which do not infiltrate the larynx or destroy the thyroid cartilage. Among the 3 subsites, the lesions of the pyriform fossa have a better prognosis and ladies and younger age are the two good host prognostic factors. The post-cricoid lesions carries the worst prognosis and especially so if the lesions are over 5 cm in length, and have bilateral nodes. It is in these groups of patients that the role of neoadjuvant chemotherapy has been studied extensively and has been found to be more beneficial than radical external radiation alone. However, it can be concluded that among the head and neck sites, the lesions of the hypopharynx carries the worst prognosis when compared stage to satge.[28–30]

Salivary gland tumours

The major salivary glands are the parotid, submandibular and sublingual glands. Malignant tumours of this region make up only 0.4% of all cancers and 3%–4% of all HNCs. The most common histologies are those of adenomas, adenoid cystic carcinomas and muco-epidermoid carcinomas, though other histologies may also be rarely met with.

Surgery remains the mainstay of treatment of all salivary gland tumours and depending upon indications radiation is mostly given as an adjuvant treatment, except in a small group of patients in whom surgery could not be done due to medical reasons. Most of the salivary glands being superficial and confined diseases, rarely would the neck nodes need to be addressed in the radiation portals. The treatment volumes would include the primary tumour with a margin. The parotid would require anterior and posterior wedged beams to treat the parotid bed or more simply a combination of electrons and photons and spare the opposite parotid. The volume of irradiation may vary if there is perineural invasion of a major nerve wherein more generous fields may have to be given. Even though textbooks highlight the role of elective neck irradiation in high-grade tumours and incompletely excised tumours, it is of individual decision to do so. Usual doses of 55–60 Gy of radiation are given in the post-operative setting in conventional doses. The indication for giving post-operative radiation in cases of pleomorphic adenoma are:

- Involvement of deep lobe of parotid which would require sacrificing the facial nerve.
- Recurrent disease with deeper infiltration in successive presentations.
- Large lesions which may not allow a complete surgical removal.
- Malignant transformation in a predominantly benign tumour.

The superficial position and relatively slow growth rates have made salivary tumours a target for alternative radiotherapy approaches, such as fast neutrons. A number of trials have shown excellent control rates of 60%–81% in recurrent and inoperable cases. When using neutrons the doses of radiation used are 20–24 Gy.

References

1. Dru forrester S. Principles of cancer management part II. *Surgery, radiotherapy, hyperthermia, immunotherapy*; 1997.
2. Baumann M, Saunders M, Joiner MC. Modified fractionation. In: Steel GG (ed). *Basic Clinical Radiobiology*. 3rd ed. Hodder Arnold; 2002:147.
3. Wang CC. *Radiation therapy for head and neck neoplasms: Indications, techniques and results*. 2nd ed. 1990.
4. Kramer S, Gelber RD, Snow JB, *et al.* Combined radiation therapy and surgery in the management of advanced head and neck cancer: Final report of study 73-03 of the RTOG. *Head Neck Surg* 1987; **10**:19–30.
5. Vandenbrouk C, Sancho H, Le Fur R, *et al.* Results of a randomized clinical trial of preoperative irradiation versus postoperative in treatment of tumors of the hypopharynx. *Cancer* 1977;**39**:1445–9.
6. Peters LJ, Goepfert H, Ang KK, *et al.* Evaluation of the dose for postoperative radiation therapy of head and neck cancer: First report of a prospective randomized trial. *Int J Radiat Oncol Biol Phys* 1993;**26**:3–11.
7. Bourhis J, Pignon JP. Metaanalysis in head and neck squamous cell carcinomas. What is the role of chemotherapy? *Hemat Oncol Clin North Am* 1999;**13**:769–75.
8. Million R, Cassisi N. Oral cavity. In: Miullion R, Cassisi N (eds). *Management of head and neck cancer: A multidisciplinary approach*. Philadelphia: JB Lippincott; 1984.
9. Bachaud J, Delannes M, Allouache N, *et al.* Radiotherapy of stage I and II carcinomas of the mobile tongue and/or floor of the mouth. *Radiother Oncol* 1994;**31**:199–206.
10. Benk V, Mazeron J, Grimard L, *et al.* Comparison of curietherapy versus external irradiation combined with curietherapy in stage II squamous cell carcinoma of the mobile tongue. *Radiother Oncol* 1990;**18**:339–47.
11. Horiuchi J, Okuyana T, Shibuya H, *et al.* Results of brachytherapy for cancer of the tongue with special emphasis on local prognosis. *Int J Radiat Oncol Biol Phys* 1982;**8**:829–35.
12. Fletcher GH. *Textbook of radiotherapy*. 3rd ed. Philadelphia Lea and Febiger;1980:286–329.
13. Hamberger AD, Fletcher GH, Guillamondegui OM, *et al.* Advanced squamous cell carcinoma of the oral cavity and oropharynx treated with irradiation and surgery. *Radiology* 1976;**119**:433–8.
14. Novak A. Treatment of carcinoma of the base of the tongue and the larynx. *Laryngoscope* 1975;**89**:1332.
15. Mohan R, Wu Q, Manning M, *et al.* Radiobiological considerations in the design of fractionation strategies for intensity-modulated radiation therapy of head and neck cancers. *Int J Radiat Oncol Biol Phys* 2000;**46**:619–30.
16. Wu Q, Mohan R, Niermierko A, *et al.* Optimization of intensity-modulated radiotherapy plans based on the equivalent uniform dose. *Int J Radiat Oncol Biol Phys* 2002;**52**:224–35.
17. Fein DA, Lee WR, Amos WR, *et al.* Oropharyngeal carcinoma treated with radiotherapy: A 30-year experience. *Int J Radiat Oncol Biol Phys* 1996;**34**:289–96.

18. Lindberg RD. Distribution of cervical lymph node metastases from squamous cell carcinoma of the upper respiratory and digestive tracts. *Cancer* 1972;**29**:1446–9.

19. Fein DA, Mendenhall WM, Parsons JT, *et al*. T1–T2 squamous cell carcinoma of the glottic larynx treated with radiotherapy: A multivariate analysis of variables potentially influencing local control. *Int J Radiat Oncol Biol Phys* 1993;**25**:605–11.

20. Mendenhall WM, Parsons JT, Stringer SP, *et al*. Management of Tis, T1 and T2 squamous cell carcinoma of the glottic larynx. *Am J Otolaryngol* 1994;**15**:250–7.

21. Mendenhall WM, Parsons JT, Stringer SP, *et al*. T1–T2 vocal cord carcinoma: A basis for comparing the results of radiotherapy and surgery. *Head Neck Surg* 1988;**10**:373–7.

22. Fein DA, Nichols RC Jr, Lee WR, *et al*. T2–T3 carcinoma of the supraglottic larynx: A comparison of surgery and radiotherapy. *Radiat Oncol Investig* 1995;**2**:237–44.

23. Mendenhall WM, Parsons JT, Stringer SP, *et al*. Carcinoma of the supraglottic larynx: A basis for comparing the results of radiotherapy and surgery. *Head Neck* 1988;**10**:373–7.

24. Ogura JH, Sessions DG, Spector GJ. Conservation surgery for epidermoid carcinoma of the supraglottic larynx. *Laryngoscope* 1975b;**85**:1808–15.

25. Dubois JB, Guerrier B, DiRuggeriero JM, *et al*. Cancer of the pyriform sinus: Treatment by radiation therapy alone and after surgery. *Radiology* 1986;**160**:831.

26. EI-Badawi SA, Goepfert H, Fletcher GH. Squamous cell carcinoma of the pyriform sinus. *Laryngoscope* 1982;**92**:357.

27. Farrington WT, Weighall JS, Jones PH. Postcricoid carcinoma (a 10-year retrospective study). *J Laryngol Otol* 1986;**100**:79.

28. Clayman GL. Laryngeal preservation for advanced laryngeal and hypopharyngeal cancers. *Arch Otolaryngol Head Neck Surg* 1995;**121**:219–23.

29. McKay MJ, Bilows AM. Basiloid squamous carcinoma of the hypopharynx. *Cancer* 1989;**63**:2528–31.

30. Salvajoli JV, Morioka H, Trippe N, *et al*. A randomized trial of neoadjuvant vs concomitant chemotherapy vs radiation alone in the treatment of stage IV head and neck squmous cell carcinoma. *Eur Arch Otol Rhinol Laryngol* 1992;**249**:211–15.

6

Role of chemotherapy in head and neck cancer

CESSAL THOMMACHAN, K. RAMADAS, REJNISH KUMAR, B. RAJAN

Surgery and radiotherapy (RT) are the two main modalities of treatment in locally advanced head and neck cancer (HNC). Chemotherapy alone has no proven role in early-stage disease, and is not considered as a curative treatment in HNCs. Chemotherapy is effective in advanced HNCs, where it is used in conjunction with local modalities of treatment with the following objectives:

- To facilitate organ preservation
- To improve local control
- To improve overall survival
- To contain metastasis.

Chemotherapy is combined with local modalities of treatment in locally advanced HNC in the following ways:

- *Induction chemotherapy (neoadjuvant chemotherapy):* Chemotherapy given before local treatment (surgery/RT)
- *Concurrent chemotherapy:* Chemotherapy given along with RT (chemo-RT)
- *Induction chemotherapy followed by chemoradiation:* Two to three cycles of chemotherapy given before RT and, thereafter, with RT
- *Adjuvant chemotherapy:* Chemotherapy given after surgery or RT
- *Postoperative chemoradiation:* Radiation along with chemotherapy is given after surgical resection.

Advantages and disadvantages of combining chemotherapy with surgery/RT are given in Table 1.

Basic concepts of chemotherapy and radiation interaction

The basic aim of combining chemotherapy with radiation is to increase patient survival by improving loco-regional tumour control, decreasing or eliminating distant metastasis, or both, while preserving the organ, and tissue integrity and function. Mechanisms involved in drug–radiation interaction are:

- Increasing the initial radiation damage

Table 1. Advantages and disadvantages of combining chemotherapy with surgery/ RT

Strategy	Advantages	Disadvantages
Sequential chemo-RT (induction chemo followed by RT)	• Least toxic • Maximises systemic therapy	• Increased treatment time • Lack of local synergy
Concurrent chemoradiation	• Shorter treatment time • Potentiation of radiation effect	• Compromised systemic therapy • Increased toxicity • No cytoreduction of tumour • Response to chemotherapy cannot be assessed
Induction chemotherapy and concurrent chemoradiation	Maximises systemic therapy radiation enhancement	• Increased toxicity • Increased treatment time • Difficult to complete chemoradiation after induction chemotherapy

- Inhibition of cellular repair
- Cell cycle distribution
- Counteracting hypoxia associated tumour radio-resistance
- Inhibition of tumour cell repopulation.

Platinum compounds are the most commonly given drugs along with RT,[1-4] cisplatin being the drug of choice in most instances. It is given intravenously at a dose of 80–100 mg/m^2 once in 3 weeks.

Induction chemotherapy

In induction chemotherapy, where chemotherapy is given before local treatment, the response to chemotherapy is considered as a surrogate marker for response to subsequent RT. A number of phase III randomized clinical trials have compared induction chemotherapy followed by local treatment, with local treatment alone. The various studies are summarized in Table 2. Induction chemotherapy with cisplatin + flurouracil (PF regime) shows the following effects:

- High response rates
- No adverse effect from delay in surgery or RT
- Response seems to predict success of subsequent RT
- Decreased distant metastases
- Role in laryngeal preservation
- No improvement in local control
- No significant difference in survival.

In a recent meta-analysis,[15] incorporating 31 induction chemotherapy trials with a median follow up of 6.1 years, induction chemotherapy showed an absolute benefit of 2.4%.

Induction chemotherapy is found to be inferior to concurrent chemotherapy in terms of loco-regional control and overall survival.

The dose of PF regimen is:

Cisplatin	100 mg/m^2 i.v.
5 Flurouracil	1000 mg/m^2 D1 daily i.v.
	as 24-hour infusion D1–D5

Chemotherapy cycle is repeated once in 3 weeks.

Role of taxanes in induction chemotherapy

To improve the efficacy of induction chemotherapy, three major randomized clinical trials were conducted by adding docetaxel to cisplatin and 5-FU (TPF) schedule. TPF regimen:

Cisplatin	75 mg/m^2
Docetaxel	75 mg/m^2
5-FU	750 mg/m^2 as 24-hour infusion from D1–D5[18]

On the basis of two major randomized trials, it was found that a regimen using [Tax 323, 324] TPF is superior to PF in terms of disease-free survival and overall survival.[16,17] However, this benefit is at the expense of increased toxicity. The GORTEC study[18] showed that addition of docetaxel to the PF combination showed better laryngeal preservation rates. A summary of the induction chemotherapy regimens incorporating docetaxel is given in Table 3.

Concurrent chemotherapy and RT

Several randomized trials have tested the benefit of chemo-

Table 2. Selected trials of induction chemotherapy[24]

Study	No. of patients	Treatment	RR % (complete)	Survival % (year)	Remarks
Head and neck contracts[5] programme (1987)	152	S/RT	—	35 (5)	Insufficient chemotherapy
	140	PB x 1/S/RT	48 (8)	37	Decreased metastasis
	151	PB x 1/S/RT/P x 6		45	Survival benefit for N2 disease
Southwest oncology[6] group (1988)	76	S/RT	—	18 (median)	Difference NS, decrease in distant metastasis
	82	PBMV x 3/S/RT	70 (19)	30	
VA Larynx[7,8,13,14] (1991)	166	S/RT	—	53 (3)	Organ preservation in 64%
	166	PF x 3/RT	85 (31)	56	
Intergroup[9] (1992)	225	S/RT	—	44 (4)	Chemotherapy was given after surgery; decrease in distant metastasis
	223	S/PF x 3/RT		46	
Martin[10] (1994)	152	CPF x 3/RT	56 (31)	49 (4)	Better survival for pharyngo-laryngeal cancers with chemotherapy
	154	S/RT		38	
Paccagnella[11] (1994)	118	PF x 4/S/RT	70 (29)	37 (3)	Difference NS; Decreased metastasis
	119	S/R		33	
Richard[12] (1991)	110	S/R	48 FOM	FOM 3 (median) 7	Improved survival with chemotherapy in cancers of FOM

B Bleomycin   F-5 Flurouracil   Cp Carboplatin   M Methotrexate   P Cisplatin   S Surgery   RT Radiotherapy   RR Response rate   NS Not significant
FOM Floor of mouth   POC Posterior oral cavity and oropharynx

Table 3. Major clinical trials with docetaxel-based induction in locally advanced HNSCC

Study	No. of patients (criteria)	Primary end-point	Regimens	Result
Vermorken 2007 (EORTC 24791/TAX 323)	358 (unresectable)	PFS	PF-RT *vs.* TPF-RT	TPF led to higher PFS and OS (p<0.007)
Posner, 2007 (TAX 324)	501 (advanced)	OS	PF-CRT *vs.* TPF-RT	TPF improved OS at 3 years (p<0.007)
Calais 2006 (GORTEC 2000–01)	213 (resectable)	LxP	PF *vs.* TPF	TPF led to higher LxP, CR

Table 4. RT *versus* concurrent chemoradiation: Phase III trials

Study	No. of patients	RT vs. RT+Chemo (% of patients)	
		L/R control	Survival
Merlano, 1996	157	35 *vs.* 68	10 *vs.* 24
Wendt, 1998	270	17 *vs.* 36	24 *vs.* 48
Brizel, 1998	116	44 *vs.* 70	34 *vs.* 55 (NS)
Adelstein, 1990	100	35 *vs.* 45	55 *vs.* 52 (NS)
Calais, 1999	226	25 *vs.* 48	16 *vs.* 22
Jeremic, 2000	130	36 *vs.* 50	25 *vs.* 46
Staar, 2001	240	40 *vs.* 60	57 *vs.* 68

NS not significant

RT versus RT alone. A summary of phase III randomized trials comparing radiation versus concurrent chemo-RT is given in Table 4.

The Radiation Therapy Oncology Group (RTOG) trial 91–11 showed that concurrent chemo-RT is superior to induction chemotherapy followed by RT in terms of laryngeal preservation (88% vs 75%; p=0.005) and loco-regional control (78% vs 61%).[4]

Combined modality treatment of chemoradiation improves local control and results in better survival compared with the RT alone arm, making it the standard of care in locally advanced HNC. The majority of studies used cisplatinum 100 mg/m^2 once in 3 weeks along with RT.

Updated MACH-NC results showed that there is an absolute benefit of 6.5% at 6 years.[15] In terms of loco-regional control and overall treatment, concurrent chemoradiation is superior to induction chemotherapy followed by local treatment.

Limitations of chemoradiation include the following:
- Compliance is poor in patients having co-morbid conditions or poor performance status.
- Quality of life (QOL) assessment has not been done in various trials.
- It is unable to decrease systemic relapse.
- Benefits of chemotherapy are not proven in elderly patients.

Rationale for induction chemotherapy followed by concurrent chemo-RT

Most of the studies have shown the occurrence of lower distant metastasis in patients receiving induction chemotherapy, and improved local control in those with concurrent chemoradiation. So, induction chemotherapy followed by chemo-RT is an attractive option in advanced HNCs. Whether this strategy is superior to concurrent chemoradiation is yet to be proven.

Concurrent chemoradiation is the standard of care in locally advanced HNC. The dose of radiotherapy is 66–70 Gy over 6–7 weeks. Standard dose of chemotherapy is cisplatin 100 mg/m^2 given along with radiation. As of now, chemotherapy followed by chemoradiation is not superior to concurrent chemoradiation. Advanced oropharyngeal tumours and T3 larynx are best treated with concurrent chemoradiation. For patients who are not candidates for chemoradiation, cetuximab plus radiotherapy is a reasonable option.[19,20] Advanced oral cavity diseases are best treated by surgery followed by radiotherapy/postoperative chemoradiation. T3 hypopharynx is best treated by induction chemotherapy followed by radiation/surgery based on response to chemotherapy (GORTEC trial design). T4 larynx and T4 hypopharynx are primarily treated by surgery followed by adjuvant treatment (RT/postoperative chemoradiation).

Postoperative chemoradiation

Two major randomized trials were carried out to test the benefit in terms of outcome of chemo-RT in the postoperative setting.[21,22] Table 5 compares the criteria for selecting patients for chemoradiation related to the risk factors in these two trials. The outcome of these trials is given in Table 6.

Table 5. Comparative analysis of criteria of selection related to risk factors in EORTC trial 22931 and RTOG trial 9501[21,22]

EORTC 22931 only	RTOG 9501 only
Stage III/IV disease	Two or more positive lymph nodes
Surgical margins microscopically involved	Surgical margins micro-scopically involved
Positive lymph nodes at levels IV or V in patients with tumours arising from oropharynx or oral cavity	Extracapsular extension in positive lymph nodes
Extracapsular extension in positive lymph nodes	
Vascular emboli	
Perineural infiltration	

EORTC European Organization for Research and Treatment of Cancer RTOG Radiation Therapy Oncology Group

Table 6. Comparative analysis of treatment outcome in EORTC trial 22931 and RTOG trial 9501

Outcome end-points	EORTC trial 22931 5-year estimates	RTOG trial 9501 2-year estimates
Disease-free survival	47% *vs.* 36% (p=0.04)[a]	54% *vs.* 45% (p=0.04)[a]
Overall survival	53% *vs.* 40% (p=0.02)[a]	64% *vs.* 57% (p=0.19)[a]
Local-regional failure rates	17% *vs.* 31% (p=0.007)[a]	18% *vs.* 28% (p=0.01)[a]
Toxicity [GR$\geq$3]	41% *vs.* 21% (p=0.001)[a]	77% *vs.* 34% (p<0.0001)[a]
Late toxicity	38% *vs.* 41% (p=0.25)[b]	21% *vs.* 17% (p=0.29)[a]

[a] Chemoradiation *versus* Radiotherapy arm values; [b] Functional/objective acute reactions;
EORTC European Organization for Research and Treatment of Cancer NA data not available RTOG Radiation Therapy Oncology Group

Conclusions from postoperative chemoradiation studies

Both trials showed an improvement in loco-regional control, but at the expense of increased toxicity. However, survival benefits were observed in the European Organization for Research and Treatment of Cancer (EORTC) trial.

Palliative chemotherapy

Many chemotherapeutic agents are used in recurrent or metastatic disease. The single agents used in this clinical setting and their response rates are given in Table 7.

Table 7. Chemotherapeutic agents and their response rates in treatment of recurrent or metastatic HNSCC

Agent	RR (%)
Methotrexate	31
Bleomycin	21
Cisplatin	28
Carboplatin	22
5 Fluorouracil	15
Cyclophosphamide	36
Hydroxyurea	39
Vinblastine	29
Doxorubicin	24
Paclitaxel	38
Docetaxel	38
Ifosfamide	26

Combination chemotherapy produces an increased response rate and increases the time to tumour progression,[25] but it is associated with increased toxicity. Overall survival shows no improvement. The most commonly used chemotherapy regimens in recurrent or metastatic HNC are given in Table 8.

Table 8. Commonly used regimens for treatment of patients with recurrent or metastatic HNSCC

Agent(s)	Dose and schedule
Methotrexate	40–60 mg/m^2 i.v. weekly
Paclitaxel	80–100 mg/m^2 i.v. over I hour weekly
Docetaxel	75–100 mg/m^2 over 1 hour every 21 days
Cisplatin + Flurouracil	Cisplatin 100 mg/m^2 i.v. day 1 and fluorouracil 1,000 mg/m^2/d IVCI over days 1–4, every 21–28 days
Cisplatin + Paclitaxel	Cisplatin 75 mg/m^2 i.v. and paclitaxel 175 mg/m^2 i.v. over 3 hours, both on day 1 and every 21 days
Cisplatin + Docetaxel	Cisplatin 75 mg/m^2 i.v. and docetaxel 75 mg/m^2 i.v. over 1 hour, both on day 1 and every 21 days
Carboplatin + Paclitaxel	Carboplatin AUC 6 and paclitaxel 200 mg/m^2 i.v. over 3 hours, both on day 1, every 21 days for carboplatin AUC 2 and paclitaxel 80 mg/m^2 i.v. over 1 hour, both on day 1 and weekly

i.v. intravenous infusion IVCI intravenous continuous infusion AUC area under the concentration-time curve

Recently, cetuximab + CDDP was found to be superior to CDDP + 5-FU in terms of progression-free survival and overall survival. Overall survival benefit was minimal but statistically significant[23] (p=0.04).

Palliative chemotherapy is given either as single agent or combination chemotherapy. The response rate ranges from 20%–70% with a median survival of 8–10 months.

References

1. Marcial VA, Pajak TF, Mohiudin M, *et al.* Concomitant cisplatin chemotherapy and radiotherapy in advanced squamous cell carcinoma of the head and neck. Long-term results of the radiation therapy oncology group study 81–17. *Cancer* 1990;**66:**1861–8.

2. Haselow RE, Warshaw MG, Oken MM, *et al.* Radiation alone versus radiation plus weekly low dose cisplatinum in unresectable cancer of the head and neck. In: Fee WE, Jr, Goepfert H, Johns ME, *et al.* (eds). *Head and neck cancer* Vol. II. Philadelphia, Decker; 1990:279–81.

3. Calais G, Alfonsi M, Bardet E, *et al.* Radomized trial of radiation therapy versus concomitant chemotherapy and radiation therapy for advanced-stage oropharynx carcinoma. *J Natl Cancer Inst* 1999;**91:** 2081–6.

4. Forastiere AA, Goepfert H, Maor M, *et al.* Concurrent chemothearpy and radiotherapy for organ preservation in advanced laryngeal cancer. *N Engl J Med* 2003;**349:**2091–8.

5. Head and Neck contracts Program: Adjuvant chemotherapy for advanced head and neck squamous carcinoma. Final report. *Cancer* 1987;**60:**301–11.

6. Scheller DE, Metch B, Mattox D, *et al.* Preoperative chemotherapy in advanced resectable head and neck cancer. Final report of the Southwest Oncology Group. *Laryngoscope* 1988;**98:**1205–11.

7. Rooney M, Kish J, Jacobs J, *et al.* Improved complete response rate and survival in advanced head and neck cancer after three course induction therapy with 120-hour 5-FU infusion and cisplatin. *Cancer* 1985;**55:**1123–8.

8. Vokes EE, Moran WJ, Mick R, *et al.* Neoadjuvant and adjuvant methotrexate cisplatin and fluorouracil in multimodal therapy of head and neck cancer. *J Clin Oncol* 1989;**7:**838–45.

9. Laramore GE, Scott CB, Al-sarraf M, *et al.* Adjuvant chemotherapy for resectable squamous cell carcinoma of the head and neck. Report on Intergroup study. *Int J Radiat Oncol Biol Phys* 1992;**23:**705–13.

10. Martin M, Malaurie E, Langlet PM, *et al.* A randomized prospective study of cisplatin and 5FU as neoadjuvant chemotherapy in head and neck cancer: A final report. *Proc Am Assoc Cancer Res* 1995;**14:** A843.

11. Paccagnella A, Orlando A, Marchiori C, *et al.* Phase III trial of initial chemotherapy in stage III or IV head and neck cancers: A study by the Gruppo di Studio Sui Tomori delta Testa and del Colle. *J Natl Cancer Inst* 1994;**86:**265–72.

12. Richard JM, Kramar A, Molinari R, *et al.* Randomized EORTC head and neck co-operative group trial of pre-operative intra-arterial chemotherapy in oral cavity and oropharynx carcinoma. *Eur J Cancer* 1991;**27:**821–7.

13. The Department of Veterans Affairs Laryngeal Cancer Study Group. Induction chemotherapy plus radiation compared with surgery plus radiation in patients with advanced laryngeal cancer. *N Engl J Med* 1991;**324:**1685–90.

14. Wolf G, Hong W, Fisher S, *et al.* Larynx preservation with induction chemotherapy and radiation in advanced laryngeal cancer: Final results of the VA Laryngeal cancer study group cooperative trial [Abst]. *Proc Am Soc Clin Oncol* 1993;**12:**277.

15. Tannock IF. Combined modality treatment with radiotherapy and chemotherapy. *Radiother Oncol* 1989;**16:**83–101.

16. Grau C, Overgaard J. Effect of cancer chemotherapy on the hypoxic fraction of a solid tumor measured using a local tumor control assay. *Radiother Oncol* 1988;**13:**301–9.

17. Grau C, Agarwal JP, Jabeen K, *et al.* Radiotherapy with or without mytomycin c in the treatment of locally advanced head and neck cancer: Results of the IAEA multicentre randomized trial. *Radiother Oncol* 2003;**67:**17–26.

18. Pointreau Y. Randomized trial of induction chemotherapy with cisplatin and 5fluorouracil with or without docetaxel for larynx preservation. *J Natl Cancer Inst* 2009;**01:**498–506.

19. Bonner JA. Radiotherapy plus cetuximab for locoregionally advanced head and neck cancer: 5-year survival data from a phase 3 randomized trial, and relation between cetuximab-induced rash and survival. *Lancet Oncol* 2010;**11:**21–8.

20. Bonner JA. Radiotherapy plus cetuximab for squamous cell carcinoma of the head and neck. *N Engl J Med* 2006;**354:**567–78.

21. Cooper JS, Pajak TF, Forastiere AA, *et al.* Post-operative concurrent radiotherapy and chemotherapy for high-risk squamous-cell carcinoma of the head and neck. *N Engl J Med* 2004;**350:**1937–44.

22. Bernier J, Domenge C, Ozsahin M, *et al.* Post-operative irradiation with or without concomitant chemotherapy for locally advanced head and neck cancer. *N Engl J Med* 2004;**350:**1945–52.

23. Vermorken JB. Platinum-based chemotherapy plus cetuximab in head and neck cancer. *N Engl J Med* 2008;**359:**1116–27.

24. Ramdas K, Pandey M. Chemotherapy in head and neck cancer. In: Pandey M, Krishnan Nair M, Sebastian P. *Advances in oncology*, Vol. 2. New Delhi: Jaypee Brothers; 2002:66–88.

25. Clavel M, Vermorken JB, Cognetti F, *et al.* Randomized comparison of cisplatin, methotrexate, bleomycin and vinvristine (CABO) vs cisplatin and 5 fluorouracil (CF) vs cisplatin (C) in recurrent or metastatic squamous cell carcinoma of head and neck: A phase III study of the EORTC Head and Neck Cancer Cooperative Group. *Ann Oncol* 1994;**5:**521–6.

7

Reconstruction in head and neck cancer

SHAJI THOMAS, SUBRAMANIA IYER, SOWRABH KUMAR ARORA, BIPIN T. VARGHESE

Refinements in reconstructive techniques have improved form and function after major head and neck resections. The care, skill and planning taken to reconstruct these defects is reflected ultimately in the long-term functional outcome.

Defects of skin and mucous membrane after excision of malignant tumours of the head and neck region may be closed primarily when the defect is small and when it is suitable to do so. When the defect is too large for direct closure or when there is disfigurement or tension in the suture lines, alternate reconstructive methods may be considered. Simpler and easy reconstructive options must be considered before planning for major, complex and microvascular reconstructions.

Free skin grafts (Fig. 1)

When the defect arising from a head and neck resection cannot be closed directly, a free skin graft is the next option.

A free skin graft consists of epidermis and a variable amount of dermis. The grafts are named according to the dermal component of the skin. A full thickness skin graft contains the entire thickness of the dermis; a split skin graft contains all of the epidermis and only part of the dermis. On the basis of the amount of dermis, split skin grafts are subdivided into thin, medium and thick skin grafts. When the entire thickness of the dermis is taken along with epidermis it is called a whole skin graft or full thickness skin graft.

The full thickness skin graft is cut with a scalpel whereas a split thickness skin graft is harvested with a special instrument called a Humby knife or by using an electric dermatome. The donor defect of a whole skin graft has to be sutured. The split thickness skin graft donor area contains adnexal remnants, and pilosebaccous and sweat gland remnants from which the donor area can resurface. The time period required for the donor defect of a split thickness skin graft to heal varies according to the thickness of the graft harvested. When the skin graft is harvested from the donor area, it is potentially a dead piece of tissue and the viability varies according to the temperature. Skin grafts can be stored up to 3 weeks in a refrigerator at 4 °C when wrapped in a saline moisture gauze.

Graft take

The transplanted skin graft has to obtain a new blood supply from the recipient site for its survival. The various processes involved in achieving this are called graft take.

The transplanted skin graft gets adhered to the recipient site by fibrin and its immediate nutritional requirement is met by the plasma that exudes from the bed, referred to as

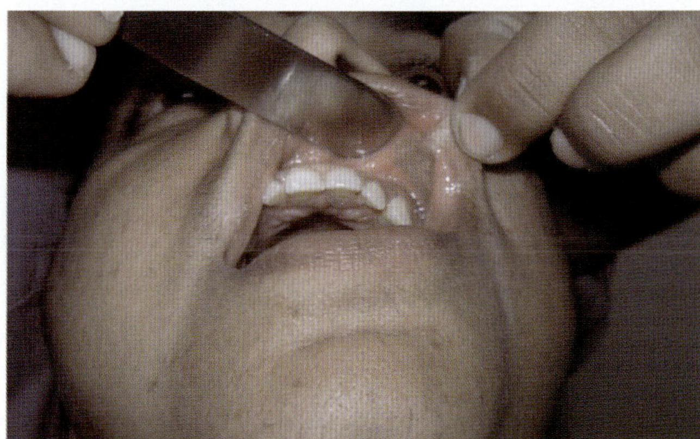

Fig. 1. Free skin grafts

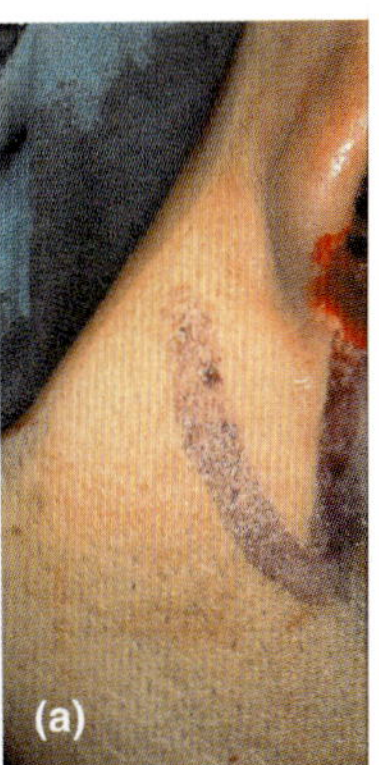

Figs 3 (a–c). Super

the donor site. Su
but can harvest a
are limited in len
The orientat
by the location
or advancement.
the needs of the
subdermal plexu
with its nerve sup
the nasolabial fla
3 weeks. Defattir
for cosmetic acce
inserted into the
the nose. The nas
procedure is sim
of the flap are th
proximity to the c
with less donor s

Forehead fla

Nasal amputatio
for various crim
a large group of
reconstruction. A
Sushruta Samita
the forehead for
Antonio Branca
the *Sushruta San*
a similar procedu

Types of foreh

- *Median:* The
  mid-forehead
  of the forehe
  supratrochlea
- *Paramedian:*
  around a nari
  over the supe

plasmatic circulation. This is followed by an outgrowth of capillaries from the recipient bed to unite with those on the deeper surface of the graft, thus establishing a circulation of blood in the graft. Meanwhile, fibres grow into the fibrin and convert the adhesive clot into a more definite fibrous tissue. The strength of attachment increases gradually, providing reasonable strength and allowing safe handling of the graft in approximately 4 days. Lymphatic link up and nervous communications are established more slowly.

The graft bed

The graft bed must have adequate blood supply to nourish the graft and should be able to provide necessary fibrin anchorage. The following recipient surfaces can take a graft:

- Healthy granulation tissue
- Muscle fascia and fat
- Soft tissues of head and neck area
- Bone covered with periosteum and cartilage with perichondrial coverage.

Bare cartilage and bone of the head and neck area usually do not take skin grafts well. The bare cortical bone of the outer table of the skull and the bare bone of the mandible lack sufficient vascularity to take skin grafts. The hard palate, the bone of the maxilla and the walls of the orbit are capable of taking grafts, although not as well as healthy soft tissue defects. Previously irradiated tissues may not take a skin graft as well as non-irradiated tissues. Previous radiotherapy is not a contraindication for grafting the defect, but the bed and tissues must be assessed at the time of surgery. Radiotherapy can cause tissue fibrosis and can lead to reduced vascularity of the tissues.

When planning to graft a granulating exposed raw area, the presence of infection with organisms that destroy fibrin and prevent adhesion of the graft to its bed should first be ruled out. The β-haemolytic *Streptococcus pyogenes* produce fibrinolysis and prevent firm adhesion of the graft to its recipient site. *Pseudomonas aeruginosa* and methicillin-resistant *Staphylococcus aureus* (MRSA) also can cause fibrinolysis, but to a lesser extent.

Donor sites for skin grafting

The usual donor sites selected for harvesting skin grafts are the thighs, the upper arm and the flat surface of abdomen.

Types of skin grafts

Full thickness skin grafts

In head and neck defects, a full thickness skin graft gives a surprisingly better appearance when compared with a split thickness skin graft. It is ideal for covering small defects after removal of tumours in areas such as the tip of the nose, parts of the pinna, and lower eye lid. The take of the graft is not as good as the take of a split skin graft. Vascularization is slower than in a split thickness graft. The common head and neck full thickness skin graft donor sites are post-auricular and pre-auricular areas, and lower neck. A full thickness skin graft cannot be used for grafting granulating surfaces, and it should be tailored accurately to fit the defect. When a full thickness skin graft is harvested, care must be taken not to include fat along with the graft. The donor site has to be closed by direct suturing.

Composite grafts (full thickness skin and cartilage)

This is used to reconstruct small and moderate-sized defects where skin and underlying cartilage are to be reconstructed. This technique is employed for defects of the nasal tip, alar rim or ear rim.

Split thickness skin grafts

In the head and neck region, split thickness skin grafts are employed for covering defects in the oral cavity, maxillectomy cavity, and so on. In these sites the graft is retained by pressure methods, either by the use of a bolus tie over the dressing, or by using a dental appliance to exert pressure on the graft. Bolus grafting is suitable where the graft bed can provide some stability, as in the buccal mucosa or floor of the mouth. When a concave surface is grafted, care should be taken to avoid tenting of the graft across the defect. Split thickness skin grafting of intraoral defects take well; however, secondary loss of the graft and contracture of the graft can lead to trismus.

FLAPS FOR HEAD AND NECK RECONSTRUCTION

A skin flap is a segment of skin and variable amount of subcutaneous tissue with a pedicle of continuing blood supply. The transfer of a flap to reconstruct the primary defect leaves a secondary defect, which is either closed primarily by direct suture or covered with a free skin graft. The flap may be local or distant, depending on the proximity of the donor site to the defect. In reconstructing defects of the face and mouth, distant flaps are often taken from the region below the lower border of the mandible.

Skin flaps may be random or axial, on the basis of their blood supply. For an axial pattern flap, a distinct blood vessel is identifiable in the pedicle, but a random pattern flap has only a dermal network for its blood supply.

When a local flap is transferred, movement takes the form of rotation, transposition or advancement.

The choice between using a transposition flap or a rotation

flap is often
When the d
flap is safer.
of the dono
Local
reconstruct
require the
inevitable b
The co
reconstruct

Nasolab

The use of
popularized
inferiorly o
is often use
based flap i

Indicatio

Superiorly t
of defects o
for reconst
nose or fo
flaps are co
commissur
Nasola
nose where
can be utili
is based on
artery), the
As the facia
raised as a
The design
redundanc

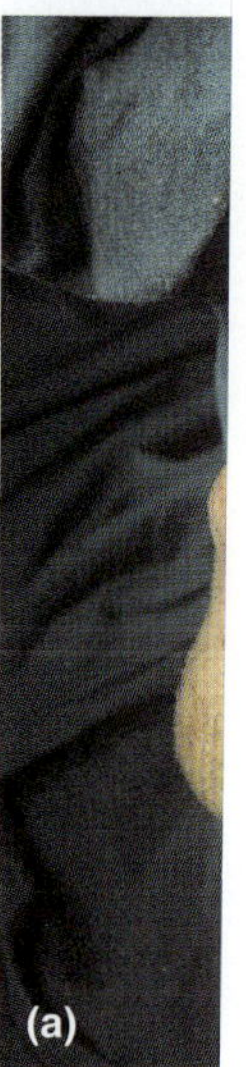
(a)

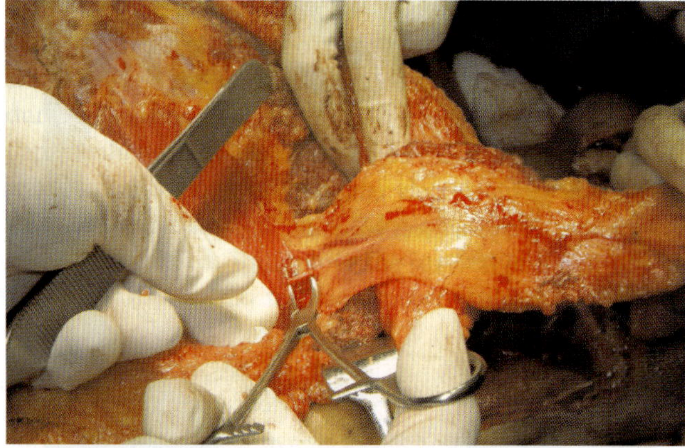

Fig. 10. PMMC flap with vascular pedicle

- For augmenting the pharyngeal closure following laryngo-pharyngectomy when there is tension in pharyngeal closure, especially in a salvage setup
- For reconstructing circumferential pharyngeal and cervical oesophageal defects.

Pectoralis major musculocutaneous flap may be elevated along with a segment of rib as an osteomyocutaneous flap for reconstructing mandibular defects along with soft tissue defects.

Technique of elevating pectoralis major flap[15,16] (Fig. 10)

Following the resection, the size of the defect is measured with the patient in the supine position. The required size of the flap is marked on the anterior chest wall. The surface marking of the acromiothoracic artery is marked. A line is drawn between the acromion and the xiphoid process. Another line is drawn from the midclavicular point at right angles to join the first line, which delineates the acromiothoracic vessel.

The skin island of appropriate size and shape is outlined, which gives adequate reach to the defect. The skin paddle is usually positioned between the lateral edge of sternum medially and nipple laterally. The point of pivot for the flap is the midclavicular point. The distance between the midclavicular point and distal portion of the surgical defect is measured. The distal portion of the skin island of the flap is positioned equidistant to the midclavicular point.

The flap should not be elevated before the surgical resection of the tumour and detailed assessment of the surgical defect. To increase the arc of rotation and reach of the flap, the skin paddle may be positioned slightly below the lower edge of the muscle to overlay the anterior rectus sheath. This part of the flap is considered as the random area of the myocutaneous flap. The survival of the random area of the flap can be improved by taking the anterior rectus sheath along with the muscle. The incision for the skin island is

extended along the anterior axillary line for exposure of the entire pectoralis major muscle.

The skin incision is deepened all around the skin island. Absorbable tacking sutures are put between the subcutaneous tissue and the anterior surface of the pectoralis major muscle to prevent shearing of the skin island from the muscle. The lateral incision is deepened and skin is elevated from the muscle to expose the entire anterior surface of the pectoralis major. In female patients, the lateral side of the skin incision in the lower part of the anterior chest wall contains the breast tissues. The lateral skin flap is elevated until the lower border of the pectoralis major muscle is identified.

The plane between the pectoralis major and pectoralis minor is now identifiable and the two muscles are separated by blunt dissection. The inferior portion of the muscle that originates from the sternum and costochondral junctions is divided. The medial side of the pectoralis major muscle is divided with diathermy.

Upon elevating the undersurface of the pectoralis major muscle from the pectoralis minor by blunt dissection, the thoracoacromial pedicle can be visualized. The muscle is divided up to the midclavicular point on the medial side. During this step, many perforating branches of the internal mammary artery will be encountered, which are divided and ligated.

This procedure makes the entire course of the thoracoacromial pedicle visible. Keeping the vascular pedicle under direct vision, the muscle is divided lateral to the vascular pedicle with scissors or diathermy. Electric diathermy reduces the bleeding when the muscle is divided. The vascular pedicle must be always under direct vision while dividing the muscle, which is done all the way up to the clavicle. If additional reach of the flap is required, the clavicular fibres of the muscle are detached from the clavicle to free up the flap completely on its vascular pedicle, and the muscle is denervated. This will improve the length of the pedicle and will avoid the unpleasant sensation in the chest when the intra-oral part of flap is stimulated. If the skin surface of the flap is to be used for intra-oral lining or for pharyngeal repair, then the flap is flipped 180° for transfer. While transferring the flap to the recipient site, care must be taken to avoid kinking or excessive tension on the vascular pedicle (Fig. 10).

When the pectoralis major muscle flap is used for head and neck reconstruction, the muscle paddle in the neck will provide additional protection to the carotid vessels. The modifications of the pectoralis major flap are:

- *Muscle only flap:* To augment the pharyngeal closure after a partial pharyngectomy, especially in irradiated patients
- *Osteomyocutaneous flap:* A segment of rib based on its periosteal supply to reconstruct mandibular defects. With the newer techniques in composite tissue transfer, this prodecure is now rarely used.[16,19]
- *Double skin paddle flap:* Two skin islands are designed in

the muscle paddle to reconstruct full thickness defects of the oral cavity. One island is used for reconstructing the lining defects and the other island for reconstructing the skin defect.

- *Folded pectoralis major skin paddle:* Instead of planning two separate skin paddles on the muscle, a larger skin island is used for reconstructing full thickness defects of the oral cavity. The lining defect is sutured first. The skin paddle is then deepithelized, or cut up to the muscle, and folded to reconstruct the outside skin defect.
- *Pectoralis major free flap:* Microvascular techniques are used to transfer the flap to a distant site.

Latissimus dorsi flap

The latissimus dorsi flap may be used as a pedicled flap or as a free flap for reconstructing major head and neck defects. This flap was initially described for resurfacing defects in the chest wall. Its use in head and neck defects was popularized by Quiller *et al.*, in 1978.

Latissimus dorsi forms part of the posterior wall of axilla as it converges on its tendinous insertion into the upper humeral shaft. The major vascular supply is from the thoracodorsal vessels, which have their origin in the subscapular artery, which in turn arises from the axillary artery. Additional vascular contributions are from the posterior intercostal arteries. The thoracodorsal artery has a constant branch to the serratus anterior muscle, and enters the latissimus dorsi muscle on its deep surface 8–10 cm from the axillary artery and 2 cm from its anterior free edge. The diameter of the proximal part of the thoracodorsal artery ranges from 2–3 mm, making it an excellent vessel for microvascular anastamosis. Venous drainage is by the venae comitantes, which accompany the thoracodorsal artery and drain into the axillary vein. The nerve supply is via the thoracodorsal nerve, which is a branch of the posterior cord of the branchial plexus.

The latissimus dorsi has a long vascular pedicle and gives a good reach to most of the head and neck sites. Large amounts of tissue are made available using this flap. Flaps measuring 10 cm × 7 cm are easily harvested and subsequent primary closure is achieved. When larger flaps are harvested, the donor site has to be skin grafted and may lead to wound healing on the back.

Technique

The skin island is fashioned as transverse or oblique. Designing the skin paddle in the lower part of the lattisimus dorsi muscle will give more length to the muscle pedicle, thus allowing a better reach to the head and neck sites. The posterior axillary fold (which forms the anterior fold of muscle), the tip of the scapula and the post iliac crest are marked. Adequate skin island is marked with particular reference to the length of the pedicle when a pedicled flap is planned. Whenever possible, a transverse flap should be harvested, which give a more acceptable scar, especially in young females.

The outline of the skin island is incised down to muscle and elevation is commenced anteriorly; when the anterior border of the muscle is reached, the plane of elevation is continued deep to it. The serratus anterior muscle is identified. (Its fibres run at right angles to the fibres of the latissimus dorsi.) The latissimus dorsi muscle is divided inferiorly. The thoracodorsal pedicle is identified and the branch to the serratus anterior muscle is divided.

With the blood vessels fully displayed, the muscle can be divided around the posterior and distal borders of the skin island. The dissection is continued up towards the tip of scapula, and the muscle is freed from the scapula. With further dissection, the junction of the thoracodorsal vessels with the circumflex scapular vessel (to form the subscapular artery), can be identified at the upper anterior end of the muscle in the axilla. If a longer pedicle is required, the circumflex scapular vessel can be ligated and the flap in the axilla on the subscapular vessel can be further elevated. The nerve also may be divided to cause later atrophy of the muscle, which will give a better contour. If a transfer of vascularized rib is planned, the perforators to rib are preserved. The latissimus myocutaneous flap is tunnelled under the pectoralis major muscle and over the clavicle. Then the flap is tunnelled through the neck to reach the recipient site. If the donor defect cannot be closed primarily, a split skin graft may be used to cover the defect.

Free flap technique

The technique for a free transfer of the latissimus dorsi is almost similar to a pedicled flap, except that the insertion of the muscle is divided as well. The dissection of the muscle is done in a retrograde fashion to identify the vascular pedicle as early as possible.

Advantages of latissimus dorsi flap
- Long pedicle, with good reach to head and neck sites
- Highly reliable
- Large amount of tissue can be transferred
- Can be used as a pedicled or free flap
- It has cosmetic advantages, especially in females.

Disadvantages of latissimus dorsi flap
- May have to change the position of the patient to lateral position for harvesting the flap
- More dissection needed to transfer latissimus dorsi flap to head and neck sites
- Functional morbidities, especially in swimmers and climbers.

Trapezius myocutaneous flap

The trapezius myocutaneous flap can be used for reconstructing defects of the head and neck region and upper back. Its location makes it the flap of choice for defects of the occipital, parotid and cervical spine regions. It may be used for intra-oral and anterior neck coverage. The posterior trapezius musculocutaneous flap should be considered as the flap of choice for defects of the posterior scalp and neck, and upper third of the posterior trunk.

Anatomy

The trapezius is a broad, flat triangular shaped muscle. It originates medially from the external occipital protuberance, the medial part of the superior nuchal line of the occipital bone, the ligamentum nuchae and the spinous processes of the seventh cervical and all the thoracic vertebrae. The muscle is inserted into the lateral third of the clavicle, acromion and to the spine of the scapula. It is divided into superior, middle and inferior fibres. The trapezius muscle overlies the splenius capitis, levator scapulae, supraspinatus, rhomboideus minor and major, and upper medial portion of the latissimus dorsi muscle.

Vascular supply[20,21]

The vascular supply consists of a dominant pedicle and several minor pedicles. The dominant blood supply originates from the transverse cervical artery and vein (a branch of the thyrocervical trunk of the subclavian artery) and associated veins. The vascular pedicle runs between the sternomastoid and scalene muscles, and enters the deep surface of the trapezius muscle at the base of the neck. The artery then divides into ascending and descending branches and forms the basis of the superior and inferior musculocutaneous flaps. The descending branch runs on the deep surface of the muscle between the spine and the scapulae, giving musculocutaneous perforators to the overlying skin. Several minor pedicles also supply the trapezius. The largest of these is a branch of the occipital artery.

Two types of trapezius myocutaneous flaps are available —the lateral and posterior vertical trapezius myocutaneous flaps. The former overlies the acromioclavicular region and has limited applications; it has a limited arc of rotation. The posterior vertical trapezius myocutaneous flap, on the other hand, is more versatile. The patient has to be positioned in a lateral position to harvest this flap. The posterior trapezius myocutaneous flap was developed in an attempt to avoid loss of function of the superior fibres and thus to maintain proper shoulder function. The skin island is positioned between the scapula and spine based on the middle and inferior portion of the trapezius muscle. The flap is best raised from distal to proximal. The lower portion of the trapezius muscle is elevated along with the skin island, dividing its vertical origin. At the level of the scapula, care must be taken to avoid raising the rhomboid muscles along with the flap, which will lead to a plane deep to the scapula. The descending branch of the vascular pedicle will be visualized on the undersurface of muscle. The muscle is divided at the lateral edge of the skin paddle taking care to preserve the upper fibres (Fig. 11).[22]

The donor defect can usually be closed primarily. The trapezius flap can be employed only when the transverse cervical artery is known to be intact, which is likely to be sacrificed in a prior neck dissection.

Platysma flap

An island myocutaneous flap based on the platysma muscle is ideal for reconstructing the superficial lining defects of the oral cavity. A turnover platysma muscle flap based superiorly, including an island of skin in its distal part, can be used for covering defects following excision of superficial diffuse lesions in the buccal mucosa and tongue. Defects in the buccal mucosa should ideally be covered with a flap, as skin grafting can lead to contractures and produce trismus.[23]

Anatomy

The platysma is a thin muscular sheet in the neck. The platysma extends from the mandible above to the clavicle below. It is well developed in men. The blood supply to the upper part of the flap comes from the submental branch of the facial artery and to the lower part from a branch of the transverse cervical artery.

Flap design and technique[23] (Fig. 12)

An elliptical skin island is designed in the lower neck above the clavicle. As the blood supply to the flap is from the submental branches of the facial artery, care should be taken in the dissection along the medial edge; also, elevating the flap beyond the lower border of the mandible should be avoided. The flap usually reaches the intra-oral defects. The skin island is now incised. The incision is extended superiorly and skin is elevated superficial to the platysma. The platysma muscle is divided below the skin paddle. The skin island is elevated along with a broad sheet of platysma muscle. The platysma is freed medially from the strap muscles and laterally from the anterior edge of the trapezius muscle. The muscle and the skin island are freed up to the level of the mandible where the marginal mandibular branch of the facial nerve is identified and preserved. A tunnel is then created in the floor of the mouth by blunt dissection to allow the passage of the flap into the oral cavity.

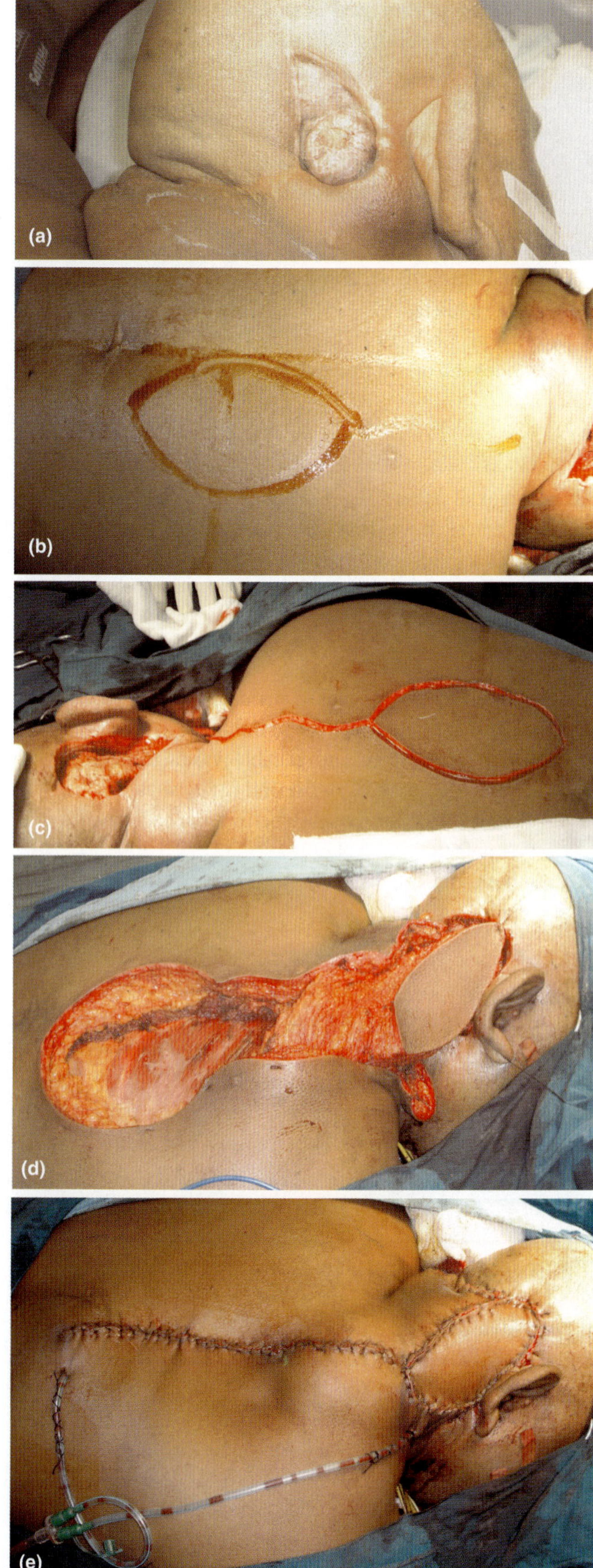

Fig. 11 (a–e). Trapezius flap for scalp reconstruction

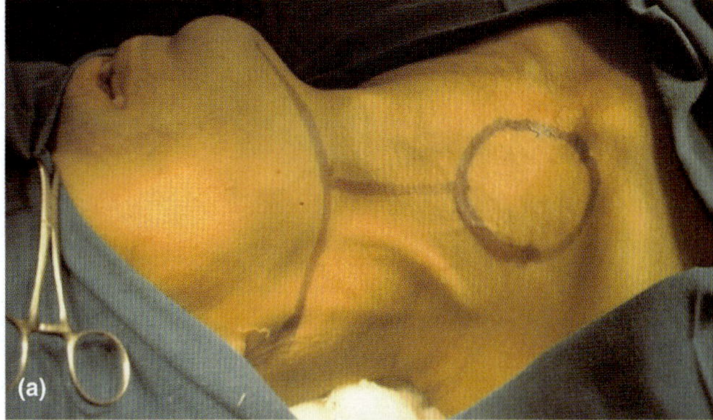

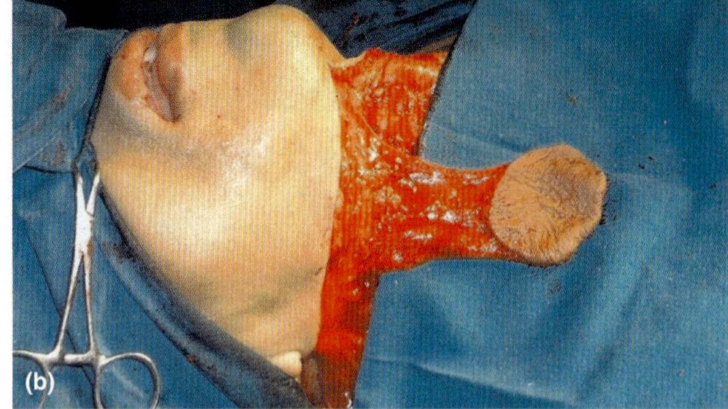

Fig. 12 (a, b). Platysma flap design and technique

Disadvantages of the platysma flap
- Blood supply can be unreliable.
- Prior neck dissection or any neck surgeries preclude the use of this flap.
- A proper neck dissection may damage the blood supply to the flap.
- Removal of the platysma interferes with the blood supply to the overlying skin and can lead to necrosis of skin.
- Platysma flap is not advisable in patients with prior irradiation to the neck.

Sternomastoid island myocutaneous flap

Owens described it in 1955 as a pedicled flap for resurfacing cheek defects. Stephan Ariyan popularized this flap as an island myocutaneous flap.

Vascular supply

The dominant blood supply is from the occipital artery. Additional blood supply is from the superior thyroid, transverse cervical and the posterior auricular artery.[24]

The sternomastoid island flap is useful in reconstructing small and medium sized intra-oral lining defects in patients with a clinically N0 neck.[24,25] It is also used for resurfacing facial and neck skin defects.[26] For reconstructing intra-oral lining defects, it is used as a superiorly based island flap. After resecting the intra-oral malignant lesion, the neck is assessed

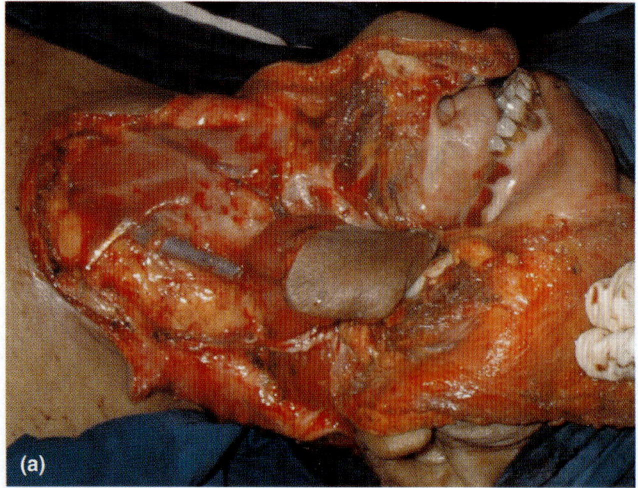

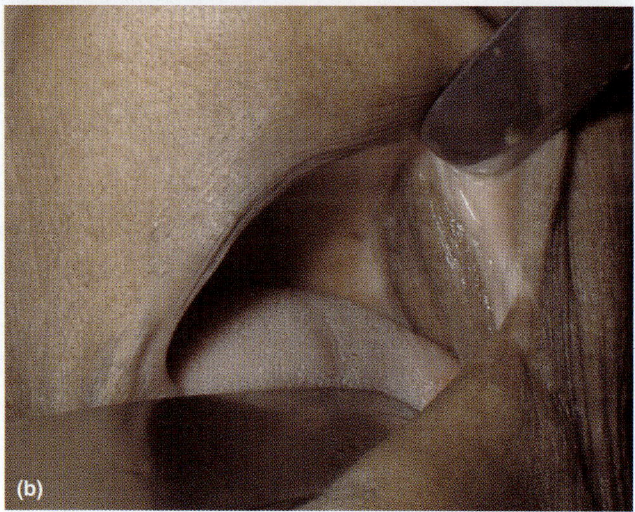

Fig. 13 (a, b). Sternomastoid island myocutaneous flap for buccal mucosa defect

for any significant nodes, especially in the level II region, after which the inferior neck skin over the origin of sternomastoid is harvested as an island. Care must be taken to avoid shearing off the skin island from the muscle. When planned as a superiorly based flap, the major blood supply from the occipital artery and that from the superior thyroid artery must always be preserved as far as possible. The sternomastoid flap may be harvested as an osteomyocutaneous flap with a segment of clavicle for mandibular reconstruction.[27] Patients who received radical radiotherapy prior to surgery were shown to have a significantly higher flap-related complication rate when compared with primary surgical resection and reconstruction (Fig. 13).

The sternomastoid flap can reach the oral cavity easily without producing tension on the suture line. The preservation of the supply from the superior thyroid artery, in addition to the branch from occipital artery, improves the flap survival.

Advantages of the sternomastoid flap
* The skin paddle of the superiorly based sternomastoid flap

is hairless and thin, and is an ideal reconstructive option for medium sized cheek defects.
* It does not produce excessive bulk in the face or mouth.
* The cosmetic defect of a segmental mandibulectomy is partly masked by the transposed muscle of the flap.
* Harvesting of the sternomastoid flap usually does not produce much functional or cosmetic deformity.

Disadvantages of the sternomastoid flap
* A proper neck dissection is likely to cause damage to the vascular pedicle.
* A previous neck surgery or concurrent lymphadenectomy precludes the use of this flap.[26]

SUBMENTAL ARTERY ISLAND FLAP

This is an axial pattern flap based on the submental branch of the facial artery. It was first described by Martin *et al.* in 1993. This flap is an ideal reconstructive option in selected defects of the head and neck region.

Advantages[28]

* Donor defect can be closed primarily on the donor site. The scar is hidden under the mandible.
* The flap has a large and reliable vascular pedicle with excellent reach to most of the oral cavity sites.
* Ideal thickness for reconstructing buccal mucosa and tongue defects
* Less bulk and less time consuming when compared with free flaps.

Disadvantages

* The submental flap is harvested with a thick surrounding fibrofatty tissue, and tissues around the facial vessels can compromise the lymphatic clearance.
* For this reason, this flap is unsuitable in patients with clinically significant nodes in levels IA and IB.

Vascular pedicle[28]

This is approximately 2 mm in size. The pedicle arises from the facial artery deep to the submandibular salivary gland. It runs forwards and medially between the anterior belly of the digastric and mylohyoid muscles, and gives cutaneous perforators (Fig. 14). The submental vein drains into the common facial vein. The submental artery island flap is also described for reconstructing defects in the larynx, cervical oesophagus and palate, and cutaneous defects of the middle and lower third of the face.

A prophylactic neck dissection can be combined with a submental flap. Being an island flap, the pedicle can be thinned as much as possible to remove lymphatic tissues.

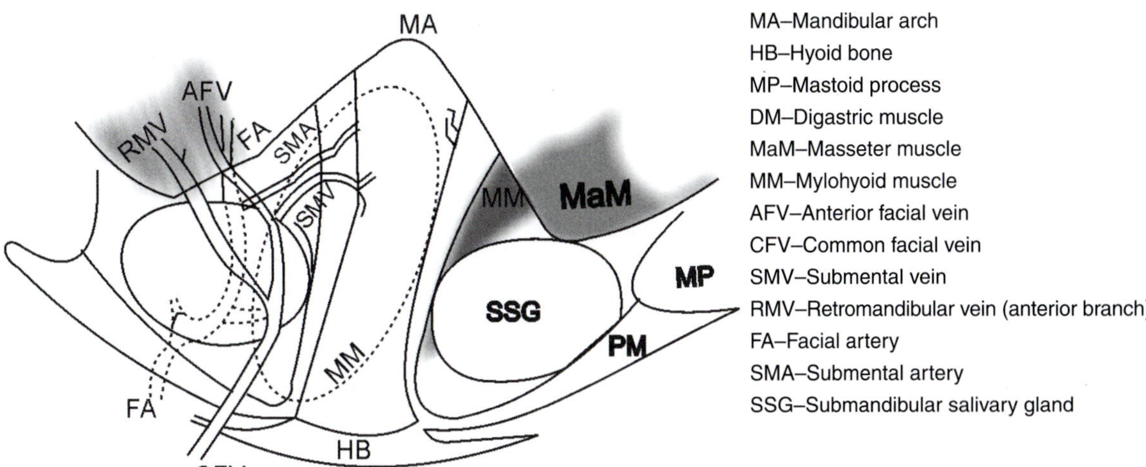

Fig. 14. Line drawing describing the vascular anatomy of SMIF [reproduced with permission, *see* reference 28]

Surgical technique (Fig. 15)

The patient is placed in a supine position with neck extended. An elliptical flap is planned in the submental area and submandibular area, allowing primary closure of the donor defect. Dissection is carried out in the subplatysmal plane. The marginal mandibular nerve is identified and preserved. The submental artery and vein are identified at the medial border of the anterior belly of the digastric muscle. The submandibular salivary gland is dissected off after identifying the submental branch of the facial artery. The branches of the facial artery to the salivary gland are ligated and divided. The submental artery is usually the second branch of the facial artery after the first salivary gland branch. The anterior belly of the digastric

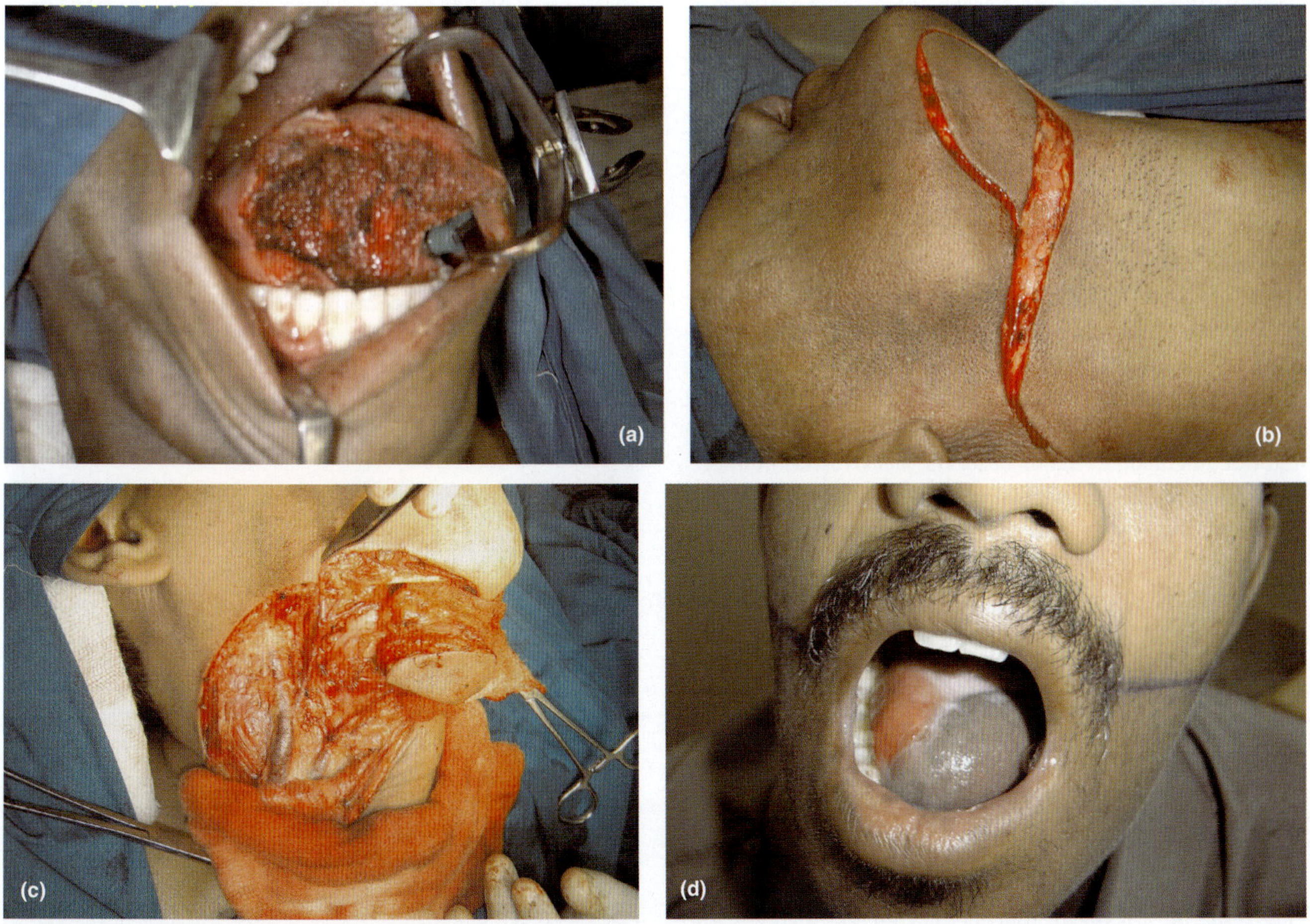

Fig. 15 (a–d). Rreconstruction of tongue defect with submental island flap [reproduced with permission, *see* reference 28]

muscle is elevated with the flap because the pedicle passes deep to the muscle. The flap is raised as an island flap based on the submental pedicle. The flap is tunnelled through the floor of the mouth into the oral cavity.

To be safer, it is better not to use the submental artery island flap in patients with prior irradiation to the neck, and in patients with clinically positive nodes in submental and submandibular levels. As the donor site is a dense hair bearing area, hair growth in the flap can cause inconvenience to male patients.

ROLE OF MICROVASCULAR FREE TISSUE TRANSFER

Since its introduction by Taylor and Daniel in the application of free flaps, reconstruction has been one of the milestones in the evolution of head and neck surgical oncology. The literature supports the advantages of free flaps over conventional flaps in the quality of life following surgery, extent of resection possible and the type of surgery performed. Reconstruction using a 'like for like' tissue is possible with the availability of composite tissue flaps, especially those containing bone. Indeed, the most important impact of the advent of microvascular free flaps has been in the transfer of vascularized bone for the mandible and reconstruction of skull base defects. This section reviews the advantages and disadvantages, basic requirements of a unint, common free flaps used, the site-wise choices, complications and their avoidance and future directions.

Advantages and disadvantages of free flaps over conventional flaps

The use of free flaps has brought in considerable improvement in the way head and neck cancers are managed. Even though the evidence so far does not support an improvement in the long-term overall survival of patients, recent reports show its positive influence on the outcome of treatment.[29] The impact of free flaps on quality of life following treatment has been well documented.[30,31] Major head and neck resection affects the three cardinal functions of speech, swallowing and nasal breathing. The use of free flaps has enabled the surgical oncologist to help in retaining these functions, or rehabilitating them, more than what was achieved with conventional methods of reconstruction. The outcome of the swallowing function following extensive oral and oropharyngeal resection resulting in mandibular discontinuity has been very different when the bone is reconstructed by free flaps.[32]

The superiority of free flaps over conventional flaps can be summarized as given below.

Single-stage transfer of most suitable tissue

The resection of head and neck cancers involves the removal of composite areas which include the skin, soft tissue, underlying bone and mucosa. Most conventional flaps provide only skin and soft tissue, which does not address the reconstruction of bone, thereby compromising on the quality of reconstruction and the function. This is because they do not compensate for the loss of mandibular continuity, which is important in the swallowing function. The impact of bony reconstruction on facial aesthesis is well appreciated, especially when the anterior mandible is involved. This effect on the appearance is however evident even in the cases of lateral mandible excision, especially if the patient is dentate and young (Figs 16, 17). Pedicle flaps are limited by their quality, quantity and manoeuvrablity of the tissues provided, thereby compromising the reconstruction.

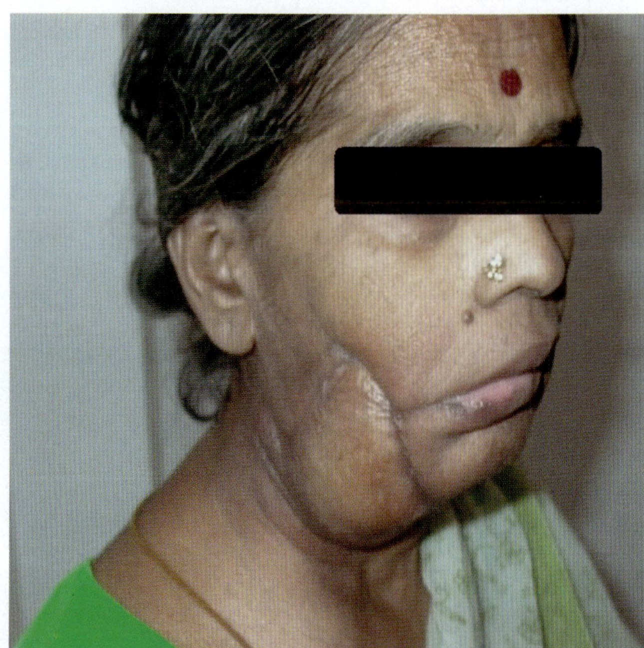

Fig. 16. Unreconstructed lateral segment of the mandible

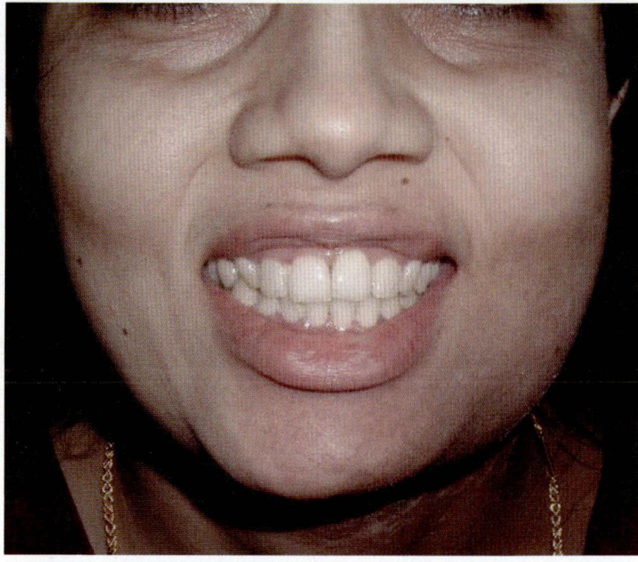

Fig. 17. Reconstructed lateral mandible maintains the occlusion

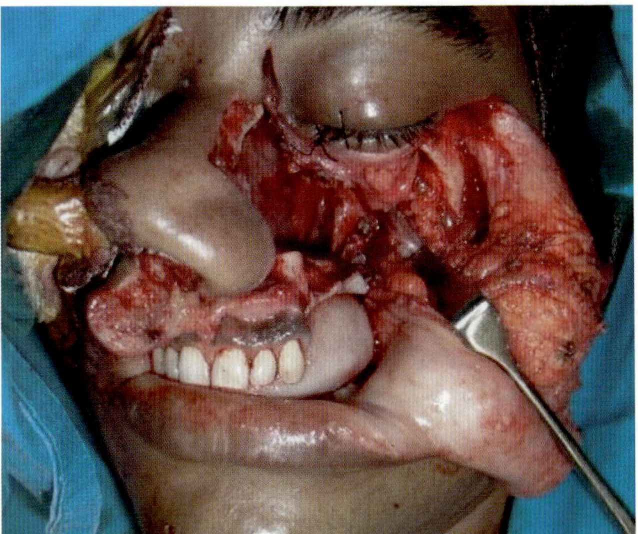

Fig. 18. Maxillectomy defect

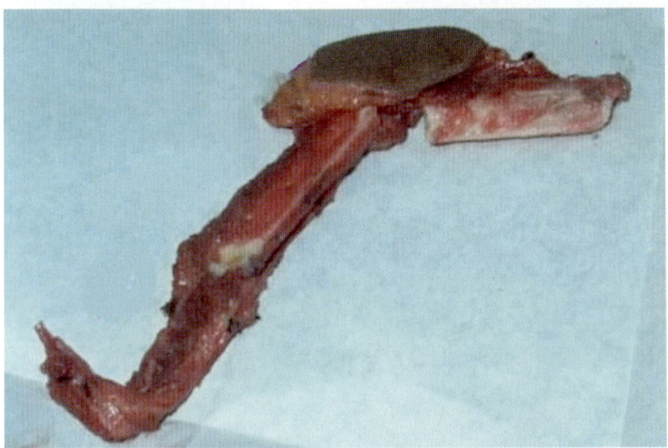

Fig. 19. Fibula fashioned for multi-axial reconstruction

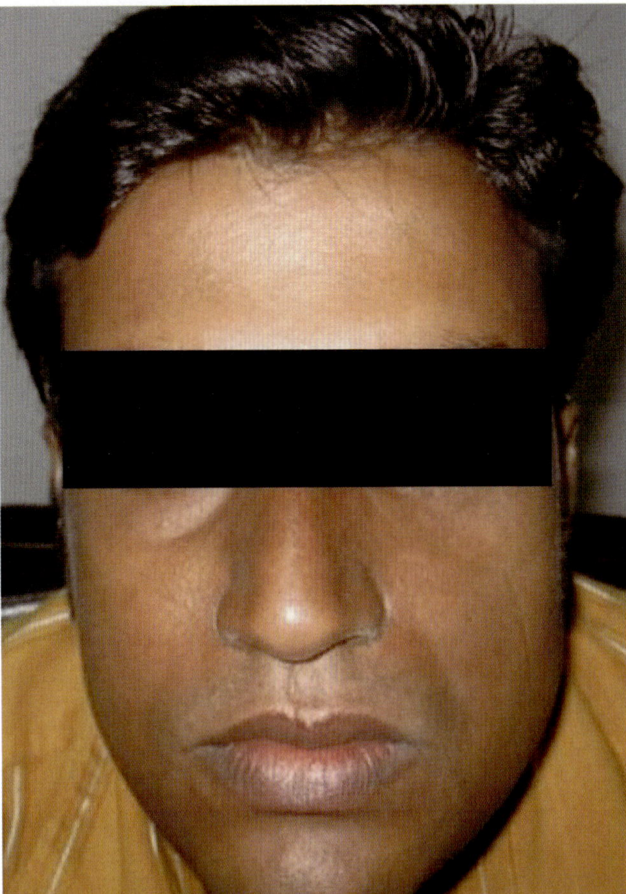

Fig. 20. Postoperative result of maxillectomy reconstruction

The reconstruction of tongue defects is qualitatively better with regard to the texture and mobility, if free flaps such as radial forearm or lateral arm flaps are used compared with the nasolabial or pectoralis major flaps.

Making multi-axial reconstruction possible

Reconstruction of defects of the oral cavity and the midface may often need tissues being provided at multiple axes. A typical example is a defect involving the orbital floor, maxilla and palate. The reconstruction here would need to provide orbital support, obturate the palatal defect and, if possible, reconstruct the upper alveolus. To achieve this with a single or combination of pedicle flaps will be difficult (Figs 18–20).

Allowing complex reconstruction of defects involving multiple sites

In defects that extend across subsites and regions in the head and neck, reconstruction of functional or aesthetic sub-units becomes important. They do not conform to simple geometric shapes; and hence reconstructing them may not be easy with a pedicle flap hampered by its fixity to the pedicle. Free flaps with their total freedom of movement with regard to their pedicle allow the reconstruction to be easier and functionally better. The availability of free flaps and the use of two free flaps simultaneously have made it possible to operate on otherwise 'seemingly inoperable' cases (Figs 21, 22).

Transferring special functions to the reconstructed area

Improving the quality of reconstruction will involve transferring special functions to the area of reconstruction in the head and neck. This may be achieved by providing sensation to the lining epithelium, bone with growth potential to the area of mandible, and secretory function to the substituted mucosal lining. Use of sensate flaps, vascularized costochondral grafts, and jejuna or gastric mucosa[34] may help in achieving these, though to a limited extent. Figures 23 and 24 show a preoperative and a 2-year postoperative picture of a young child who needed resection of the mandible for aggressive fibromatosis. The reconstruction was carried

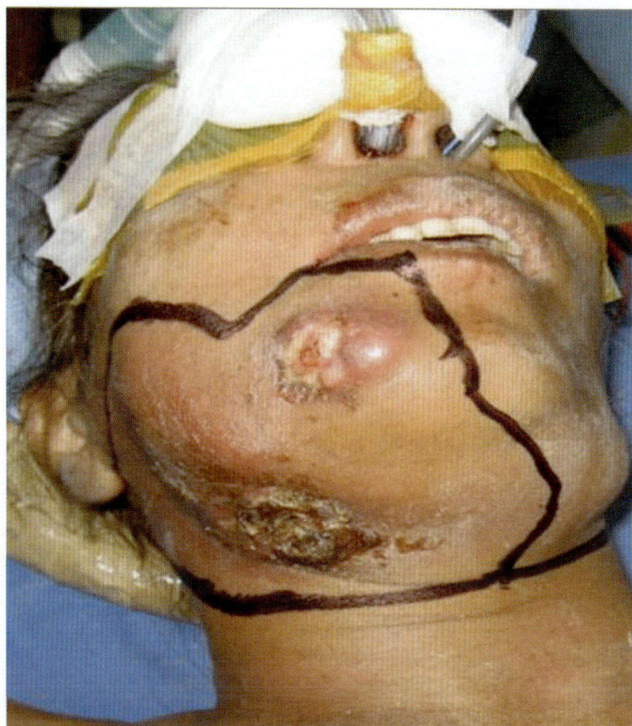

Fig. 21. Extensive resection marked in a patient

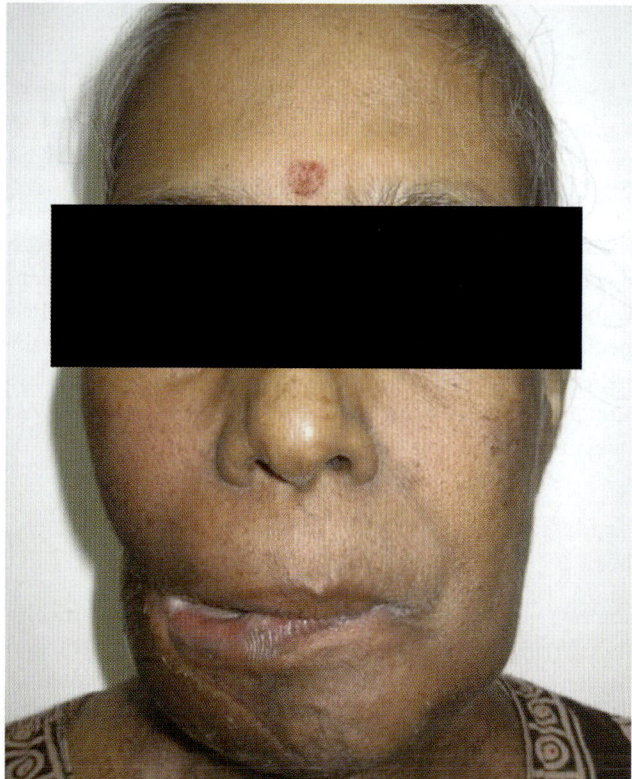

Fig. 22. Reconstruction using the ALT flap inside and the fibula outside

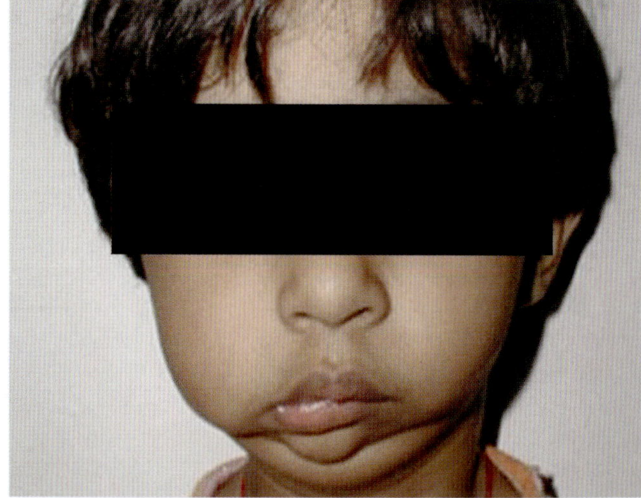

Fig. 23. Preoperative deformity after resection of the mandible

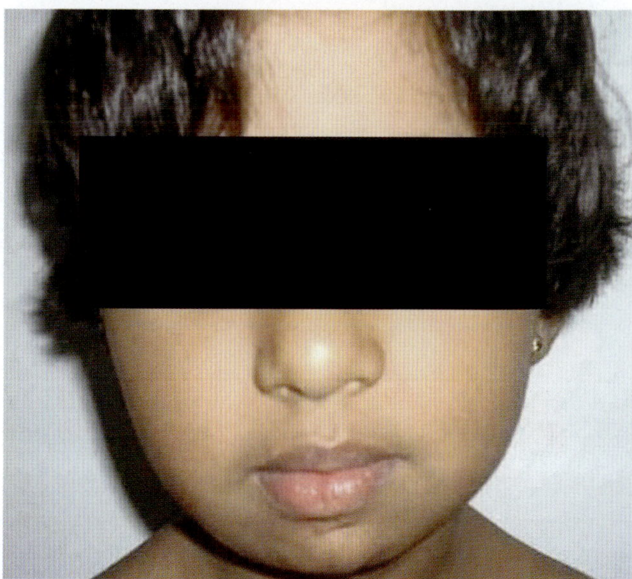

Fig. 24. The 2-year postoperative appearance shows a normal chin contour

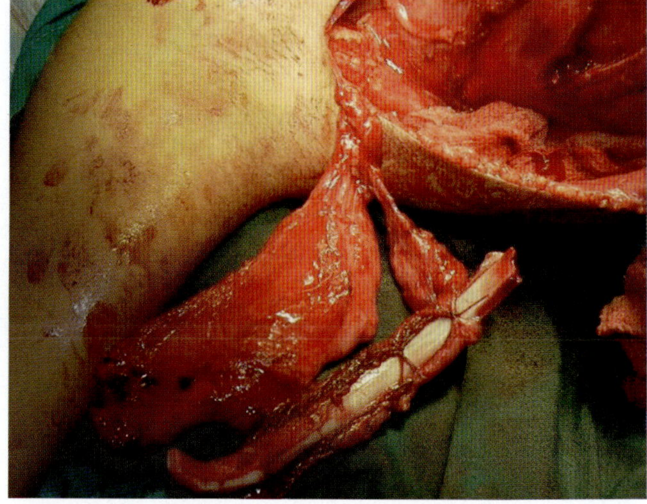

Fig. 25. Serratus/lattismus costochondral flap

out using a vascularized costochondral graft transferred along with the lattismus dorsi and serratus anterior muscle (Fig. 25).

Basic requirements of a unit

The widespread use of free flaps has been hampered in many centres with limited resources due to the fear of exhausting their resources on fewer patients. This is because more time is needed in free tissue transfer compared with that required for conventional flaps, there is need for re-exploration for free flaps, and there is fear of failure. This situation arises when the unit is not fully prepared to induct microvascular surgery into their practice. When the unit is fully equipped, the time consumed for free flaps becomes comparable, the need for re-exploration becomes less, and failures become fewer. A successful unit should have a couple of reconstructive microsurgeons interested in head and neck reconstruction. The head and neck ablation team should also be acquainted with the reconstructive surgeon's needs, especially the need for preserving the donor blood vessels for anastomosis in the neck and leaving back a clean bloodless field. The anaesthesiologists and the ICU team should also be cognizant of the special needs of these patients, especially the need to maintain the blood volume, detect the compromised blood supply to flap, etc. A two-team approach in resection and reconstruction will help in reducing the time of the procedure. Monitoring of the flaps is made easy if the ICU staff is acquainted with the pin-prick method of monitoring. Studies of cost-effectiveness of these procedures have been reported from developed countries, which clearly show the superiority of free flaps compared to pedicled flaps.[34–36]

Common free flaps used

For reconstructive requirements in head and neck surgery, only a few free flaps need to be mastered and practised. These include radial forearm, anterolateral thigh (Figs 26, 27), fibula, jejunum and rectus abdominis. Other flaps such as deep circumflex iliac artery (DCIA)-based iliac crest (Fig. 28); lateral arm and osteocutaneous radial forearm may become handy in select cases.

A radial forearm flap can be raised as a faciocutaneous, facial (Fig. 29) or bone-containing flap. This flap is suitable in

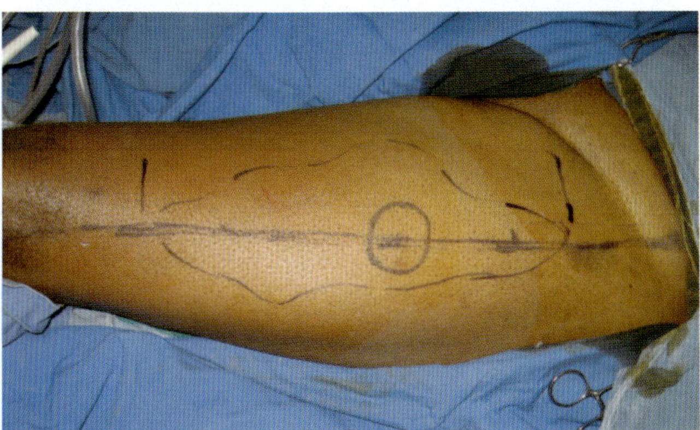

Fig. 26. Anterolateral thigh flap marked

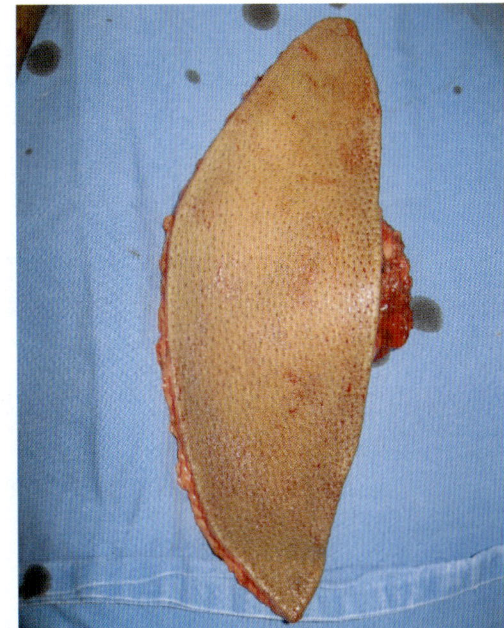

Fig. 27. Anterolateral thigh flap harvested

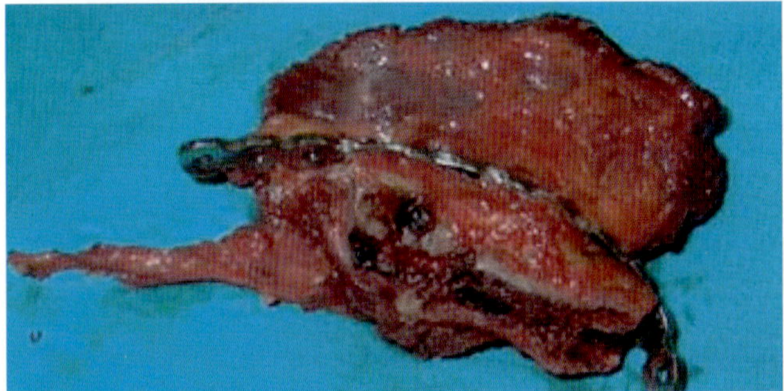

Fig. 28. DCIA flap harvested

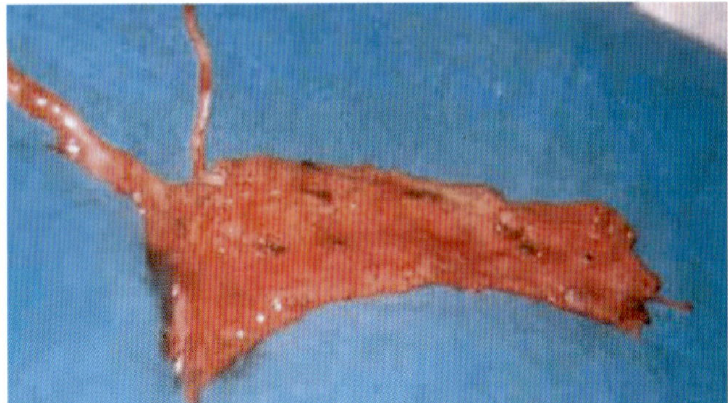

Fig. 29. Radial forearm facial flap

defects requiring soft and pliable tissue, such as defects of the tongue and cheek. It is also good in providing partial or full lumen reconstruction of pharyngeal defects. The availability of the bone is limited; hence its use in mandibular reconstruction is not common. The donor site morbidity is of concern, which has tarnished the reputation of this otherwise sturdy and safe free flap. This can be controlled to a great extent by suprafacial dissection as well as by utilizing the modified design suggested by Matev (Figs 30, 31, 32).

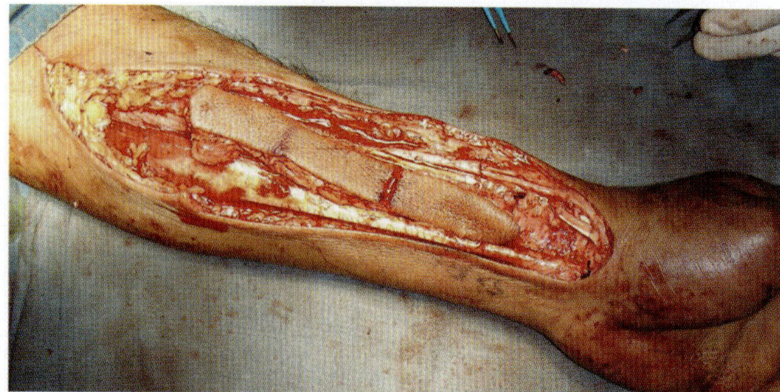

Fig. 30. The modified design of RFF

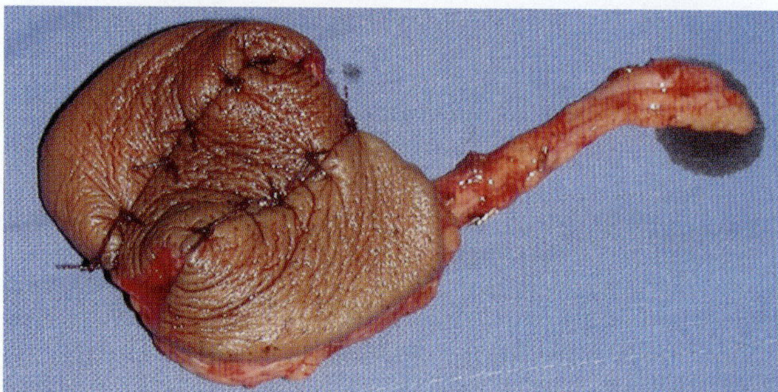

Fig. 31. Flap fashioned to form the tongue

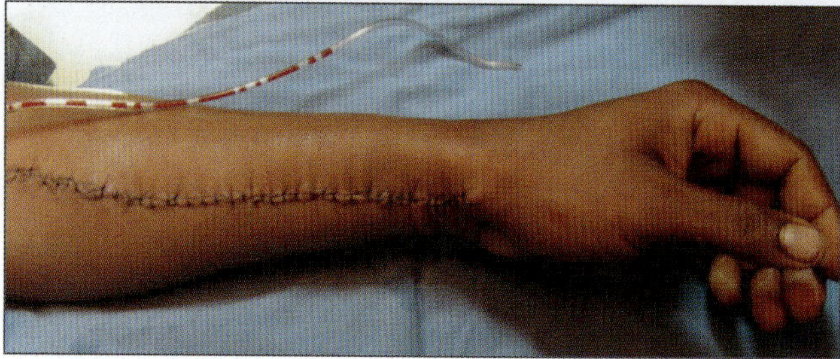

Fig. 32. Resultant scar in the forearm after harvesting the flap with the modified design

Site-wise indications

Reconstructive needs differ in various subsites of the head and neck. The suitability of using free flaps also differs accordingly.

Skull base defects

One of the foremost reasons why skull base excisions are safer, hence making it more practised, is the advent of free flaps to aid its reconstruction. Complications of dural leak, encephalocele and meningitis can be controlled to a great extent if free vascularized tissue is used. Rectus abdominis and anterolateral thigh flaps have been the common choices. Pedicled flaps are limited by their volume (temporalis) and reach (pectoralis major, latismus dorsi).

Maxillectomy defects

Reconstruction after maxillectomy is increasing in practice due to its advantages over obturator placement. Pedicled flaps lag behind badly when reconstruction of these complex three-dimensional defects is undertaken. Fibula, deep circumflex iliac artery DCIA and tensor facia lata–iliac crest (TFL-IC) (Fig. 33) flaps are more robust and suitable in these cases.

Mandibular reconstruction

No other areas of head and neck reconstruction have been as positively influenced by the advent of free flaps as the reconstruction of mandibular defects. Reconstruction with alloplastic materials, free bone grafts and pedicled flaps has been found to be unsatisfactory while reconstructing these defects. The main drawback of these methods is their poor ability to withstand the effects of radiation therapy either in the pre- or post-operative period. Free vascularized bone flaps have been found to be a dependable method and have become the method of choice for bone reconstruction. The exception of using soft tissue pedicled flaps would be the reconstruction of lateral mandibular defects in an oedentulous and elderly person where bony reconstruction is not mandatory. The free bone flaps used in this scenario would be fibula, DCIA or scapula. Figure 34 shows a fibula flap in position after mandibulectomy.

Oral cavity defects

Reconstruction of tongue and cheek defects need provision of a soft, thin and pliable epithelial surface to enable mobility to the reconstructed part. Thick flaps such as pectoralis major, temporalis or nasolabial flaps are ill-suited due to their bulk and lack of mobility. Free flaps such as radial forearm, lateral arm or thinned anterolateral thigh (ALT) flaps have become the optimal choices in cheek and tongue reconstruction. Figure 35 shows a tongue reconstructed using a radial forearm flap.

Laryngopharyngeal defects

Gastric pull-up has been the mainstay of reconstruction of full

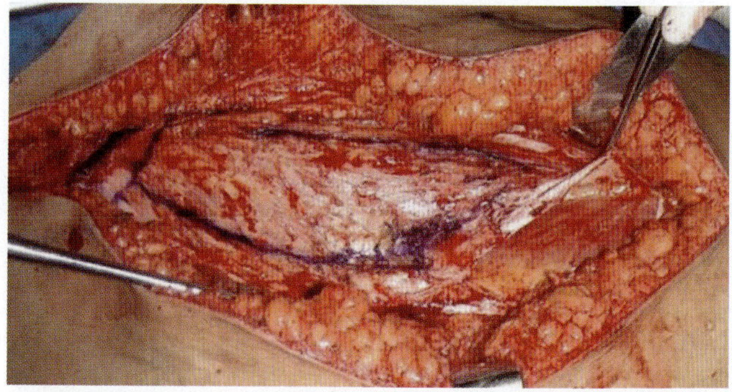

Fig. 33. Tensor facia lata–iliac crest (TFL-IC) flap for orbitomaxillary reconstruction

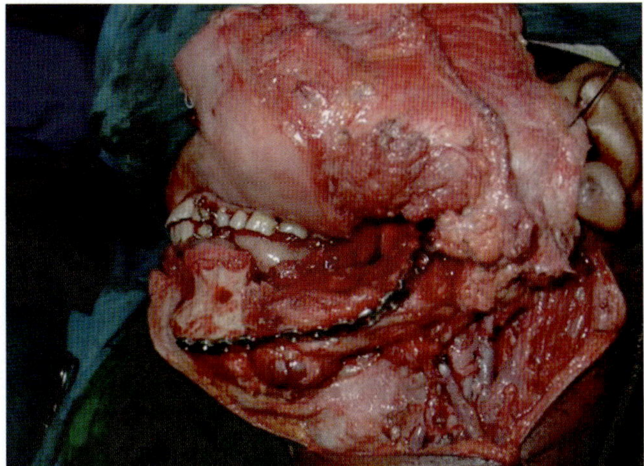

Fig. 34. A fibula flap in place for the resected mandible

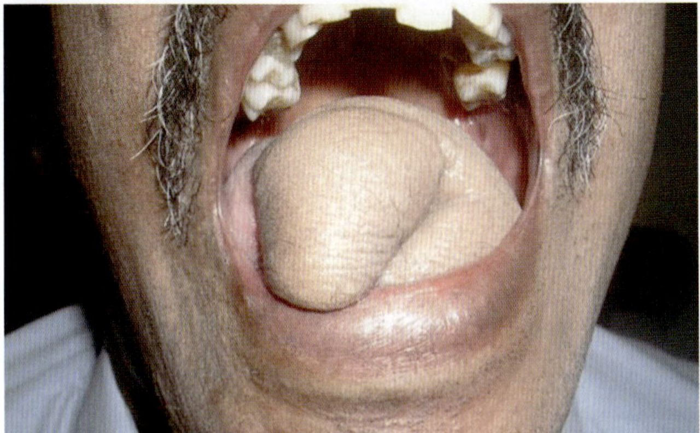

Fig. 35. Tongue reconstructed using a radial forearm flap

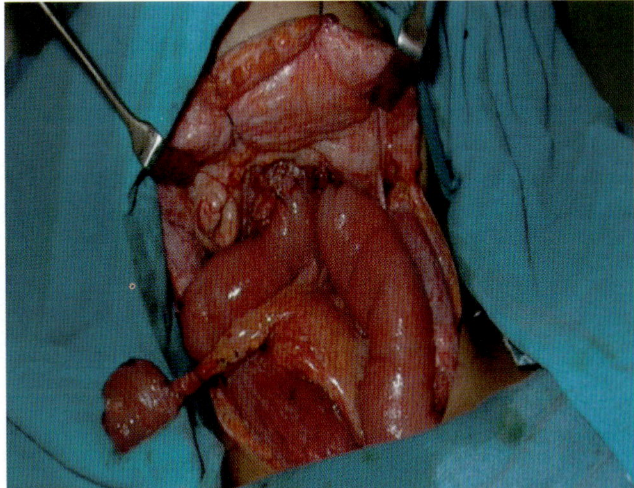

Fig. 36. Jejuna flap in place

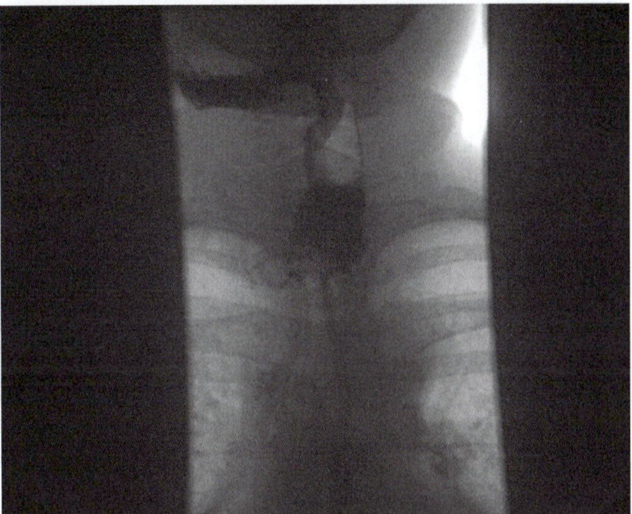

Fig. 37. Barium swallow through a reconstructed pharynx using the jejunum

luminal defects of the laryngopharynx. Even though effective, the procedure is associated with a very high morbidity as well as significant mortality due to extensive abdominal and thoracic manipulations. The dumping syndrome and poor quality of speech following a tracheogastric puncture also are negative points regarding gastric pull-up. Free tissue transfer has helped in reducing this morbidity and providing a good food passage with better speech rehabilitation. The flaps used include free jejunum (Figs 36, 37), tubed ALT or radial forearm skin flaps. The lower extent of the tumour will decide whether a free flap is a feasible alternative, since gastric pull-up has the advantage of removing the entire oesophagus in the resected specimen.

neck cancer surgery that adversely affect the success of free tissue transfer include the effects of radiation in patients of salvage surgery and the lack of recipient vessels in the neck due to the extent of resective surgery. The safety of free flaps in heavily irradiated fields has been proven.[37–39] Various methods have been described to overcome the problems of vessel depleted neck by the use of transposition of cephalic vein, use of transverse cervical vessels and vein grafts.

Complications and pitfalls

Free tissue transfer has become a very safe method with predictable success rates ranging from 90% to 98%.[37–39] To achieve uniform results, meticulous attention has to be paid during the stages of planning, execution and after-care. Besides the surgeon's experience, the availability of support staff of experienced anaesthesiologists, theatre and ICU personnel also contributes to successful outcomes. Factors in head and

Future directions

Developments continue to occur in microsurgery, which in turn affect head and neck reconstruction. A better understanding of the skin vascularity of flaps, evolution of super microsurgery and the possibility of using sutureless techniques in microvascular anastomosis will make the use of free flaps more effective and useful in head and neck reconstruction. Recent advances in osseo-integration have made functional rehabilitation of these patients a reality, which will improve with the advent of newer materials and techniques. Tissue engineering has made rapid strides and its integration with reconstructive surgery is set to revolutionize the field of reconstruction. Prelamination and prefabrication, transfer of suitable tissue engineered constructs and the use of bioinductive materials will have a considerable impact on the reconstruction of these complex defects.

References

1. Kaplan I. Reconstruction of a columella. *Br J Plast Surg* 1972;**25**:37.
2. Cameron RR. Nasolabial and cheek flaps. In: Straunch B, Vanconez LO, Hall-Findlay EJ (eds). *Grabb's encyclopedia of flaps.* 2nd ed. Philadelphia: Lippincott-Raven; 1998;**1**:56–61.
3. Kaluzinski, E Crasson F. Nasolabial flap reconstruction of the columella Rev. *Stomatol Chi Maxillofac* 2004;**105**:171.
4. Varghese BT, Sebastian P, Cherian MK, *et al*. Nasolabial flaps in oral reconstruction: An analysis of 224 cases. *Br J Plast Surg* 2001;**54**:499–503.
5. Kleintjes WG. Forehead anatomy: Arterial variations and venous link of the midline forehead flap. *J Plast Reconstr Aesthet Surg* 2007;**60**:593–606.
6. McGregor JA, Reid WH. The use of the temporal flap in the primary repair of full-thickness defects of the cheek. *Plast Reconstr Surg* 1966;**38**:1–9.
7. Chiarelli A, Forcignano R, Boatto D, *et al*. Reconstruction of the inner canthus region with a forehead muscle flap: A report on three cases. *Br J Plast Surg* 2001;**54**:248–52.
8. Watkinson JC, Gaze M, Wilson JA, *et al*. *Stell and Maran's head and neck surgery.* 4th ed. Oxford: Butterworth-Heinemann; 2000.
9. Little SC, Hughley BB, Park SS. Complications with forehead flaps in nasal reconstruction. *Laryngoscope* 2009;**119**:1093–9.
10. Blackwell KE, Buchbinder D, Biller HF, *et al*. Reconstruction of massive defects in the head and neck: The role of simultaneous distant and regional flaps. *Head Neck* 1997;**19**:620–8.
11. Andrews BT, McCulloch TM, Funk GF, *et al*. Deltopectoral flap revisited in the microvascular era: A single-institution 10-year experience. *Ann Otol Rhinol Laryngol* 2006;**115**:35–40.
12. Stewart IV CE, Urken ML. *Flaps and reconstructive surgery.* 2009; 193–205.
13. Chung-Ho Chen A, Gau-Tyan Lin, Yin-Chih Fu, *et al*. Comparison of deltopectoralis flap and free radial forearm flap in reconstruction after oral cancer ablation. *Oral Oncol* 2005;**41**:602–6.
14. Mortensen M, Genden EM. Role of the island deltopectoral flap in contemporary head and neck reconstruction. *Ann Otol Rhinol Laryngol* 2006;**115**:361–4.
15. Ariyan S. The pectoralis major myocutaneous flap. A versatile flap for reconstruction the head and neck. *Plast Reconstr Surg* 1979;**63**:73–81.
16. Baeeg Son, Lawsar W, Biller HF. An analysis of 133 pectoralis major myocutaneous flaps. *Plast Reconst Surg* 1982;**69**:460–9.
17. Coleman JJ. Recontruction of pharynx after resection for cancer, a comparison of methods. *Ann surg* 1989;**209**:554–61.
18. Shah JP, Haribhakti V, Loree TR, *et al*. Complication of the pectoralis major myocutaneous flap in head and neck reconstruction. *Ann J Surg* 1990;**160**:352–55.
19. Cuono CB, Ariyan S. Immediate reconstruction of a composite mendibular defect with a regional osteomusculocutaneous flap. *Plast Reconstr Surg* 1980;**65**:477.
20. Bertolti JA. Trapezius musculocutaneous island flap in the repair of major head and neck cancer. *Plast Reconstr Surg* 1980;**65**:16.
21. Horch RE, Doz P, Stark GB. The contralateral bilobed trapezius myocutaneous flap for closure of large defects of the dorsal neck permitting primary donor site closure. *Head Neck* 2000;**22**:513–19.
22. Haas F, Weiglein A. Trapezius flap. In: Wei FC, Mardini S (eds). *Flaps and Reconstructive Surgery.* Philadelphia: Saunders Elsevier; 2009:249–69.
23. Eutrell J W. Platysma myocutaneous flap for intra oral reconstruction. *Am J Surg* 1978;**136**:504.
24. Ariyan S. One stage reconstruction for defects of the mouth using a sternomastoid myocutaneous flap. *Plast Reconstr Surg 1979*;**63**:618–25.
25. Sebastian P, Cheriyan T, Ahmed I. Sternomastoid island myocutaneous flap for oral reconstruction. *Arch Otolaryngo Head and Neck Surg* 1994;**120**:629–32.
26. Glenwood A. Charles MD, Ronald C, *et al*. Sternocluidomastoid myocutaneous flap. *Larynyngoscope* 2009;**97**:970–4.
27. Bertolti JA. Trapezius musculocutaneous island flap in the repair of major head and neck cancer. *Plast Reconstr Surg* 1980;**65**:16.
28. Sebastian P, Thomas S, Varghese BT, *et al*. The submental island flap for reconstruction of intraoral defects in oral cancer patients. *Oral Oncol* 2008;**44**:1014–18.
29. Hanasono MM, Friel MT, Klem C, *et al*. Impact of reconstructive microsurgery in patients with advanced oral cavity cancers. *Head Neck* 2009;**31**:1289–96.
30. Schusterman MA, Miller MJ, Reece GP, *et al*. A single center's experience with 308 free flaps for repair of head and neck cancerdefects. *Plast Reconstr Surg* 1994;**93**:460–9.
31. Hidalgo DA, Disa JJ, Cordeiro PG, *et al*. A review of 716 consecutive free flaps for oncologic surgical defects: Refinement in donor-site selection and technique. *Plast Reconstr Surg* 1998;**102**:722–32.
32. Urken ML, Buchbinder D, Weinberg H, *et al*. Functional evaluation following microvascular oromandibular reconstruction of the oral cancer patient: A comparative study of reconstructed and non-reconstructed patients. *Laryngoscope* 1991;**101**:935–50.
33. Colangelo LA, Logemann JA, Pauloski BR, *et al*. T-stage and functional outcome in oral and oropharyngeal cancer patients. *Head Neck* 1996;**18**:259–68.
34. Sharma M, Iyer S, Kuriakose MA, *et al*. Functional reconstruction of near total glossectomy defects using composite gastro-omental-dynamic gracilis flaps. *J Plast Reconstr Aesthet Surg* 2009;**62**:1277–80. Epub 2008.
35. Tsue TT, Desyatnikova SS, Deleyiannis FWB, *et al*. Comparison of cost and function in reconstruction of the posterior oral cavity and oropharynx: Free vs Pedicled soft tissue transfer. *Arch Otolaryngol Head Neck Surg* 1997;**123**:731–7.
36. Chepaha DB, Annich G, Pynnonen MA, *et al*. Pectoralis major myocutaneous flap vs. revascularized free tissue transfer: Complications, gastrostomy tube dependence and hospitalization. *Arch Otolaryngol Head Neck Surg* 2004;**130**:181–6.
37. Kroll SS, Evans GRD, Goldberg D, *et al*. A comparison of resource costs for head and neck reconstruction with free and pectoralis major flaps. *Plast Reconstr Surg* 1997;**99**:1282–6.
38. Blackwell KE. Unsurpassed reliability of free flaps for head and neck reconstruction. *Arch Otolaryngol Head Neck Surg* 1999;**125**:295–9.
39. Wei FC, Demirkan F, Chen HC, *et al*. The outcome of failed free flaps in head and neck extremity reconstruction: What is next in the reconstructive ladder? *Plast Reconstr Surg* 2001;**108**:1154–60.
40. Eckardt A, Fokas K. Microsurgical reconstruction in the head and neck region: An 18-year experience with 500 consecutive cases. *J Craniomaxillofac Surg* 2003;**31**:197–201.

8

Management of cervical metastases

JOHANNES J. FAGAN

More than 90% of cancers of the head and neck are mucosal squamous cell carcinomas (SCCs) of the upper aerodigestive tract. Hence, this chapter will focus on the management of cervical metastases from SCCs.

Cervical metastases reduce the survival of patients with mucosal SCCs of the upper aerodigestive tract by approximately half.[1] The prognosis of patients with cervical metastases depends on *inter alia* the number of metastases,[2–5] the cervical level,[3,6,7,8] the tumour burden in the neck,[7,9,10] the presence of extracapsular spread (ECS),[3,4,7,10–13] whether the nodal metastases were resectable and whether the neck had previously been treated with surgery or irradiation.[6] These patients are also more likely to have distant metastases[7] and, possibly, are more prone to developing a recurrence of the primary tumour.[13] Patients with cervical metastasis may die from persistent or recurrent carcinoma in the neck, or from complications of treatment. Uncontrolled cancer metastasis to cervical nodes carries considerable morbidity. Surgical treatment of cervical metastases also has morbidity related principally to shoulder function. Hence, the management of the cervical lymphatics always requires careful consideration so that both over- and under-treatment are minimized.

Treating patients in developing countries presents its own unique challenges in terms of limited resources, limited availability of imaging and cytology modalities, false-positive results with PET scans in patients with tuberculous adenopathy, the availability of radiation therapy and chemotherapy, and frequently, unreliable patient follow-up. Hence doctors who treat patients with cancers of the head and neck need to adapt their diagnostic and therapeutic approaches to the neck by taking all such factors into account.

Surgical treatment of cervical metastases commenced in the 19th century. The first successful radical *en bloc* surgical dissection was performed in 1888 by Franciszek Jawdyński, a Polish surgeon. In the early 20th century George Crile recognized that excision of individual lymph nodes did not effect a cure and popularized radical *en bloc* neck dissection. *En bloc* dissection was designed to control cervical metastases by completely clearing the involved lymph nodes and associated neck structures from the base of the skull to the clavicle.[14] The classic operation involved *en bloc* resection of the cervical nodes, sternocleidomastoid muscle (SCM), internal jugular vein (IJV), spinal accessory nerve (XIn), submandibular gland and cervical plexus. The underlying principle was that once a metastasis had occurred to one node, subclinical metastases to other cervical nodes would possibly follow. Crile subsequently introduced the concept of modified neck dissection (MND), as he recognized that the spinal accessory nerve (SAN) could be preserved if there was no gross tumour close by.[14]

Anatomical studies by Suarez illustrated that cervical lymphatics are contained within well defined fascial spaces; and that investing, visceral and deep layers of cervical fascia envelop muscles, nerves, blood vessels, the thyroid gland and the aerodigestive tract, and thus partition these structures from the lymph node bearing tissues of the neck. He proposed that muscles, nerves and blood vessels could be preserved in neck dissections if the disease was limited, without adversely affecting regional control.[15] This initiated a change in the surgical approach to cervical metastases and the evolution of MND, which spared the IJV, sternocleidomastoid muscle (SCM) and SAN. Outcome studies have confirmed the efficacy of MND.[15,16]

An improved understanding of lymphatic drainage patterns based on the location of the primary cancer, and a quest to reduce morbidity of comprehensive neck dissections, subsequently led to the employment of selective neck dissection (SND), either electively for the N0 neck, or for clinically apparent, but limited, cervical metastases.

Numerous imaging modalities, such as ultrasound (US), US-guided fine-needle aspiration cytology (USGFNAC), CT, MRI and FDG PET scanning, as well as sentinel node mapping, were subsequently employed to improve accuracy of nodal staging, and to improve selection of patients who might benefit from neck dissection. However, because some of these diagnostic techniques are expensive and/or labour-intensive, and because their sensitivity to detect subclinical metastases is not always deemed adequate, many surgeons rely on elective neck dissection (END), both as a staging and as a therapeutic tool.

Chemoradiation is the preferred treatment for cervical metastases originating from nasopharyngeal carcinoma, and it is favoured by some surgeons for advanced oropharyngeal SCC, with surgery reserved for salvage. Radiation is also known to be an effective treatment for subclinical metastases,[17] and is an important adjunct to neck dissection in patients with markers of increased regional recurrence, such as ECS or multiple cervical metastases.

Anatomy of cervical lymphatics

Cervical nodes are part of a continuum, with parotid, occipital, facial, parapharyngeal and retropharyngeal / prevertebral nodes present superiorly, and axillary and mediastinal nodes inferiorly. The cervical lymphatics are enveloped by deep and superficial cervical fasciae. Lymph nodes do not occur within the muscles of the neck or within the carotid sheath. From a practical and clinical perspective, cervical lymphatics are divided into six 3-dimensional lymphbearing levels called Levels I–VI. The Committee for Neck Dissection Classification, American Head and Neck Society, refined the previous classification of cervical levels in 2008 (Fig. 1, Table 1).[18,19]

Patterns of lymphatic drainage

The lymphatic drainage pathways for cancers of the head and neck have been documented by retrospective clinicopathological studies.[20-22] Cancers involving midline structures naturally have bilateral drainage, as do cancers of the soft palate, base of tongue, supraglottic larynx and medial wall of the pyriform fossa.[23] Although lymphatic drainage patterns are generally predictable, they may be altered by previous surgery or radiation therapy, or when there is extensive nodal metastasis. The anterior oral cavity, including the oral tongue, may exhibit skip metastases/fast

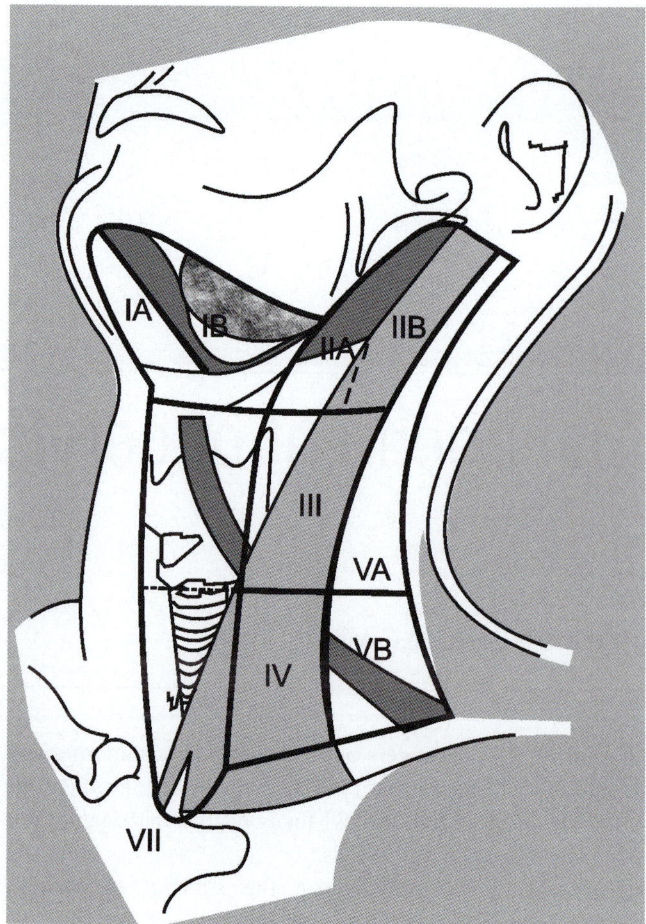

Fig. 1. Anatomical diagram depicting the boundaries of the six neck levels and three neck sublevels (adapted from reference 19)

tracking to Level IV of the neck on account of lymphatic channels bypassing the nodes in the higher cervical levels.[22] Lymphoscintigraphy may occasionally reveal unexpected contralateral lymphatic drainage that is not in keeping with conventional drainage patterns.

Neck dissection

Neck dissection refers to surgical removal of lymph-node-bearing tissue from the neck. The superficial boundary of neck dissection is represented by the investing layer of cervical fascia that lines the deep aspect of the platysma muscle. The deep boundary is formed by the deep and visceral layers of cervical fascia. In 1991, the American Academy of Otolaryngology-Head and Neck Surgery standardized the terminology for neck dissection and classified neck dissection as radical, modified radical, extended radical and selective.[24] Radical neck dissection (RND) refers to *en bloc* resection of lymph-bearing tissue in Levels I–V, SCM, IJV and SAN. MND entails resection of lymph-bearing-tissue from Levels I–V, with preservation of one or more non-lymphatic structures, i.e. SAN, IJV and SCM. It is common practice to

Table 1. Anatomical boundaries of cervical levels

Level	Anatomical boundaries			
	Superior	**Inferior**	**Anterior (Medial)**	**Posterior (Lateral)**
1A	Symphysis of mandible	Body of hyoid	Anterior belly of contralateral digastric muscle	Anterior belly of ipsilateral digastric muscle
1B	Body of mandible	Posterior belly of digastric muscle	Anterior belly of digastric muscle	Posterior border of submandibular salivary gland
2A	Skull base	Horizontal plane at inferior border of hyoid bone	Posterior border of submandibular salivary gland	Vertical plane defined by SAN
2B	Skull base	Horizontal plane at inferior border of hyoid bone	Vertical plane defined by SAN	Posterior border of sternocleidomastoid muscle
3	Horizontal plane at inferior border of hyoid bone	Horizontal plane at inferior border of cricoid cartilage	Sternohyoid muscle or medial aspect of common carotid artery when viewing the neck in an axial plane radiologically	Posterior border of sternocleidomastoid muscle or sensory branches of cervical plexus
4	Horizontal plane at inferior border of cricoid cartilage	Clavicle		
5A	Apex of convergence of sternocleidomastoid and trapezius muscles	Horizontal plane at inferior border of cricoid cartilage	Posterior border of sternocleidomastoid muscle or sensory branches of cervical plexus	Anterior border of trapezius muscle
5B	Horizontal plane at inferior border of cricoid cartilage	Clavicle		
6	Hyoid bone	Suprasternal	Common carotid artery	Common carotid artery
7	Suprasternal	Innominate artery		

refer to preservation of the SAN as MND Type 1, the SAN and IJV as MND Type 2, and SAN, IJV and SCM as MND Type 3. SND refers to resection of selected cervical lymph-bearing levels (Fig. 2). SNDs that are frequently performed include supraomohyoid (Levels I, II, III), lateral (Levels II, III, IV), posterolateral (Levels II, III, IV, V, suboccipital and retroauricular nodes) and anterior (Level VI). Extended neck dissection is a RND with resection of lymphatic and/or non-lymphatic structures not normally included in a RND, such as parotid, suboccipital, paratracheal or mediastinal nodes. Non-lymphatic structures might include muscle, nerve, skin, carotid artery and visceral structures.

The choice of neck dissection should take into account a number of factors, such as the clinical stage of cervical metastasis, operative findings, prior treatment of the neck, the site of the primary tumour, the need for donor vessels for free tissue transfer flaps, reliability of follow up and surgical bias. Although some authorities advocate SND for selected N+ cancer, it is generally reserved for the clinically N0 neck.

Morbidity associated with neck dissection includes the 'shoulder syndrome' (shoulder weakness, deformity, pain, 'winging' of the scapula, and adhesive capsulitis), cosmetic deformity resulting from loss of the SCM and anaesthesia in the cutaneous distribution of the cervical plexus. Although MND encompasses the same lymphatic levels (1–5) of the neck as RND, it reduces morbidity by preserving non-lymphatic structures, such as the IJV, SCM and SAN. The SAN innervates the SCM and trapezius muscles. The superior part of the trapezius muscle is innervated by the SAN, whereas the inferior and middle parts also receive branches from C3 and C4. The SAN also receives contributions from one or two branches from C2 and C3 in Level 5. It is possible that these cervical contributions may have proprioceptive and motor functions, but there is inadequate clinical evidence

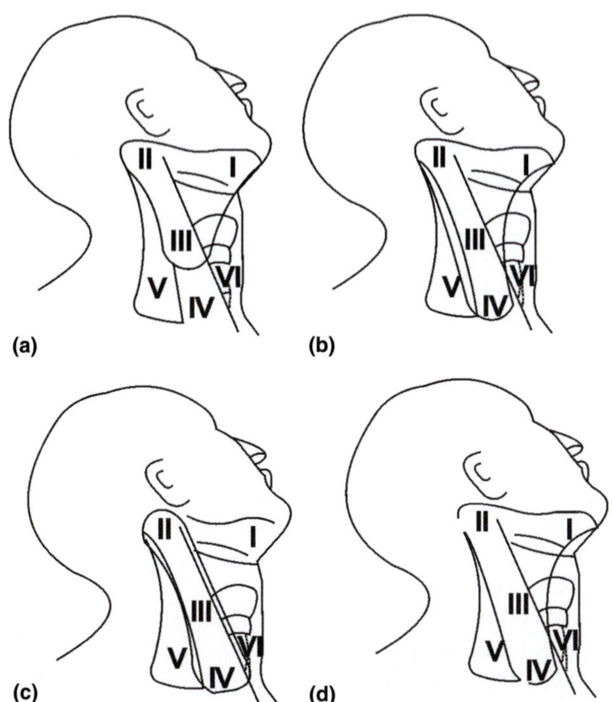

Fig. 2. Types of neck dissection: (a) Supraomohyoid: Levels I–III, (b) Levels I–IV; (c) Lateral: Levels II–IV; (d) Radical/Modified: Levels I–V

that preserving these branches contributes to preservation of shoulder function.[25] Leipzig *et al.* reported shoulder drop and/or pain in 60% of RND patients, 50% of patients that had undergone MND Type 1 with SAN preservation, and 30% of patients that had had the SAN, IJV and SCM preserved (SND and MND Type 3).[26] SAN dysfunction after dissection of only the proximal segment of the nerve, as in supraomohyoid and lateral SND, may result from stretching of the nerve during dissection and delivery of the supraspinal accessory lymph node pad of Level 2B, or it may be a consequence of devascularization of the nerve from ligation of the occipital artery.[26] Therefore, even patients that have only had an SND should have their shoulder function monitored, as they may require physiotherapy to minimize morbidity. Preservation of the SCM (MND type 3) is of questionable benefit because, although the muscle still contracts, significant SCM atrophy occurs, particularly in the caudal and middle portions of the muscle. This is thought to be related to damage to the segmental blood supply in these parts of the muscle, as well as injury to SAN innervation.[27]

The N0 neck

How best to manage the N0 neck is a controversial topic. Management varies from centre to centre and from country to country. Occult nodal metastasis will generally become clinically apparent if left untreated, as the incidence of histologically positive nodes in electively treated necks corresponds with the nodal conversion rate of untreated N0 necks.[5] Understaging, and hence under-treatment of the occult positive neck, is therefore likely to adversely affect regional control and survival. The central issue pertaining to the various staging modalities is the sensitivity, or the false-negative rate, in the N0 neck. Specificity only assumes importance when the treatment of the false-positive neck has significant associated morbidity.

It is generally accepted that greater than 15%–20% incidence of occult cervical metastasis necessitates elective treatment, as the benefits are then considered to outweigh the morbidity of neck dissection. Yet it does mean that 80%–85% of necks might be treated unnecessarily, and that those that have been electively irradiated might be compromised in the future, should a second primary tumour be diagnosed within the irradiated field. The following points need to be considered when deciding on how to manage the N0 neck:

- *What is the likelihood of occult metastases being present?*
  The likelihood of occult metastases being present depends on tumour site, T-stage, depth/thickness,[28] presence of perineural invasion (PNI)[29] and the sensitivity of the method employed to evaluate the neck. Twelve per cent of tumour-positive neck dissections contain only micrometastases (<2 mm), and of clinically N0 necks with occult metastases, 25% contain only micrometastases.[30]

- *What diagnostic means are employed to evaluate the neck?*
  The N0 neck may be evaluated clinically, or by US, USGFNAC, CT, MRI, PET scan, sentinel node mapping, or intra-operatively by the surgeon, with or without frozen section. END provides the opportunity for pathological evaluation and for staging of the neck. It should be noted that studies of the accuracy of imaging for cervical metastases use histopathological staging of the neck dissection as the reference point, and do not take cognisance of the presence of micrometastases, which would reduce sensitivity.[30,31] In centres that routinely employ END in patients with >15% chance of having occult nodal metastasis, diagnostic imaging is of questionable benefit and is likely to change management of the neck only if nodes are detected outside the expected lymphatic drainage area, e.g. the contralateral neck or retropharyngeal nodes.

  CT scanning, MRI and US rely principally on nodal size as a criterion for malignancy. There is, however, a trade-off between sensitivity and specificity when reliance is placed on nodal diameter alone, i.e. the smaller the nodal diameter used as a criterion for malignancy, the greater the sensitivity but the lower the specificity, and vice versa. A minimum nodal size criterion for a malignancy of 10 mm is generally recommended. Yet the majority of lymph node metastases in the N0 neck are smaller than 10 mm[32] and non-malignant nodes may vary in size between 2 mm and 2 cm.[33] Central necrosis is another marker of malignancy. Although 74% of lymph node metastases have central necrosis, this percentage is much reduced with smaller nodes found in the N0 neck.[32] Central necrosis may also be confused with caseous necrosis of tuberculous lymphadenopathy.

  USGFNAC has overcome problems relating to specificity associated with CT, MRI and ultrasound, and has a specificity approaching 100%.[34] Yet the sensitivity of USGFNAC in the N0 neck ranges between 44% and 73%.[30]

  Tuberculous nodes have similar FDG PET features to metastases. Specificity of PET scanning for cervical metastasis therefore presents problems in countries where tuberculosis is endemic, and the diagnosis of metastatic disease should be confirmed by cytological/pathological examination before the initiation of a definitive treatment.[35]

  The role of sentinel node biopsy, although a well established technique for staging breast cancer and the N0 neck with melanoma, still needs to be elucidated with SCC of the upper aerodigestive tract, and studies are ongoing.

- *Is electively treating the N0 neck likely to improve regional control and/or survival?*
  Intuitively, treating the N0 neck before cervical metastases become clinically apparent should improve patient outcome for the following reasons: larger metastases are more

likely to exhibit ECS; the metastases are more likely to be confined to the upper neck; and the tumour burden is likely to diminish. Van den Brekel reported an 18% failure rate in the neck, with a 71% salvage rate, for early oral cavity carcinomas staged and followed by USGFNAC.[32] One could postulate that END might have avoided some of these failures and improved overall outcome.

ECS is an important prognostic indicator of regional and distant failure and survival, and timely identification of patients with ECS is important as they may benefit from adjuvant radiation and chemotherapy.[36] The likelihood of ECS parallels nodal diameter, and occurs with 23% of nodes <1 cm, 44% with nodes measuring 1–2 cm, 53% with 2–3 cm, and 74% with >3 cm.[7] If left untreated, small nodes will increase in size and may subsequently manifest ECS. Should imaging alone be relied upon to decide on who requires elective treatment, a significant number of patients with ECS would remain untreated until cervical metastases become clinically apparent. On the other hand, by intervening early in the course of the disease, END may theoretically prevent progression to ECS, and permit earlier detection of patients with ECS who may benefit from adjuvant therapy.

Yet, clinical evidence to support END is tenuous. Lydiatt *et al.* reported a survival benefit for END in a non-randomized study of carcinoma of the oral tongue.[37] Two prospective randomized studies of END versus watchful waiting reported no significant survival benefit.[38,39] In the study by Vandenbrouck *et al.*, 45% of deaths were unrelated to regional failure.[38] The study by Fakih *et al.* did not control for ECS, tumour margins and contralateral regional failure, and median follow up was only 20 months.[39] These studies are therefore flawed, and neither study had adequate power to detect a significant difference in outcome.[40,41]

- *Does the possibility of improved oncological outcome outweigh the morbidity and cost of electively treating the N0 neck?*
- *Does the neck need to be explored as part of the oncological/reconstructive procedure for the primary tumour?*
When free tissue transfer flaps are utilized to reconstruct oral or pharyngeal defects, then the neck, usually Levels I and IIa, have to be dissected anyway to do the microvascular anastomosis to the internal jugular vein and, usually, either the facial or superior thyroid artery. It makes sense to do at least a supraomohyoid neck dissection in such cases. Similarly, the neck has to be entered and the SCM resected to provide space for pectoralis major or latissimus dorsi flaps. It is sensible to do a MND under such circumstances.

- *Does the primary tumour need to be irradiated?*
Single modality therapy is always desirable in terms of convenience and cost. In patients in whom the primary is to be treated with radiation therapy and the neck needs to be treated electively, the high-risk N0 neck may be treated with radiation therapy.[17]

- *Is the patient likely to present for regular follow up?*
Patient follow up may be unreliable for socio-economic reasons, particularly in developing world communities. For these patients it may be advisable to lower the threshold for END.

- *How will the neck be monitored at follow up?*
Should the neck not be electively treated, then follow up should ensure early detection of cervical metastases while it is still operable. However, even with regular follow up by USGFNAC in a controlled study situation, many patients present with inoperable cervical metastases.[32] Therefore, unless a very intensive follow-up regime is possible, a more proactive approach to the N0 neck is warranted.

- *What is the level of surgical expertise, availability and quality of irradiation, and physician and patient bias?*
Ultimately, the management of the N0 neck should be individualized according to patient factors and bias, as well as the level of surgical expertise, availability of theatre time, availability and quality of irradiation therapy and the philosophy of the oncology team.

- *What type of END should be performed?*
Neck dissections, either elective or therapeutic, should include at least the cervical levels that are statistically most likely to contain metastases. Although practices do vary, Table 2 outlines an approach to the choice of elective neck dissection.

- *When should an SND be converted to a comprehensive neck dissection?*
A possible dilemma for the surgeon is whether to convert

Table 2. Commonly performed SNDs

Location of primary cancer	Levels of neck	Type of SND
Oral cavity (except anterior tongue and floor of mouth), skin cancers of lateral and anterior face	I, II, III	Supraomohyoid
Anterior tongue, floor of mouth	I, II, III, IV	Anterolateral
Oropharynx, larynx, parotid	II, III, IV	Lateral
Hypopharynx, subglottis	II, III, IV, VI	
Thyroid	VI	Anterior
Skin cancers of posterior and postauricular scalp	II, III, IV, V	Posterolateral

an SND to a MND when lymphadenopathy is encountered at the time of END. A surgeon's ability to accurately determine whether suspicious nodes represent metastatic disease is not very good (sensitivity 44%, specificity 63%), although adding frozen section improves sensitivity to 71%.[36] In a study in a developing world setting in which the lymphadenopathy may have been due to previously untreated dental and tonsillar infections, HIV and tuberculosis, the sensitivity and specificity of intra-operative staging of the N0 neck were reported as 72% and 33%, respectively.[42] Although incorporating a frozen section into the intra-operative assessment would not improve sensitivity unless nodes are sampled, which would otherwise not have been considered to be metastatic, the frozen section should improve specificity. Therefore, when cervical nodes are discovered at the time of END, histological (frozen section) confirmation of the presence of cervical metastasis should ideally be obtained before converting an END to a therapeutic comprehensive neck dissection with its attendant morbidity.[36,43]

- *Pathologically N+ END*
  Pathological examination of a SND specimen may reveal cervical metastases. This raises the dilemma whether the patient should undergo completion MND or whether the undissected levels of the neck should be irradiated, or whether the neck should simply be closely followed. In a patient who requires radiation for the primary tumour, or because of the number of metastases present, or the ECS status of the cervical nodes, it may be appropriate for the radiation to include the undissected levels in the neck.

The N+ neck

Clinically apparent cervical lymph node metastases are generally treated with a neck dissection, with adjuvant therapy reserved for selected cases. Neck dissection is inadequate when employed as sole treatment for patients with advanced disease or with metastasis with adverse histological features, such as ECS and perineural invasion.[29] Hence, a combination of surgery and radiation therapy is required for such patients. Cervical metastases from a nasopharyngeal carcinoma respond well to chemoradiation therapy, and neck dissection is indicated only when radiation therapy has controlled the primary, but there are persistent or recurrent cervical nodes. Similarly, advanced oropharyngeal carcinoma, particularly HPV+ cases, appear to respond favourably to chemoradiation.[44]

Specificity of clinical staging of N+ neck

Palpable cervical nodes in patients with a primary cancer of the upper aerodigestive tract are assumed to be metastases. Some surgeons consider patients with bilateral cervical metastases to be incurable. Therefore, specificity of clinical palpation of enlarged cervical lymph nodes is important, as a false-positive diagnosis of cervical metastasis may, on the one hand, lead to an unnecessary comprehensive neck dissection, but on the other hand may deprive a patient with bilateral non-malignant nodal hypertrophy of the opportunity to be cured. Cervical nodes of up to 2 cm are found in normal adults.[33] False-positive rates for cervical metastases of 20%,[33] 22%,[6] and 31%[45] have been reported for patients with squamous cancer of the upper aerodigestive tract with palpable cervical nodes, and a 21% false-positive rate for patients with clinically N1 and N2 supraglottic carcinoma.[46] Even with nodes of >3 cm, a false-positive rate of 17% was reported, although all fixed nodes were malignant.[6] Enlarged, non-cancerous nodes are more likely in cancer patients with poor oral hygiene, concurrent tuberculosis, and with HIV. Although specificity may be improved by use of fine-needle aspiration cytology (FNAC) or ultrasound-guided FNAC, sampling error may still yield false-negative results.

Preoperative cytological or histological confirmation of a suspected cervical metastasis is generally advisable when palpable nodes occur outside the normal lymphatic drainage area of the primary tumour, when a primary tumour cannot be found, when there has been a long time-interval between the treatment of a tumour and detection of cervical adenopathy, or when doubt exists about the malignant nature of the nodes. Excision biopsy of a lymph node for histological examination does not appear to be deleterious, provided the incision is placed along incision lines of a neck dissection and the neck is appropriately treated with irradiation, in case there was tumour spillage or an incisional nodal biopsy had been done.[47–50]

Type of neck dissection

The choice of neck dissection is influenced by a number of factors, such as clinical stage of the neck, intra-operative findings, prior treatment of the neck, the site of the primary tumour and surgical bias. Comprehensive neck dissection (MND types 1/2/3, or RND) is the standard of care for the clinically N+ neck. RND is rarely required, and both the SAN and IJV can generally be preserved to reduce morbidity related to shoulder function and facial swelling. Sparing Level V of the neck to reduce the shoulder syndrome is debatable. However, 5%–10% of patients with oro- and hypo-pharyngeal carcinoma (and less frequently with laryngeal and oral cavity carcinoma) undergoing comprehensive neck dissection have histological evidence of nodes in Level V.[21,51,52] This might be an underestimation as these studies did not employ immunohistochemistry to look for micrometastases. Some authorities advocate SND for selected patients with cervical metastases.[53–56]

Cystic cervical metastases

Cystic nodal metastases typically occur with primary cancers of the oropharynx, papillary carcinoma of the thyroid gland, carcinoma of the oesophagus and SCC of the skin. The diagnosis is not uncommonly made when an unsuspecting surgeon removes a suspected branchial cyst. Cystic metastases may grow rapidly, and appear overnight. The differential diagnosis also includes a tuberculous cold abscess, and hydatid, thyroglossal duct and thymic cysts. Cystic metastases are usually well circumscribed and surrounded by a fibrous capsule. Unlike metastases that undergo cystic degeneration, the fluid aspirate of cystic metastases is thin and straw coloured, and may later become thicker and brown or haemorrhagic. Unlike excellent sensitivity for FNAC of solid cervical metastases, FNAC of cystic metastases has reported sensitivities of only 33%–80%.[57] A positive result for HPV-16 on *in situ* hybridization of the aspirate is suggestive of an oropharyngeal primary.[57,58] If FNAC is unhelpful, and the primary cancer is not apparent, then the neck node should be excised. If it is proven to be cancerous, then panendoscopy and tonsillectomy, and guided biopsies of the base of tongue, are required; or a PET scan may be employed to look for a primary cancer in the oropharynx.

The N+ neck with adverse histological features

Perineural invasion, ECS and vascular invasion are associated with an adverse prognosis.[4] PNI is associated with increased risk of local recurrence and reduced survival.[29] Adjuvant therapy should be considered in all such cases.

The contralateral N0 neck

For the reasons previously discussed, and even though its efficacy has not been subjected to a properly designed prospective randomized trial, contralateral END or irradiation should be considered for midline tumours and tumours with bilateral lymphatic drainage, such as cancers of the base of the tongue, soft palate, supraglottic larynx and medial wall of the pyriform fossa.

Bilateral nodes and the second jugular vein

Jones reported that survival of patients with nodes <6 cm was not affected by laterality, whereas it was for patients with massive nodes.[59] Therefore, bilateral mobile nodes should not preclude patients from treatment with curative intent. Simultaneous ligation of both IJVs causes venous congestion and oedema of the face and neck, raised intracranial pressure, and syndrome of inappropriate antidiuretic hormone secretion (SIADH). When both IJVs are infiltrated with carcinoma, the therapeutic options are to stage the second neck dissection, or to proceed with bilateral IJV resection, with or without IJV reconstruction. The IJV may be reconstructed with the saphenous vein, a segment of the contralateral (resected) IJV, polytetrafluoroethylene, or the external jugular vein.

The carotid artery

Adherence to, or invasion of, the carotid artery is associated with a poor prognosis.[60] Invasion of the carotid sheath is clinically suspected when nodes are fixed in the vertical axis, but mobile in the transverse axis of the neck, and by the presence of vagus nerve paralysis. US, CT and MRI scans may be helpful in evaluating the degree of carotid artery involvement.

If <180° of the carotid artery circumference is involved, then peeling the tumour off the artery in a subadvential plane should be considered,[60] even though stripping the tumour off the artery does not provide adequate oncological margins, and may be complicated by carotid artery blow-out.

Invasion of the external carotid artery can be simply managed by resection of the involved arterial segment. The options for common or internal carotid artery invasion are: No treatment, debulking with adjuvant therapy, or irradiation therapy; for carotid encasement, carotid artery resection with or without revascularization may be considered. Carotid artery resection and ligation has high rates of neurological complications (45%) and mortality (31%–41%). Carotid artery resection and ligation has significant risks of neurological complications and mortality. Snyderman reported that carotid artery resection was associated with a 2-year disease-free survival of 22%.[61] Cerebral blood flow studies before surgery might identify patients who will benefit from revascularization.

Fixed nodes

The meaning of the term 'fixed node' varies from clinician to clinician. Reports of treatment outcome are, therefore, subject to selection bias. Patients with fixed nodes have a poor prognosis.[1] This is probably due to the association of fixed nodes with the presence of ECS, and incomplete resections. Some patients may still be cured or palliated with surgery and/or radiation therapy.[62] A fixed mass may be resectable, depending on the anatomical structure it is attached to, e.g. tumours fixed to the mandible, larynx, sternocleidomastoid and prevertebral muscles; and mastoid process can be resected with a margin of normal tissue. Postoperative radiation therapy is essential to treat a microscopic residual tumour. Stell reported a 5-year survival rate of 15% for patients treated with surgery and postoperative radiation therapy.[62] Radiation therapy followed by salvage surgery (7% survival at 2 years) did not significantly improve survival compared with untreated patients (3% survival at 1 year).[62] The concept of preoperative irradiation to 'make an inoperable tumour operable' by reducing tumour size and improving tumour mobility is therefore questionable. Cutaneous involvement does not preclude surgery, as long-term survival has been reported with wide resection of carcinoma invading skin.[62,63] Postoperative radiation therapy should be administered to the surrounding skin as recurrence frequently occurs in the surrounding skin, possibly due to involvement of subdermal lymphatics.

Retropharyngeal nodes

Tumours situated in the nasopharynx, soft palate and lateral and posterior walls of the oropharynx and hypopharynx may metastasize to retropharyngeal nodes. Although clinically apparent retropharyngeal nodes can be resected, lymphadenectomy is unlikely to be complete. Hence, such patients should have the pharyngeal lymphatic plexus irradiated.

Unknown primary

This refers to the situation when a cervical metastasis is diagnosed, but a primary carcinoma is not found. The location of the node may point to the most likely location of the primary tumour. A cystic and/or HPV-positive node is suggestive of an oropharyngeal carcinoma. The detection rate with FDG PET of the primary tumour does not exceed 25%.[64] Panendoscopy and guided biopsies of the nasopharynx, base of tongue, hypopharynx and tonsillectomy may therefore be required to attempt to identify the primary tumour. Although there is some debate about whether and to what extent to treat potential primary sites with radiation, the principles of treating the neck are the same as for the other SCC metastases.[64]

Neck dissection after chemoradiation

The management of the post-chemoradiation neck, suspected of possibly harbouring persistent cervical metastases, is still evolving; and no consensus exists on the need for neck dissection. A watchful, waiting approach, with surgery for recurrence, reduces the therapeutic efficacy of surgery, whereas the morbidity of surgical treatment increases. Early neck dissection of patients at high risk of nodal recurrence provides an opportunity for regional control. Some centres rely on CT, MRI and/or PET evidence to determine the presence of persistent cervical metastatic disease, whereas others perform planned neck dissections 4–12 weeks after completion of radiation. How extensive neck dissections should be is a matter of debate.[65]

Salvage neck dissection

Long-term survival in patients with recurrence in the neck after

comprehensive neck dissection is <5%.[66] Tumours that recur appear to be biologically more aggressive, although inadequate clearance of lymph-bearing tissue may also account for the recurrence. RND or extended RND is generally performed for recurrence. Previous skin incisions should be excised. Radiation damage may necessitate resurfacing of the neck with regional or free flaps, particularly if a second course of adjuvant irradiation (external beam or brachytherapy) is to be employed.[67] In patients with fixed nodes that are to have salvage surgery following previous irradiation, adjuvant therapy should be planned before surgery, as such patients may benefit from interstitial irradiation.[67,68] Nodes fixed to the skin should be resected in continuity with the affected skin. Frequently, a regional or free flap will be required to replace resected skin.

Adjuvant radiation therapy/chemotherapy

Neck dissection alone is an effective treatment for patients with N1 and limited N2 disease without ECS, but has limited value in patients with multiple cervical metastases, ECS, N3 disease, fixed nodal metastasis and carotid or perineural invasion. Such patients require postoperative radiation therapy and/or chemotherapy. Postoperative radiation therapy has been shown to reduce the recurrence rate in patients with multiple cervical metastases or ECS. Postoperative chemoradiation may improve survival of patients with ECS by treating systemic metastases.[69]

Palliative treatment of the N+ neck

If left untreated, cervical metastasis may ultimately ulcerate through skin, erode into major blood vessels, and may cause brachial plexus and other neuropathies, thoracic inlet syndrome and obstruction of the upper aerodigestive tract. Therefore, patients with distant metastases, and those considered to have incurable regional cervical nodal metastases should be carefully considered for palliative treatment. Since the aim of such treatment would be to maximize the quality of life, the morbidity and mortality of treatment needs to be carefully weighed against the potential benefits of treatment. Treatment options include surgery, external beam radiation, brachytherapy, chemotherapy, or combinations thereof. Patients should be evaluated and managed by a team that includes a surgeon, a medical oncologist, a radiotherapist, a dietitian and a social worker.

References

1. Myers EN, Fagan JJ. Treatment of the N+ neck in squamous cell carcinoma of the upper aerodigestive tract. *Otolaryngol Clin North Am* 1998;**31**:671–86.
2. DeSanto LW, Holt JJ, Beahrs OH, *et al.* Neck dissection: Is it worthwhile? *Laryngoscope* 1982;**92**:502–9.
3. Kalnins IK, Leonard AG, Sako K, *et al.* Correlation between

prognosis and degree of lymph node involvement in carcinoma of the oral cavity. *Am J Surg* 1977;**134**:450–4.

4. Olsen KD, Caruso M, Foote RL, *et al*. Primary head and neck cancer: Histopathologic predictors of recurrence after neck dissection in patients with lymph node involvement. *Arch Otolaryngol Head Neck Surg* 1994;**120**:1370–4.

5. Snow GB, Patel P, Leemans CR, *et al*. Management of cervical lymph nodes in patients with head and neck cancer. *Eur Arch Otorhinolaryngol* 1992;**249**:187–94.

6. Grandi C, Alloisio M, Moglia D, *et al*. Prognostic significance of lymphatic spread in head and neck carcinomas: Therapeutic implications. *Head Neck Surg* 1985;**8**:67–73.

7. Leemans CR, Tiwari R, Nauta JJP, *et al*. Regional lymph node involvement and its significance in the development of distant metastases in head and neck carcinoma. *Cancer* 1993;**71**:452–6.

8. Van den Brekel MW, Snow GB. Assessment of lymph node metastases in the neck. *Oral Oncol, Eur J Cancer* 1994;**30B**:88–92.

9. Ellis ER, Mendenhall WM, Rao PV, *et al*. Does node location affect the incidence of distant metastases in head and neck carcinoma? *Int J Radiation Oncol Biol Phys* 1989;**17**: 293–7.

10. Grandi C, Mingardo M, Guzzo M, *et al*. Salvage surgery of cervical recurrences after neck dissection or radiotherapy. *Head Neck* 1993;**15**:292–5.

11. Johnson JT, Barnes EL, Myers EN, *et al*. The extracapsular spread of tumors in cervical node metastases. *Arch Otolaryngol* 1981;**107**: 725–9.

12. Johnson JT, Myers EN, Bedetti CD, *et al*. Cervical lymph node metastases: Incidence and implications of extracapsular carcinoma. *Arch Otolaryngol* 1985;**111**:534–7.

13. Leemans CR, Tiwari R, Nauta JJ, *et al*. Recurrence at the primary site in head and neck cancer and the significance of neck lymph node metastases as a prognostic factor. *Cancer* 1994;**73**:187–90.

14. Ferlito A, Johnson JT, Rinaldo A, *et al*. European surgeons were the first to perform neck dissection. *Laryngoscope* 2007;**117**:797–82.

15. Gavilan J, Gavilan C, Herranz J. Functional neck dissection: Three decades of controversy. *Ann Otol Rhinol Laryngol* 1992;**101**:339–41.

16. Bocca E, Pignataro O, Oldini C, *et al*. Functional neck dissection: An evaluation and review of 843 cases. *Laryngoscope* 1984;**94**:942–5.

17. Fletcher GH. Elective irradiation of subclinical disease in cancers of the head and neck. *Cancer* 1972;**29**:1450–4.

18. Robbins KT, Clayman G, Levine PA, *et al*. Committee for Head and Neck Surgery and Oncology, American Academy of Otolaryngology–Head and Neck Surgery, Neck Dissection Classification Update. Revisions Proposed by the American Head and Neck Society and the American Academy of Otolaryngology–Head and Neck Surgery. *Arch Otolaryngol Head Neck Surg* 2002;**128**:751–8.

19. Robbins KT, Shaha AR, Medina JE, *et al*. Committee for Neck Dissection Classification, American Head and Neck Society. *Arch Otolaryngol Head Neck Surg* 2008;**34**:536–8.

20. Lindberg R. Distribution of cervical nodal metastases from squamous cell carcinoma of the upper respiratory and digestive tracts. *Cancer* 1972;**229**:1446–9.

21. Shah JP. Patterns of cervical lymph node metastasis from squamous carcinoma of the upper aerodigestive tract. *Am J Surg* 1990;**60**: 405–9.

22. Woolgar JA. Histological distribution of cervical lymph node metastases from intraoral/oropharyngeal squamous cell carcinomas. *Br J Oral Maxillofac Surg* 1999;**37**:175–80.

23. Johnson JT, Bacon GW, Myers EN, *et al*. Medial vs lateral wall pyriform sinus carcinoma. *Head Neck* 1994;**16**:401–5.

24. Robbins KT, Medina JE, Wolfe GT, *et al*. Standardizing neck dissection terminology: Official report of the Academy's Committee for Head and Neck Surgery and Oncology. *Arch Otolaryngol Head Neck Surg* 1991;**117**:601–5.

25. El Ghani F, Van den Brekel MWM, De Goede CJT, *et al*. Shoulder function and patient well-being after various types of neck dissections. Preservation of the SAN does not guarantee normal shoulder function. *Clin Otolaryngol* 2002;**27**:403–8.

26. Leipzig B, Suen JY, English JL, *et al*. Functional evaluation of the spinal accessory nerve after neck dissection. *Am J Surg* 1983;**146**:526–30.

27. Cuccia G, Shelley OP, Stagno F, *et al*. Evidence of significant sternocleidomastoid atrophy following modified radical neck dissection type III. *Plast Reconstr Surg* 2006;**117**:227–32.

28. Spiro RH, Huvos AG, Wong GY, *et al*. Predictive value of tumor thickness in squamous carcinoma confined to the tongue and floor of the mouth. *Am J Surg* 1986;**152**:345–50.

29. Fagan JJ, Collins R, Johnson JT, *et al*. Perineural invasion in squamous cell carcinoma of the head and neck. *Arch Otolaryngol* 1998;**124**:637–40.

30. Van den Brekel MW, van der Waal I, Meijer CJ, *et al*. The incidence of micrometases in neck dissection specimens obtained from elective neck dissections. *Laryngoscope* 1996;**106**:987–91.

31. Rhee D, Wenig BM, Smith RV. The significance of immuno-histochemically demonstrated nodal micrometastases in patients with squamous cell carcinoma of the head and neck. *Laryngoscope* 2002;**112**:1970–4.

32. Brekel MWM van den, Castelijns JA, Snow GB. Diagnostic evaluation of the neck. *Otol Clin North Am* 1998;**31**:601–20.

33. Ali S, Tiwari RM, Snow GB. False positive and false negative neck nodes. *Head Neck* 1985;**8**:78–82.

34. Brekel MWM van den, Stell HV, Castelijns JA, *et al*. Lymph node staging in patients with clinically negative neck examinations by ultrasound and ultrasound-guided fine needle aspiration cytology. *Am J Surg* 1991;**162**:362–6.

35. Ataergin S, Arslan N, Ozet A, *et al*. Abnormal FDG uptake on 18F-fluorodeoxyglucose positron emission tomography in patients with cancer diagnosis: Case reports of tuberculous lymphadenitis. *Inter Med* 2009;**48**:115–19.

36. Myers EN, Fagan JJ. Management of the neck in cancer of the larynx. *Ann Otol Rhinol Laryngol* 1999;**108**:828–32.

37. Lydiatt DD, Robbins KT, Byers RM, *et al*. Treatment of stage 1 and 11 oral tongue cancer. *Head Neck* 1993;**15**:308–12.

38. Vandenbrouck C, Sancho-Garnier H, Chassagne D, *et al*. Elective versus therapeutic radical neck dissection in epidermoid carcinoma of the oral cavity. *Cancer* 1980;**46**:386–90.

39. Fakih AR, Rao RS, Borges AM, *et al*. Elective vs therapeutic neck dissection in early carcinoma of the oral tongue. *Am J Surg* 1989;**158**:309–13.

40. Davidson J, Biem J, Detsky A. The clinically negative neck in patients with early oral cavity carcinoma: A decision-analysis approach to management. *J Otolaryngol* 1995;**24**:323–9.

41. Steiner W, Hommerich CP. Diagnosis and treatment of the N0 neck of carcinomas of the upper aerodigestive tract. Report of an International Symposium, Gottingen, Germany, 1992. *Eur Arch Otorhinolaryngol* 1993;**250**:450–6.

42. De Waal PJ, Fagan JJ, Isaacs S. Pre- and intra-operative staging of the neck in a developing world practice. *J Laryngol Otol* 2003;**117**: 976–8.

43. Rassekh CH, Johnson JT, Myers EN. Accuracy of intra-operative staging of the N0 neck in squamous cell carcinoma. *Laryngoscope* 1995;**105**:1334–6.

44. Gillison M. Unpublished data presented at 2009 Annual Meeting of American Society of Clinical Oncology, and at 2009 Meeting of International Association of Oral Oncology.

45. Byers RM. Modified neck dissection. A study of 967 cases from 1970 to 1980. *Am J Surg* 1985;**150**:414–21.

46. Bocca E, Pignataro O, Oldini C. Supraglottic laryngectomy: 30 years of experience. *Ann Otol Rhinol Laryngol* 1983;**92:**14–18.

47. Mack Y, Parsons JT, Mendenhall WM, *et al.* Squamous cell carcinoma of the head and neck: Management after excisional biopsy of a solitary metastatic neck node. *Int J Radiat Oncol Biol Phys* 1993;**25:**619–22.

48. Robbins KT. Detrimental effects of diagnostic cervical node biopsy: Dogma vs science [Editorial]. *Head Neck* 1991;**13:**175–6.

49. Robbins KT, Cole R, Marvel J, *et al.* The violated neck: Cervical node biopsy prior to definitive treatment. *Otolaryngol Head Neck Surg* 1986;**94:**605–10.

50. Ellis ER, Mendenhall WM, Rao PV, *et al.* Incisional or excisional neck-node biopsy before definitive radiotherapy, alone or followed by neck dissection. *Head Neck* 1991;**13:**177–83.

51. Davidson BJ, Kulkarny V, Delacure MD, *et al.* Posterior triangle metastases of squamous cell carcinoma of the upper aerodigestive tract. *Am J Surg* 1993;**166:**395–8.

52. Lim YC, Koo BS, Lee JS, *et al.* Level V lymph node dissection in oral and oropharyngeal carcinoma patients with clinically node-positive neck: Is it absolutely necessary? *Laryngoscope* 2006;**116:**1232–5.

53. Ambrosch P, Freudenberg L, Kron M, *et al.* Selective neck dissection in the management of squamous cell carcinoma of the upper digestive tract. *Eur Arch Otorhinolaryngol* 1996;**253:**329–35.

54. Medina JE, Byers RM. Supraomohyoid neck dissection: Rationale, indications, and surgical technique. *Head Neck* 1989;**11:**111–22.

55. Pellitteri PK, Robbins KT, Neuman T. Expanded application of selective neck dissection with regard to nodal status. *Head Neck* 1997;**19:**260–5.

56. Traynor SJ, Cohen JI, Gray J, *et al.* Selective neck dissection and the management of the node-positive neck. *Am J Surg* 1996;**172:**654–7.

57. Goldenberg D, Begum S, Westra WH, *et al.* Cystic lymph node metastases in patients with head and neck cancer: An HPV-associated phenomenon. *Head Neck* 2008;**30:**898–903.

58. Zhang MQ, El-Mofty SK, Davila RM. Hybridization in fine-needle aspiration biopsies of cervical metastasis. A tool for identifying the site of an occult head and neck primary. *Cancer (Cancer Cytopathol)* 2008;**114:**118–23.

59. Jones AS, Stell PM. Is laterality important in neck node metastases in head and neck cancer? *Clin Otolaryngol* 1991;**16:**261–5.

60. Yoo GH, Hocwald E, Korkmaz H, *et al.* Assessment of carotid artery invasion in patients with head and neck cancer. *Laryngoscope* 2000;**110:**386–90.

61. Snyderman CH, D'Amico F. Outcome of carotid artery resection for neoplastic disease: A meta-analysis. *Am J Otolaryngol* 1992;**13:**373–80.

62. Stell PM, Dalby JE, Singh SD, *et al.* The fixed cervical lymph node. *Cancer* 1984;**53:**336–41.

63. Bakamajian VY, Cervino L, Miller S, *et al.* The concept of cure and palliation by surgery in advanced cancer of the head and neck. *Am J Surg* 1973;**126:**482–7.

64. Patel RS, Clark J, Wyten R, *et al.* Squamous cell carcinoma from an unknown head and neck primary site: A 'Selective Treatment' approach. *Arch Otolaryngol Head Neck Surg* 2007;**133:**1282–7.

65. Lango MN, Myers JN, Garden AS. Controversies in surgical management of the node-positive neck after chemoradiation. *Semin Radiat Oncol* 2008;**9:**24–8.

66. Ridge JA. Squamous cancer of the head and neck: Surgical treatment of local and regional recurrence. *Semin Oncol* 1993;**20:**419–29.

67. Stafford N, Dearnaley D. Treatment of inoperable neck nodes using surgical clearance and postoperative interstitial irradiation. *Br J Surg* 1988;**75:**62–4.

68. Lee DJ, Liberman FZ, Park RI, *et al.* Intraoperative I-125 seed implantation for extensive recurrent head and neck carcinomas. *Radiology* 1992;**178:**879–82.

69. Johnson JT, Wagner RL, Myers EN. A long-term assessment of adjuvant chemotherapy on outcome of patients with extracapsular spread of cervical metastases from squamous carcinoma of the head and neck. *Cancer* 1996;**77:**181–5.

Cancer of the lip and oral cavity

PAUL SEBASTIAN, ELIZABETH MATHEW IYPE, SAJITH BABU, BIPIN T. VARGHESE

Oral cancers

Introduction

Oral cancer is the sixth most common cancer worldwide, constituting approximately 5% of all cancers and accounting for over half a million new cancers diagnosed each year. The incidence of oral cancer has significant geographical variation. Southeast Asia, Brazil, southern and eastern Europe, and parts of France and Australia report a significantly high incidence of oral cancer with estimates exceeding 40 in 100,000 populations.

In India, oral cancer is the most common malignancy among men, accounting for approximately 35% of all newly diagnosed cancers, and the third most common cancer among women.[1] Squamous cell carcinomas (SCCs) account for 90% of all oral cancers in India. The current discussion is about oral cancers in general, oral cancer in young adults and management of the mandible in oral cancer.

Epidemiology

Subgroup analyses of various head and neck cancers (HNCs) have shown that low socioeconomic status (SES) is significantly associated with increased risk of oral cancers in high and low income countries across the world, even after adjusting for potential behavioural confounders. Risk association of oral cancers with low SES is significant and comparable to risk factors pertaining to lifestyle.[2]

These results signify that, despite the declining long-term trends in the incidence of oral cancer and mortality globally, there are localized geographical areas where the incidence and mortality from oral cancers has been increasing. These areas represent sites where specific populations can be targeted for public health education and preventative measures so that cancer treatment outcomes can improve and disparities within these populations are reduced.[3,4]

A review of the literature on the epidemiology and natural history of potentially malignant disorders (PMDs), detailing characteristics of the patients and lesions associated with future development of oral SCC (OSCC), shows that older patients, particularly women, are at greater risk than younger patients, and that the duration of PMDs may be important. Those who have never used tobacco in this subgroup seem to be at greater risk than smokers in general. OSCC is more likely with a PMD on the lateral and ventral tongue, floor of mouth and retromolar/soft palate complex than with that elsewhere.[5]

Anatomy

Sites of oral cancers

Lip: Upper lip, lower lip, commissure
Oral cavity: Buccal mucosa, upper alveolus, lower alveolus, hard palate, anterior two-thirds of the tongue up to the line of circumvallate papillae, floor of mouth, the retromolar trigone, gingivae and the buccogingival sulcus.

Lymphatic drainage

The upper and lower lips have cutaneous and mucosal

lymphatics. The lower lip has medial and two lateral lymphatic collecting trunks. The middle third of the lip drains to the submental group (Level IA) of lymph nodes, the lateral third of the lower lip to the submandibular group (Level IB), and the upper lip to the preauricular, intraparotid, submandibular and submental groups.

The tip of the tongue drains to the submental group and to the upper deep cervical, the mid deep cervical and the lower deep cervical groups (levels II, III and IV). The lateral border of the tongue drains to level IB group, then to levels II, III and IV groups.

The buccal mucosa drains to the submandibular group and from there to the upper deep cervical group and the subparotid group.

The anterior part of the floor of mouth drains directly to the inferior glands of the superior deep cervical group, or indirectly through the submental group. The rest of the floor of mouth drains into the submandibular group and then into the superior deep cervical group.

Aetiology of oral cancers

Alcohol and tobacco consumption are the most common aetiological factors worldwide. In South-East Asia, chewing tobacco and betel quid are the most common aetiological factors.[6] Smoking and other types of tobacco use are associated with approximately 75% of oral cancer cases, probably because of the irritation to the mucous membranes of the mouth from smoke and the heat of cigarettes, cigars and pipes, and the exposure of the mucosa to carcinogens in tobacco. These effects can be compounded by the tumour promoting effects of alcohol. Tobacco smoke and alcohol act synergistically in their carcinogenic effects in the oral cavity.[7] The relative risk of oral cancer for heavy smokers is 7 times that of non-smokers, and for heavy drinkers it is 6 times that of non-drinkers. The risk for patients abusing both alcohol and tobacco is 38 times that of those who abstain from both. Chewing betel quid also increases the risk of oral cancer. Tobacco contains over 19 known carcinogens; its combustion and the resulting by-products are the primary mode of carcinogenesis.

In the past decade, infection with human papilloma virus (HPV) has emerged as a common factor associated with oral cancers in non-smoking and non-drinking young individuals of both sexes. HPV, particularly type 16 (there are >120 types), is not only a known risk factor, but is an independent aetiological factor in oral cancer.[8] Although it is much commoner in men, the sex distribution over the past several decades shows a rising incidence of oral cancer in women. In 1930, the men to women ratio was 10:1, whereas it has dropped to 2:1 in the present decade. The ratio between men and women with cancer of the lip is approximately 15:1. Those with light-coloured skin or with prolonged exposure to sunlight are most prone to developing lip carcinoma.

Chronic irritation by dentures, teeth and poor dental hygiene are the other known aetiological factors in oral cancers. Oral premalignant conditions that can turn malignant are leukoplakia, erythroplakia and submucous fibrosis.

Chronic carcinogen exposure creates a field effect and the entire mucosa of the upper aerodigestive tract is at risk of malignancy in smokers and drinkers. After successful treatment of oral cancer, the risk of a second primary cancer is 3.7% per year, which increases to 24% at 10 years. Cessation of alcohol and tobacco exposure reduces the risk of a second aerodigestive carcinoma.

Although the data on incidence and sex distribution is conflicting, studies suggest that the physiological response to risk factors by men and women and the clinical behaviour of these cancers in the younger population may differ from the normal variant. An effort is being made currently to elucidate the aetiology and pathogenesis of oral cancer in the younger population. HNC in young adults is addressed separately in this chapter.

Carcinogenesis

Essential steps involved in carcinogenesis are:
- Accumulation of genetic/epigenetic alterations
- Pre-malignancy
- Carcinoma.

At the molecular level, oral carcinoma is characterized by acquisition of proliferative autonomous signalling, inhibition of growth inhibitory signals, evasion of apoptosis (programmed cell death), angiogenesis (acquisition of nutrient blood supply), tissue invasion and metastasis.

Pathology

There are three types of SCC, viz. exophytic, verrucous and ulcerative. These tumours may occur in three grades—well differentiated, moderately differentiated and poorly differentiated.

Premalignant lesions

Some oral cancers begin as leukoplakia, which is a white patch (lesion), or erythroplakia (red patch), or non-healing sores that have existed for more than 14 days. A biopsy should be performed in case of clinical suspicion of malignancy, as indicated by a sudden change in size, appearance or development of induration. Clinical variants of leukoplakia include homogenous leukoplakia (leukoplakia simplex) and non-homogenous leukoplakia, which is subdivided into ulcerative leukoplakia, nodular (speckled) leukoplakia, verrucous (exophytic) leukoplakia and erythro leukoplakia.

Clinical features and presentation of oral malignancies

History and physical examination

These lesions present mostly as chronic non-healing ulcers and rarely as a swelling underneath an intact mucosa. An indurated swelling in the tongue is a common finding, and inspection of all the sites of the oral cavity should be done meticulously to avoid missing any lesions. The sites usually missed are floor of mouth, retromolar area and gingivobuccal sulcus. Frequent palpation of these sites with a gloved finger is necessary to identify the lesions and to confirm their extent. Measurements of the lesion are recorded for clinical staging of the tumours.

Histopathological tissue diagnosis

All suspicious lesions need to be punch biopsied. Deep-seated submucosal lesions may require an incisional biopsy. It is generally not advisable to do an excisional biopsy as it might compromise margins and interfere with the definitive management later. Accurate diagnosis of premalignant or malignant oral lesions depends on the quality of the biopsy, adequate clinical information and correct interpretation of the biopsy results.[9]

Imaging

Evaluation of the deep extent of oral cancer requires the use of imaging modalities. Plain radiographs, such as panorex, dental films or a submental occlusal film, may demonstrate gross bone involvement but they do not show early cortical invasion. Computed tomography (CT) is the most common imaging modality for assessing the extent of oral cancers, including extension into the mandible or maxilla, or the invasion of the masticator space and nodal involvement. Advantages of CT include good soft tissue discrimination, identification of blood vessels and excellent definition of bone–soft tissue interfaces. Magnetic resonance imaging (MRI) may be useful in delineating the soft tissue extents of the disease in selected situations.

Endoscopic examination

Endoscopy is performed as an office procedure with a fibreoptic nasopharyngolaryngoscope to identify any second primary in the susceptible region, or to look for extension into the tongue base, pharynx or larynx.

Differential diagnosis

Although a majority of persistent indurated tongue lesions are squamous carcinomas, the following conditions need to be ruled out: (i) Aphthous ulcer, (ii) Tuberculous ulcer, (iii) Traumatic ulcer, and (iv) Pyogenic granuloma.

Salivary gland tumours and other rare benign tumours of the oral cavity include papilloma, fibroepithelial polyps, juvenile fibroma, pregnancy tumours, haemangioma, lymphangioma, plexiform neurofibromatosis, lipoma, osteoma, chondroma and granular cell myoblastoma.[10]

Classification, Staging

Spread of the disease can be by local extension, regional nodal involvement through lymphatics and haematogeneous distant metastsis, such as the lungs, brain and bone.

TNM staging (AJCC 7th ed, 2010)[11] [Figs 1–11]

Primary Tumour (T)

TX   Primary tumour cannot be assessed

T0   No evidence of primary tumour

Tis   Carcinoma *in situ*

T1   Tumour 2 cm or less in greatest dimension

T2   Tumour more than 2 cm but not more than 4 cm in greatest dimension

T3   Tumour more than 4 cm in greatest dimension

T4a   Moderately advanced local disease.*
(lip) Tumour invades through cortical bone, inferior alveolar nerve, floor of mouth, or skin of face, i.e. chin or nose
(oral cavity) Tumour invades adjacent structures only (e.g., through cortical bone [mandible or maxilla] into deep [extrinsic] muscle of tongue [genioglossus, hyoglossus, palatoglossus, and styloglossus], maxillary sinus, skin of face)

T4b   Very advanced local disease
Tumour invades masticator space, pterygoid plates, or skull base and/or encases internal carotid artery

Note: Superficial erosion alone of bone/tooth socket by gingival primary is not sufficient to classify a tumour as T4.

Regional Lymph Nodes (N)

NX   Regional lymph nodes cannot be assessed

N0   No regional lymph node metastasis

N1   Metastasis in a single ipsilateral lymph node, 3 cm or less in greatest dimension

N2   Metastasis in a single ipsilateral lymph node, more than 3 cm but not more than 6 cm in greatest dimension; or in multiple ipsilateral lymph nodes, none more than 6 cm in greatest dimension; or in bilateral or contralateral lymph nodes, none more than 6 cm in greatest dimension

N2a   Metastasis in single ipsilateral lymph node more than 3 cm but not more than 6 cm in greatest dimension

N2b   Metastasis in multiple ipsilateral lymph nodes, none more than 6 cm in greatest dimension

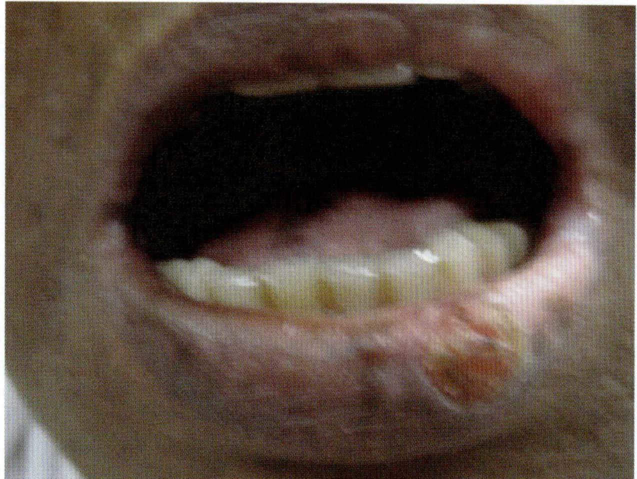

Fig. 1. Carcinoma lip T1 lesion

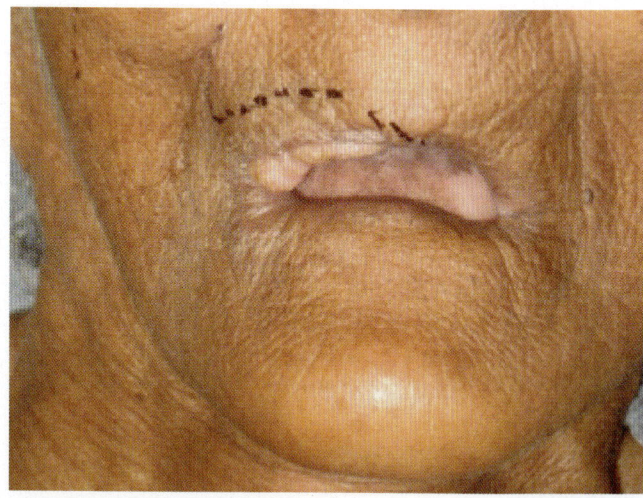

Fig. 2. Carcinoma lip T2 lesion

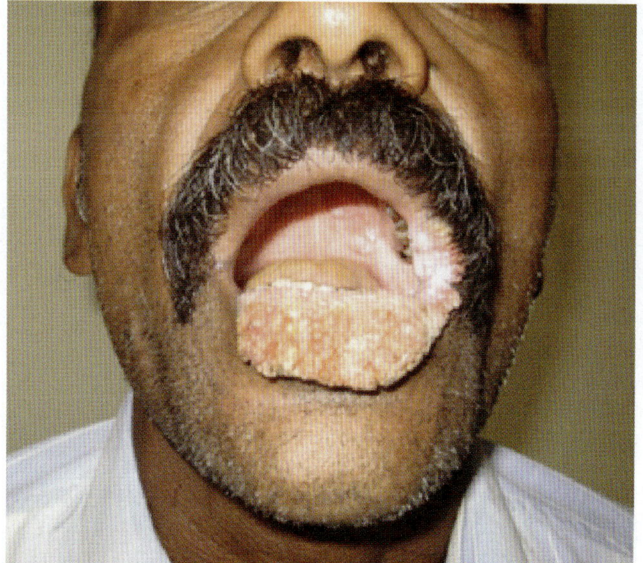

Fig. 3. Carcinoma lip T3 lesion

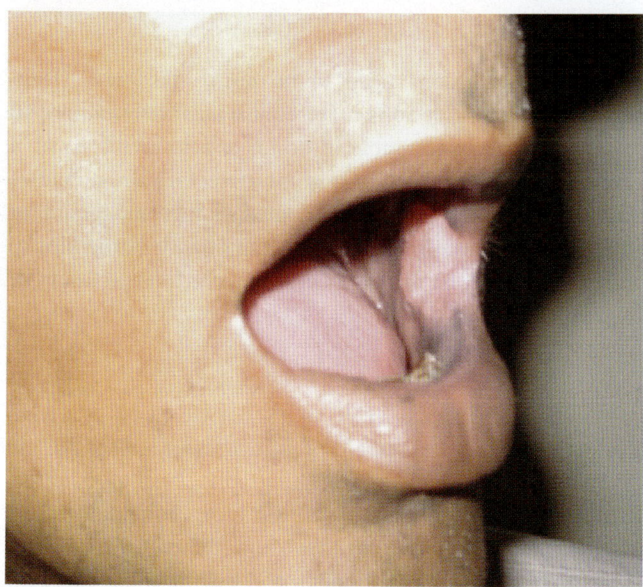

Fig. 4. Carcinoma buccal mucosa T2

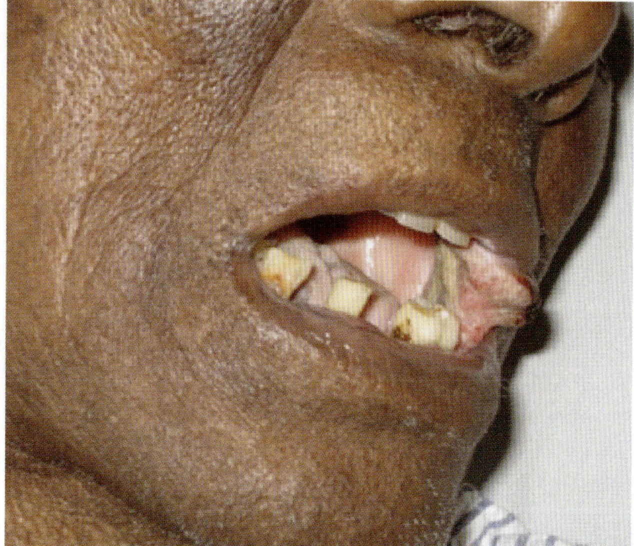

Fig. 5. Carcinoma buccl mucosa T3 lesion

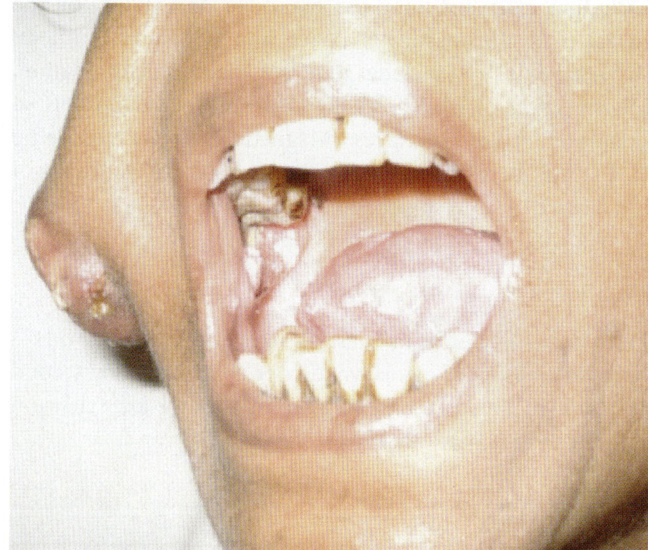

Fig. 6. Carcinoma buccal mucosa T4 lesion

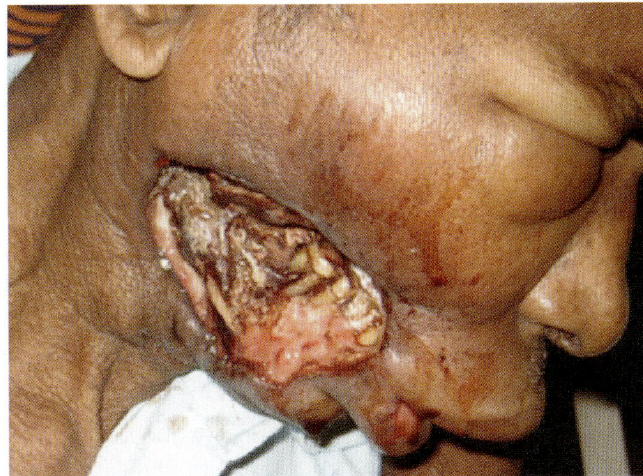

Fig. 7. Advanced inoperable carcinoma of buccal mucosa

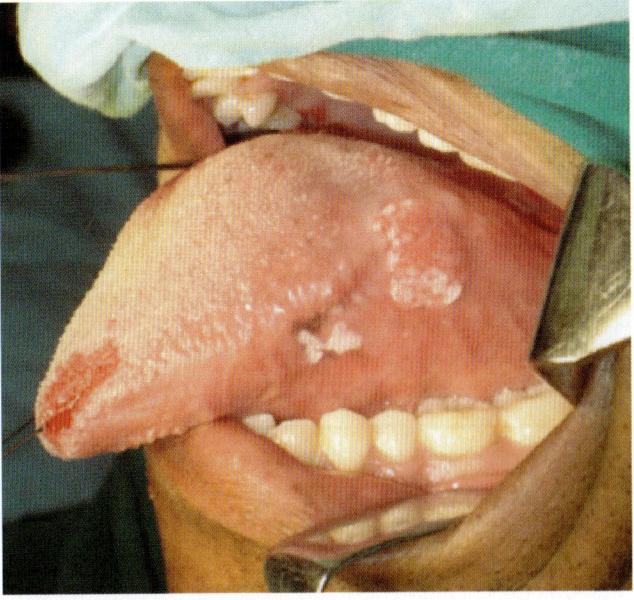

Fig. 8. Carcinoma tongue T1 lesion

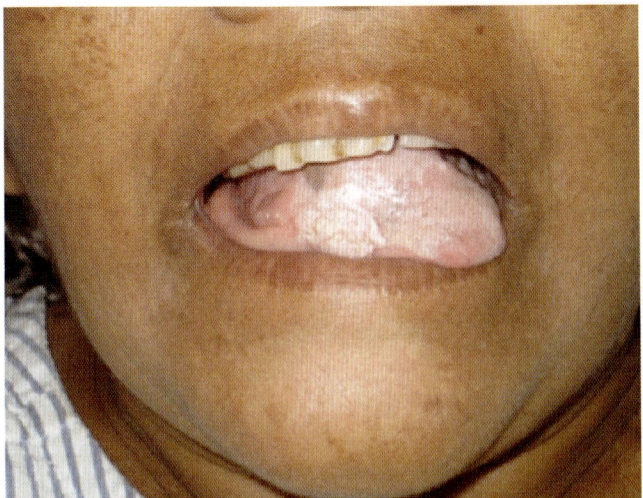

Fig. 9. Carcinoma tongue T2 lesion

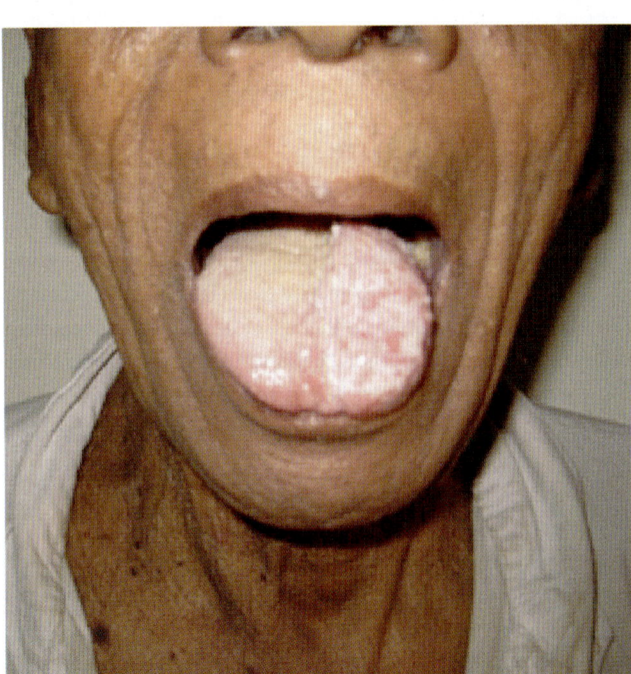

Fig. 10. Carcinoma tongue T3 lesion

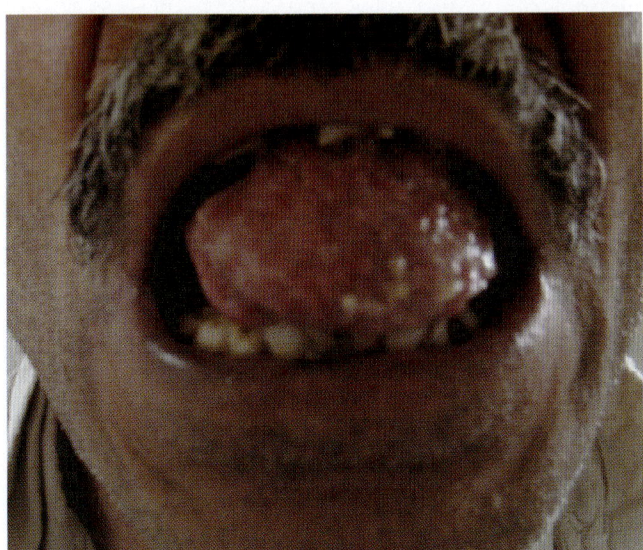

Fig. 11. Carcinoma tongue T4 lesion

N2c Metastasis in bilateral or contralateral lymph nodes, none more than 6 cm in greatest dimension

N3   Metastasis in lymph node more than 6 cm in greatest dimension

Distant metastasis (M)

M0   No distant metastasis

M1   Distant metastasis

(Used with the permission of the American Joint Committee on Cancer (AJCC), Chicago, Illinois. The original source for this material is the *AJCC Cancer Staging Manual*, Seventh Edition (2010) published by Springer Science and Business Media LLC, www.springer.com.)

Treatment

The treatment goals for oral cancer are to eradicate the cancer, preserve or restore form and function, avoid or minimize the sequelae of treatment and prevent second primary tumours. The treatment modalities for achieving these goals are surgery, radiotherapy chemotherapy and molecular targeted therapy, either alone or in combination.

The factors influencing the choice of initial treatment for primary carcinomas of the oral cavity are dependent on the characteristics of the primary tumour (tumour factors) such as site, size, location, proximity to bone, histological characteristics and tumour morphology; the status of cervical lymph nodes; and presence or absence of distant metastasis. In addition, factors related to the patient (patient factors) and those related to the treatment team providing care to the patient (physician factors or resource factors) are important. In general, oral cancer is primarily treated with surgery as the initial definitive treatment, either alone or in combination with radiotherapy or chemoradiotherapy. Patient factors include the patient's age, profession, co-morbidities, convenience, rehabilitation potential and the patient's wishes. Resource factors include the availability of a well-trained surgeon or radiotherapist with a dedicated interest in HNC, availability of advanced hardware for the planning and delivery of radiation, and the availability of funds to pay for the treatment.

The size of the primary tumour has a clear impact on the decision regarding the choice of initial treatment. Small and superficial primary tumours of the oral cavity are easily accessible for surgical resection through the open mouth. On the other hand, larger tumours will require more extensive surgical approaches for exposure and excision. Certain primary sites in the oral cavity are easily amenable to initial treatment with radiotherapy, such as primary tumours of the lip, in contrast to those that are situated in close proximity to bone, such as tumours of the gum and hard palate. Similarly, with increasing size (T-stage) of the primary lesion, the risk of regional lymph node metastases increases, bringing into consideration the need for elective treatment of the neck, even when the neck is staged N0 after clinical examination and imaging. Moreover, certain primary sites have a higher risk of nodal metastases compared with other sites in the

oral cavity. For example, primary tumours of the oral tongue and floor of the mouth have an increased risk of lymph node metastases compared with similar-staged lesions of the hard palate or upper gum. Apart from these, primary tumours located anteriorly in the oral cavity have a lesser risk for dissemination to the regional lymph nodes compared with similar-staged tumours in the posterior part of the oral cavity and oropharynx.

The principles of treatment

Early lesions

Early lesions are treated by a single modality. Surgical excision with good margins or radiotherapy with standard dose-delivery techniques is sufficient as a single modality. However, the mainstay of treatment of early oral cancer is surgery. Advantages of surgery for T1 and T2 oral cancer compared with radiation include decreased cost, decreased time of treatment, generation of a surgical specimen for examination of potential prognostic features and, in some instances, an opportunity to sample the regional clinically negative nodes for occult disease. Potential advantages of radiation therapy for early lesions are preservation of tissue and the avoidance of general anaesthesia or hospital admission.

The thickness of the tumour measured by an optical micrometer is an important predictor of lymph node metastasis of oral malignancies, especially the tongue. In cancers of the tongue and floor of the mouth, for which prophylactic neck dissections (PNDs) are advocated for even T1 and T2 lesions, evidence is accruing that, for a small subset of these tumours (<4 mm), it is preferable to observe than to perform a PND immediately.[12] However, if the subsequent histopathology report shows perineural or lymphovascular invasion, in spite of clear margins, a PND or irradiation may be warranted. PND is traditionally considered therapeutically equivalent to a prophylactic irradiation with an efficiency of approximately 90% of the control. Taking all these caveats into consideration, those patients with a low-volume T1 or early T2 cancer may be considered for transoral laser excision in conjunction with a PND.[13,14]

Brachytherapy can sometimes be employed for oral cancers (especially tumours of the tongue) utilizing after-loading catheters. Tumour factors that limit the use of brachytherapy for oral cavity cancers are their close proximity to the mandible, their complex surface anatomy and uncertainty of their margins.

Locally advanced lesions

Multimodality treatment is preferred for locally advanced lesions. Tumours of the oral cavity are poorly responsive to traditional organ-sparing approaches that combine chemotherapy and radiation therapy, either sequentially or

Table 1. Important prognostic factors in oral cancers

- Status of cervical lymphnodes: The pathological status of neck nodes, their levels of involvement, perinodal invasion and the number of nodes involved
- T-stage
- Tumour thickness
- Surgical margins
- Pattern of tumour invasion
- Presence of perineural/lymphovascular invasion

Table 2. Advantages of surgery for early disease

- Simple method of treatment
- Short treatment time
- No significant functional or cosmetic defects
- Repeated procedures possible
- Cost-effective

Table 3. Indications for treatment modalities

Indications for postoperative radiotherapy
When lesion is more than T3 or if nodes are +ve

Indication for postoperative chemotherapy
Positive margins and perinodal or extracapsular spread of nodal disease

Role of neoadjuvant chemotherapy
In very limited situations to down-stage the tumour

concomitantly. The control rates for oral cavity cancers using these regimens are the lowest of all head and neck sites.[15]

Preoperative chemotherapy for oral cancers is usually not helpful because resection margins do not shrink with the clinical response of the tumour. Studies show that microscopic tumour foci exist where the previous gross tumour has been shrunk by chemotherapy treatment. It is therefore not ordinarily possible to reduce the extent of surgical resection and the morbidity of oral cancer surgery by tumour shrinkage with preoperative chemotherapy. Contrary to this, Licitra and co-workers[16] in their randomized controlled trial on 195 patients with T2–T4 (>3 cm) and N0–N2 resectable SCC of the oral cavity, showed that patients who received three cycles of induction chemotherapy with cisplatin and 5-fluorouracil were less likely to undergo mandibular resection (31% *vs.* 52%) and to require postoperative radiation therapy (33% *vs.* 46%). However, there was no improvement in locoregional control, distant relapse, or survival. Unpublished data from the Regional Cancer Centre, Thiruvananthapuram, Kerala also supports this view.

The modern reconstructive options available have made surgery the primary treatment modality in most situations, as it offers good organ and function preservation, even when the resection is extensive. All T3 and T4 tumours require planned postoperative radiotherapy. Recent evidence shows that addition of chemotherapy to postoperative irradiation may be required in the presence of a positive tumour margin or extracapsular spread of nodes in the neck dissection.

Important prognostic factors in oral cancers are given in Table 1.

Surgery

Surgery for primary disease

A wide three dimensional excision with negative margins has to be attained. The access can be per oral, or with cheek flaps, or by a mandibulotomy approach. A mandibulectomy required to get a three dimensional margin can be either marginal or segmental. Marginal mandibulectomy is indicated when the tumour closely abuts the mandible without cortical invasion. If cortical involvement is suspected, either segmental or arch mandibulectomy is needed. Reconstruction is required to restore form and function.

To reduce morbidity, it is now possible to limit the extent of selective neck dissection (SND) for mucosal SCC of the head and neck (HNSCC) by sparing selected lymphatic levels. SND (with dissection of levels I–III) is a sound and effective procedure in the management of the clinically negative (N0) neck in SCC of the oral cavity. A clinically N0 but pathologically N+ neck requires adjuvant radiation therapy. This treatment probably has a therapeutic role in selected cases of SCC of the oral cavity with a N1 neck. In these cases an extension of dissection to levels IV and V is beneficial.[17] Any N status above N1 warrants a comprehensive neck dissection. Except in superficial tumours of <4 mm, PND is indicated in all cases of tongue and floor of mouth cancers. With regard to the alveolus, buccal mucosa, retromolar trigone and lip tumours, a PND is warranted only for those cases above T3, when the neck is clinically N0.[18] Generally, in a supraomohyoid neck dissection the pathological specimen should yield at least six nodes, and in a comprehensive neck dissection it should yield at least 10 nodes.

Advantages of surgery for early disease are given in Table 2.

Postoperative radiotherapy

All T3 and T4 tumours require planned postoperative radiotherapy. Recent evidence shows that addition of chemotherapy to post-operative irradiation may be required in the presence of a positive tumour margin or extracapsular spread of nodes in the neck dissection.

Indications for treatment modalities are given in Table 3.

Advanced oral cancers

Advanced disease can be classified as locally advanced operable, locally advanced inoperable, and metastatic.

Treatment of locally advanced operable lesions

These patients are treated with a combined modality. Tumours in such cases are usually treated by surgery followed by radiotherapy or chemoradiation.

Locally advanced inoperable and metastatic disease

A complete resection cannot be achieved if there is extension to the vertebrae or brachial plexus, or if the carotid artery is encased by the tumour. The goal of treatment in such patients is essentially palliation.

Gene therapy

Gene therapy essentially consists of introducing specific genetic material into target cells without producing toxic effects on the surrounding tissues. Advances in recent decades in the surgical, radiotherapeutic and chemotherapeutic treatment of oral cancer have not produced a significant improvement in patient survival. Increasing interest is being shown in developing novel therapies to reverse oral epithelial dysplastic lesions. A combination of gene therapy with chemotherapy (e.g. 5-fluorouracil) and immunotherapy has shown promising results, such as using adenovirus to act at an altered gene level (e.g. p53). Other techniques, such as suicide gene therapy and the use of oncolytic viruses or antisense RNA, have shown positive, although very preliminary, results.[19]

Survival[20]

The median survival for cancers of the lip is >120 months for tumours of stage I, 99 months for stage II, 50 months for stage III and 37 months for stage IV.

The median survival for tongue cancer patients is 95 months, 58 months, 32 months, and 22 months for stages I, II, III and IV, respectively.

Floor of mouth cancer patients have median survival in months, ranging from 93 to 18 (93, 63, 29, 18) for stages I–IV.

Cancers of the buccal mucosa have better survival. Stage I tumours have a median survival of 95 months, which is comparable to other sites, whereas higher stage tumours also show good median survival, i.e. stage II has 90 months, stage III has 76 months and stage IV has 70 months of median survival.[20]

Oral cancer in young adults

Young adults (defined as adults of <45 years of age) have shown an increasing incidence of carcinoma of the tongue. These cancers tend to occur in the oral cavity and oropharynx.[21,22] The reason for this trend remains unclear, although marijuana use and HPV infection are likely explanations. The most common histology is SCC, but other histological types, such as adenocarcinoma and Kaposi sarcoma, are also seen. Several reports have indicated a female preponderance in this group, unlike in the general trend of HNC.

According to reports of the Surveillance Epidemiology and End Results (SEER) from the USA, Schantz and Yu[22] found that younger patients were more likely to present with localized disease than older patients.[22] Similarly, Funk et al.[23] reviewed the 1985–1996 National Cancer Database (NCDB) and found that younger patients, when analysed only for SCC, presented at an earlier stage across all types of histology, and had a higher proportion of stage I disease that was statistically significant. Contrary to these findings, both Verschuur et al.[24] and Veness et al.[25] independently found that a higher rate of nodal metastases was seen in younger patients at presentation, albeit in small, single institution studies. Byers[21] found a high percentage (almost 50%) of high-grade histology in his young patients (<30 years old) with oral tongue SCC. Atula and colleagues[26] reviewed 34 Finnish patients of <40 years of age with SCC of the tongue, and found the vast majority (70%) to have well differentiated tumours. Similarly, Sasaki and colleagues[27] found 66% of tumours in young patients (<40 years of age) to be well differentiated compared with only 33% in their older cohort.

Aetiology and risk factors

Tobacco and alcohol

Studies in young patients have found a variable and sometimes absent relationship with traditional risk factors, such as smokeless tobacco. Interestingly, in a series on young patients with OSCC, Llewellyn et al.[28] highlighted a caveat regarding the connection between tobacco and cancer by reporting that young patients with cancer who did not use tobacco delayed seeking medical care for their cancer-related symptoms. Thus, the treating physician and the young patients themselves who do not have any risk factors may not suspect cancer, despite the worrisome signs and symptoms.

Diet

In the series by Llewellyn and colleagues,[29] a significant reduction in risk was found in subjects who reported consumption of three or more portions of fresh fruit or vegetables per day. Generally, a diet high in fruits and vegetables is inversely related to a risk of oral cancer and, on the basis of Lewellyn and co-workers[29] studies, this fact can be applied also to young patients.

HPV

Perhaps the most widely studied virus in the literature on

HNC in recent years is HPV, a virus initially linked to cervical carcinogenesis that has now gained interest for its connection to cancer of the oropharynx, particularly the lingual and palatine tonsils.[29] The increasing incidence of tongue and tonsil cancer among young patients has led some authors[30] to suggest that HPV may be responsible for this trend, although the connection between oral (versus oropharyngeal) cancer and HPV is controversial.[31]

In a multi-institutional, prospective phase II trial of chemoradiation for advanced HNSCC (ECOG 2399), which included analysis of HPV status in the primary biopsy, the mean age of 38 patients with HPV-positive tumours was <58 years whereas in 56 HPV-negative tumours it was 60 years (58 versus 60, respectively), but the difference was not statistically significant. However, this study did find a significantly better response and survival in the HPV-positive group, even when adjusted for age, tumour stage and performance status.[32]

Sisk *et al.*[33] likewise found HPV positivity to be linked to a better overall prognosis, which has been corroborated by several other studies, although none of these studies specifically addressed young patients. Interestingly, improved survival was also seen with increasing copy number of HPV-16 in 35 patients with tonsil carcinoma in one study, suggesting that the connection between HPV status and response to treatment may be quite strong.[33]

Human immunodeficiency virus (HIV)

Infection with HIV and progression to AIDS is positively correlated with malignancies of the upper aerodigestive tract, particularly Kaposi sarcoma and non-Hodgkin lymphoma and, to a lesser extent, SCC.[34]

Genetics

Young patients are likely to have some genetic component in developing cancer, particularly those patients with no recognized risk factors. These patients have been shown to have increased DNA fragility, which may make them more susceptible to developing genetic abnormalities. However, studies examining specific genetic alterations in HNSCC as a function of patient age, including mutations in p53, p21, Rb, MDM2,[35] and microsatellite instability,[36] have failed to find an increase in these abnormalities in young patients. Likewise, Koch and colleagues found tumours of non-smokers with HNSCC to have fewer genetic abnormalities than those of their smoking counterparts, leading them to conclude that the genetic alterations in tumours from non-smoking patients remain undiscovered. In a larger series, Llewellyn and colleagues[29] reported a positive family history of cancer in 75% of women and 59% of men younger than 45 years of age with HNSCC, suggesting that genetics, immunology or some common environmental exposure may predispose young

adults to developing HNSCC.[36]

A rare, inherited cancer syndrome associated with HNSCC is Fanconi anaemia (FA), an autosomal recessive syndrome caused by defects in DNA repair. FA carries a high risk of development of malignancy at a young age, with a median age at presentation of 31 years, and a cumulative incidence of HNSCC of 14% by age 40 years. Patients with FA and HNSCC are more likely to be women (2:1), with very few reporting tobacco use. The oral cavity is the most common site and the outcome is poor, with a 63% rate of second primaries and a 2-year overall survival of 49%.[27,37]

Prognosis and outcome

The vast majority of publications on young patients with HNSCC address outcome, and yet debate in the literature continues on whether age at presentation has any effect on prognosis. An analysis by Shiboski and colleagues[30] of the 1973–2001 SEER database revealed an overall increased 5-year survival for patients with HNSCC who were younger than 45 years. An analysis of Scandinavian cancer registries by Annertz and colleagues[38] similarly found an increased 5-year survival among patients younger than 40 years. Lacy and colleagues[39] found, in a similar study, that young patients also had a lower recurrence rate and a lower incidence of second primaries than their older counterparts.

However, several other studies are contradictory, and have indicated poorer survival.[37,40] Several small case series have been published reporting young patients with a high rate of locoregional recurrence. Whereas these case series may be subject to publication or referral bias, they highlight a subset of young patients that may have more aggressive disease. Another explanation for the higher local recurrence rate could be a lack of appropriate initial surgical treatment. Because of their young age, these patients may not have been as aggressively treated as their older counterparts, although in the absence of details about margin assessment and extent of resection, this is speculative.

Two small, matched control studies and one retrospective institutional series found high locoregional recurrence in younger patients compared with older patients, but none demonstrated a corresponding difference in 5-year survival. On the contrary, Von Doersten[41] and colleagues found that age did not affect recurrence in a multivariate analysis on 155 patients, of whom 23 were under the age of 40. Thus, whether young patients, or a subset thereof, have a higher propensity for locoregional recurrence is yet to be confirmed.

Mandible in oral cancer

Mandibular invasion of OSCCs

Mandibular involvement in oral cancers can occur in several

ways. The tumour can invade the mandible from the oral cavity through the upper surface of the mandible (occlusal route), or through the periodontal membrane.[42] In the edentulous mandible, the tumour appears to enter through the crest of the alveolus or through cortical perforations. In addition, secondary tumours in the neck can also involve the lower border of the mandible. Non-occlusal foramina provide an additional site of entry (i.e. mental and mandibular foramina).

In a prospective study to assess the histological patterns of tumour invasion and routes of tumour entry into the mandible of 100 consecutive, previously untreated patients, Brown *et al.*[43] found that the most common location for tumour invasion is at the junction of attached and free mucosa in both the dentulous and edentulous mandible. They also noted that spread in the non-irradiated mandible occurs along the medullary cavity, with fibrosis replacing haemopoietic tissue, and hence the presence of haemopoietic marrow at the lateral resection margin would indicate clear margins. Within the medullary cavity, the inferior alveolar nerve provides a ready pathway for spread in the proximal and distal directions. In the irradiated mandible, because the mucoperiosteum is not an effective barrier for tumour spread, it can invade the mandible at multiple places of abutment, making marginal resections unsafe.

The orthopantogram (OPG) evaluation is similar to the standard X-rays in all respects, except that it reduces overlap of bone images in the ramus and the body, making evaluation of demineralization better. In spite of this, it can detect bony erosion only after 30% mineral loss, resulting in high false-negative results. The symphysis is sometimes difficult to image accurately by OPG, due to overlap of the spine. The dentascan, which is a formatted high resolution tool for the mandible, has a sensitivity of 95% and a specificity of 79%.[44] However, clinical examination combined with direct per operative visualization and periosteal stripping has the greatest accuracy in assessing mandibular invasion.[45]

The most sensitive investigations are the single photon emission computerized tomography (SPECT) (97%) and isotope bone scan (93%); and the most specific investigations are CT scan (88%) and MRI (86%).

In 1971, Marchetta *et al.*[46] had shown that malignancies in the oral cavity spread through locoregional lymphatics and that there is a rationale for performing a marginal mandibulectomy in tumours that abut the mandible. Until then the rationale for doing a segmental mandibulectomy had been subperiosteal lymphatic spread from oral cancers.

In a recent series of 136 patients, Wolff and Hassfeld[47] found no significant difference in survival rates between those who had undergone segmental and marginal mandibulectomy. Careful case selection by clinical assessment and imaging is therefore the key to a successful mandible conserving surgery.

Surgical significance of the mandible in oral cancer

The management of the mandible is of utmost importance in surgical treatment of oral cancers. Surgery for the mandible is considered in instances when a tumour that abuts the mandible is resected, or when accessing tumours in the oral cancers, in which case a mandibulotomy is done and swung laterally after incising the mucosa on the lingual side and dividing the mylohyoid muscle. For approach to the oropharynx it may be necessary to release the temporalis muscle from the coronoid process.

Mandibular resections can be divided broadly into marginal mandibulectomy, the rim resections, and the segmental resections, which include the hemimandibulectomy, i.e. resection of the body or the arch of the mandible. Lateral segmental resections can be left alone without much cosmetic and functional impairment if adequate soft tissues are available for a primary closure or if they are adequately filled by soft vascularized tissues, whereas a central defect involving the arch mandibulectomy will require reconstruction to prevent an unsightly Andy Gump deformity and tongue fall-back, causing airway obstruction and impaired swallowing.

Conclusion

The most important factor affecting long-term outcome after initial treatment of cancer of the oral cavity is the stage of the disease at the time of presentation. Early stage tumours offer excellent cure rates; however, once regional lymph node metastases have taken place, a significant drop in the cure rate is to be expected. Early diagnosis and implementation of appropriate treatment based on tumour and patient factors, selective management of regional lymph node metastases at risk, and involvement of multidisciplinary teams for implementation of adjuvant radiotherapy or chemo-radiotherapy, have all contributed to improvements in survival of patients with oral cancers.

References

1. Parkin DM, Whelan SL, Ferlay J, *et al. Cancer incidence in five continents.* Vol. VII. Lyon: IARC Scientific Publications No. 143; 1997.
2. Conway DI, Petticrew M, Marlborough H, *et al.* Socioeconomic inequalities and oral cancer risk: A systematic review and meta-analysis of case–control studies. *Int J Cancer* 2008;**122**:2811–19.
3. Kingsley K, O'Malley S, Ditmyer M, *et al.* Analysis of oral cancer epidemiology in the US reveals state-specific trends: Implications for oral cancer prevention. *BMC Public Health* 2008:87.
4. Sankaranarayanan R, Ramdas K, Thomas G, *et al.* Effect of screening on oral cancer mortality in Kerala, India: A cluster–randomized controlled trial. *Lancet* 2005;**365**:1927–33.
5. Napier SS, Speight PM. Natural history of potentially malignant oral lesions and conditions: An overview of the literature. *J Oral Pathol Med* 2008;**37**:1–10.

6. Franceschi S, Bidoli E, Herrero R, *et al.* Comparison of cancers of the oral cavity and pharynx worldwide: Aetiological clues. *Oral Oncol* 2000;**36**:106–15.

7. Cancela MC, Ramadas K, Fayette JM, *et al.* Alcohol intake and oral cavity cancer risk among men in a prospective study in Kerala, India. *Community Dent Oral Epidemiol* 2009;**37**:342–9.

8. Gillison ML. Current topics in the epidemiology of oral cavity and oropharyngeal cancers. *Head Neck* 2007;**29**:779–92.

9. Poh CF, Ng S, Berean KW, *et al.* Biopsy and histopathologic diagnosis of oral premalignant and malignant lesions. *J Can Dent Assoc* 2008;**74**:283–8.

10. Thomas S, Varghese BT, Sebastian P, *et al.* Intramuscular lipomatosis of tongue. *Postgrad Med J* 2002;**78**:295–7.

11. Edge SB, Byrd DR, Compton CC (eds). *AJCC Cancer Staging Manual.* 7th ed. New York, NY: Springer; 2010:33

12. Sparano A, Weinstein G, Chalian A, *et al.* Multivariate predictors of occult neck metastasis in early oral tongue cancer. *Otolaryngol Head Neck Surg* 2004;**131**:472–6.

13. Steiner W, Fierek O, Ambrosch P, *et al.* Transoral laser microsurgery for squamous cell carcinoma of the base of the tongue. *Arch Otolaryngol Head Neck Surg* 2003;**129**:36.

14. Mendenhall WM, Parsons JT, Stringer SP, *et al.* Squamous cell carcinoma of the head and neck treated with irradiation: Management of the neck. *Semin Radiat Oncol* 1992;**2**:163.

15. Hill BT, Price LA, MacRae K. Importance of primary site in assessing chemotherapy response and 7-year survival data in advanced squamous cell carcinomas of the head and neck treated with initial combination chemotherapy without cisplatin. *J Clin Oncol* 1986;**4**:1340–7.

16. Licitra L, Grandi C, Guzzo M, *et al.* Primary chemotherapy in resectable oral cavity squamous cell cancer: A randomized controlled trial. *J Clin Oncol* 2003;**21**:327.

17. Iype EM, Sebastian P, Mathew A, *et al.* The role of selective neck dissection (I–III) in the treatment of node negative (N0) neck in oral cancer. *Oral Oncol* 2008;**44**:1134–8. PMID: 18486527.

18. Fitzpatrick PJ. Cancer of the lip. *J Otolaryngol* 1984;**13**:32.

19. ón-Barbellido S, Campo-Trapero J, ánchez J, *et al.* Gene therapy in the management of oral cancer: Review of the literature. *Med Oral Patol Oral Cir Bucal* 2008;**13**:E15–E21.

20. Piccirillo JF, Costas I, Reichman ME. Cancers of the head and neck. In: Reis LAG, Young LF, Keel GE, *et al.* (eds). *SEER survival monograph: Cancer survival among adults: US SEER Program, 1988–2001, patient and tumor characteristics.* Bethesda, MD: National Cancer Institute, SEER Program, NIH Pub. No. 07-6215, 2007:7–22.

21. Byers RM. Squamous cell carcinoma of the oral tongue in patients less than thirty years of age. *Am J Surg* 1975;**130**:475–8.

22. Schantz SP, Yu GP. Head and neck cancer incidence trends in young Americans, 1973–1997, with a special analysis for tongue cancer. *Arch Otolaryngol Head Neck Surg* 2002;**128**:268–74.

23. Funk GF, Karnell LH, Robinson RA, *et al.* Presentation, treatment, and outcome of oral cavity cancer: A national cancer data base report. *Head Neck* 2002;**24**:165–80.

24. Verschuur HP, Irish JC, O'Sullivan B, *et al.* A matched control study of treatment outcome in young patients with squamous cell carcinoma of the head and neck. *Laryngoscope* 1999;**109**:249–58.

25. Veness MJ, Morgan GI, Sathiyaseelan Y, *et al.* Anterior to cancer and the incidence of CLN mets. *ANZ J Surg* 2005;**75**:101–5.

26. Atula S, Grenman R, Laippala P, *et al.* Cancer of the tongue in patients younger than 40 years. A distinct entity? *Arch Otolaryngol Head Neck Surg* 1996;**122**:1313–19.

27. Sasaki T, Moles DR, Imai Y, *et al.* Clinico-pathological features of squamous cell carcinoma of the oral cavity in patients <40 years of age. *J Oral Pathol Med* 2005;**34**:129–33.

28. Llewellyn CD, Linklater K, Bell J, *et al.* Squamous cell carcinoma of the oral cavity in patients aged 45 years and under: A descriptive analysis of 116 cases diagnosed in the South-East of England from 1990 to 1997. *Oral Oncol* 2003;**39**:106–14.

29. Llewellyn CD, Johnson NW, Warnakulasuriya KA. Risk factors for squamous cell carcinoma of the oral cavity in young people—a comprehensive literature review. *Oral Oncol* 2001;**37**:401–18.

30. Shiboski CH, Schmidt BL, Jordan RC. Tongue and tonsil carcinoma: Increasing trends in the US population ages 20–44 years. *Cancer* 2005;**103**:1843–9.

31. Miller CS, Johnstone BM. Human papilloma virus as a risk factor for oral squamous cell carcinoma: A meta-analysis, 1982–1997. *Oral Surg Oral Med Oral Pathol Oral Radiol Endod* 2001;**91**:622–35 ECOG.

32. Carole F, William HW, Signi L, *et al.* Improved Survival of patients with human papilloma virus—positive head and neck squamous cell carcinoma in a prospective clinical trial. *J Natl Cancer Inst* 2008;**100**:261–9.

33. Sisk EA, Bradford CR, Jacob A, *et al.* Human papilloma virus infection in "young" versus "old" patients with squamous cell carcinoma of the head and neck. *Head Neck* 2000;**22**:649–57.

34. Epstein JB, Silverman S Jr. Head and neck malignancies associated with HIV infection. *Oral Surg Oral Med Oral Pathol* 1992;**73**:193–200.

35. Regazi JA, Dekker NP, McMillan A, *et al.* P53, p21, Rb, and MDM2 proteins in tongue carcinoma from patients <35 versus >75 years. *Oral Oncol* 1999;**35**:379–83.

36. Koch WM, Lango M, Sewell D, *et al.* Head and neck cancer in non-smokers: A distinct clinical and molecular entity. *Laryngoscope* 1999;**109**:1544–51.

37. Kutler DI, Auerbach AD, Satagopan J, *et al.* High incidence of head and neck squamous cell carcinoma in patients with Fanconi anemia. *Arch Otolaryngol Head Neck Surg* 2003;**129**:106–12.

38. Annertz K, Anderson H, Biorklund A, *et al.* Incidence and survival of squamous cell carcinoma of the tongue in Scandinavia, with special reference to young adults. *Int J Cancer* 2002;**101**:95–9.

39. Lacy PD, Piccirillo JF, Merrit MG, *et al.* Head and neck squamous cell carcinoma: Better to be young. *Otolaryngol Head Neck Surg* 2000;**122**:253–8.

40. Kolker JL, Ismail AI, Sohn W, *et al.* Trends in the incidence, mortality, and survival rates of oral and pharyngeal cancer in a high-risk area in Michigan, USA. *Community Dent Oral Epidemiol* 2007;**35**:489–99.

41. Von Doersten PG, Cruz RM, Rasgon BM, *et al.* Relation between age and head and neck cancer recurrence after surgery: A multivariate analysis. *Otolaryngol Head Neck Surg* 1995;**113**:197–203.

42. McGregor AD, MacDonald DG. Routes of entry of squamous cell carcinoma to the mandible. *Head Neck* 1988;**10**:294–301.

43. Brown JS, Lowe D Kalavrezo N, *et al.* Patterns of invasion and routes of tumor entry into the mandible by oral squamous cell carcinoms. *Head Neck* 2002;**24**:370–83.

44. Van der Brekel MW, Runne RW, Smeele LE, *et al.* Assessment of tumour invasion into mandible: The value of different imaging techniques. *Eur Radiol* 1998;**8**:1552–7.

45. Genden EM, Rinaldo A, Jacobson A. Management of mandibular invasion: When is marginal mandibulectomy appropriate? *Oral oncology* 2005;**41**:777.

46. Marchetta FC, Sako K, Murphy JB. The periosteum of the mandible and intraoral carcinoma. *Am J Surg* 1971;**122**:711–13.

47. Wolff D, Hassfeld S. Influence of marginal and segmental mandibular resection on the survival rate in patients with squamous cell carcinoma of the inferior parts of the oral cavity. *Craniomaxillofac Surg* 2004;**34**:318–23.

10

Cancer of the oropharynx

N. KANNAN, BIPIN T. VARGHESE, K. CHANDRAMOHAN, PAUL SEBASTIAN

Introduction

Squamous cell carcinomas of the head and neck (HNSCC) are by far the commonest type of cancer in the Indian subcontinent. The factors that predispose to HNSCC are the use of tobacco products, alcohol and malnutrition. Oropharyngeal cancers can arise from the lining epithelium, lymphoid tissues present in the tonsils and base of tongue (BOT), or the minor salivary glands located in the soft palate uvula and BOT. Almost half of the epithelial tumours are formed by those arising from the tonsils and its pillars (50%), followed by BOT or vallecula (30%), soft palate (10%) and posterior pharyngeal wall (5%). By virtue of the unique location and dual role of a conduit to both food and air, successful management of the tumours at this site poses functional and rehabilitative problems that require a multidisciplinary management team, including a surgeon, radiation oncologist, medical oncologist, physiotherapist, dental surgeon and prosthodontist. Failed therapy, unfortunately, results in poor survival and a poorer quality of life. Whereas the histology and biological characteristics of oropharyngeal tumours are no different from tumours of other sites of the head and neck, certain anatomical factors make their presentation, symptomatology and overall behaviour different. According to American Joint Committee on Cancer (AJCC), overall observed survival is 50%, 47.5%, 37.9%, and 26.1% for stages 1, 2, 3 and 4, respectively. Similarly, relative survival at 5 years is 57.3%, 53.7%, 43.2% and 29.6%, for stages 1, 2, 3 and 4, respectively.[1]

Anatomy

The oropharynx is a hollow muscular, epithelium-lined tube situated at the junction of the nasopharynx, oral cavity and hypopharynx. It is a part of pharynx that extends from the plane of the superior surface of the soft palate to the superior surface of the hyoid bone (or floor of the vallecula). At the superior boundary the ciliated columnar mucosa gives way to stratified squamous mucosa. Anteriorly, it extends to the plane of the junction of the hard and soft palate and the circumvallate papillae of the tongue. Laterally, it is bounded by the anterior and posterior tonsillar pillars, tonsillar fossae, superior constrictor and the parapharyngeal spaces. The inferior limit is the plane of the hyoid bone. Posteriorly, the orophyarynx is bounded by the posterior pharyngeal wall, buccopharyngeal fascia and the prevertebral fascia covering the prevertebral muscles and ligaments (Fig. 1). The sites at which a mucosal/sub-mucosal lesion occur in this anatomical area are the soft palate and uvula, tonsillar pillars, tonsil, pharyngo-epiglottic fold, posterior third of the tongue, tonsillolingual or glosso-tonsillar sulci and the lateral and posterior pharyngeal walls.

Parapharyngeal and retropharyngeal lesions, such as salivary neoplasms, schwannoma and lymph nodes, may also present in the site by projecting into the lumen of the oropharynx with an intact mucosa.

The region is densely innervated, with nerves often causing referred pain along their distribution in the ear and temporal region. A rich network of lymphatics and their draining nodes

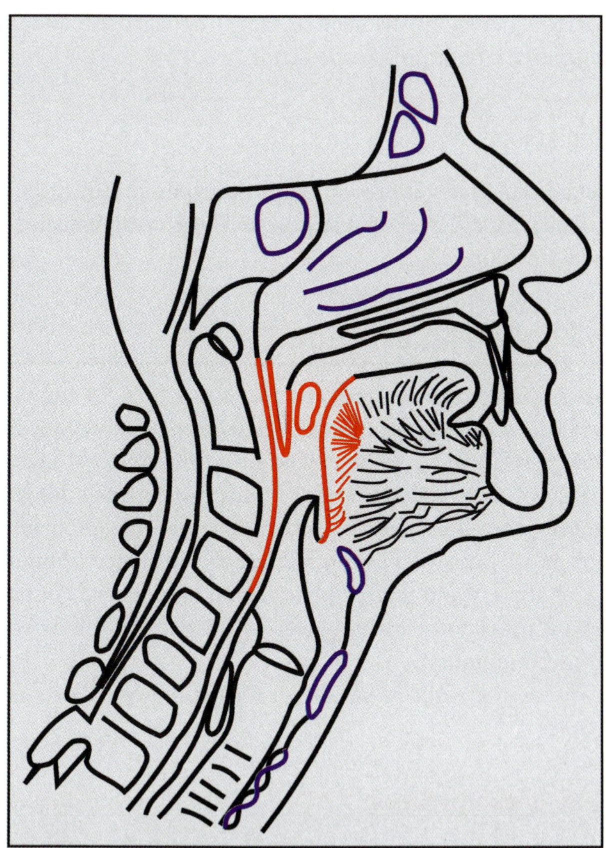

Fig. 1. Anatomical limits of oropharynx (marked in red)

are present in the oropharynx because of which lymph node spread is quite common. Superficial lymphoid follicles are present in the BOT in close relationship to the mucosa. In addition, the palatine tonsils (part of the Waldeyer ring) are situated laterally.

Cancers of the oropharynx are aggressive, apart from tumours of the soft palate. As tumours spread deeper they progressively involve the posterior segment of the mandible, pterygoid muscles and pharyngeal musculature leading to trismus, and swallowing and speech difficulties. Invasion of the buccopharyngeal fascia leads to fixity with the prevertebral fascia and spread in the longitudinal axis. Perineural spread of the tumour along tissue planes often produces involvement of cranial nerves IX–XII and extension to the base of skull.

Pathology

Whereas tumours of the head and neck continue to be the commonest type of malignancy in India, the developed world is presently witnessing a rise in the incidence of HNSCC, especially of the oropharynx, which is possibly related to an increase in chewing tobacco, sexual practices, human papilloma virus (HPV) and human immunodeficiency virus (HIV) infection.[2] Squamous cell carcinoma and its uncommon variants—verrucous, spindle cell and adenosquamous

carcinomas—account for >90% of all tumours of the oropharynx. Diagnostic difficulty is usually encountered with the verrucous carcinoma and often a clinical call needs to be taken after repeated biopsies are analysed as hyperkeratosis.

The entire mucosa of the oropharynx is studded with salivary glands—both mucous and serous in equal proportion. So it is not surprising that salivary gland tumours are the next most common lesions of the oropharynx. The incidence of malignancy in minor salivary tumours is high and all salivary gland tumours need to be assessed for malignancy, especially adenoid cystic carcinoma which has a high potential for distant metastasis.

Many lymphomas may present with proliferation of the lymphoid tissue of Waldeyer ring in isolation or associated with lymphadenopathy. This is one of the most common extranodal sites for non-Hodgkin lymphoma in the head and neck region. Some parapharyngeal tumours, notably those from the deep lobe of the parotid gland, the rare carotid body tumours and schwannoma arising from the cranial nerves or its branches may present with a bulge in the soft palate region.

Precancerous changes, such as leukoplakia, erythroplakia and hyperkeratosis, which are likely to be precursors to frank invasive squamous cell carcinoma, are however often not noted because of the inaccessibility of the oropharynx, which makes routine inspection difficult.

Tobacco use in any form has been linked strongly, along with alcohol intake, to the development of carcinomas of the oral cavity and oropharynx. The association is multiplicative rather than merely additive.[3] HPV is known to be associated with HNSCC in approximately 25% of cases. It induces carcinogenesis by inhibition of p53 and pRb by the viral oncogenes E6 and E7. Evidence supports the role of HPV as a co-agent even in the absence of expression of these proteins.[4,5]

Presentation of tumour spread

These tumours usually present with sore throat or odynophagia, earache and a muffled, plummy or a hot-potato quality of voice. In up to 75% of cases the patient may present with an enlarged cervical node. Gross appearance of the tumour may be exoplytic, ulcerative or smooth surfaced. The patterns of its spread are important in planning the limits of treatment.

Pattern of tumour spread

Local

Tumours of the oropharynx tend to spread either to the masticator space or downwards to the larynx, either of which makes the tumour a bad candidate for upfront surgery. The recent tumour, node, metastasis (TNM) classification stages them as T4b.[1]

All squamous cell cancers spread in the submucosal plane to varying distances, usually 5–10 mm from the primary site. Invasion thereafter occurs to deeper tissues and the tumour spreads along natural tissue planes and areas of fascial deficiency, resulting in involvement of adjacent sites.

BOT lesions are typically burrowing and infiltrating, usually causing involvement of deeper tongue muscles and leading to impaired mobility. Lateral tongue lesions invade the tonsillolingual sulcus and spread of tumour into the neck posterior to the myelohyoid muscle allows the tumour to be palpable in the neck. Vallecular lesions have a propensity to spread submucosally and involve the pre-epiglottic space.

Lesions of the anterior tonsillar pillar usually present early with erythroplakia or leucoplakia. They spread superiorly to the maxillary gingival, posterior to the hard palate and soft palate and inferiorly to the tonsillo-lingual sulcus and tongue. Anterior spread can also occur to the buccal mucosa and retromolar trigone. Deeper invasion results in involvement of the medial pterygoid, extension to base of skull and invasion of the mandible, which produces trismus and temporal pain.

Lesions of the tonsillar fossa are usually infiltrative and ulcerative, spreading to the posterior tonsillar pillar, lateral pharyngeal wall and lateral BOT. Whereas advanced lesions invade the parapharyngeal space, involvement of the cranial nerves is uncommon. These lesions tend to spread along the palatopharyngeus muscle to the middle constrictor and the thyroid cartilage.

Lesions of the soft palate are almost always on the oral side. Multiple premalignant lesions may coexist along with a frank malignancy. Spread is usually to the hard palate, tonsillar pillars and further lateral extension leads to invasion of the superior constrictor and base of skull.

Nodal

The first echelon nodes are the subdigastric level 2 nodes. The progression of nodal involvement is fairly orderly and proceeds downwards along the jugular vein. Involvement of levels 1 and 5 nodes are infrequent. However, a higher degree of invasion of the nodes in level 2b is seen. Well lateralized lesions, such as tonsil and anterior tonsillar pillar, have a 10% incidence of contralateral disease compared to the high propensity for bilaterality in BOT and soft palate lesions.

The mapping studies by the Anderson group[6] reveal that 75% of patients with cancers in BOT have clinically positive nodes on admission. Thirty per cent have bilateral nodes and the risk of occult positivity is close to 50%. Anterior tonsillar pillar lesions have a lower nodal positivity of 45% compared with tonsillar lesions, which are almost always diagnosed with a neck node. Tonsillar lesions have a low (10%) incidence of contralateral nodes. Posterior tonsillar pillar lesions are more likely to have nodes along the spinal accessory nerve. Involvement of the retropharyngeal nodes is considered a poor prognostic factor.

Metastasis

Distant metastasis at presentation is uncommon (in <10% of patients), except in case of large lesions with a high degree of nodal invasion.

Evaluation and staging

The AJCC staging[7] is used, according to which T1 tumours are those within 2 cm in longest diameter, T2 between 2 and 4 cm, T3 >4 cm or those extending to the mucosal lingual surface of the epiglottis and T4 showing extrinsic tongue/ medial pterygoid muscle, larynx, adjacent mandibular or hard palate invasion (T4a or moderately advanced tumours) or lateral pterygoid muscle/plate, lateral nasopharynx or base of skull invasion or carotid artery encasement (T4b or very advanced tumours).

N staging is the same as that for lip and oral cavity (*see* Chapter 9).

Clinical examination

Good clinical examination is the cornerstone for successfully diagnosing lesions early in patients presenting with non-specific symptoms of throat pain, nasal speech, dysarthria, ill fitting dentures, blood in sputum, halitosis, otalgia, headache, nasal regurgitation, aspiration, dysphagia, odynophagia, or enlarged lymph nodes. It is equally important to evaluate the local extent of disease spread to the nodes and second primary which includes a panendoscopy, digital examination, examination under anaesthesia, and biopsy of suspicious areas.

The recent increase in incidence of oropharyngeal cancers in the West, especially in younger patients, has prompted adjunctive diagnostic aids in the form of screening with toluidine blue and autofluroscence technology,[8] although data from these methods are yet not robust for implementation in clinical practice.

Imaging

All patients who are diagnosed with an oropharyngeal tumour will benefit from a high quality contrast-enhanced computerized tomography (CT) scan, which defines the anatomy of the tumour and its extent in all dimensions, and reveals the involvement of nodes, bony structures, parapharyngeal spaces and vascular spaces. The CT scan is essential for treatment volume planning when the patient is to be treated by radiotherapy (RT).

A contrast-enhanced magnetic resonance imaging (MRI)

defines the soft tissue detail with better clarity than the CT scan. CT and MRI are complimentary investigations and are useful in planning surgery.

The introduction of positron emission tomography-CT (PET-CT) in the last decade has made functional evaluation of the primary site and involved nodes possible. The sensitivity of PET-CT in picking up second primary or involved nodes is >90%, but coexisting infections accompanying oral cancers make the specificity lower. The utility of PET standardized uptake values (SUVs) has been demonstrated in prediction of response to therapy,[9] outcome of treatment,[10] mapping of disease for planning RT fields and follow up of treated cases for detection of recurrence.[11]

Principles of treatment

Conservation surgery and radical RT are equally effective in treating T1 and T2 oropharyngeal tumours. Good exposure and adequate clearance are the key factors determining success of surgical management. Surgical access to the site of the tumour is gained by a lip split and paramedian mandibulatomy approach with a mandibular swing. The mandible is swung laterally after incising the mucosa on the lingual side and dividing the mylohyoid muscle. For approach to the oropharynx, it may be necessary to release the temporalis muscle from the coronoid process.

Those T1 and T2 tumours limited to BOT can be excised and the defect closed primarily. Similar lesions in the uvula can be excised in the form of a wedge with primary closure of the defect (uvulectomy). Tumours confined to tonsils can be dealt with an extended tonsillectomy.

Superficial T1 and T2 tumours can be excised with the help of lasers. The best form of reconstruction of an oropharyngeal defect after excision of T3 and T4 tumours is free-flap repair, as it offers the best tissue match.

For more advanced tumours (T3 and T4), combination treatment offers the best chance for the patient. Primary surgery followed by RT or chemo-RT is probably the best form of treatment, but in practice it carries a high degree of morbidity and complications. Hence, non-surgical means of treatment in the form of chemotherapy, radiation, or targeted therapy with biological agents in combination with RT is used.

In view of the general belief that oropharyngeal tumours are quite radiosensitive and that surgery carries a high morbidity, most of the patients are treated by RT with or without chemotherapy or molecular targeted therapy. Moreover, anatomical proximity of the oropharynx to the internal carotid artery, prevertebral space and larynx, often restricts good surgical tumour clearance. Surgery is, therefore, often reserved as a salvage option when disease residue is limited after a non-surgical treatment regime or for early recurrence after non-surgical treatment.

Primary surgery as a treatment option is decided on the basis of (i) the location of the tumour, (ii) when there is a possibility of three-dimensional clearance of at least 0.5 cm, (iii) the histology and type of the tumour (salivary gland tumours) and (iv) the availability of good reconstructive options.

Deciding on the optimal therapy for patients with oropharyngeal cancers is crucial to ensure desirable quantity and quality of life and to prevent them from being condemned to the life of an oropharyngeal and airway cripple. Many of the patients present with advanced cancers, and in addition have significant co-morbidity related to pre-treatment nutritional deprivation, and cardiac and pulmonary compromise secondary to the ravages of tobacco and alcohol abuse. Whereas it may be possible to do an oncologically sound surgery, the possibility of the patient being able to cope with the procedure is often limited.

Patients who are nutritionally challenged due to the pre-existing dysphagia and odynophagia often need correction of deficits of macro- and micronutrients prior to the start of therapy.[12] Co-morbidity relating to cardiac and pulmonary compromise needs to be optimized by drug therapy and physiotherapy. Education of measures to prevent aspiration will aid in prevention of soiling of lungs pre- and post-operatively.

When surgery is considered, a thorough discussion of the extent of the procedure, resultant cosmetic deformity, functional disability and post-surgical rehabilitation after treatment needs to be made with the patient to ensure adequate compliance from the patient and relatives during the recovery. Often, a patient, especially in India, will opt for a treatment that may have less physical and financial constraints.

Treatment options

The choice of therapy is usually between surgery and RT. Generally, for early-stage lesions, i.e. T1 and T2, the functional morbidity of surgical procedures and the need to address both sides of the neck make RT an acceptable and preferred modality of treatment by virtue of similar control rates, ease of treatment and lesser morbidity.[13] An exception may, however, be made in the case of young patients in whom RT can be reserved for a recurrence. Many studies have shown that the results in terms of disease-specific survival, overall survival and recurrence rates are similar for RT alone and in combination with surgery.[14]

For large lesions (T3 and T4), surgery needs to be included in the multidisciplinary treatment planning if any attempt to achieve long-term control is desired. The use of novel treatment schedules, i.e. neoadjuvant therapy with radiation, and chemotherapy[15] alone or in combination with radiation,[16] may be used to make lesions surgically manageable and achieve R0 resection. The morbidity of resections in terms of healing, fistulation, swallowing and speech impairment is high and the loss of the mandible worsens the recovery. The complex and massive procedures needed for large lesions also carry a significant mortality of 5%–7%.[17]

Many large lesions of BOT that extend inferiorly would need resection of the supraglottic larynx. In such patients the decision to operate would depend on the age of the patient, general health, pulmonary status and whether or not it will be possible to save at least 50% of the tongue base with its vasculature and nerve supply for ensuring adequate swallowing and laryngeal protection. The patients in whom a large portion of BOT would be resected, or those who are unlikely to be able to protect their airway, may need a total or near total laryngectomy or a laryngoplasty[18] procedure to prevent aspiration and pulmonary sepsis.

Surgery

Surgery for oropharyngeal cancers is usually indicated in the following situations:

- Lateralized lesions of BOT, when the excision is likely to leave behind one lingual artery and at least 50% of the tongue base
- Lesions of the tonsil alone, or with minimal extensions to the palate, retromolar trigone or tongue (Fig. 2)
- Superficial lesions of the palate, uvula, vallecula and anterior tonsillar pillar
- Small midline lesions of BOT, usually salivary neoplasms
- As a salvage procedure for residual disease after RT or small-volume recurrent disease (Fig. 2).

Approach to the primary lesion

Transoral excision: This is an approach usually used for small and possibly very early cancers or leucoplakia in easily approachable sites, such as the tonsillar pillar, tonsil, soft palate and posterior pharyngeal wall, which are clinically superficial; complete resection is possible with clear margins. Often, this excision can be performed using a CO_2 laser, although excision with cold knife or electrocautery is equally feasible. The ipsilateral neck, which is likely to be N0 clinically, is addressed either by a staged approach or concurrently. Eckel and colleagues have demonstrated >80% disease-specific survival and 78% of locoregional control at 5 years using CO_2 laser for the primary and discontinuous neck dissection in carefully selected oropharyngeal cancer patients.[19] The need to incorporate adjuvant multimodality therapy is essential when using such an approach to achieve good disease control in addition to preservation of organ and function.[20]

Mandibular swing approach by anterior mandibulotomy/ lateral mandibulotomy: Contrary to the previously held belief that the mandible needs to be sacrificed to ensure that the lymphatics are adequately addressed, studies by Marchetta and colleagues have found that the periosteal lymphatics

of the mandible do not contain malignant cells.[21] This has paved the way for mandibular preservation strategies, which improve the quality of cosmesis and function. Mandibular preservation is possible in most cases in the absence of previous irradiation and a disease-free periosteum. In general, no imaging modality has accurately predicted mandibular periosteal invasion. Clinically, the mandible is presumed to be uninvolved if the periosteum strips easily during surgery.

Mandibular division for access to the pharynx was first suggested by Trotter in 1931.[22] The approach is usually through an anterior midline lip split or a visor flap. The anterior midline split accords excellent exposure of the tonsillar and BOT areas, and is preferred whenever the posterior segment of the mandible can be preserved.

The mandibulectomy approach, usually a posterior segment mandibular excision, is used for tonsillar lesions that have extended to the retromolar trigone area and/or invaded the mandible (Figs 2 and 3). The mandibular incision is placed anterior to the area to be resected, taking care not to enter the tumour by mistake.

Midline translingual pharyngotomy is a procedure usually used for small, purely midline tumours of BOT. The approach bisects the tongue in the midline; the tongue is reconstructed following resection. Usually, tongue tumours are large owing to the long period of dormancy and non-specific complaints leading to a delay in diagnosis. This procedure is hence used only in the occasional small salivary neoplasms of BOT.

Transcervical transhyoid pharyngotomy is more popular than the midline translingual approach and is used for small non-squamous lateral BOT tumours via a vallecular entry

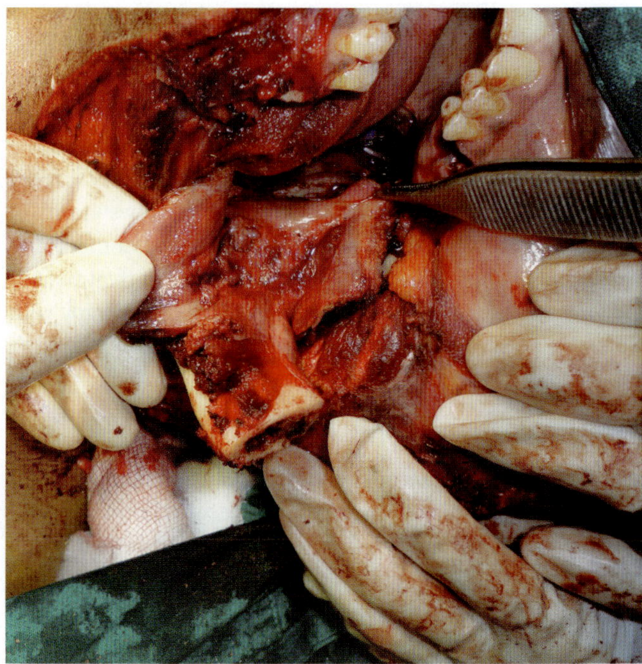

Fig. 2. Radioresidual advanced cancer of the tonsil being resected with the affected portion of the mandible [commando procedure]

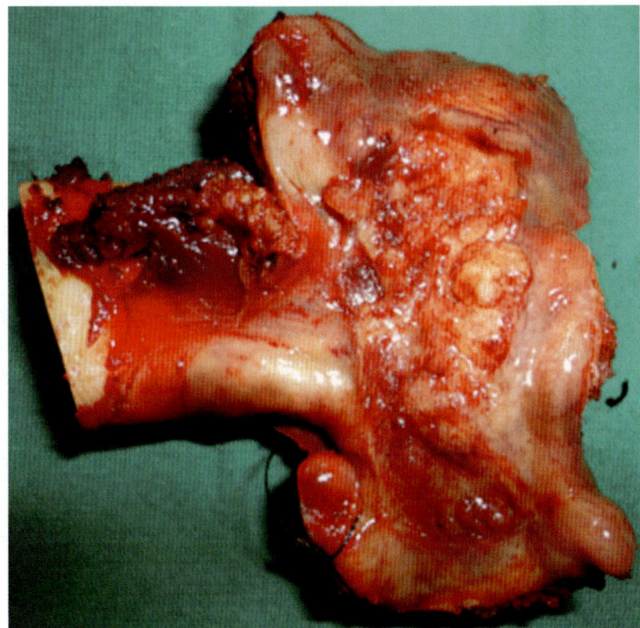

Fig. 3. Resected specimen

by resecting the lateral part of the hyoid.[23,24] Adequate care needs to be taken to protect the lingual artery and hypoglossal nerve.

Management of the neck

Approximately 50% of patients have clinically apparent nodes at presentation. The incidence of occult nodal deposits in a clinically negative neck (N0) increases with the tumour size. Whereas incidence of truly T1 (<2 cm) lesions that have an occult N+ status is approximately 10%–15%, the incidence for T2 and beyond is >50%.[25] The incidence of contralateral nodal disease is also similarly high in lesions in the midline, like BOT and vallecula. Upstaging happens in 40%–50% of cases after elective dissection of the neck.[26] This incidence of occult disease makes a wait-and-watch policy for neck dissection a dangerous one, except for the very small anterior pillar, soft palate, or uvular lesion.

The type of neck dissection has been substantially debated, much of which is addressed at length in a different section. Modified radical neck dissection is the standard of care and the surgeon performing a bilateral neck dissection needs to preserve at least one jugular vein. Preservation of the accessory nerve and/or the sternomastoid muscle in the presence of involved nodes needs to be weighed against the oncological completeness of the surgery. Whereas there is no doubt about the need for neck dissection on the side of the disease, in the presence of pathologically involved nodes, RT for a clinically negative neck (N0), especially on the opposite side, is amply supported in the literature with a view to reducing morbidity.[27]

Reconstruction

Special attention needs to be paid to the physiology of the oropharynx and the way the surgical defect will alter it. When reconstruction of oropharyngeal defects is planned, there needs to be a special attention to the physiology of the region. During deglutition, the oropharynx is important for bolus formation, propulsion down the cricopharyngeal sphincter and prevention of nasal regurgitation or laryngeal aspiration. For speech to occur, the closure of the nasopharynx by the soft palate and mobility of the pharynx and tongue are important to prevent dysarthria. The aim of resection and reconstruction is to close the wound in a leak-poof manner. This prevents pooling and retention of secretions and food and aids the remaining oropharynx to perform the native functions adequately. Most patients almost invariably need about 1 year to speak intelligibly and eat in public without aspiration. These are important aspects of evaluation of a successful treatment.[28] Reconstruction methods include the following:

Primary closure and local flaps: When the defect is small, or consequent to resection of the posterior mandible, the tissues collapse and allow approximation of the cut edges. This situation is often encountered during resection of the tonsil with a small portion of BOT and the mandible. Functional results are good with this procedure. However, larger defects thus treated increase the risk of fistula formation and result in tethering of the tongue, leading to speech and swallowing difficulty.[29] The tongue flap is a local flap available to line such a defect of the tonsillar region.[30]

Skin grafts: These are rarely used in oropharyngeal surgery owing to the difficulty in maintaining them in position and their limited use in composite tissue loss. Defects of the lateral tongue base and tonsil may be treated with skin grafts to prevent tethering of the tongue and ensure a primary closure.

Pedicled flaps: Various flaps, such as the forehead flap and delto-pectoral flap, had been the workhorse of the head and neck oncologist. Despite being robust flaps they have fallen out of favour due to their lack of bulk, resulting cosmetic defect and need for a second procedure for insetting them.

Ariyan first described the pectoralis major myocutaneous (PMMC) flap in 1980 and since then this has become one of the most commonly used flaps in head and neck surgery. The advantage of myocutaneous flaps is that they have excellent blood supply, skin and muscle available to line the defect and provide bulk and single-stage dependable reconstruction (Fig. 4).[31] The other commonly used flap is the latissmus dorsi flap. Other conventional options are sternomastoid myocutaneous flap and the submental artery island flap.

Free tissue transfer: The state of the art since the late 1970s is to use composite free tissue transfer, which provides tissues with adequate bulk, vascularity and minimal cosmetic

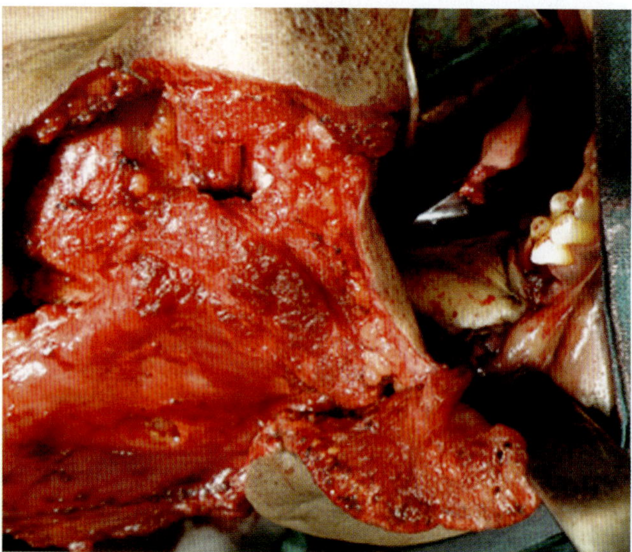

Fig. 4. Reconstruction of the defect with pectoralis major myocutaneous (PMMC) flap

deformity and donor site dysfunction. The common donor sites are the radial forearm, groin, latissmus dorsi and anterolateral thigh. The radial forearm flap is by far the most popular, and modifications have been made to the flap to make reconstruction of BOT more physiological and the functional results more superior.[32] Alternatively, a free jejunal segment or a free gastro-omental flap, which can provide lining and bulk *vis-a-vis* the jejunal flap, can also be used for the defects.[33]

Photodynamic therapy (PDT)

The use of laser to excite photoporphyrin derivatives for destroying cancer cells has been under investigation for the past 2 decades. The major drawback, despite being an appealing concept, has been drug development for PDT and their side-effects. Newer photochemicals with fewer side-effects and lesser light precaution guidelines have been developed. PDT is highly effective and has the advantage of repeatability, temporary morbidity, and minimal organ dysfunction.[33,34] It is still an experimental tool with a role in recurrent tumours and is useful as an alternative modality when conventional therapy is not possible.

Radiotherapy and chemo-radiotherapy

For early oropharyngeal cancer, RT is an acceptable and often the preferred modality of treatment with loco-regional control rates and disease-specific survival in approximately 80% of cases at 5 years. The advantages of RT include the following:
- Avoidance of surgical complications
- Preservation of appearance and, potentially, the function of the treated organ
- Advantage of including irradiation of lymph nodes, with little added morbidity compared with the added morbidity of extensive neck dissection
- Better tolerance than surgery by medically unfit patients.

For post-operative patients, RT is essential in the presence of high-risk factors, such as margin positivity, perineural or lymphovascular space invasion, multiple positive nodes and extracapsular spread of tumour from the nodes. RT reduces the risk of recurrence in these poor risk cases.[35] Gourin *et al.* reported a 56% disability status scale for cases treated by surgery followed by RT in a group with 50% T1 and T2 lesions.[16] Similar results are echoed in other studies.[12,13] The risk reduction is better when the adjuvant RT is combined with chemotherapy.[36]

Conventional RT with a total dose of 66–70 Gy imparts a locoregional control of about 50% at 2 years and an overall survival of 40% at 3 years for all stages combined. Recent efforts to improve this figure by altered fractionation of RT improves locoregional control by about 10%.[37] This comes with added toxicity and a small but significant mortality, and no change to the distant recurrence rates.

Intensity-modulated RT (IMRT): Newer technology and precise image-guided collimation of radiation by means of multi-leaf collimators makes it possible to deliver a tumoricidal radiation dose to a specified target consisting of the tumour and its margins, while at the same time sparing the normal unaffected tissues from radiation effects. This technology makes it possible to spare vital structures, such as the spinal cord, blood vessels and salivary glands from the effect of RT, thus improving post-treatment quality of life. Comparison with conventional RT shows equivalent if not better control.[38] IMRT results in a significant reduction of patient- and observer-rated head and neck symptoms compared with standard 3D-chemo-RT.[39]

Head and neck cancers exhibit moderate sensitivity to chemotherapy. Commonly used chemotherapeutic regimes are platinum-based, using cisplatin or carboplatin alone or in combination with 5-FU (fluorouracil), and/or taxanes, with response rates of 50%–60%, including complete responses in approximately 10%–15% of patients.[37] Chemotherapy has the potential to improve the result of treatment by reducing distant metastasis, mopping up microscopic local and regional disease, and sensitizing the tumour to the effect of RT. More importantly, the use of chemotherapy is likely to increase organ preservation and improve overall quality of life.

Chemotherapy in conjunction with RT is the modality which has the support of numerous randomized controlled trials and is the standard of care[40] for unresectable disease as primary definitive therapy, with improvement of 5-year overall survival from 25% to 50%.[41,42] Various combinations of therapy are under investigation and they include the use of chemotherapy as induction therapy, chemotherapy with altered fractionation of RT, adjuvant chemoradiation following surgery, RT with epidermal growth factor receptor inhibitors and adjuvant chemotherapy. This subject is described in detail elsewhere in the book.

Rehabilitation

A significant number of patients report speech and swallowing problems in addition to xerostomia, pain and shoulder syndrome after surgery, radiation, or both for treatment of oropharyngeal cancer. The degree of difficulty and extent of impairment reflects on the volume of tissue loss, stage and site of disease, and whether or not RT was used. Younger patients have lesser coping up issues than older patients. A successful rehabilitation programme includes participation of a physiotherapist, prosthodontist and speech therapist, supported by clinicians.

It is well known that most patients lose weight secondary to the treatment effects of surgery and RT. The standard policy is to advise nutritional supplementation to enable adequate nutrition and energy intake to be able to tolerate therapy. Often, this is ensured by tube feeding or percutaneous gastrostomy, which guarantees adequate caloric and protein intake with less weight loss than if patients were to rely solely on oral feeding.[43] Usage of the standardized protocols designed by the American Dietetic Association makes nutritional therapy easier.[44,45]

Conclusion

In general, stages 1 and 2 tumours may be managed by surgery or RT alone with excellent response and long-term survival. The incidence of upstaging is high—to the tune of 40%–50%; hence most patients are categorized as stage 3 or 4 and need combined modality therapy.[11] Deciding what is best for a patient with oropharyngeal cancer is a surgeon's dilemma. The morbidity of surgery can often be classified as unacceptable,[46] and often this results in patients opting for RT in its various modifications as a first-line therapy. Salvage of a post-radiation failure is often a difficult if not an impossible task, both surgically and for rehabilitation, thereby making the choice and extent of procedure and reconstruction crucial to avoid unacceptable morbidity.

References

1. Green FL, Page DL, Fleming ID, *et al*. Pharynx (including base of tounge, soft palate, and uvula). In: Fritz A, Balch CM (eds). *AJCC cancer staging handbook*. 6th ed. New York: Springer–Verlag; 2002:47–60.
2. Curado MP, Hashibe M. Recent changes in epidemiology of head and neck cancer. *Curr Opinion Oncol* 2009;**21**:194–200.
3. Znaor A, Brennan P, Gajalakshmi V, *et al*. Independent and combined effects of tobacco smoking, chewing and alcohol drinking on the risk of oral, pharyngeal and esophageal cancers in Indian men. *Int J Cancer* 2003;**105**:681–6.
4. Ragin CC, Modugno S, Gollin SM. The epidemiology and risk factors of head and neck carcinoma: Focus on HPV. *J Dental Res* 2007;**86**:104–14.
5. Chocolatewala MN, Chaturvedi P. Role of human papilloma virus in oral carcinogenesis: An Indian perspective. *J Cancer Res Ther* 2009;**5**:71–7.
6. Lindberg RD. Distribution of cervical lymphnode metastasis from squamous cell carcinoma of the upper respiratory and digestive tracts. *Cancer* 1972;**29**:1446.
7. Edge SB, Byrd DR, Compton CC (eds). *AJCC Cancer Staging* Manual. 7th ed. New York, NY: Springer; 2010:44–5.
8. Cohan DM, Popat S, Kaplan SE, *et al*. Oropharyngeal carcinoma: Current understanding and management. *Curr Opinion Otolaryngol Head Neck Surg* 2009;**17**:83–94.
9. Sang Yoon Kim, Jong-Lyel Roh, Mi Ra Kim, *et al*. Use of 18F-FDG PET for primary treatment strategy in patients with squamous cell carcinoma of the oropharynx. *J Nucl Med* 2007;**48**:752–7.
10. Schwartz DL, Rajendran J, Yueh B, *et al*. FDG-PET prediction of head and neck squamous cell cancer outcomes. *Arch Otolaryngol Head Neck Surg* 2004;**130**:1361–7.
11. Höder H, Fury M, Lee N, Kraus D. PET monitoring of therapy response in head and neck squamous cell carcinoma. *J Nucl Med* 2009;**50** (Suppl 1):74S–88S. Epub 2009 Apr 20.
12. Bassett MR, Dobie RA. Patterns of nutritional deficiency in head and neck cancer. *Otolaryngol Head Neck Surg* 1983;**91**:119.
13. Sessions DG, Lenox J, Sector GJ, *et al*. Analysis of treatment results for base tongue cancer. *Laryngoscope* 2003;**113**:1252–61.
14. Layland MC, Sessions DG, Lenox J. Influence of Lymphnodal metastasis in treatment of squamous cell carcinoma of oral cavity, oropharynx, larynx and hypopharynx: Node negative vs node positive. *Laryngoscope* 2005;**115**:629–33.
15. Domenge C, Hill C, Lefebvre JL, *et al*. Randomized trial of neoadjuvant chemotherapy in oropharyngeal carcinoma. French Groupe d'Etude des Tumeurs de la Tête et du Cou (GETTEC). *Br J Cancer* 2000;**83**:1594–8.
16. Malone JP, Stephens JA, Greaula JC, *et al*. Disease control, survival and functional outcomes after multimodal treatment for advanced stage tongue base cancer. *Head Neck* 2004;**26**:561–72.
17. Gourin CG, Johnson JT. Surgical treatment of squamous cell cancer of the base tongue. *Head Neck* 2001;**23**:653–60.
18. Biller HF, Lawson W, Baek S. Total glossectomy: A technique of reconstruction eliminating laryngectomy. *Arch Otolaryngol* 1983;**109**:69.
19. Eckel HE, Volling P, Potoschnig C, *et al*. Trans oral laser resection with staged discontinuous neck dissection for oral cavity and oropharyngeal cancers. *Laryngoscope* 1995;**105**:53–60.
20. Panje WR, Scher N, Karnell N. Transoral CO_2 laser ablation for cancers, tumours and other diseases. *Acta Otolaryngol Head Neck Surg* 1989;**115**:681–8.
21. Marchetta FC, Sako K, Murphy JB. The periosteum of mandible in intraoral carcinoma. *Am J Surg* 1971;**122**:711–13.
22. Trotter W. Some principles in the surgery of the pharynx. *Lancet* 1931;**2**:833.
23. Civantos F, Wening BL. Transhyoid resection of tongue base and tonsil tumours. *Otolaryngol Head Neck Surg* 1994;**111**:59.
24. Weber PC, Johnson JT, Meyers EM. The suprhyoid approach for squamous cell carcinoma of the base of the tongue. *Laryngoscope* 1992;**102**:637.
25. Vartanian JG, Pontes E, Agra IMG, *et al*. Distribution of metastatic lymphnodes in oropharyngeal carcinoma and its implications for elective treatment of the neck. *Arch Otolaryngol Head Neck Surg* 2003;**129**:729–32.

26. Walvekar RR, Li RJ, Gooding WE, *et al*. Role of surgery in limited T1-2 N0-1 carcinoma of the oropharynx. *Laryngoscope* 2008;**118**:2129–34.

27. Flecher GH. Elective irradiation of subclinical disease in cancers of the head and neck. *Cancer* 1972;**29**:1450.

28. Suarez Cunqueiro MM, Schramm A, Schoen R, *et al*. Speech and swallowing impairment after treatment of oral and oropharyngeal carcinoma. *Arch Otolaryngol Head Neck Surg* 2008;**34**:1299–304.

29. Conley JJ. The crippled oral cavity. *Plast Reconstr Surg* 1962;**30**:469.

30. DeSantoLW, Whicker JH, DeVine KD. Mandibular osteotomy and lingual flaps-use in patients with cancer of the tonsil and tongue base. *Arch Otolaryngol* 1975;**101**:652.

31. Schuller D. Myocutaneous flaps in reconstructive surgery of the head and neck. In: Wolf G (ed). *Head and neck oncology*. Boston: Martinus Nijhoff; 1984:107–28.

32. O'Connel DA, Rieger J, Harris JR, *et al*. Swallowing function in patients with base of tongue cancer treated by primary surgery and reconstruction with modified radial forearm free flap. *Arch Otolaryngl Head Neck Surg* 2008;**134**:857–74.

33. Bayles SW, Hayden RE. Gastro-omental free flap reconstruction of the head and neck. *Arch Facial Plast Surg* 2008;**10**:255–9.

34. Schweitzer UG, Sommers ML. PHOTOFRIN-mediated photo-dynamic therapy for treatment of early statge (Tis-T2 N0M0) squamous carcinoma of oral cavity and oropharynx. *Lasers Surg Med* 2010;**42**:1–8.

35. Ringual NR, Thankappan K, Cooper M, *et al*. Photodynamic therapy for head and neck dysplasia and cancer. *Arch Otolaryngol Head Neck Surg* 2009;**135**:784–8.

36. Bernier J, Cooper JS, Pajak TF, *et al*. Defining risk levels in locally advanced head and neck cancers: A comparative analysis of concurrent postoperative radiation plus chemotherapy trials of the EORTC (#22931) and RTOG (#9501). *Head Neck* 2005;**27**:843–50.

37. Bachaud JM, Cohen-Jonathan E, Alzieu C, *et al*. Combined postoperative radiotherapy and weekly cisplatin infusion for locally advanced head and neck carcinoma: Final report of a randomized trial. *Int J Radiat Oncol Biol Phys* 1996;**36**:999–1004.

38. Choong N, Everett V. Expanding role of the medical oncologist in management of head and neck cancer. *CA Cancer J Clin* 2008;**58**:32–53.

39. Huang K, Xia P, Chuang C, *et al*. Intensity modulated radiotherapy for treatment of Stage 3 and 4 oprpharyngeal cancer: University of California Sanfransisco Experience. *Cancer* 2008;**113**:497–507.

40. Vergeer MR, Doornaert PA, Rietveld DH, *et al*. IMRT reduces radiation induced morbidity and improves health related quality of life: Results of non-randomized prospective study using a standardized follow-up program. *Int J Oncol Rad Biol Phys* 2009;**74**:1–8.

41. Bourhis J, Amand C, Pignon J-P. Update of MACH-NC (meta-analysis of chemotherapy in head and neck cancer) database focused on concomitant chemoradiotherapy. *Proc Am Soc Clin Oncol* 2004;**22**:14s. Abstract 5505.

42. Pignon JP, Bourhis J, Domenge C, *et al*. Chemotherapy added to locoregional treatment for head and neck squamous-cell carcinoma: Three meta-analyses of updated individual data. MACHNC Collaborative Group. Meta-analysis of chemotherapy on head and neck cancer. *Lancet* 2000;**355**:949–55.

43. Browman GP, Hodson DI, Mackenzie RJ, *et al*. Choosing a concomitant chemotherapy and radiotherapy regimen for squamous cell head and neck cancer: A systematic review of the published literature with subgroup analysis. *Head Neck* 2001;**23**:579–89.

44. Daly JM Hearne B, Dunaj J, *et al*. Nutritional rehabilitation in patients with advanced head and neck cancer receiving radiotherapy. *Am J Surg* 1984;**148**:514–20.

45. Isenring EA, Bauer ID, Capra S. Nutritional support using the American Dietetic Association Medical Nutrition Therapy protocol for radiation oncology patients improves dietary intake compared to standard practices. *J Am Diet Assoc* 2007;**107**:404–12.

46. Kreeft A, Tan IB, van der Brekel MWM, *et al*. The surgical dilemma of 'functional inoperability' in oral and oropharyngeal cancer: Current consensus on operability with regard to functional status. *Clin Otolaryngol* 2009;**34**:140–6.

11

Cancer of the larynx—early stage

ALBERTO STAFFIERI, GINO MARIONI, BIPIN T. VARGHESE

Laryngeal cancer forms approximately 2% of all cancers. Seen predominantly in men, the men to women ratio of the prevalence of these tumours is 9:1.[1] Smoking and alcoholism are common aetiological factors specific to laryngeal cancer. Chronic laryngitis with hyperplasia of the vocal cords can also lead to laryngeal cancer. Approximately 90% of laryngeal malignancies are squamous cell carcinomas (SCCs). The rare types of malignancy are outlined in Table 1. Most of laryngeal malignancies are treated primarily by surgery (conservative/total) with or without adjuvant radiotherapy (RT) or by radical radiotherapy.

Anatomical considerations

The larynx is formed by its bony cartilaginous frame, adjacent ligaments, membranes, the investing mucosal lining and the folds formed by it.

The bony component is the hyoid bone, and cartilaginous components include the unpaired thyroid and cricoid cartilages and the paired arytenoids. The arytenoid cartilages are in turn formed by the cuneiform and corniculate cartilages.

The connecting ligaments include the medial and lateral thyrohyoid ligament, cricothyroid ligament, cricovocal ligament or conus elasticus and the quadrangular ligament. The free lower edge of the quadrangular ligament forms the ventricular band, and free upper edge of the conus elasticus forms the vocal cords. The folds of the larynx include the medial and lateral glossoepiglottic folds (or the pharyngo epiglottic fold) and the aryepiglottic folds. The anatomical division between the supraglottis and glottis is the arcuate line located at the apex of the ventricle, which marks the change from respiratory to squamous epithelium. The anatomical extent of the vocal cord is from the superior arcuate line to the inferior arcuate line, which has a vertical height of 5 mm (Figs 1a and 1b).

The vocal folds consist of an outer squamous epithelial layer, a middle layer of lamina propria and a deep muscular layer formed by the vocalis muscle, which is the free upper edge of the thyroarytenoid muscle and which forms the main bulk of the vocal cord. The lamina propria consists of a superficial layer of loose fibres and matrix, which is clinically referred to as the Reinke space. The intermediate layer contains elastic and collagenous fibres at a higher concentration and the deep layer has the highest density of collagen fibres. The intermediate and deep layer together forms the vocal ligament. Reinke space is an avascular space, which avoids the spread of glottic cancers. The interior of the larynx (or the endolarynx), as visualized through the endoscope, shows the laryngeal vestibule, ventricular bands or the false vocal cords, the vocal cords and the subglottis (Figs 2a and 2b).

Sites of the larynx

The larynx is divided into the supraglottis and glottis by the ventricle, which is the space between the ventricular band and the vocal cord itself. The subglottic region conventionally begins 5 mm below the free edge of the true vocal folds extending to the lower border of the cricoid cartilage (Figs 1a and 1b). Supraglottis and subglottis are richly supplied by lymphatics, whereas the glottis is virtually free of any lymphatic drainage. Laryngeal cancers generally spread by the mucosal or submucosal route, direct infiltration, lymphatic or vascular

Table 1. Laryngeal malignancies

Epithelial tumours	Squamous cell carcinoma Verrucous squamous cell carcinoma Spindle cell carcinoma Adenoid squamous cell carcinoma Basaloid squamous cell carcinoma Adenocarcinoma Acinic cell carcinoma Mucoepidermoid carcinoma Adenoid cystic carcinoma Carcinoma in pleomorphic adenoma Epithelial–myoepithelial carcinoma Clear cell carcinoma Adenosquamous carcinoma Giant cell carcinoma Salivary duct carcinoma Carcinoid tumour Atypical carcinoid tumour Small cell carcinoma Lymphoepithelial carcinoma
Soft tissue tumours	Fibrosarcoma Malignant fibrous histiocytoma Liposarcoma Leiomyosarcoma Rhabdomyosarcoma Angiosarcoma Kaposi sarcoma Malignant haemangiopericytoma Malignant nerve sheath tumour Alveolar soft part sarcoma Synovial sarcoma Ewing sarcoma
Tumours of bone and cartilage	Chondrosarcoma Osteosarcoma
Malignant lymphomas	
Miscellaneous tumours	Malignant melanoma Malignant germ cell tumours
Secondary tumours	
Unclassified tumours	

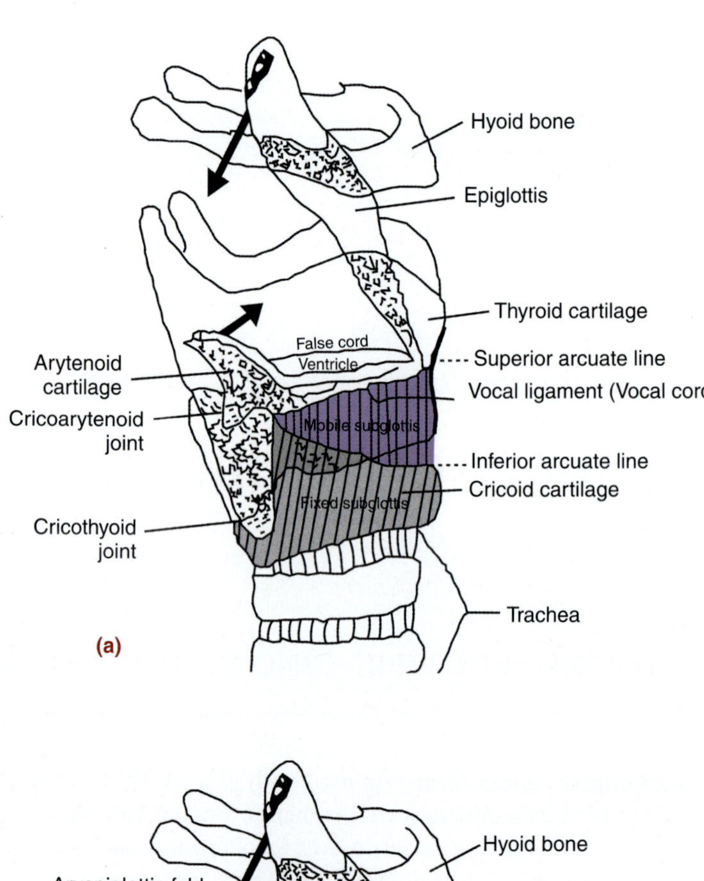

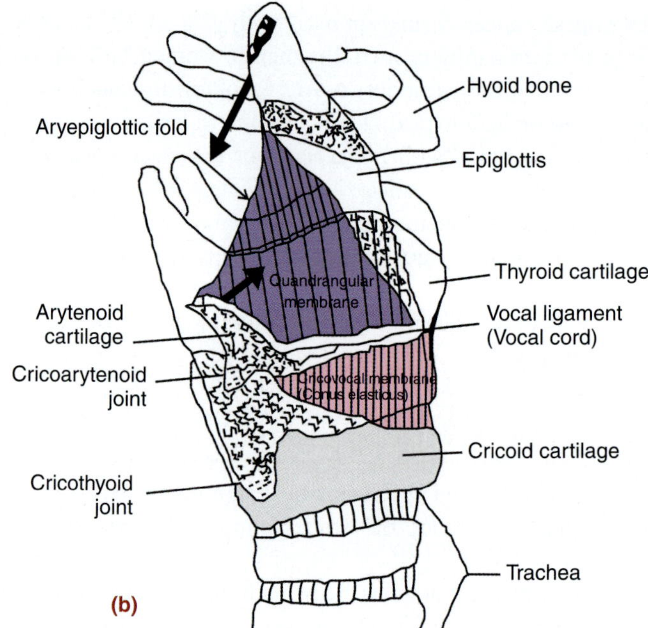

Figs 1 (a, b). Anatomy of the laryngeal skeletal framework

permeation, or perineural spread. Partial laryngectomies of small (confined) tumours are possible because the fibroelastic membranes compartmentalize the larynx into defined areas.

Pattern of tumour spread

Glottic cancers

In situ, glottic carcinoma is limited by the basement membrane. Invasive cancers are initially limited by the conus elasticus and the vocal ligament. The anterior limiting barrier is the weak Broyle tendon after which it is the inner perichondrium of the laryngeal cartilage. Once the conus elasticus is breached, the paraglottic space is invaded and the thyroarytenoid muscle infiltrated, leading to vocal fold fixity (Fig. 3).

Supraglottic tumours

These tumours are divided into those that involve the suprahyoid and those that involve the infrahyoid epiglottis, for the purpose of characterizing their spread. The former spreads to the base of tongue and shows early invasion of the pre-epiglottic space, whereas the latter is prone to early involvement of false cords and spreads to the medial wall of the pyriform fossa by circumferential growth.

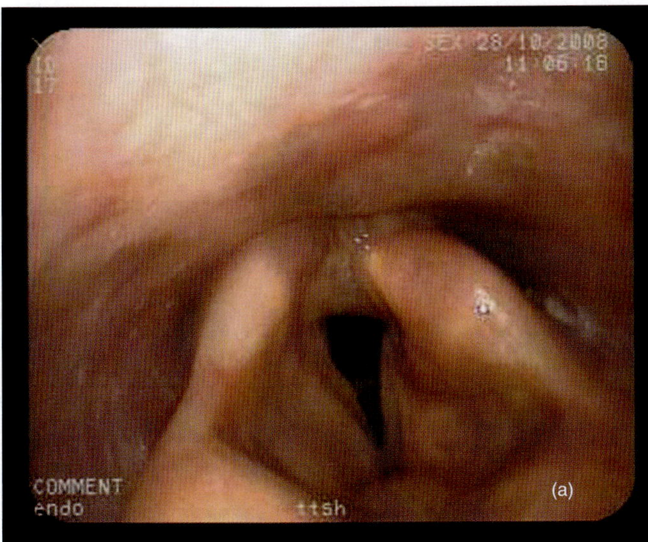

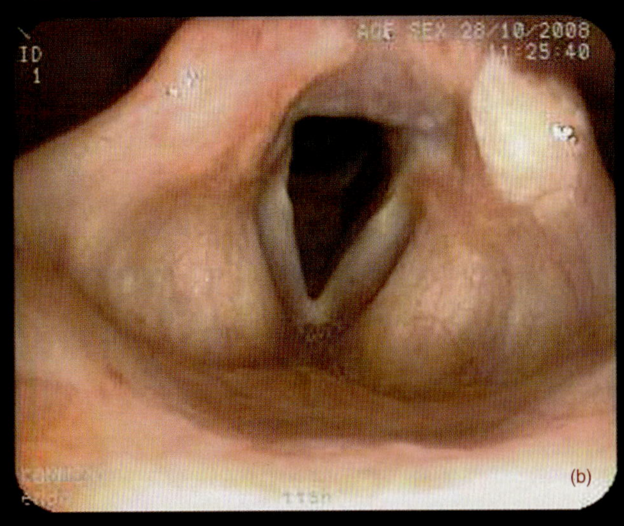

Figs 2 (a, b). Endoscopic views of the laryngeal inlet

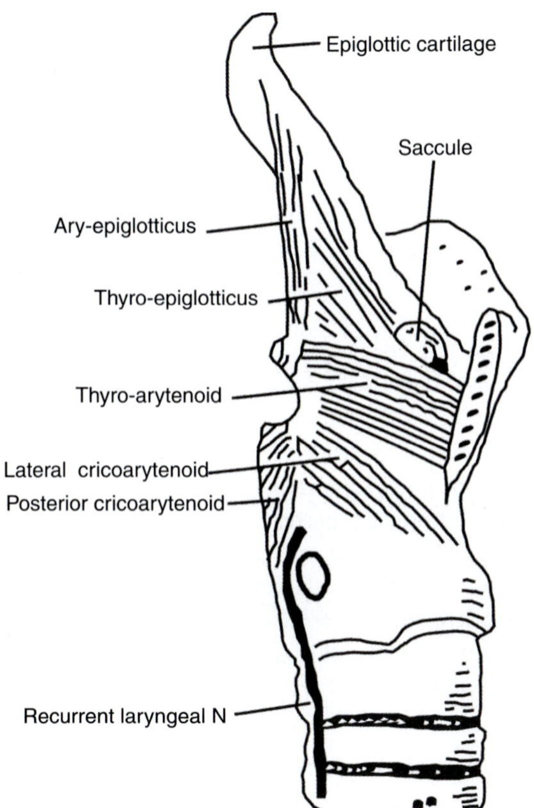

Fig. 3. Musculature of the larynx

Subglottic tumours

These form <1% of all laryngeal cancers. Bilateral circumferential growth and early cricoid invasion are the characteristic features.

Transglottic tumours

Cancer involving both the glottic and supraglottic regions in association with fixation of the true vocal cords is termed transglottic. Kirchner and Som's work[2-4] suggests that transglottic cancer has a single rather than a multi-focal point of origin, which is most likely to be located deep within the ventricle. Most (65%) of the transglottic cancers invade the laryngeal framework and are usually not amenable to conservation laryngectomies.

A detailed knowledge of sub-sites of the larynx is of utmost importance for understanding the surgical management of the larynx. In 1956,[5,6] Pressman and his team, while experimenting on cadavers, showed that the supraglottis has bilateral lymphatic drainage, which correlates with its midline origin from the buccopharyngeal anlage from the 4th and 5th branchial arches. They also showed that glottis, due to its bilateral origin from the tracheobronchial anlage, has unilateral lymphatic drainage. These studies have also formed the basis for horizontal and vertical partial laryngectomies. The supraglottis is delineated by the ventricle, which permits oncologically sound resections of the supraglottic larynx (supraglottic or horizontal laryngectomies), and the glottis is divided into 2 halves by the midline (anteroposteriorly)—giving room for hemilaryngectomies or vertical partial laryngectomies.[5-7]

Management principles for early laryngeal cancer

Early disease, or limited stage laryngeal cancer, constitutes a wide spectrum and it demands a sound judgement to choose the appropriate treatment. Factors that may influence treatment modality include the extent and volume of tumour, involvement of the anterior commissure, lymph node metastasis, age, occupation, preference and compliance of the patient and previous history of head and neck malignancy.

Treatment options for stage T1–T2 N0 glottic laryngeal carcinoma include transoral laser excision, RT and open partial laryngectomy (OPL).[7] Endoscopic laser surgery has nowadays gained increasing popularity. The major advantages of this procedure are the preservation of the thyroid cartilege and significant resource savings. However, it is now well recognized that the likelihood of local control without preservation of function increases with tumour volume.[8,9]

OPL is primarily used to salvage local recurrences amenable to laryngeal preservation. If primary RT fails in T2 laryngeal cancers, survival is inversely affected even with salvage surgery.[8–10] If surgery is done first for an early laryngeal or hypopharyngeal cancer, complete excision is mandatory for local control. Likewise, failure of RT also has been attributed to volume of the early-staged supraglottic cancers and anterior commissure involvement in early glottic cancers.[8–10]

This situation lent support to a new wave of surgical research that has veered towards either open partial surgery or endoscopic laser surgery with CO_2 laser, using the same principles of resections.[11,12] Surgical advances and refinements in these techniques allowed integration of surgery in the armamentarium of laryngeal preservation.[13,14] Larynx conservation surgeries practiced currently include endoscopic laser excision, OPL (vertical and horizontal), supracricoid partial laryngectomies and near total laryngectomy (NTL).[7]

Selection of a treatment option will depend on patient factors, local expertise, and the availability of appropriate support and rehabilitation services. Surgical patients will need complete evaluation for suitability of larynx preservation including pulmonary function tests and patient appraisal of their treatment options, their effects, and their complications. These patients are generally selected for a single modality treatment although adjuvant radiation or chemoradiation treatment becomes mandatory in the presence of positive neck nodes, positive margins (where further re-excision is not feasible), or extracapsular extension of nodes.

Surgical conservation options for early glottic carcinoma:
- Transoral laser excision, preferably with a CO_2 laser for Tis, T1 and T2 tumours
- Laryngofissure cordectomy for T1 glottic tumours, which are not amenable to laser excision (e.g. exophytic bulky lesions, no acceptable glottic exposure) (Fig. 4).
- Vertical partial laryngectomy (VPL)—suitable for more advanced T1 and T2 glottic tumours. At least two-thirds of contralateral cord needs to be preserved for a successful VPL. If this is not possible, VPL has to be converted to a supracricoid partial laryngectomy.

Surgical conservation options for supraglottic laryngeal carcinoma:
- Transoral laser excision
- OPL (horizontal partial or supracricoid partial laryngectomy with cricohyoidopexy [CHP]).

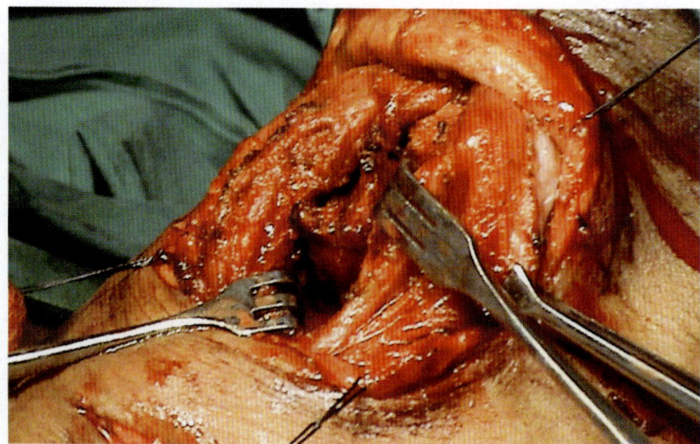

Fig. 4. Exposure of tumour by laryngofissure approach

Other options for supraglottic laryngeal carcinoma:
- Definitive RT
- Chemo-RT.

Low-volume tumours are favorable for definitive RT or OPL alone. Relatively high-volume tumours with a good airway and minimal neck disease are generally considered for definitive RT and concomitant chemotherapy, if not for OPL. Hypopharygeal conservation or partial laryngopharyngectomies can be combined with preservation of the entire larynx or conservation of the larynx (in any one of its permutations), depending on the laryngeal invasion of the tumour.

Horizontal laryngectomies

These procedures range from simple epiglottectomy to supracricoid partial laryngectomy (Table 2). Whereas a simple resection of an early lesion is affected by a transvallecular approach, partial resection of the thyroid cartilage framework and a thyrohyoidopexy may be required for more advanced lesions; at the extreme end of the spectrum are the supracricoid resections with cricohyoidoepiglottopexy (CHEP) and in particular the subtotal laryngectomies with tracheohyoidopexy.

Supracricoid partial laryngectomy (SCL)

Although the concept of supracricoid partial laryngectomy (SCL) was mooted by two Austrian surgeons in 1959, the French[15,16] in the 1970s innovated it to the present form, and in the 1990s it was documented in the English literature. It was in 1980 that Laccourreye[17,18] standardized supracricoid partial laryngectomies and their reconstructions as either CHP or CHEP. The classical indications for the procedure are glottic and supraglottic tumours with paraglottic spread, with or without pre-epiglottic invasion in the presence of free pyriform sinuses. The operation entails removal of the

Table 2. Open partial laryngeal surgery for glottic and supraglottic carcinomas

Vertical partial conservation procedures for early glottis cancers
• Laryngofissure cordectomy (via thyrotomy) • Hemilaryngectomy • Frontolateral partial laryngectomy • Anterior frontal vertical partial laryngectomy • Extended frontolateral laryngectomy (vertical hemilaryngectomy) • Extended hemilaryngectomy with cricoid excision
Horizontal conservation procedures for early supraglottis cancers and intermediate glottis cancers
• Epiglottectomy • Supraglottic laryngectomy (with partial resection of upper portion of thyroid cartilage) • Extended supraglottic laryngectomy • Supraglottic subtotal laryngectomy • Supraglottic subtotal laryngectomy with resection of arytenoid cartilage • Subtotal laryngectomy (subtotal glottic supraglottic laryngectomy, three-quarter laryngectomy) • Supracricoid laryngectomy with cricohyoidopexy or cricohyoidoepiglottopexy

thyroid cartilage, true vocal cords, epiglottis with or without pre-epiglottic space, false vocal cords and only one arytenoid, if necessary (Figs 5a and 5b).

Classically, contraindications for SCL include fixation of both arytenoids, subglottic extension, involvement of cricoid cartilage or posterior commissure, extensive extra-laryngeal spread, or base of tongue involvement.

Procedure

In SCL, at least one arytenoid has to be spared to preserve phonetic and sphincter functions. In a classical supraglottic horizontal laryngectomy with partial resection of the upper portion of thyroid cartilage, the hyoid is stitched to the thyroid cartilage. In the supracricoid partial laryngectomies, the vocal cords are sacrificed additionally and the larynx is reconstructed with a cricohyoid impaction, referred to as CHEP or CHP, making use of the crico-arytenoid unit(s), which is the fundamental unit of laryngeal function. This reconstruction preserves the airway, speech and swallowing even when one arytenoid needs to be sacrificed. Careful preservation of the unaffected superior laryngeal nerve and cartilaginous, muscular and mucosal structures is the key to successful surgery. In some selected cases the anterior arch of the cricoid can be resected and a tracheocricohyoidoepiglottopexy created.[19]

Apart from ensuring the resection of both the membranous vocal cords, this procedure affords comprehensive clearance of both paraglottic spaces, the lower third of the epiglottis and pre-epiglottic space and, when indicated, one arytenoid. It can also be used in selected anteriorly confined T4 cancers. Tension-free CHP is facilitated by a cervicomediastinal release of the trachea by finger dissection down to the level of the carina, staying in the midline on the anterior wall of the trachea.

Omohyoid and sternohyoid are divided at their upper attachment, and the sternothyroid muscle is divided at its insertion along the oblique line of the thyroid cartilage to partially release the bony cartilagenous laryngeal framework. The inferior constrictor muscle is now detached from the lateral insertion to the thyroid cartilage on both sides and the cricothyroid joint is disarticulated bilaterally at the level of the lesser horn of the thyroid cartilage, avoiding injury to the recurrent laryngeal nerves. The endolarynx can now be entered through the cricothyroid membrane, thereby permitting visualization of the inferior glottic mucosal margin. An endotracheal tube is then placed through the cricothyrotomy and the rest of the resection continued.

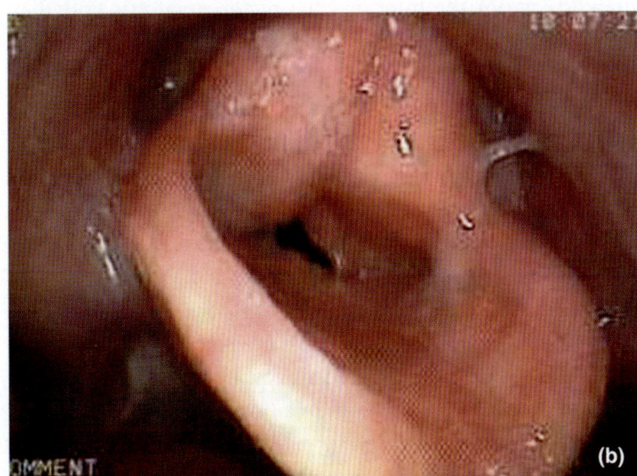

Figs 5 (a, b). Endoscopic views of glottis in a case of supracricoid laryngectomy with cricohyoidoepiglottopexy for selected T4 carcinoma glottis (a, during abduction and b, during adduction of the preserved arytenoids).

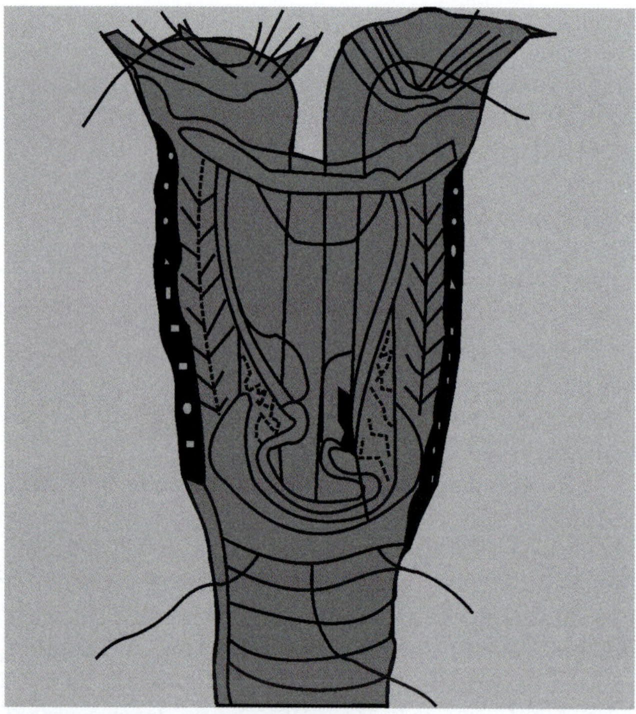

Fig. 6. Supracricoid partial laryngectomy

A transepiglottic laryngotomy is performed for a CHEP, a transvallecular pharyngotomy is performed for a CHP, and the aryepiglottic folds are divided with scissors.

After this resection, the arytenoids fall posteriorly because it is the thyroarytenoid muscles that position the arytenoids anteriorly (Figs 1a, 1b and 3) against the posterior pharyngeal wall. Appropriate stitches may be placed to pull the arytenoids anteriorly off of the posterior pharyngeal wall, thereby creating a T-shaped valve that will close against the epiglottis or the base of tongue (Fig. 6). Three stitches are placed approximately 8–10 mm apart along the anterior surface of the cricoid cartilage in the midline to prevent hypoglossal injury.[20] For CHEP, the stitch is passed submucosally through the cartilage of the inferior edge of the epiglottis and then into the pre-epiglottic space just below the hyoid bone for the impaction.

Pulling the lateral pharyngeal walls more anteriorly by placing two approximating 3-0 vicryl stitches in the fascia of the released inferior constrictor muscle helps to restore the symmetry, physiological position and function of the inferior constrictors and the pyriform sinuses, and enhances swallowing outcomes.

To prevent an air-leak and consequent postoperative subcutaneous emphysema, stitches are placed to approximate the tracheotomy to the skin. This can be supplemented with pressure dressings. Early cuff deflation or the use of cuffless tracheotomy tubes may prevent the downregulation of the infraglottic receptors and improve the chances for successful de-cannulation, besides diminishing the effects of tracheotomy on laryngeal closure reflex.[21]

In summary, the remnant laryngeal structures after an SPL are sutured in such a way that the larynx occupies a position attained by the larynx in the final pharyngeal phase of swallowing in order to minimize post-operative aspiration to the extent possible (Figs 1a and 1b).

Conservative salvage surgery after failed RT for laryngeal carcinoma

The past two decades have seen an increase in the non-surgical treatment of laryngeal cancer.[22] The aim of these treatments is tumour control with maximal preservation of function. RT is the primary treatment for patients with limited laryngeal carcinomas in most centres in northern Europe and North America.[23] Hoffman *et al.*[22] reviewed the National Cancer Data Base (NCDB), and revealed 158,426 cases of laryngeal squamous cell carcinoma (SCC) (excluding verrucous carcinoma) diagnosed between the years 1985 and 2001 in the United States of America. RT alone was the more frequent initial treatment modality chosen for a percentage of patients, ranging from 32.2% to 36.0%. Reported irradiation failure rates have been in the range of 9%–21% for T1 and 28%–37% for T2 glottic carcinomas. In supraglottic laryngeal cancer, the reported failure rates for T1 and T2 lesions are 24%–30% and 25%–45%, respectively.[24]

How to manage laryngeal carcinoma recurring after primary RT has failed remains a debated issue.[25] Also, recent reviews[26] have failed to give unambiguous guidelines on rational salvage laryngeal surgery after irradiation failure. Salvage surgery aims to remove the tumour with an adequate margin of healthy tissue. Small nests of neoplastic cells lying deep below intact mucosa are characteristic of the histological pattern of presentation of laryngeal recurrences after irradiation. However, these islands follow mucous glands and blood vessels into areas of the larynx otherwise unaffected by the carcinoma, some distance from the site of the original lesion.[27] Zbären *et al.*[28] recently observed a marked perineural infiltration in recurrent laryngeal carcinomas, supporting the hypothesis that tumours also grow along nerves, consequently involving previously unaffected areas. This pathological evidence (which poses significant clinical problems regarding the proper restaging of the tumour after irradiation) justifies the classical choice of total laryngectomy as the salvage treatment in cases of carcinoma recurrence after failed RT.[29] Total laryngectomy is also often chosen for salvage surgery in the belief that partial laryngectomy of irradiated cartilage is associated with a higher rate of complications.[30] Young *et al.*[31] stated that the difference in survival after salvage total laryngectomy for radiation or chemoradiation failure is nil. On the other hand, recent evidence has confirmed that selected laryngeal cancer recurrences may be treated successfully with partial laryngectomy even after high-dose radiation therapy.[32] For partial laryngectomy to replace conventional salvage surgery, it has to achieve survival rates comparable to those of total laryngectomy, with an acceptable morbidity, tracheostomy closure, effective swallowing, and satisfactory voice intelligibility. Here, we critically analyse the available data on the indications, and the oncological and functional results of partial laryngectomy in the treatment of laryngeal carcinoma recurring after radiation failure.

Staging laryngeal carcinoma recurrence

Advances in functional salvage surgery and the tendency to avoid total laryngectomy for recurrent carcinoma, if possible, have emphasized the importance of the early diagnosis of laryngeal carcinoma recurrences after the failure of RT. In patients with symptoms (progressive hoarseness, dysphagia, pain, respiratory distress) or clinical signs, such as severe oedema or necrosis, it is often clinically and radiologically difficult to differentiate between recurrent laryngeal carcinoma and the sequelae of RT because the tumour may involve multiple sites without affecting the surface epithelium.[33–35] Sites such as the laryngeal ventricle and subglottic region are difficult to examine in the presence of severe oedema.[34] Other critical sites for the purposes of indicating conservative salvage surgery are the crico-arytenoid and inter-arytenoid regions, and the thyroid and cricoid cartilages.[34] Endoscopic evaluation and biopsy sampling may exacerbate post-RT changes and initiate superimposed infections, leading to perichondritis, healing defects and further oedema.[33] Using positron emission tomography (PET) with 18-fluorodeoxyglucose (FDG) seems to have promise for distinguishing locally recurrent carcinoma (in the submucosa in particular) from the sequelae of RT due to the fact that FDG-PET focuses on the neoplastic cells' metabolic function.[33]

A comprehensive diagnostic approach is needed before organ preserving surgery can be indicated for cases of laryngeal carcinoma in which RT has failed. It may be difficult to assess accurately the extent of the recurrence because of the residual inflammatory, anatomical or functional changes associated with radiation therapy.[28] Endoscopic and radiological investigations underestimate the true extent of the recurrent carcinoma in a high percentage of cases. In a limited series, Zbären *et al.*[34] found a 50% accuracy of clinical/endoscopic/radiological findings; most tumours were under-classified. It is mandatory to consider reviewing the patient's clinical records with regard to their prior diagnosis and treatment, related staging, pathological slides and clinical findings. Previous radiotherapeutic measures (method, doses and courses) should also be considered. Patients should be examined using fibre-optic laryngoscopy and videolaryngostroboscopy. Direct laryngoscopy under general anaesthesia is useful for precisely defining the extent of the recurrence and exploring sub-sites, e.g. the anterior commissure, laryngeal ventricle, subglottis and pyriform sinus (using 30°, 45° and 90° angled

rigid endoscopes may improve the preoperative staging),[36] and for obtaining biopsies of the lesion. In cases of advanced recurrence, a fibroscopic evaluation of the oesophagus is mandatory to rule out any synchronous malignancy of the upper digestive tract.[32] Nowadays, computerized tomography (CT) or magnetic resonance imaging (MRI) are considered necessary radiological procedures for recurrent laryngeal carcinoma staging; both provide information on its volume, cartilage involvement, invasion of the pre-epiglottic space, and extension beyond the larynx. Laryngeal CT scanning can supply significant details of the carcinoma's local submucosal extension and it is also crucial for investigating the laryngeal areas most influencing the planning of surgical treatment. The main questions that head and neck surgeons and radiologists have to bear in mind are: (i) whether a conservative surgical approach is oncologically reasonable, and (ii) which conservative surgical modality is best.[37] MRI seems to be more sensitive than CT in detecting cartilage invasion.[38,39] When considering the conservative surgical options for laryngeal carcinoma recurrences, the importance of the patient's general condition, medical co-morbidities, and pulmonary and swallowing functions have to be emphasized.[40] Ultrasonography of the neck is needed in patients with clinically evident neck metastases (using fine-needle aspiration cytology; FNAC), or carcinomas at high risk of occult lymph node metastases. Reported figures for the accuracy of FNAC guided by ultrasonography range between 89% and 97%.[41] The accuracy of CT scanning in neck staging is reportedly 87%–93%; MRI of cervical node metastases seems to have a comparable sensitivity and specificity.[42] The diagnosis of distant metastases will obviously influence the planning of any laryngeal surgery.[40] The salvage surgical options should be discussed with the patient and their willingness to accept a potentially lengthy rehabilitation has to be considered before deciding on partial laryngeal surgery.[43] Given the likelihood of clinical and radiological investigations having underestimated the extent of the recurrence after RT, patients should be prepared for a total laryngectomy and the surgical staff should have obtained their informed consent to the procedure.

Conservative surgical strategies after failure of RT

Although larger series are needed to confirm preliminary evidence, conservative salvage surgery definitely seems promising for the treatment of recurrent laryngeal carcinoma after primary irradiation.[44]

Transoral laser surgery

The most appealing feature of transoral laser-assisted surgery in this scenario is the chance to perform a tumour-tailored excision, while retaining the opportunity to switch intra-operatively to an OPL if the carcinoma proves to be more extensive than expected. Good functional results have been reported in terms of voice quality and swallowing, with lower complication rates, lower costs and shorter hospital stays.[45] The criteria for establishing whether transoral laser surgery is appropriate after RT has failed, include a complete endoscopic visualization of the carcinoma of tumours extending not more than 3 mm into the contralateral vocal fold, no arytenoid involvement (apart from the vocal process), a subglottic extension not exceeding 5 mm, a supraglottic involvement reaching no further than the lateral extension of the Morgagni sinus, mobile vocal folds, no cartilage involvement, and a strict correlation between the site and extension of the recurrent lesion and those of the primary tumour before irradiation.[46]

Although anterior commissure involvement is not a contraindication for endoscopic laser resection after irradiation has failed, extreme caution should be used because of the potential persistence of deep nests of carcinoma invading visceral compartments or focally involving the laryngeal framework. In cases of macroscopic anterior commissure involvement by recurrent carcinoma, several authors prefer a supracricoid laryngectomy (SCL), which allows for wider resection margins.[45,47] In 2001, de Gier et al.[48] reviewed the records of 40 patients treated with the CO_2 laser for recurrent glottic carcinoma at the University Hospital in Rotterdam and the Dr Daniel den Hoed Cancer Center between 1980 and 1996 (mean follow up 77 months): 23 patients (58%) had another recurrence after laser surgery, and 3 of them were cured by a second laser procedure. Ultimately, laser surgery was successful in 20 patients (50%). In 2006, Motamed et al.[46] reviewed the available literature on endolaryngeal salvage laser surgery after irradiation had failed, considering 145 cases in all, with a mean follow up of approximately 24 months (range 3–132). More than one laser-assisted surgical procedure was needed in 40% of cases and the mean local control rate was 65% (range 51%–87%). Total laryngectomy was subsequently necessary in 25% of cases due to residual/recurrent disease or refractory dysphagia. Motamed et al.[46] calculated that the mean overall local control rate (including patients who subsequently required total laryngectomy) was 83% (range 80%–100%). The review by Motamed et al.[46] also considered the Steiner et al.[49] series of 34 patients with both early and advanced recurrent glottic carcinomas (rT1–rT4) who had previously undergone RT. Steiner et al.[49] said that extensive and specific surgical experience is essential for the CO_2 laser excision of advanced recurrent cancers. The University of Göttingen experience of salvage surgery with the CO_2 laser was updated in 2009 by Roedel et al.[50] Piazza et al.[45] have reported on 22 cases of laryngeal carcinoma recurrence (rT1–rT2) after irradiation that were treated with CO_2 laser-assisted excision. Their analysis of the oncological results identified 5-year disease-specific and disease-free

survival, and laryngeal preservation rates of 95%, 63%, and 75%, respectively. In 2007, Ansarin et al.[51] also retrospectively analysed the results of CO_2 laser excision in 37 consecutive patients with recurrent glottic cancer after RT; their 5-year actuarial recurrence-free and overall survival rates were 58% and 86%, respectively, and the larynx was preserved in 26 patients (70%). Most authors report experiencing greater difficulty identifying recurrent carcinoma in irradiated tissues; frozen sections should hence be used routinely. All margins should also be confirmed postoperatively on permanent sections. It is important to emphasize the need for a strict follow up, with fibroscopic examination and serial imaging to ensure early detection and treatment of recurrence. That CO_2 laser excision of laryngeal carcinoma recurring after irradiation has failed does not preclude its further use for persistent or multiple recurrent disease.[36] Tracheostomy and a nasogastric feeding tube are not required routinely in the laser excision of recurrent laryngeal carcinoma. Complications are reported in <5% of cases,[46] the most common being granuloma formation and laryngeal oedema. Laryngeal stenosis and chondronecrosis have also been described.[46,49]

Supracricoid laryngectomy

The surgical technique for SCL was first described in the early 1950s and better defined in the 1970s.[52] A Medline-based review of available studies on SCL (1970 to October 2009) showed an increasing diffusion of this surgical approach[53] (Fig. 7). Most reported experiences with SCL were conducted by European groups, but the last decade has seen an increasing interest in SCL by American and Chinese surgeons[53] (Fig. 8). Nowadays, the local control and 5-year survival rates are considered similar for patients undergoing either total laryngectomy or SCL for the treatment of selected T2–T3 supraglottic/glottic laryngeal SCCs.[52] SCL with CHP is deemed to be a suitable surgical approach for supraglottic carcinomas involving the glottis, ventricle, or anterior commissure. It involves removing the whole thyroid cartilage, both true and false cords, the ventricles, the epiglottis, and the paraglottic and pre-epiglottic spaces. At least one arytenoid has to be spared. SCL with CHEP is used to treat advanced glottic carcinomas. It involves resecting the infra-hyoid part of the epiglottis and the pre-epiglottic space; and again, at least one arytenoid must be spared. By preserving a crico-arytenoid unit, SCL allows for the creation of a neolarynx, enabling swallowing and speech. The tracheostomy can be closed in most cases, thereby eliminating a cause of extreme discomfort. Contraindications to SCL include the following: infiltration of both arytenoid cartilages, or of the crico-arytenoid joint, or inter-arytenoid region; a subglottic extension >1 cm below the vocal fold's free margin at anterior commissure level; extension to the glosso-epiglottic vallecula; major pre-epiglottic space invasion; hyoid bone invasion; invasion of the outer perichondrium

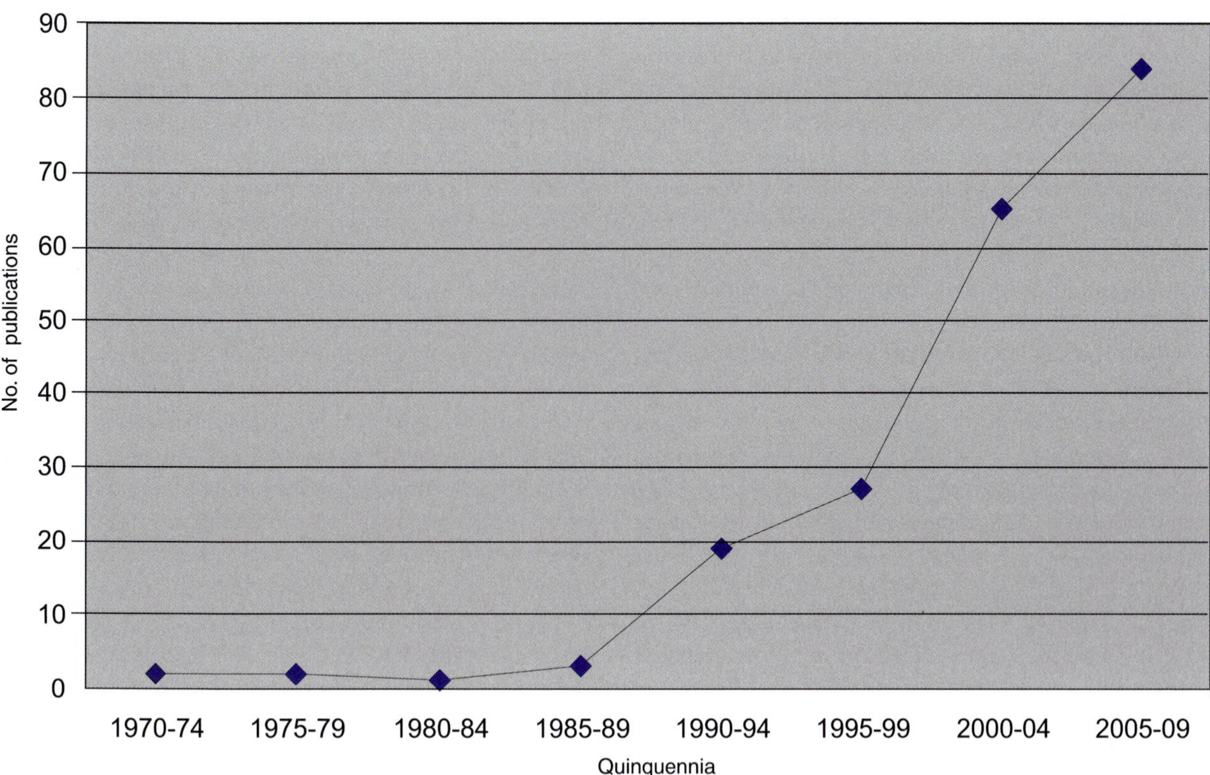

Fig. 7. Medline-indexed studies involving supracricoid laryngectomy from 1970 to October 2009.[53]

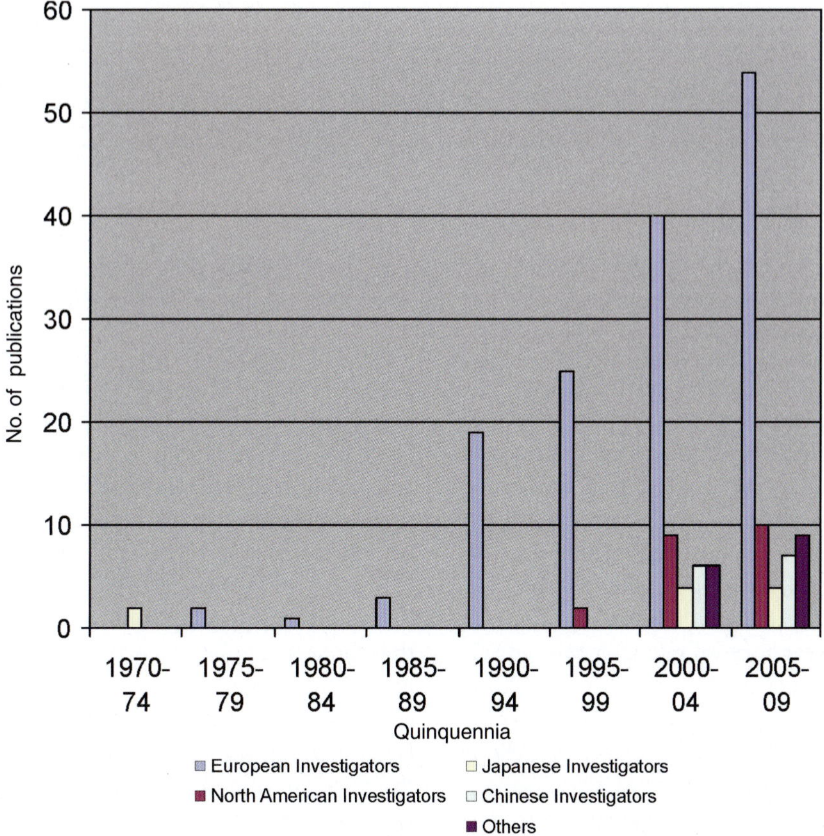

Fig. 8. Medline-indexed studies regarding supracricoid laryngectomy from 1970 to October 2009: Nationality of the institutions involved.[53]

of the thyroid cartilage; and extra-laryngeal spread. Subtotal laryngectomy with tracheohyoidopexy seems to represent a promising approach to extend the laryngeal resection beyond the limits adopted for SCL. Tracheohyoidopexy enables glottic carcinomas extending subglottically to be treated, i.e. not only laryngeal carcinomas invading one crico-arytenoid joint, but also locally advanced laryngeal carcinomas extending anteriorly through the thyroid cartilage. Available data on the oncological and functional results of this approach are currently extremely limited.[54]

In 1950, Hofmann-Saguez[55] first reported a 'subtotal conservative laryngectomy', a precursor of SCL, in a 65-year-old patient who had refused total laryngectomy and in whom laryngeal carcinoma recurred after RT. SCL is a fascinating alternative to total laryngectomy in the treatment of selected laryngeal carcinomas failing to respond to irradiation, because it preserves laryngeal functions.[56,57] Increasing international interest in SCL as a salvage procedure is evident[53] (Fig. 9). In 2006, Marioni *et al.*[56] reviewed the available reports on salvage SCL after the failure of RT in glottic carcinoma (103 cases in all) and, more recently, Pellini *et al.*[58] reported on a multi-institutional series of 78 cases of salvage SCL

19.4% of cases died of their disease. Laryngeal functions were restored in 89.3% of patients. In the previously mentioned review of 103 cases, Marioni *et al.*[56] evaluated the available functional results of SCL in carcinomas recurring after irradiation; decannulation was feasible in all but two cases after a range of 12–28 days. Swallowing disorders were the most common short-term complications of SCL.[52] Laccourreye *et al.*[62] performed percutaneous endoscopic gastrostomy before salvage SCL in 10 out of 12 patients and a cricopharyngeal myotomy on one patient. Their overall swallowing results seemed to be good, but previously irradiated patients took longer to recover from SCL than non-irradiated patients. Voice quality, as determined by psychoacoustic methods, was 'hoarse' or 'rough and breathy', but reasonably intelligible. Aspiration pneumonia was the most frequent complication of SCL for carcinoma recurrences after RT (17.5% of the cases with sufficient data) and it was the cause of death in two cases. Neo-laryngeal oedema was another quite common postoperative complication of SCL for carcinoma recurrences after RT.[56] Pellini *et al.*[63] retrospectively compared postoperative complications and functional outcomes of two groups of patients who had SCL with CHP, one comprising

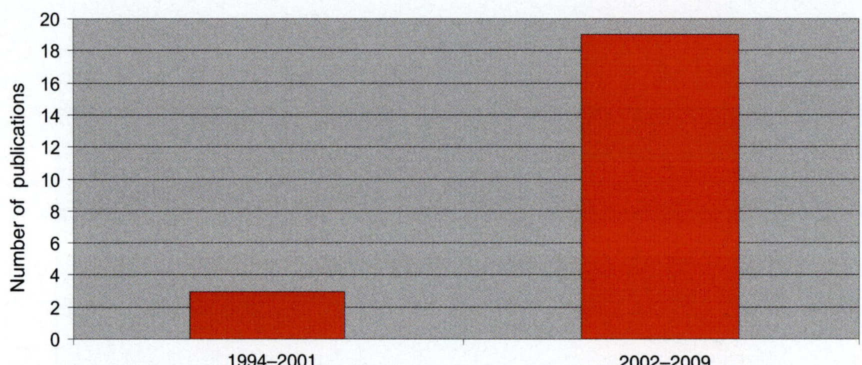

Fig. 9. Medline-indexed studies investigating supracricoid laryngectomy as a salvage procedure after laryngeal carcinoma recurrence (1994 to October 2009).[53]

for supragottic/glottic carcinoma after RT (many of which had been reported in single-institution experiences and considered in the previous review[56]). Marioni *et al.*[56] found that 84.5% of the cases of salvage SCL, after irradiation had failed, experienced no new local recurrence. Judging from the available data, laryngeal recurrences after salvage SCL (15.5%) were successfully treated with total laryngectomy in 66.7% of patients. The 3-year survival rate after salvage SCL ranged from 80% to 100%, and the 5-year survival rate from 69% to 100%.[30] Other experiences of salvage SCL after RT were reported more recently.[59–61] In particular, Deganello *et al.*[60] described 31 patients who underwent SCL as a salvage procedure after RT had failed. The locoregional control rate was 75%, with a 60% 5-year overall survival rate, whereas

previously-untreated laryngeal carcinomas (65 cases), and the other comprising laryngeal recurrences after RT (17 cases). No statistical differences were found between the functional results in the two groups, but the proportion of early surgical complications was significantly higher among the patients who had previously received RT.[63]

While still awaiting confirmation from larger series, SCL thus far seems to be an oncologically safe surgical approach, enabling laryngeal functions to be preserved in selected cases of recurrence after RT has failed.[64] As for subtotal laryngectomy with tracheohyoidopexy, available data on the oncological and functional results of this approach for carcinomas failing to respond to irradiation are limited, but this procedure seems to have potential for all locally advanced laryngeal carcinomas, except for those extending to the pharynx and trachea, or involving both arytenoids and/or the posterior commissure.[54] Looking at the future prospects of salvage surgery, the flexibility of the SCL approach in locally extending laryngeal carcinoma was recently pragmatically confirmed.[65] The authors reported on a patient whose planned SCL was intra-operatively converted to an extended partial laryngectomy with tracheo-hyoidoepiglottopexy for a carcinoma involving the cricoid cartilage.[65]

Other open partial laryngectomys (OPLs)

Selected laryngeal recurrences after RT can also be appropriately treated using other open partial surgical procedures.[44]

Vertical partial laryngectomy

The contraindications for vertical partial laryngectomy in recurrences after irradiation has failed can be summarized as follows: large T3 or any T4 lesions; inter-arytenoid or crico-arytenoid joint involvement; bilateral arytenoid cartilage involvement or a diminished motility of both vocal folds; thyroid cartilage penetration; supraglottic extension exceeding the lateral wall of the ventricle; subglottic extension beyond 10 mm at the anterior commissure or 5 mm at the vocal process of the arytenoid; and poor lung function. In 2003, Yiotakis *et al.*[24] reviewed the reported outcomes of vertical partial laryngectomy after RT had failed in cases of glottic carcinoma (462 patients). The considered series contained from 3 to 61 cases. The median local control rate was 82% (mean 78%; range 50%–100%), and 66 of 424 patients with available data needed their laryngectomy to be completed due to a second recurrence. Intra-operative frozen sections should be used in partial laryngectomies for maximum safety,[23] after which all margins have to be confirmed postoperatively on permanent sections. Should salvage vertical partial laryngectomy fail, total laryngectomy remains a reasonable option, without apparently jeopardizing ultimate local control.[46]

Horizontal supraglottic laryngectomy

For horizontal supraglottic laryngectomy after RT has failed, the contraindications are: involvement of the vocal fold, thyroid cartilage, or posterior commissure; a more than minimal involvement of the base of tongue or the medial wall of the pyriform sinus; and poor lung function. Yiotakis *et al.*[24] reviewed the few available series describing the oncological results of horizontal supraglottic laryngectomy for supraglottic carcinoma failing to respond to irradiation (49 patients in total). The median local control rate was 77% (mean 61%; range 0%–100%). Such a wide variability in the oncological outcome of salvage horizontal supraglottic laryngectomy may be reasonably attributed to patient selection, clinical evaluation of the lesions and the limited size of the series considered.

Complications and functional results of partial laryngectomies after the failure of RT

Morbidity in patients undergoing partial laryngectomy after a full course of RT is a controversial issue. The complications usually reported are delayed wound healing, infections, fistula formation and aspiration pneumonia.[46] Other less common complications include laryngeal stenosis, laryngeal oedema, or granuloma formation, perichondritis and surgical emphysema.

According to Yiotakis *et al.*,[24] the use of bipedicled flaps of strap muscle to replace the excised intralaryngeal soft tissue after vertical partial laryngectomy seems to facilitate rehabilitation in selected patients. From a functional viewpoint, swallowing impairment, aspiration and delayed decannulation are frequently described. In patients treated with vertical partial laryngectomy, the mobile cord succeeds in compensating, with time, and adequately protects the airway during swallowing; whereas patients treated with horizontal supraglottic laryngectomy reportedly have a high rate of delayed swallowing and recurrent aspiration.

Treating neck lymph node metastases

Neck dissection is needed in all cases of recurrent laryngeal carcinoma with clinical/cytological evidence of regional metastatic disease. The indication for elective neck dissection in patients staged as cN0 before salvage laryngeal surgery remains controversial.[66,67] According to Ganly *et al.*,[30] the choice of elective neck dissection has to be based on rT-staging, supraglottic or subglottic extent and extra-laryngeal involvement. In the near future, specific biological markers might be investigated as hallmarks of laryngeal carcinomas at higher risk of developing neck metastases. Convincing evidence is mandatory before suggesting that elective neck dissection should be considered for cN0 patients with laryngeal carcinomas showing a significant modification (presence/absence, pattern of localization, expression, etc.) of such markers.[44]

Conclusion

With the growing acceptance of non-surgical, organ sparing therapies, it has become increasingly important to define the surgical treatment strategies for patients with recurrent laryngeal carcinoma. Although 70%–80% of laryngeal carcinoma recurrences after RT are staged as rT3/T4 and total laryngectomy is considered the treatment of choice in the majority of such cases,[31,43,56] several studies have been published with the results of various conservative options for selected patients after irradiation has failed. Properly selected recurrent laryngeal cancer cases may be candidates for conservative laryngectomies, preserving laryngeal functions with no loss of oncological efficacy, even after high-dose radiation therapy has failed.

Endoscopic CO_2 laser-assisted, partial and reconstructive laryngectomy techniques should be familiar to the oncological laryngeal surgeon because these approaches are becoming increasingly interesting for the modern treatment of laryngeal carcinoma recurring after RT has failed.

References

1. Parkin DM, Whelan SL, Ferlay J, *et al*. *Cancer incidence in five continents, Vol 8*. International Agency for Research on Cancer (IARC). Scientific publication no. 155. Lyon: IARC; 2002:60.

2. Kirchner JA, Som ML. The anterior commissure technique of partial laryngectomy: Clinical and laboratory observations. *Laryngoscope* 1975;**85**:1308–17.

3. Kirchner JA, Som ML. Clinical and histological observations on supraglottic cancer. *Ann Otol Rhinol Laryngol* 1971;**80**:638–45.

4. Kirchner JA, Som ML. Clinical significance of fixed vocal cord. *Laryngoscope* 1971;**81**:1029–44.

5. Pressman J, Dowdy A, Libby R, *et al*. Further studies upon the submucosal compartments and lymphatics of the larynx by the injection of dyes and radioisotopes. *Ann Otol Rhinol Laryngol* 1956;**65**:963–80.

6. Pressman JJ. Submucosal compartmentation of the larynx. *Ann Otol Rhinol Laryngol* 1956;**65**:766–71.

7. Silver CE, Levin RJ. The larynx. In: Silver CE, Ferlito A (eds). *Surgery for cancer of larynx and related structures*. 2nd ed. London: WB Saunders; 1996.

8. Lee SC, Shores CG, Weissler MC. Salvage surgery after failed primary concomitant chemoradiation. *Curr Opin Otolaryngol Head Neck Surg* 2008;**16**:135–40.

9. Mancuso AA, Mukherji SK, Schmalfuss I, *et al*. Preradiotherapy computed tomography as a predictor of local control in supraglottic carcinoma. *J Clin Oncol* 1999;**17**:631–7.

10. Garden AS, Forster K, Wong PF, *et al*. Results of radiotherapy for T2N0 glottic carcinoma: Does the '2' stand for twice-daily treatment? *Int J Radiat Oncol Biol Phys* 2003;**55**:322–8.

11. Strong MS, Jako GJ. Laser surgery in the larynx. Early clinical experience with continuous CO2 laser. *Ann Otol Rhinol Laryngol* 1972;**81**:791–8.

12. Steiner W, Ambrosch P. *Endoscopic laser surgery of the upper aerodigestive tract—with special emphasis on cancer surgery*. New York: Thieme; 2000.

13. National Comprehensive Cancer Network (NCCN), USA. *Clinical practice guidelines in oncology, Head and Neck Cancers*. Vol. 1. 2007. Available at www.nccn.org.

14. National Comprehensive Cancer Network (NCCN), USA. *Clinical practice guidelines in oncology, Head and Neck Cancers*. Vol. 1. 2007. Available at www.nccn.org.

15. Labayle J, Bismuth R. Total laryngectomy with reconstitution. *Ann Otolaryngol Chir Cervicofac* 1971;**88**:219–28.

16. Piquet JJ, Desaulty A, Decroix G. Crico-hyoido-epiglotto-pexy. Surgical technic and functional results. *Ann Otolaryngol Chir Cervicofac* 1974;**91**:681–6.

17. Laccourreye H, Laccourreye O, Weinstein G, *et al*. Supracricoid laryngectomy with cricohyoidoepiglottopexy: A partial laryngeal procedure for glottic carvinoma. *Ann Otol Thinol Laryngol* 1990;**99**:421–6.

18. Laccourreye H, Laccourreye O, Weinstein G, *et al*. Supracricoid laryngectomy with cricohyoidopexy: A partial laryngeal procedure for selected supraglottic and transglottic carcinomas. *Laryngoscope* 1990;**100**:735–41.

19. Laccourreye O, Ross J, Brasnu D, *et al*. Extended supracricoid partial laryngectomy with tracheocricohyoidoepiglottopexy. *Acta Otolaryngol* 1994;**114**:669–74.

20. Lauretano AM, Li KK, Caradonna DS, *et al*. Anatomic location of the tongue base neurovascular bundle. *Laryngoscope* 1997;**107**:1057–9.

21. Sasaki CT, Suzuki M, Horiuchi M, *et al*. The effect of tracheostomy on the laryngeal closure reffflex. *Laryngoscope* 1977;**87**:1428–33.

22. Hoffman HT, Porter K, Karnell LH, *et al*. Laryngeal cancer in the United States: Changes in demographics, patterns of care, and survival. *Laryngoscope* 2006;**116** (Suppl 111):1–13.

23. Sewnaik A, Meeuwis CA, Van Der Kwast TH, *et al*. Partial laryngectomy for recurrent glottic carcinoma after radiotherapy. *Head Neck* 2005;**27**:101–7.

24. Yiotakis J, Stavroulaki P, Nikolopoulos T, *et al*. Partial laryngectomy after irradiation failure. *Otolaryngol Head Neck Surg* 2003;**128**:200–9.

25. Jørgensen K, Godballe C, Hansen O, *et al*. Cancer of the larynx – treatment results after primary radiotherapy with salvage surgery in a series of 1005 patients. *Acta Oncol* 2002;**41**:69–76.

26. Silver CE, Beitler JJ, Shaha AR, *et al*. Current trends in initial management of laryngeal cancer: The declining use of open surgery. *Eur Arch Otorhinolaryngol* 2009;**266**:1333–52.

27. Brandenburg JH, Condon KG, Frank TW. Coronal sections of larynges from radiation-therapy failures: A clinical-pathologic study. *Otolaryngol Head Neck Surg* 1986;**95**:213–18.

28. Zbären P, Nuyens M, Curschmann J, *et al*. Histologic characteristics and tumour spread of recurrent glottic carcinoma: Analysis on whole-organ sections and comparison with tumour spread of primary carcinomas. *Head Neck* 2007;**29**:26–32.

29. Marchese-Ragona R, Marioni G, Chiarello G, *et al*. Supracricoid laryngectomy with cricohyoidopexy for recurrence of early-stage glottic carcinoma after irradiation. Long-term oncological and functional results. *Acta Otolaryngol (Stockh)* 2005;**125**:91–5.

30. Ganly I, Patel SG, Matsuo J, *et al*. Results of surgical salvage after failure of definitive radiation therapy for early-stage squamous cell carcinoma of the glottic larynx. *Arch Otolaryngol Head Neck Surg* 2006;**132**:59–66.

31. Young VN, Mangus BD, Bumpous JM. Salvage laryngectomy for failed conservative treatment of laryngeal cancer. *Laryngoscope* 2008;**118**:1561–8.

32. Marioni G, Marchese-Ragona R, Cartei G, *et al*. Current opinion in diagnosis and treatment of laryngeal carcinoma. *Cancer Treatment Rev* 2006;**32**:504–15.

33. de Bree R, van der Putten L, Hoekstra OS, *et al*. On behalf of the RELAPS Study Group. A randomized trial of PET scanning to improve diagnostic yield of direct laryngoscopy in patients with suspicion of recurrent laryngeal carcinoma after radiotherapy. *Contemp Clin Trials* 2007;**28**:705–12.

34. Zbären P, Christe A, Caversaccio MD, *et al*. Pretherapeutic staging of recurrent laryngeal carcinoma: Clinical findings and imaging studies compared with histopathology. *Otolaryngol Head Neck Surg* 2007;**137**:487–91.

35. Zbären P, Caversaccio M, Thoeny HC, *et al*. Radionecrosis or tumour recurrence after radiation of laryngeal and hypopharyngeal carcinomas. *Otolaryngol Head Neck Surg* 2007;**135**:838–43.

36. Bradley PJ, Ferlito A, Suárez C, *et al*. Options for salvage after failed

initial treatment of anterior vocal commissure squamous carcinoma. *Eur Arch Otorhinolaryngol* 2006;**263**:889–94.

37. Lucioni M, Marioni G, Bertolin A, *et al*. Conservative surgery planning in laryngeal carcinoma: The role of CT investigation of critical anatomic subsites. (Submitted).

38. Thoeny HC, Delaere PR, Hermans R. Correlation of local outcome after partial laryngectomy with cartilage abnormalities on CT. *AJNR Am J Neuroradiol* 2005;**26**:674–8.

39. Becker M. Neoplastic invasion of laryngeal cartilage: Radiologic diagnosis and therapeutic implications. *Eur J Radiol* 2000;**33**:216–29.

40. Esclamado R, Day T, Flint P, *et al*. Recurrent glottic cancer. *Head Neck* 2007;**29**:609–14.

41. Knappe M, Louw M, Gregor RT. Ultrasonography-guided fine needle aspiration for the assessment of cervical metastases. *Arch Otolaryngol Head Neck Surg* 2000;**126**:1091–6.

42. Session RB, Picken CA. Malignant cervical adenopathy. In: Cummings CW, Fredrickson JM, Harker LA, *et al*. (eds). *Otolaryngology head and neck surgery*. St Louis: Mosby-Year Book; 1998:737–57.

43. Holsinger FC, Funk E, Roberts DB, *et al*. Conservation laryngeal surgery versus total laryngectomy for radiation failure in laryngeal cancer. *Head Neck* 2006;**28**:779–84.

44. Marioni G, Marchese-Ragona R, Lucioni M, *et al*. Organ-preservation surgery following failed radiotherapy for laryngeal cancer. Evaluation, patient selection, functional outcome and survival. *Curr Opinion Otolaryngol Head Neck Surg* 2008;**16**:141–6.

45. Piazza C, Peretti G, Cattaneo A, *et al*. Salvage surgery after radiotherapy for laryngeal cancer: From endoscopic resections to open-neck partial and total laryngectomies. *Arch Otolaryngol Head Neck Surg* 2007;**133**:1037–43.

46. Motamed M, Laccourreye O, Bradley PJ. Salvage conservation laryngeal surgery after irradiation failure for early laryngeal cancer. *Laryngoscope* 2006;**116**:451–5.

47. Rifai M, Heiba MH, Salah H. Anterior commissure carcinoma II: The role of salvage supracricoid laryngectomy. *Am J Otolaryngol* 2002;**23**:1–3.

48. de Gier HH, Knegt PP, de Boer MF, *et al*. CO2-laser treatment of recurrent glottic carcinoma. *Head Neck* 2001;**23**:177–80.

49. Steiner W, Vogt P, Ambrosch P, *et al*. Transoral carbon dioxide laser microsurgery for recurrent glottic carcinoma after radiotherapy. *Head Neck* 2004;**26**:477–84.

50. Roedel RM, Matthias C, Wolff HA, *et al*. Transoral laser microsurgery for recurrence after primary radiotherapy of early glottic cancer. *Auris Nasus Larynx* 2009 Dec 21 [Epub ahead of print].

51. Ansarin M, Planicka M, Rotundo S, *et al*. Endoscopic carbon dioxide laser surgery for glottic cancer recurrence after radiotherapy: Oncological results. *Arch Otolaryngol Head Neck Surg* 2007;**133**:1193–7.

52. Marioni G, Marchese-Ragona R, Ottaviano G, *et al*. Supracricoid laryngectomy. Is it time to define guidelines to evaluate functional results? A review. *Am J Otolaryngol* 2004;**25**:98–104.

53. Staffieri A. Supracricoid laryngectomies in the treatment of radiotherapy failures. International Meeting of the European Study Group for Rehabilitation and Functional Surgery following Laryngectomy, Lisbon (Portugal), October 21–24, 2009.

54. Rizzotto G, Succo G, Lucioni M, *et al*. Subtotal laryngectomy with tracheohyoidopexy: A possibile alternative to total laryngectomy. *Laryngoscope* 2006;**116**:1907–17.

55. Hofmann-Saguez MR. Laryngectomie subtotale conservatrice. *Ann Otolaryngol* 1950;**67**:811–16.

56. Marioni G, Marchese-Ragona R, Pastore A, *et al*. The role of supracricoid partial laryngectomy for glottic carcinoma recurrence after radiotherapy failure. A critical review. *Acta Otolaryngol (Stockh)* 2006;**126**:1245–51.

57. Farrag TY, Koch WM, Cummings CW, *et al*. Supracricoid laryngectomy outcome: The John Hopkins experience. *Laryngoscope* 2007;**117**:129–32.

58. Pellini R, Pichi B, Ruscito P, *et al*. Supracricoid partial laryngectomies after radiation failure: A multi-institutional series. *Head Neck* 2008;**30**:372–9.

59. León X, López M, García J, *et al*. Supracricoid laryngectomy as salvage surgery after failure of radiation therapy. *Eur Arch Otorhinolaryngol* 2007;**264**:809–14.

60. Deganello A, Gallo O, De Cesare JM, *et al*. Supracricoid partial laryngectomy as salvage surgery for radiation therapy failure. *Head Neck* 2008;**30**:1064–71.

61. Luna-Ortiz K, Pasche P, Tamez-Velarde M, *et al*. Supracricoid partial laryngectomy with cricohyoidoepiglottopexy in patients with radiation therapy failure. *World J Surg Oncol* 2009;**7**:101.

62. Laccourreye O, Weinstein G, Naudo P, *et al*. Supracricoid partial laryngectomy after failed laryngeal radiation therapy. *Laryngoscope* 1996;**106**:495–8.

63. Pellini R, Manciocco V, Spriano G. Functional outcome of supracricoid laryngectomy with cricohyoidopexy. Radiation failure vs previously untreated cases. *Arch Otolaryngol Head Neck Surg* 2006;**132**:1221–5.

64. Marioni G, Marchese-Ragona R, Staffieri C, *et al*. *A critical review of the results of supracricoid laryngectomy for glottic carcinoma recurrence after radiotherapy failure*. International Meeting of the European Study Group for Rehabilitation and Functional Surgery following Laryngectomy, 8–10 June 2007; Rome.

65. Marchese-Ragona R, Calgaro N, Tregnaghi A, *et al*. Intraoperative modification of a supracricoid laryngectomy to a subtotal laryngectomy with tracheohyoidoepiglottopexy. *Eur Arch Otorhinolaryngol* 2009;**266**:2005–8.

66. Weber RS, Forastiere A, Rosenthal DI, *et al*. Controversies in the management of advanced laryngeal squamous cell carcinoma. *Cancer* 2004;**101**:211–19.

67. Farrag TY, Lin FR, Cummings CW, *et al*. Neck management in patients undergoing post-radiotherapy salvage laryngeal surgery for recurrent/persistent laryngeal cancer. *Laryngoscope* 2006;**116**:1864–6.

12

Cancer of the larynx—advanced stage

UMANATH NAYAK, REHAN KAZI

The management of locally advanced cancer of the larynx has undergone a paradigm shift in the past two decades. Total laryngectomy was the earlier standard of care in the management of this disease. With the proven success of various trials in recent times, chemoradiation has become an acceptable alternative for a majority of these cancers. Total laryngectomy, however, continues to have an important role in the management of T4 cancers with a non-functioning larynx, and for patients in whom chemoradiation has failed or is not a therapeutic option. The addition of total laryngectomy as a salvage procedure following the failure of chemoradiation has optimized the survival of patients undergoing various larynx preservation protocols. The newer generation voice prostheses are notable in having greatly improved post-laryngectomy rehabilitation and have resulted in better acceptability of total laryngectomy as the surgical procedure of choice for these patients. Overall, 5-year survivals in excess of 60%, even in the advanced stages, make laryngeal cancer one of the more curable cancers of the head and neck.[1–5]

Anatomy

The larynx is an important organ, not only for speech and respiration, but also for swallowing, on account of its intimate relationship with the pharynx during the pharyngeal phase of swallowing. The larynx has a cartilaginous framework composed of the thyroid, cricoid, arytenoid, cuneiform and corniculate cartilages. In addition, the epiglottic cartilage and the hyoid bone also form part of the larynx, along with the mucous lining, the fibro-elastic membranes (that form a barrier to cancer spread), and the connective tissue spaces beyond these membranes. The quadrangular membrane and the conus elasticus, which are fibro-elastic membranes deep to the submucosa, limit the initial spread of the cancer. However, once these membranes are breached, the tumour gains access to the pre-epiglottic and paraglottic spaces and spreads along the internal framework of the larynx.

In view of the potential for extensive spread of the disease, involvement of these spaces is, therefore, a relative contraindication for larynx conservation surgery. The pre-epilgottic space is triangular and bounded by the thyrohyoid membrane anteriorly, the vallecula superiorly, and the epiglottis posteriorly; it is commonly involved in supraglottic cancers. A connective tissue barrier usually separates it inferiorly from the paraglottic space, thus forming the basis for performing a horizontal partial (supraglottic) laryngectomy. The paraglottic space is bounded by the thyroid cartilage laterally, the quadrangular membrane and the conus elasticus medially, and the pre-epiglottic space superiorly. Glottic cancers that breach through the membranes and enter this space spread rapidly in all directions within the laryngeal framework, as well as outside the larynx via the crico-thyroid membrane and the pre-epiglottic space.[6] Extension into this space also results in vocal cord immobility due to involvement of the thyro-arytenoid muscle and the terminal branches of the recurrent laryngeal nerve.

The larynx is sub-divided into three regions: (i) supraglottic, (ii) glottic, and (iii) subglottic, each of which is anatomically and embryologically distinct and with separate lymphatic channels. Tumours arising from each of these regions are, therefore, different in terms of presentation, pattern of spread, treatment and prognosis.

Supraglottis

The supraglottis consists of the epiglottis, the aryepiglottic folds and the arytenoid cartilages on both sides, and the false cords and ventricle inferiorly. The lymphatics of the supraglottis are extensive and drain bilaterally to nodes in Levels II, III and IV. This has to be borne in mind while treating supraglottic cancers.[7]

Glottis

The glottis consists of the true cords and the anterior commissure. The vocal cords are membranous in the anterior two-thirds, consisting of the mucous membrane and the vocalis muscle, and cartilaginous in the posterior one-third, containing the vocal process of the arytenoid cartilage. The lymphatics of the true vocal cord are sparse and nodal involvement in tumours restricted to the true cord is rare. However, once tumours extend into the supraglottis, regional node involvement is common. Tumours that extend from the glottis to the supraglottis are termed transglottic cancers.

Subglottis

The subglottis is the part of the larynx from below the margin of the vocal cords up to the lower border of the cricoid cartilage. Primary tumours of this region are rare and are mostly extensions from glottic cancers. The lymphatics from this area drain predominantly into pretracheal and paratracheal nodes, which accounts for their involvement in glottic cancers that have extended into the subglottis.

The overall incidence of supraglottic cancers is higher in Indians than glottic cancers. However, in the West, the ratio is reversed, with glottic cancer being more common than supraglottic cancer. This variation in demographics is due to the higher prevalence of chewing tobacco rather than smoking in the Indian subcontinent, which results in tobacco-rich saliva coming in contact with the supraglottis. In contrast, smoke from tobacco smoking has more contact with the glottis on the way to the lungs.

Diagnosis and evaluation

Patients with tumours of the larynx present with hoarseness of voice, dysphagia or odynophagia and, occasionally, haemoptysis. Associated referred otalgia or cervical lymphadenopathy may be present. Hoarseness of voice is an early symptom in glottic cancers, which explains why more glottic cancers present in the early stages than supraglottic cancers. Advanced cancers may be accompanied with visible stridor due to respiratory obstruction. Examination with a mirror or a Hopkin telescope will usually indicate the exact location of the growth and its local extensions, as well as the status of vocal cord mobility, which has an important bearing on

management. A direct laryngoscopy under general anaesthesia is necessary for histopathological confirmation and more detailed assessment. In certain cases, microlaryngoscopy may assist in the evaluation of early glottic cancers before planning conservation laryngeal surgery.

High-resolution CT scans of the larynx are necessary in the routine evaluation of both early-stage and advanced laryngeal cancers.[8] In early cancers, they may demonstrate early involvement of the thyroid cartilage, especially in lesions extending to the anterior commissure and the presence of sub-clinical neck secondaries in supraglottic cancer. In advanced cancers, they indicate spread to paraglottic and pre-epiglottic spaces, as well as invasion into the thyroid cartilage and soft tissues of the neck. MRI is useful to assess subglottic extension of the tumour, as well as to detect sub-clinical nodal disease. PET-CT scan has a limited role in the routine evaluation of laryngeal cancer; however, it is invaluable in the assessment of a patient after radiotherapy to detect residual or recurrent cancer (Fig. 1).

Management

As mentioned in the beginning of this chapter, larynx preservation protocols with chemoradiation have had a significant impact on the way advanced laryngeal cancers are managed today.

Chemoradiation for cancer of the larynx

The Veterans Administration Larynx Preservation Trial in 1991 highlighted the feasibility of preserving the larynx by

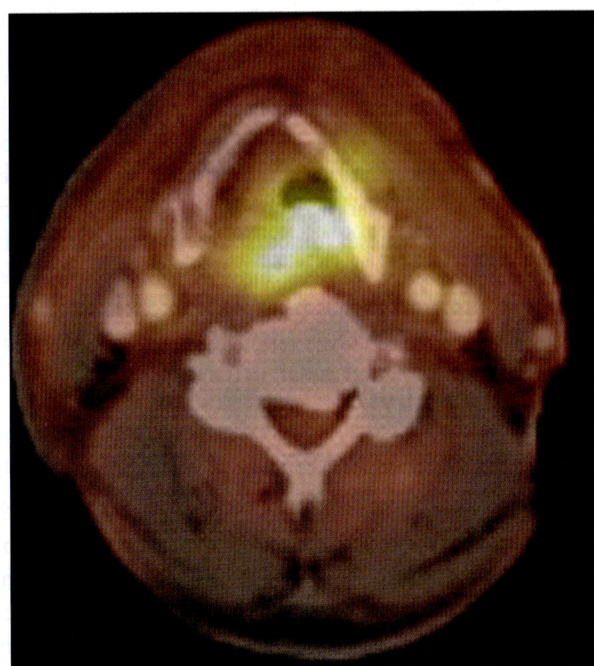

Fig. 1. PET-CT scan showing post RT recurrent glottic cancer

Posterior pharyngeal wall

The posterior pharyngeal wall of the hypopharynx is a continuation of the posterior wall of the oropharynx. The level of the hyoid bone is considered as the anatomical landmark dividing the two. Inferiorly, it continues as the posterior wall of the cricopharynx and from there as the cervical oesophagus, with the anatomical landmark being the lower border of the cricoid cartilage. Laterally, it is continuous with the lateral walls of the pyriform sinus on both sides. Primary posterior pharyngeal wall malignant tumours are uncommon, and most of them are either an extension of the pyriform sinus cancers or superior extensions of cervical oesophagus cancers.

Post-cricoid region

The post-cricoid region refers to the region of the hypopharynx behind the cricoid cartilage and is surrounded by the cricopharyngeus muscle. Being the narrowest part of the pharynx and also a relatively rigid muscular tube with the cricoid cartilage in front, tumours of this area tend to cause dysphagia early. The post-cricoid region continues inferiorly into the cervical oesophagus.

The lymphatic network of the hypopharynx is quite rich, and involvement of regional nodes occurs early in the course of the disease. Nearly two-thirds of patients with cancer of the hypopharynx present with neck secondaries.[4] Whereas pyriform sinus cancers metastasize mainly to Levels II, III and IV, posterior pharyngeal wall and post-cricoid cancers additionally metastasize to retropharyngeal nodes.

Diagnosis and evaluation

The principal signs and symptoms of cancer of the hypopharynx are dysphagia or odynophagia, referred otalgia, hoarseness of voice and a palpable neck mass because of secondaries. The presence of these symptoms usually indicates an advanced stage of the disease. Pyriform sinus and posterior pharyngeal wall cancers are notoriously silent in their early stages and the only symptom may be a foreign body sensation in the throat. In advanced stages, stridor may also be present due to the involvement of the larynx in pyriform sinus cancer, or due to bilateral abductor paralysis, as in the case of post-cricoid carcinoma. Examination of the hypopharynx with a Hopkin telescope may show the tumour in the pyriform sinus with its extensions. Often, there may be only pooling of saliva in the pyriform sinus and fixity of the ipsilateral cord, indicating a need for further examination under anaesthesia. A direct laryngoscopy and oesophagoscopy under general anaesthesia are mandatory for a proper assessment of the disease and for deciding on the plan of management, as well as for histological confirmation.

All patients with hypopharyngeal cancer should preferably

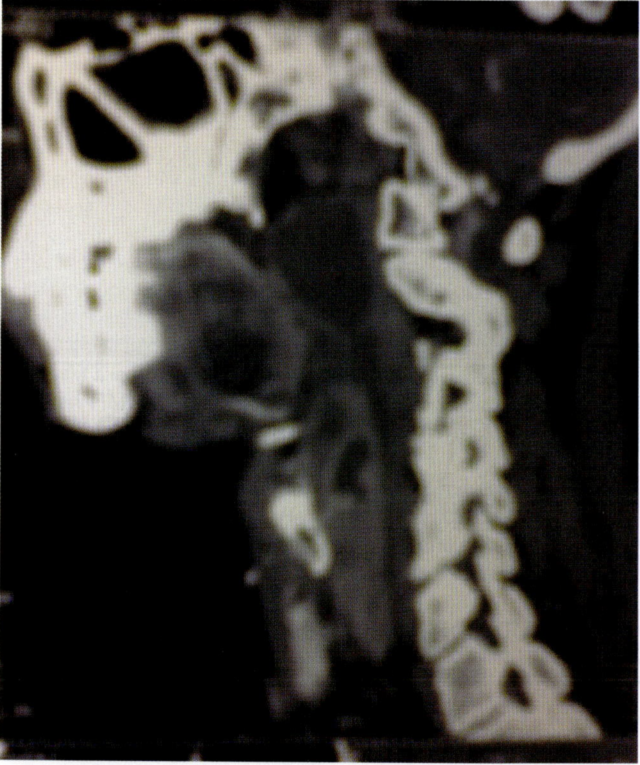

Fig. 2. Carcinoma hypopharynx with retropharyngeal node

have a CT scan or MRI for full assessment of the disease and its extensions. A CT scan is particularly useful to assess extensions into the larynx and the presence of unsuspected regional nodes. The detection of retropharyngeal nodes or invasion of pre-vertebral soft issues on CT scan may alter the decision for surgical management (Fig. 2). PET-CT is being increasingly used in the initial evaluation of the patient as well as in the early detection of residual or recurrent disease after radiotherapy, when other modalities of investigation may not be accurate.[5,6] It should be noted that the incidence of distant metastasis in advanced hypopharyngeal cancers is high (approximately 60%), unlike in other head and neck cancers.[7]

In the evaluation of a patient with hypopharyngeal cancer, performance status and nutritional status are as important as tumour factors. Patients with poor performance status are not candidates for major surgical resection or concurrent chemoradiation, and this may adversely affect their chances of a cure. Additionally, patients who have lost a significant amount of weight (>10% of their total weight within the past 6 months) require nutritional support before they can be taken up for surgery or chemoradiation.[8] Serious consideration may be given for a nasogastric feeding tube or PEG tube for these patients. In patients undergoing chemoradiation for cancer of the hypopharynx, a routine PEG tube insertion before the start of treatment is highly recommended and will improve compliance with the treatment.

TNM staging (AJCC 7th ed, 2010)[9]

Primary Tumour (T)

TX Primary tumour cannot be assessed

T0 No evidence of primary tumour

Tis Carcinoma *in situ*

T1 Tumour limited to one subsite of hypopharynx and/or 2 cm or less in greatest dimension

T2 Tumour invades more than one subsite of hypopharynx or an adjacent site, or measures more than 2 cm but not more than 4 cm in greatest dimension without fixation of hemilarynx

T3 Tumour more than 4 cm in greatest dimension or with fixation of hemilarynx or extension to oesophagus

T4a Moderately advanced local disease
Tumour invades thyroid/cricoid cartilage, hyoid bone, thyroid gland, or central compartment soft tissue*

T4b Very advanced local disease
Tumour invades prevertebral fascia, encases carotid artery, or involves mediastinal structures

Note: Central compartment soft tissue includes prelaryngeal strap muscles and subcutaneous fat.

*Regional Lymph Nodes (N)**

NX Regional lymph nodes cannot be assessed

N0 No regional lymph node metastasis

N1 Metastasis in a single ipsilateral lymph node, 3 cm or less in greatest dimension

N2 Metastasis in a single ipsilateral lymph node, more than 3 cm but not more than 6 cm in greatest dimension, or in multiple ipsilateral lymph nodes, none more than 6 cm in greatest dimension, or in bilateral or contralateral lymph nodes, none more than 6 cm in greatest dimension

N2a Metastasis in single ipsilateral lymph node more than 3 cm but not more than 6 cm in greatest dimension

N2b Metastasis in multiple ipsilateral lymph nodes, none more than 6 cm in greatest dimension

N2c Metastasis in bilateral or contralateral lymph nodes, none more than 6 cm in greatest dimension

N3 Metastasis in lymph node more than 6 cm in greatest dimension

Note: Metastases at level VII are considered regional lymph node metastases.

Distant metastasis (M)

M0 No distant metastasis

M1 Distant metastasis

(Used with the permission of the American Joint Committee on Cancer (AJCC), Chicago, Illinois. The original source for this material is the *AJCC Cancer Staging Manual*, Seventh Edition (2010) published by Springer Science and Business Media LLC, www.springer.com.)

MANAGEMENT

The results of treatment of cancer of the hypopharynx vary considerably, depending on whether the cancer is early or advanced. The general principles of treatment are also different in these two groups.

Early cancer of the hypopharynx (T1/T2 N0)

Results following treatment for early cancer of the hypopharynx are gratifying and most centres report 5-year survival rates of 70%–80%.[10,11] However, patients who present in this stage are few, since early cancer of the hypopharynx is basically asymptomatic. Single modality of treatment (either surgery or radiation) is usually sufficient to treat these patients successfully and chemotherapy is rarely used.

Surgery

Laser endoscopic surgery is the standard method of surgical resection of early hypopharyngeal cancer. Open surgery is rarely performed in this situation except for occasional lesions of the superior aspect of the pyriform sinus, which may be excised using the technique of partial laryngopharyngectomy.[12,13] Partial laryngopharyngectomy is an extension of the supraglottic laryngectomy for supraglottic cancer (*see* Chapter 10) and involves additional excision of the pyriform sinus. Postoperative aspiration is a serious problem with this surgery and many of these lesions are now treated with radiation therapy.

Steiner has pioneered the procedures for laser excision of hypopharyngeal cancers, basically as an extension of laser resection of laryngeal cancers.[14] Lesions of only the pyriform sinus and posterior pharyngeal wall are amenable to this procedure and case selection is important. This procedure can only be practised by expert hands and by those who are already familiar with laser resection of laryngeal cancer. The special endoscopic instruments designed by Steiner make it possible to expose areas of the hypopharynx amenable to laser resection, which otherwise would not have been possible with conventional instruments. Again, many of these lesions can be successfully treated with radiation therapy, which also has the advantage of addressing the neck which is at significant risk in early hypopharyngeal cancers. Laser excision is probably a good method to salvage post-radiotherapy failures, provided the disease is accessible and is still limited in size and depth.

Radiotherapy for early hypopharyngeal cancer

Radiotherapy is the primary mode of treatment for most early hypopharyngeal cancers. The overall 5-year survival rates vary from 70% to 85% in different centres.[10,11] Advances in radiation, such as intensity-modulated radiation therapy (IMRT), has made it possible to irradiate limited areas of the hypopharynx and avoid radiation to surrounding tissues. The neck can also be addressed simultaneously. In general, results are much better in cancer of the pyriform sinus than that for posterior pharyngeal wall and post-cricoid cancers.

Locally advanced cancer of the hypopharynx (T3/T4 N+)

Locally advanced cancer of the hypopharynx presents challenges, both in view of the complexity of treatment as well as the poor outcomes. Large tumours significantly affect swallowing function, and nutritional management can be a major issue. The following are the various options of treatment with curative intent:

- Concurrent chemoradiation
- Surgery followed by postoperative radiotherapy.

Concurrent chemoradiation

The gratifying results obtained with concurrent chemoradiation for laryngeal cancer has resulted in it being tried for hypopharyngeal cancer; however, results have been mixed.[15] Certain sub-sites (such as pyriform sinus) have shown better responses as compared to other sub-sites (pharyngeal wall, post-cricoid). Additionally, results for T4 tumours have been unsatisfactory, such that chemoradiation may not be considered as the first option for the management of resectable T4 hypopharyngeal cancer.

Most chemoradiation protocols use cisplatinum at a dose of 100 mg/m^2 administered every 3 weeks, along with 68–72 Gy of radiation. Tolerance of this regimen can sometimes become an issue and many radiation oncologists substitute with weekly cisplatinum (30 mg/m^2), which is better tolerated. The performance status of the patient is an important factor in determining which patients can be subjected to this treatment, and the routine insertion of a PEG tube may improve compliance with the treatment. Patients with poor performance status and advanced age may have to be subjected to radiation alone; albeit with inferior results. In selected cases, targeted therapy with monoclonal antibodies (e.g. Cetuximab) may have a role in improving responses to radiotherapy.[16] Recently, sequential therapy utilizing three-drug chemotherapy with docetaxel (75 mg/m^2), cisplatinum (100 mg/m^2) and 5-FU (750 mg/m^2) (referred to as TPF regimen), followed by chemoradiation, has shown encouraging results and may hold some promise in improving responses in the future.[17]

Surgery

Surgery is the treatment of choice for T4 resectable cancers of the hypopharynx. Additionally, for certain sub-sites of T3 tumours (infiltrative lesions, those involving the post-cricoid region and large bulky tumours), surgery may give better results than chemoradiation. However, the decision to operate should be balanced against the functional outcome achievable with respect to both speech and swallowing. In view of the intimate relationship of the larynx to the hypopharynx, surgery for locally advanced hypopharyngeal cancer almost always includes a total laryngectomy, and the ability to provide satisfactory voice rehabilitation is an integral part of the decision-making process for treatment. Many of these patients require reconstruction of the pharyngo-oesophagus and the availability of these reconstructive methods has a major bearing on the decision to operate. It should be noted that almost all these patients require postoperative radiation therapy for maximizing the cure rates. The various surgical procedures practised for cancer of the hypopharynx are:

- Near total laryngopharyngectomy
- Total laryngectomy with partial or sub-total pharyngectomy
- Total laryngopharyngectomy
- Total laryngopharyngo-oesophagectomy.

Near total laryngopharyngectomy

This procedure is advocated for T3 and selected T4 well lateralized cancers of the pyriform sinus.[18,19] It is a semi-conservative procedure that combines the radicality of a total laryngectomy with the conservation of voice by creating a myomucosal shunt between the trachea and the pharynx. The patient breathes through an anterior tracheostomy, which is permanent. Its advantage over a total laryngectomy is that it avoids the necessity for the insertion of a voice prosthesis with its attendant additional costs and maintenance and, therefore, is popular in some centres in developing countries, such as India.[20] However, careful case selection and familiarity with the intrinsic anatomy of the larynx is mandatory for performing the procedure (*see* Chapter 11).

Total laryngectomy with partial/sub-total pharyngectomy

This procedure is usually performed for cancer of the pyriform sinus and involves resection of the involved pharynx with a 1 cm margin, along with total laryngectomy. When the disease in the pyriform sinus is limited and the residual mucosa after resection is sufficient for comfortable and tension-free closure of the pharynx, the procedure is termed laryngectomy with partial pharyngectomy (Fig. 1). However, when more extensive resection of the pharynx is necessary and sufficient mucosa is not available for comfortable closure, the procedure is termed laryngectomy with subtotal pharyngectomy. In general, a 5 cm width of the mucosa is necessary for closure without stricture formation. If the residual mucosa is less than this, it is necessary to augment it with a flap. The various options of flaps for augmentation of the pharynx after laryngectomy with subtotal pharyngectomy are:

- Pectoralis major myocutaneous flap
- Radial forearm free flap
- Antero-lateral thigh flap
- Gastro-omental free flap.

The last three are micro vascular free tissue transfers and are generally preferable because they are less bulky and more pliabile, thus providing better swallowing and speech function. The gastro-omental flap also has the advantage of being mucous secreting.

Total laryngopharyngectomy

This procedure, involving circumferential resection of the pharynx in addition to total laryngectomy, is indicated for post-cricoid and posterior pharyngeal wall cancers, as well as extensive pyriform sinus cancers that have extended to involve the post-cricoid region or the posterior pharyngeal wall (Fig. 3). Circumferential reconstruction of the pharynx becomes necessary in these situations and the same flaps mentioned earlier under laryngectomy with sub-total pharyngectomy may be utilized for the purpose. The pectoralis major myocutaneous flap, however, has a high incidence of stricture formation and should be avoided for circumferential reconstruction of the pharynx. Microvascular free jejunal transfer is also popular in these cases (Fig. 4).[21,22] Common sequelae following reconstruction of circumferential defects of the pharynx is the development of a lower anastomotic stricture, especially common with skin flaps due to the constricting effect of the suture line. This may be obviated by making a cut in the posterior wall of the oesophagus and inserting a wedge-like portion of the skin flap into this gap to break the suture line.

Total laryngopharyngo-oesophagectomy

When post-cricoid or posterior pharyngeal wall cancers extend into the cervical oesophagus to an extent that sufficient cervical oesophagus is not left in the neck for comfortable anastamosis, total oesophagectomy becomes necessary in addition to laryngopharyngectomy. This decision can usually be made preoperatively on the basis of imaging and endoscopic

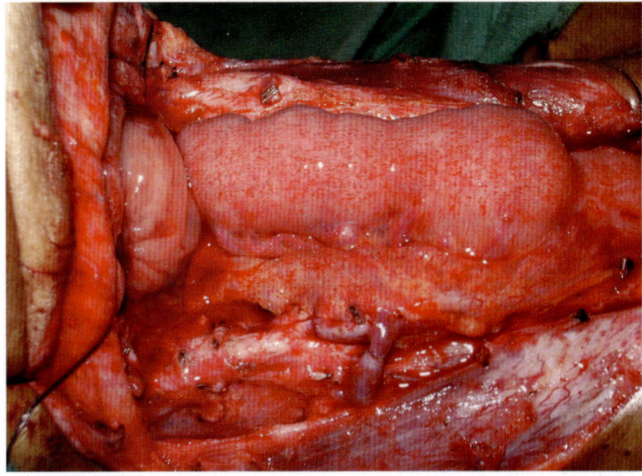
Fig. 4. Jejunal free flap

studies. Rarely, one may have to resort to this method during surgery on finding extensive submucosal spread of the disease into the cervical oesophagus. Following a laryngopharyngo-oesophagectomy, the stomach is pulled into the neck through the posterior mediastinum after converting it into a tube and is anastomosed to the base of tongue (Fig. 5).[21] The morbidity

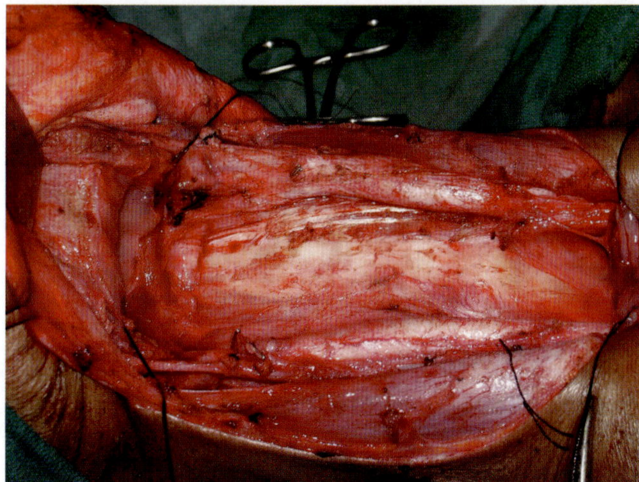
Fig. 3. Completed laryngo pharyngectomy

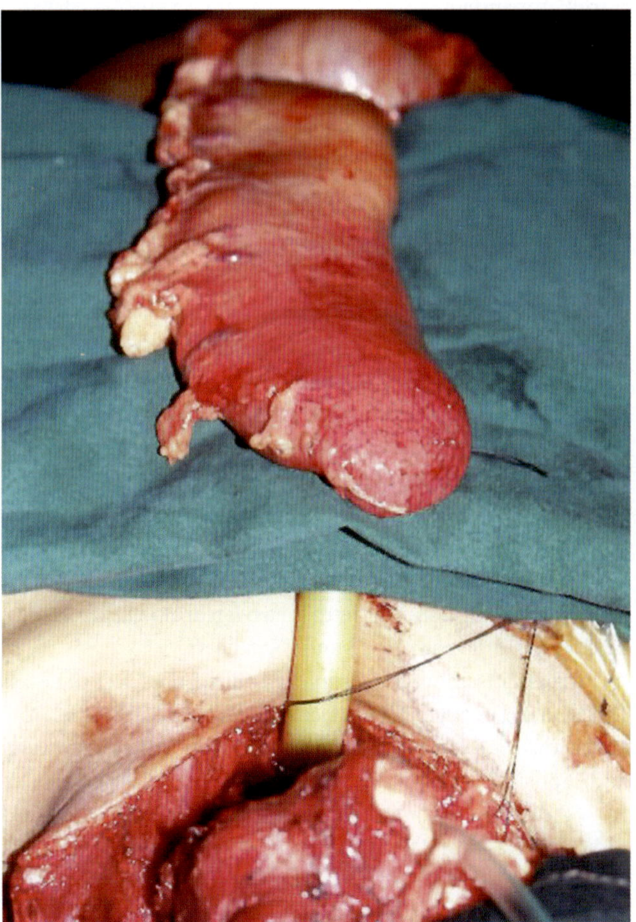
Fig. 5. Gastric transposition following laryngopharyngo-oesophagectomy

of this procedure is considerable and it is resorted to only when laryngopharyngectomy alone is not possible.[23]

Surgery after radiotherapy failure

With the increasing popularity of chemoradiation for larynx preservation, more and more patients are being treated with this modality. However, unlike in case of the larynx, failures are more when treating hypopharyngeal cancers and surgical salvage remains the only option for these patients. Not all of these patients are salvageable and the overall results are also inferior compared with that following upfront surgery and post-operative radiotherapy. Postoperative complications, such as wound breakdown and pharyngo-cutaneous fistula, are also much higher in this group of patients. However, despite these drawbacks, salvage surgery should be offered to these patients in resectable cancers after paying attention to the following issues:

- An interval of 2–3 months is preferable after completion of chemoradiation, as surgery immediately following chemoradiation has higher complications.
- Tight mucosal closures are to be strictly avoided and will almost always result in fistula. Liberal use of flaps is recommended.
- Always buttress the pharyngeal closure with non-radiated tissue if a flap is not being used; the pectoralis major myofacial flap is ideal for this purpose.
- Always cover the carotid artery with locally available soft tissue or soft tissues from the flap.

Management of the neck in cancer of the hypopharynx

Adequate treatment of the neck forms an integral part of the management of cancer of the hypopharynx. Even in early cancers, the incidence of subclinical neck disease is significant enough to warrant elective neck treatment. In patients undergoing radiation therapy, neck nodes in Levels II, III and IV have to be covered bilaterally even when they are clinically N0. Full ipsilateral/bilateral neck irradiation is required for N+ disease, depending on whether the nodes are unilateral or bilateral. In addition, the retro-pharyngeal nodes are also to be covered, especially in T3 and T4 cancers.

In patients undergoing surgery, routine clearance of Levels II, III and IV bilaterally is performed for N0 disease. Any suspicious nodes have to be checked with a frozen section; and, if positive, a comprehensive neck dissection is performed. In N+ disease, a comprehensive neck dissection (modified radical or classical RND) is performed on the side of the neck disease. Often, in patients undergoing chemoradiation, neck disease can persist after completion of the treatment, even though the primary disease has completely responded. This can happen especially when the neck disease was advanced before the start of the treatment. In these situations, after confirming the absence of primary disease both by imaging and endoscopy, patients may be subjected to neck dissection alone if the neck nodes are resectable.

Voice rehabilitation after surgery for hypopharyngeal cancer

Voice rehabilitation forms an integral part of the surgical management of cancer of the hypopharynx.[24] As in laryngeal cancer, primary voice restoration is the method of choice and the voice prosthesis is inserted at the time of surgery. The new generation voice prostheses (indwelling Provox™, Blom–Singer) have made this possible to the convenience of both the patient and the surgeon. The earlier method of prior stenting of the tracheo-oesophageal fistula, followed by insertion of the prosthesis at a later stage, is no longer required and a single-stage insertion of the voice prosthesis is practised at the time of the surgery.

The quality of voice following surgical voice restoration is satisfactory in patients who have undergone laryngectomy and partial pharyngectomy for pyriform sinus cancer. In patients who have undergone subtotal pharyngectomy or laryngopharyngectomy, the quality of voice acquired may be determined by the type of flap used for pharynx reconstruction. In general, skin flaps provide better speech quality than mucosa-lined flaps. In jejunal-free flaps, the quality of the speech may be further compromised by the copious mucous discharge produced by the jejunum, giving it a 'wet' quality. In laryngopharyngo-oesophagectomy and gastric pull-up, only secondary prosthesis insertion is possible to allow the transposed stomach and posterior tracheal wall to adhere to each other.

Salvage surgery following recent chemoradiation may be a relative contraindication to the use of primary voice restoration because of the increased incidence of wound breakdown. In these situations, it may be preferable to perform a secondary voice restoration procedure at a later date after the patient has fully recovered from the surgery.

References

1. Shah JP. *Head and neck surgery*. 2nd ed. St Louis: Mosby-Wolfe; 1996.
2. Carpenter RJ III, DeSanto LW, Devine KD, *et al*. Cancer of the hypopharynx. Analysis of treatment and results in 162 patients. *Arch Otolaryngol* 1976;**102**:716–21.
3. Pradhan S. *Voice conservation surgery for laryngeal and hypophanryngeal Cancer*. Mumbai: Lloyds Publishing House; 2006.
4. Lefebvre JL, Castelain B, De la Torre JC, *et al*. Lymph node invasion in hypopharynx and lateral epilarynx carcinoma: A prognostic factor. *Head Neck Surg* 1987;**10**:14–18.
5. Maylee K, Catherine C, Patrick F. 18 Fluoro-2-deoxy D-glucose positron emission tomographic imaging: Recent developments in head and neck cancer. *Curr Opin Oncol* 2005;**17**:249–53.

6. Schöder H, Yeung HWD, Gonen M, *et al*. Head and neck cancer: Clinical usefulness and accuracy of PET-CT image fusion. *Radiology* 2004;**231**:65–72.

7. Kotwall C, Sako K, Razack MS, *et al*. Metastatic patterns in squamous cell cancer of the head and neck. *Am J Surg* 1987;**154**:439–42.

8. Van Bokhorst-de van der Schueren MA, van Leeuwen PA, Sauerwein HP, *et al*. Assessment of malnutrition parameters in head and neck cancer and their relation to post-operative complications. *Head Neck* 1997;**19**:419–25.

9. Edge SB, Byrd DR, Compton CC (eds). *AJCC Cancer Staging Manual*. 7th ed. New York, NY: Springer; 2010:44–45.

10. Garden AS, Morrison WH, Clayman GL, *et al*. Early squamous cell carcinoma of the hypopharynx: Outcomes of treatment with radiation alone to the primary disease. *Head Neck* 1996;**18**: 317–22.

11. Garden AS, Morrison WH, Ang KK, *et al*. Hyperfractionated radiation in the treatment of squamous cell carcinomas of the head and neck: A comparison of two fractionation schedules. *Int J Radiat Oncol Biol Phys* 1995;**31**:493–502.

12. Ogura, JH, Jurena AA, Watson RK. Patial laryngopharyngectomy and neck dissection for pyriform sinus cancer. *Laryngoscope* 1960;**70**: 1399–417.

13. Ogura JH, Marks ME, Freeman RB. Results of conservation surgery for cancers of the supraglottis and pyriform sinus. *Laryngoscope* 1980;**90**:591–600.

14. Steiner W, Aabrosch P, Steiner W, *et al*. Organ preservation by transoral laser micro surgery in pyriform sinus carcinoma. *Otolaryngol Head Neck Surgery* 2001;**124**:58–67.

15. Yu L, Vikram B, Malamud S, *et al*. Chemotherapy rapidly alternating with twice-a-day accelerated radiation therapy in carcinomas involving the hypopharynx or esophagus: An update. *Cancer Invest* 1995;**13**:567–72.

16. Bonner JA, Harari PM, Giralt J, *et al*. Radiotherapy plus cetuximab for squamous cell carcinoma of the head and neck. *N Engl J Med* 2006;**354**:567–78.

17. Posner M. Paradigm shift in the treatment of head and neck cancer: The role of neoadjuvant chemotherapy. *The Oncologist* 2005;**10** (suppl 3):11–19.

18. Pradhan SA, D'Cruz AK, Pai PS, *et al*. Near total laryngectomy in advanced laryngeal and pyriform cancers. *Laryngoscope* 2002;**112**:375–80.

19. Dumich PS, Pearson BW, Weiland LH. Suitability of near-total laryngopharyngectomy in pyriform carcinoma. *Arch Otolaryngol Head Neck Surgery* 1984;**110**:664.

20. Shenoy AM, Plinkert PK, Nanjundappa N, *et al*. Functional utility and oncologic safety of near-total laryngectomy with tracheopharyngeal speech shunt in a Third World oncologic center. *Eur Arch Otorhinolaryngol* 1997;**254**:128–32.

21. Kato H, Watanabe H, Iizuka T, *et al*. Primary esophageal reconstruction after resection of the cancer in the hypopharynx or cervical esophagus: Comparison of free forearm skin tube flap, free jejunal transplantation and pull-through esophagectomy. *Jpn J Clin Oncol* 1987;**17**:255–61.

22. Bradford CR, Esclamado RM, Carroll WR, *et al*. Analysis of recurrence, complications, and functional results with free jejunal flaps. *Head Neck* 1994;**16**:149–54.

23. Cahow CE, Sasaki CT. Gastric pull-up reconstruction for pharyngo-laryngo-esophagectomy. *Arch Surg* 1994;**129**:425–9.

24. Nayak U, Kazi R. Voice restoration after total laryngectomy—Current science and future perspectives. Delhi: Byword Books; 2009.

14

Cancer of the nose and paranasal sinuses

RANJIT RAJAN, ALOK THAKAR, DAN FLISS, BIPIN T. VARGHESE

Introduction

Neoplasms of the nose and paranasal sinuses (PNS) are uncommon tumours. They tend to present late. The initial symptoms of a nasal–PNS neoplasm may not be different from those of chronic sinusitis and may be overlooked until the disease becomes advanced. Their treatment has the potential to produce considerable disfigurement of the most exposed part of the body—the face. This can deter surgeons from appropriately and aggressively treating these neoplasms surgically, leading to suboptimal treatment and unsatisfactory outcomes.

The treatment of these cancerous growths requires the close interdisciplinary co-operation of the specialties of otolaryngology—head and neck surgery, radiodiagnosis, radiation oncology, pathology and dental prosthodontics. Surgery remains the mainstay of treatment.

Surgical anatomy

The nasal fossa and PNS, located in the mid-face, have a complex anatomy and relationship to various important structures such as the orbit and its contents, the optic nerve, the anterior and middle cranial fossae, the pterygomaxillary and infra-temporal fossae, the palate and the superior alveolar process with its dentition.

The maxilla is a three-sided, pyramid-shaped hollow bone with its base directed medially and its apex supero-laterally. In the context of PNS tumours, the term 'maxilla' refers to the maxillary–zygomatic complex, which consists of the conjoint maxillary and the zygomatic bones, and which also incorporates the lacrimal, inferior turbinate and palatine bones. In the adult, the maxillary sinus occupies all of the maxillary bone and, in its supero-lateral limit, extends into the body of the zygomatic bone.

The maxilla has three surfaces—the orbital, facial and infra-temporal; the base comprises the nasal surface, which forms part of the lateral wall of the nose. All of its surfaces are thin and, hence, easily breached by neoplasms.

The facial or anterior surface, directed antero-laterally, is the palpable aspect of the maxilla, especially intra-orally. The infra-orbital nerve exits here. Erosion of this surface is palpable intra-orally before the swelling becomes obvious externally. The anterior–superior alveolar nerve fibres descend in this surface to supply the superior incisors. Numbness of these teeth indicates invasion of this surface by a tumour. The canine ridge on this surface corresponds to the lateral wall of the nose.

The superior surface is the orbital surface. Its anterior edge forms the medial half of the infra-orbital margin, the lateral half being formed by the zygomatic bone. Its posterior margin forms the inferior margin of the infra-orbital fissure, which leads to the infra-temporal fossa from the orbit. The maxillary nerve enters posteriorly via a groove on this surface that gradually deepens into a canal (the infra-orbital canal) when traced anteriorly. It lodges the nerve bearing the same name. The posterior–superior alveolar nerves branch off from this nerve as it enters the groove and descend through the infra-temporal surface of the maxilla. These nerves are affected by tumour invasion of this wall, leading to numbness of the upper molars and premolars, as well as the buccal aspect of the posterior part of the superior alveolus.

Tumours on the nasal or medial surface of the maxilla are the most accessible for examination and biopsy. This is the preferred site for biopsy as the biopsy site can be removed easily with the surgical specimen. A tumour extending to involve the greater palatine nerve that runs vertically downwards in the posterior part of the medial surface in the greater palatine canal causes hemipalatal anaesthesia. Tumours arising from the medial wall of the antrum in its posterior and superior part are likely to present late because of their distant location from the teeth and cheek. Hence, they are unlikely to produce warning dental symptoms or cheek swelling.

Posteriorly, where its medial and infra-temporal surfaces merge, the maxilla is related to the pterygopalatine fossa. The pterygopalatine fossa communicates in all directions with all major structures of the midface and has, therefore, been described as the 'Piccadilly Circus of the midface'. It has pathways to the middle cranial fossa posteriorly through the foramen rotundum and the vidian canal, the nasal fossa medially via the sphenopalatine foramen, the orbit superiorly through the inferior orbital fissure, and the infra-temporal fossa laterally. Invasion of the pterygopalatine fossa by cancer from the maxillary sinus opens up avenues of spread along these pathways and results in a poorer prognosis. As parasympathetic secretomotor fibres to the lacrimal gland traverse this fossa, decreased lacrimation may be a sign of invasion of this region.

The cavity of the sinus extends into the alveolar process. The roots of the teeth protrude into this part of the sinus cavity, especially those of the second pre-molar and first two molars. Dental symptoms are, therefore, not unusual with cancer of the maxillary sinus.

On its superomedial aspect, the maxilla fuses with the ethmoid labyrinth, a complex honeycomb-like collection of cells between the orbit and the superior nasal cavity. The ethmoid labyrinth is separated from the orbit by the papery thin lamina papyracea. The ethmoid is roofed by the thick fovea ethmoidalis, which is a part of the frontal bone. Just medial to this, the ethmoid roof slopes abruptly inferiorly as a thin plate of bone to join the thin cribriform plate which roofs the olfactory cleft of the nose and is perforated by the olfactory nerve fibres. Ethmoid neoplasms extending to the bone's superior aspect find their way intra-cranially, breaching the thin bone at this location. The medial canthal ligament serves as an external landmark to the level of the cribriform plate. During surgery, the frontoethmoid suture on the medial wall of the orbit also serves a guide to the level of the cribriform plate. Its anterior limit is indicated by the position of the anterior ethmoid artery. Posteriorly, the jugum of the sphenoid borders the cribriform plate and constitutes the posterior limit of a craniofacial resection.

The bony walls of the PNS may be thin and lamellar, offering little resistance to the spread of neoplasms, as with the orbital floor and lamina papyracea, or thick and spongy like the alveolar process and the zygomatic bone. Although these thicker walls are less likely to be breached by a tumour, they may sometimes be affected by osteoradionecrosis consequent to radiation as they are relatively less vascularized.

Lymphatic pathways

The anterior nasal mucosa and vestibular skin drain to the facial, parotid and submandibular nodes (Level I) and, then, onto the deep cervical nodal chain (Level II). The remaining posterior nasal fossa drains to a lymphatic plexus anterior to the torus tubarius, which then drains to the lateral retropharyngeal nodes of Rouviere, which in turn drain to the superior deep cervical nodes (Level II). The lymphatic drainage of the maxillary sinus is via its ostium to the middle meatus, from where it drains along the above-mentioned posterior lymphatic pathways to the retropharyngeal node and thereon to the deep cervical nodes. Resection of maxillary cancers should, therefore, include the middle meatus and the middle turbinate if the lymphatic pathways have to be encompassed.

As involvement of the retropharyngeal node is not clinically obvious, the first clinical sign of lymphatic spread along the posterior lymphatic pathways is often an enlargement of the second echelon Level II nodes. This is believed to signify grave prognostic import and can be taken as an indication for non-curative treatment. Anterior tumour extension to the subcutaneous tissues of the cheek, the dentoalveolar ridge, or the buccal mucosa, however, traverses the anterior lymphatic pathways directly to the facial and submandibular nodes (first echelon), and their involvement does not necessarily signify a similar dismal prognosis.

Aetiology

Environmental and occupational carcinogens have a significant role in the genesis of sinonasal malignant neoplasms and may effect carcinogenesis in a synergistic fashion.

Woodworkers have long been known to be particulary affected, and both hard woods (e.g. mahogany—ethmoidal adenocarcinoma) and soft woods (e.g. pine—maxillary squamous cell carcinoma) have been implicated.[1,2] The carcinogenic effect may, additionally, be consequent to other carcinogens commonly used in the industry, including formaldehyde, polycyclic aromatic hydrocarbon-containing solvents, and wood preservatives that contain arsenic.

Cadmium, chromium and silica dust have also been implicated as carcinogens. An increased incidence of PNS tumours is seen in workers in the leather industry. Chromium is present in leather tanning solutions. Tannins and phenolic compounds that are used to manufacture leather from animal hides are also carcinogenic. Radium dial workers and metal industry workers have a higher risk of developing these tumours because of their exposure to carcinogenic nitrosamines in cutting oils. Exposure to heavy metals such as nickel is associated with sinonasal tumours.[3] Thorotrast (25% solution of thorium dioxide), a radioactive agent previously used as a contrast agent for sinus radiography, has also been implicated. Exposure to mustard gas is associated with PNS neoplasms.

Cigarette smoke—a ubiquitously implicated carcinogen for most upper aerodigestive cancer sites—is not commonly believed to have a significant aetiological role. However, it is interesting to note that one of the earliest recorded observations on the carcinogenic effect of environmental agents pertains to the role of the immoderate use of snuff in the causation of ulcerated nasal tumours, as described by John Hill in 1761. This observation preceded even the well known connection between scrotal cancer and chimney soot made by Sir Percival Pott in 1775.

Pathology

In contrast to other locations in the upper aerodigestive tract, a wide histological variety of tumours occur at this site. The nasal and PNS mucosa (*aka* Schneiderian mucosa) is of ectodermal origin, and is a pseudostratified, ciliated, columnar epithelium (respiratory epithelium) with serous and mucous glands. Minor salivary glands are present, especially around the sinus ostia. The superior-most portion of the nasal fossa—the olfactory cleft or olfactory recess—is lined by olfactory mucosa, which is markedly less vascular and contains the olfactory receptor cells, supporting cells and Bowman (olfactory) glands.

Tumours of the nose and PNS may be considered broadly under the categories of epithelial and non-epithelial, either of which may be benign or malignant. Epithelial tumours may arise from the respiratory epithelium or metaplastic squamous epithelium, or they may be glandular tumours originating from the mucus gland epithelium (adenocarcinoma) or salivary gland components (adenoid cystic carcinoma). Mesodermal tumours are encountered relatively rarely. A more comprehensive listing of the types of neoplasms at this location is given in Table 1.

Benign non-epithelial tumours

Osteomas

In the sinonasal tract, osteomas are more usually seen in the fronto-ethmoid region and need only be resected if they are symptomatic. Symptoms can occur secondary to obstruction of the frontal sinus outflow tract, or may be consequent to extension into the orbit or compression of the optic nerve. Surgical excision requires an external fronto-ethmoidectomy/ lateral rhinotomy or an osteoplastic flap. Small, medially located osteomas may be removed endoscopically.

Table 1. Histological classification of neoplasms of nose and paranasal sinuses

---

I. EPITHELIAL
- Benign Epithelial Neoplasms
  —Papillomas
  —Adenomas
- Malignant Epithelial Neoplasms
  —Squamous cell carcinoma
  —Non-epidermoid carcinomas
    1. Adenoid cystic carcinoma
    2. Adenocarcinoma
- Olfactory neuroblastoma
- Malignant melanoma
- Sinonasal undifferentiated carcinoma

II. NON-EPITHELIAL
- Benign non-epithelial neoplasms
  —Osteoma
  —Fibroma
  —Chondroma
  —Schwannoma (neurilemmoma)
- Malignant non-epithelial neoplasms
  —Sarcomas
    1. Malignant nerve sheath tumours
    2. Osteosarcoma
    3. Chondrosarcoma
    4. Fibrosarcoma
    5. Rhabdomyosarcoma
  —Haemangiopericytoma
  —Lymphoreticular neoplasms
    1. Lymphoma
    2. Plasmacytoma

III. METASTATIC NEOPLASMS

Chondromas

They are extremely rare and are treated by local excision.

Neurogenic tumours

These rare and slow growing tumours may present as very large nasal masses. Approximately two-thirds are neurilemmomas/ schwannomas and the rest are neurofibromas. Treatment is by complete resection. Immunohistochemical staining with S-100 confirms the diagnosis.

Benign epithelial tumours

Sinonasal papillomas

The most common of the benign neoplasms of the PNS, sinonasal papillomas account for 0.4%–4.7% of all sinonasal tumours. The tumour arises from the sinonasal mucosa (Schneiderian mucosa) and is often referred to as a Schneiderian papilloma. Evidence is mounting for an aetiological role of human papilloma virus types 6 and 11 in these neoplasms.[4–6]

Hyams sub-divided Schneiderian papillomas into three categories—inverted, fungiform and cylindrical cell (or oncocytic).[7] Inverted papillomas, also called transitional cell papillomas, constitute ~75% of Schneiderian papillomas, fungiform papillomas comprise ~20%, and the cylindrical cell papilloma is the least frequently encountered (3%–8%). The tumours, although histologically benign, demonstrate locally aggressive behaviour with a tendency to erode bone. They may also harbour a co-existent malignancy, or may manifest subsequent malignant change. The tumour has a tendency to recur, especially with incomplete resection.

Inverted papillomas originate from the lateral nasal wall and appear as a unilateral pinkish, polypoidal mass. The tumour is called 'inverted' due to its invaginating surface growth pattern, wherein the epithelial cover tends to grow down into the underlying stroma and may lead to a wrinkled surface appearance. As opposed to this, an exophytic or outward growth pattern is seen in the fungiform variety. These tumours present as a warty mass arising from the septum. The cylindrical cell variety may show a mixture of exophytic and inverted growth patterns and it typically presents as a pinkish, fleshy, papillary mass arising from the lateral nasal wall.

The tumour is seen most often in middle-aged and elderly men and presents with unilateral nasal obstruction, nasal discharge and epistaxis. Headache, proptosis and diplopia may be seen in advanced cases. Pain should lead to suspicion of malignant transformation.

Radiologically, an inverted papilloma appears as a soft tissue density occupying the nasal fossa and adjacent sinuses. The sinuses may show bony expansion and, later, bone erosion caused by pressure necrosis. Extensive bone erosion should evoke the suspicion of a carcinoma arising in the papilloma.

The treatment of sinonasal papillomas is by complete resection. Resection of inverted papillomas has been achieved conventionally by utilizing a lateral rhinotomy with medial maxillectomy. However, with the ability to precisely determine the disease extent by pre-operative computerized tomography (CT) and magnetic resonance imaging (MRI), and with the advent of endoscopic sinus surgery, endoscopic resection for anatomically suitable tumours is now being increasingly advocated.[8,9] The tumour is usually pedunculated with a relatively small site of origin from the lateral nasal wall, which is usually in the area of the ascending plate of the palatine bone in the posterior lateral nasal wall. Special attention has to be directed to this area with resection or drilling of its surface. Approximately 10% of inverted papillomas may harbour a coexistent carcinoma. Even after resection of an inverted papilloma, a carcinoma can again develop in the same area. The number of times an inverted papilloma recurs has no bearing on the propensity toward malignant transformation. Increased keratinization of the papilloma is considered to be one of the histological features that may predict the risk of recurrence.

Adenomas

These arise frequently from the nasal septum and are treated by complete excision, after which they rarely recur.

Malignant non-epithelial tumours

Neurogenic sarcomas

Neurogenic sarcomas are rare and locally aggressive neoplasms. Often, they present with distant metastasis. Treatment is primarily surgical. Radiation and chemotherapy are used for unresectable and recurrent disease.

Osteosarcoma

A rare neoplasm, it presents as a painful, hard swelling of the upper jaw, more often in young adults. Prior exposure to ionizing radiation is considered an important aetiological factor. Radical resection is the recommended treatment. The prognosis is often poor.

Chondrosarcoma

A rare, slow growing tumour, it may demonstrate varying degrees of aggressiveness (histological grades I–IV), and has a tendency to recur. Wide local excision is the treatment of choice. These tumours are not radiosensitive.

Rhabdomyosarcoma

Among the commonest malignant tumours of the PNS in the paediatric age group, rhabdomyosarcomas are composed of small, round, hyperchromatic cells with desmin positivity on immunohistochemistry. Three varieties occur—embryonal, botryoid and alveolar. The tumour presents as rapidly growing polypoidal masses with proptosis and aggressive growth. Treatment is primarily by radiation and chemotherapy. Surgery may be undertaken as part of the initial treatment if the tumour is considered to be resectable, or it may be undertaken subsequently for residual or recurrent disease following radiation and chemotherapy.

Haemangiopericytoma

These uncommon sinonasal neoplasms arise from the pericytes of Zimermann. Benign and malignant varieties have been described but histological differentiation is not easy. They are highly vascular neoplasms. This neoplasm behaves less aggressively in the nose and PNS than elsewhere. Wide excision is the mainstay of treatment.

Lymphoma

Lymphomas in the nose and sinuses are usually of the non-Hodgkin type. They are rarely seen in the sinonasal region. Radiotherapy is the treatment advocated for localized disease and chemotherapy for disseminated disease and recurrence.

Extramedullary plasmacytoma

Although a plasmacytoma may be isolated, it may also be the initial manifestation of a multiple myeloma. Initial screening investigations should include a search for bony lesions elsewhere in the skeleton, a bone marrow biopsy, serum electrophoresis and urinalysis for Bence–Jones proteins. Treatment may be by surgical resection or by radiation therapy.

Malignant epithelial tumours

Olfactory neuroblastoma

This is an exceedingly rare tumour which arises from the olfactory epithelium in the upper third of the nasal fossa. It has a bimodal age distribution with two peaks of incidence, one at 10–20 years of age and another at 50–60 years of age.

The initial presentation may be with nasal obstruction and a blood-stained nasal discharge consequent to an exophytic nasal mass with ulceration. The tumour may erode the nasal septum and present bilaterally. Typically, these neuroblastomas involve the olfactory fossa and often erode the cribriform plate to involve the anterior cranial fossa and the adjoining dura. The diagnosis is suggested by the presence of typical olfactory rosettes on histopathological examination. These are acinar spaces containing mucin and are lined by columnar cells. On other occasions, however, these typical histological features may not be seen and only sheets of round cells may be visualized, leading to histological confusion with undifferentiated carcinoma, lymphoma and rhabdomyosarcoma. The presence of neuron-specific enolase positivity on immunohistochemistry then becomes essential to confirm the diagnosis.

These neoplasms are staged clinically, either on the basis of the Kadish staging system[10] or the UCLA (University of California, Los Angeles) Classification.[11]

Kadish staging system[10]

Stage A—Tumour confined to nasal cavity
Stage B—Tumour extends to PNS
Stage C—Tumour extends to orbit, base of skull, cranial cavity, or with cervical/distant metastasis.

UCLA staging system[11]

T1   Tumour involves nasal cavity and/or PNS, excluding sphenoid and most superior ethmoidal cells
T2   Tumour involves nasal cavity and/or PNS, including sphenoid with extension to or erosion of cribriform plate
T3   Tumour extends into orbit/protrudes into anterior cranial fossa
T4   Tumour involves brain.

These tumours behave aggressively and have a pronounced tendency for local recurrence. They can metastasize regionally to the cervical lymph nodes or distantly to the lungs and bones. The treatment is primarily surgical and entails a craniofacial resection followed by radiation therapy. Chemotherapy is advised for Kadish Stage C, especially in the presence of metastasis.

Malignant melanoma

They are uncommon in the nose and PNS. They are aggressive neoplasms and those arising in the PNS are much worse prognostically. The maxillary sinus is more often involved than the other sinuses. These tumours are most commonly seen in the elderly. Amelanotic melanomas may present as unilateral nasal polyps. They have a tendency to spread via the blood and lymphatics. Although radical surgery is recommended, this is often not feasible. Radical radiotherapy may be offered in such cases for palliation. The role of chemotherapy is not well-established. Local recurrence is often the cause of treatment failure.

Adenocarcinoma

Constituting 5%–15% of nasal and paranasal malignant epithelial tumours, they arise mostly from the ethmoid sinuses and nasal cavity. They are associated with exposure to wood dust and leather processing and are, hence, seen more frequently in wood and leather workers. These neoplasms are classified into high- and low-grade on the basis of their histopathology and clinical behaviour, with the former having a tendency for distant metastasis and the latter for local recurrence.

Adenoid cystic carcinoma

These salivary carcinomas exhibit a marked tendency for perineural spread, which is their hallmark. Spread is likely to occur along the infra-orbital nerve and, further posteriorly along the maxillary nerve. Spread can also be submucosal. Adenoid cystic carcinomas often present with advanced disease. These tumours arise mostly from the lower parts of the nasal fossa. Low-grade adenoid cystic carcinoma has <30% solid architecture and demonstrates either a cribriform or tubular pattern. High-grade tumours have >30% solid architecture and behave more aggressively with a greater tendency for local recurrence and metastasis.

Sinonasal undifferentiated carcinoma

These tumours present at an advanced stage and involve multiple sinuses. They tend to progress rapidly with marked local invasion. They are composed of small and medium cells and are likely to be mistaken histologically for olfactory neuroblastoma, lymphoma and squamous cell carcinoma. Combined treatment is recommended, but surgery may not be feasible because of the advanced stage at presentation.

Squamous cell carcinoma

This is the most common type of malignant neoplasm of the nose and PNS, constituting ~75% of sinonasal neoplasms. The majority of squamous cell carcinomas are of the keratinizing type, which is usually moderately differentiated. Like other malignant neoplasms of the PNS and nose, affected patients present in an advanced stage.

Metastatic tumours

The sinuses are rarely a site for metastatic tumours. The maxillary sinus is the one most often affected. The common primary sites are the kidneys, breasts and lungs.

Clinical features

Malignant lesions of the PNS typically present with unilateral nasal obstruction and nasal discharge, which may be blood-stained or purulent. The mass may be visible on anterior rhinoscopy or may be discerned on nasal endoscopy. Granulomatous lesions of the PNS (Wegener granulomatosis, tuberculosis, rhinoscleroma, rhinosporiodosis) may present similarly and constitute the differential diagnosis.

Presentation, however, is often delayed and these tumours may only manifest clinically when they extend beyond the confines of the PNS. Anterior extension results in a cheek swelling or fullness and numbness of the upper teeth due to involvement of the anterior alveolar nerves. When much advanced, the patient may present with cheek ulceration. Orbital extension of the growth is not uncommon and leads initially to involvement of the infra-orbital nerve and, then, to proptosis and diplopia. The infra-orbital rim may be blunted and, on insinuating a finger into the orbit beneath the globe, a vague mass may be felt in the orbital floor. Obstruction of the nasolacrimal duct in the medial maxillary wall gives rise to epiphora. Downward extension from the antrum to involve and expand the alveolar process results in loosening of teeth, ill-fitting dentures, or discomfort and pain while using dentures. Other symptoms include palatal swelling and dental pain.

Advanced ethmoid involvement produces swelling of the medial canthal area, widening of the nasal bridge and hypertelorism. Anosmia can result from mechanical obstruction of the olfactory cleft. Erosion of the cribriform plate and fovea ethmoidalis with meningeal involvement causing headache can also develop in advanced disease, although this is not common. In advanced maxillary neoplasms with extension to the infra-temporal fossa and involvement of the pterygoid musculature, trismus is an important feature.

Metastasis to the neck is unusual and occurs in ~10% of cases. This is more common with neoplasms that invade the oral cavity and cheek.

As the early features of maxilloethmoid neoplasms are indistinguishable from those of chronic sinusitis, persistent features of chronic sinusitis not responding to appropriate treatment should trigger suspicion and merit radiological investigations, especially in the middle-aged and elderly patient.

Assessment

Clinical assessment

The symptoms and signs resulting from these neoplasms may offer clues to the extent of disease. Many of the clinical signs signifying specific extensions have been included in the 'anatomy' section of this chapter. Although it sounds clichéd, a thorough physical examination continues to be of paramount importance—even in this era of CT and MRI when radiology is the dominant modality for evaluating disease extent.

A complete ENT and endoscopic examination is essential, with stress being placed on adequate visualization of the nasal fossae and nasopharynx. Examination should include the following: evaluation of the oral cavity, especially the palate, maxillary teeth and upper alveolus; palpation of the superior gingivobuccal sulcus for any swelling; evaluation of the infra-orbital margin for expansion or blunting; palpation of the orbital floor for any palpable mass; and orbital examination for proptosis and assessment of ocular movements. Expansion of the medial canthus region indicates ethmoidal involvement and puckering of the skin overlying the maxillary sinus (or an inability to pinch it up) indicates skin involvement. Anaesthesia of the infra-orbital nerve or the teeth indicates involvement of the anatomically relevant neural canal. Secretory otitis media may indicate nasopharyngeal extension. Trismus indicates extension to the pterygoid muscles and is a sign of advanced disease. The neck needs to be palpated for metastatic neck nodes.

Radiological assessment

CT scan and MRI have completely replaced plain radiographs in the assessment of nasal and PNS neoplasms. CT and

MRI offer complementary information, and in the ideal and unlimited resource setting, both should be undertaken.

CT scan is done in both axial and coronal views. Bone window setting in CT scans is better in demonstrating bone erosion, which is a feature of malignant neoplasms. Coronal sections are better in demonstrating involvement of the fovea ethmoidalis and cribriform plate as well as extension from the PNS to the orbit. MRI is superior in assessing soft tissue extension. It is particularly useful in distinguishing sinus opacification resulting from pent-up secretions from that due to tumour extension into the sinus. T_2-weighted images show an increased signal intensity in inflammatory conditions as opposed to most cellular tumours which have intermediate signal intensity. MRI is also better in demonstrating perineural spread, dural invasion and intracranial extension, but is incapable of demonstrating bone invasion. MRI also has less artifact effect in the presence of dental fillings, unlike CT.

Most of the tumours show mild, uniform enhancement with contrast on both CT and MRI. Schwannomas appear hyperintense on T_2-weighted MRIs. Tumour calcification may be seen in neurogenic tumours on CT. Sectional imaging may also be undertaken for evaluation of neck metastasis. Lung metastases are unusual but, nevertheless, need to be excluded by an X-ray or CT of the chest. For mesenchymal tumours, which spread haematogenously, CT of the chest and abdomen is advisable. Positron emission tomography (PET)-CT is more sensitive for metastatic evaluation but is not entirely specific.

Histological evaluation

Tissue for biopsy is best obtained by nasal endoscopy. Sublabial biopsy by a Caldwell–Luc approach is best avoided as it may lead to seeding of the soft tissues of the cheek by the tumour tissue. Immunohistochemistry is useful in differentiating between undifferentiated carcinoma, rhabdomyosarcoma, olfactory neuroblastoma and lymphoma.

Other

Olfactory neuroblastomas may be associated with severe hyponatraemia secondary to the inappropriate secretion of antidiuretic hormone.[12]

Classification

Classification by site

In 1906, Sebileau classified maxilloethmoid neoplasms into those involving the suprastructure, mesostructure and infrastructure. This was done by dividing the maxilloethmoid complex into three by means of two imaginary horizontal lines, one drawn across the orbital floor (infra-orbital rim) and another across the floor of the nose. In the adult, the floor of the fully pneumatized maxillary sinus is below the floor of the nose and this constituted the infrastructure.

In 1969, Lederman added a pair of vertical lines to the original lines of Sebileau.[13] These passed along the medial orbital wall on both sides and separated the ethmoidal and nasal tumours from the maxillary tumours.

In 1933, Ohngren divided the facial skeleton into posterosuperior and anteroinferior parts by means of a line (or a plane) extending from the angle of the mandible to the medial canthus. This line (plane) is called the 'Ohngren line' or the 'plane of malignancy'. Tumours below the Ohngren line are believed to have a better prognosis than those above it—largely because of the propensity for orbital and infra-temporal fossa invasion of the latter.

Carcinoma of the nasal cavity

This is an uncommon disease, which is most frequently seen in middle-aged and elderly men. The vast majority of these cancers are squamous cell carcinomas, which arise from the lateral nasal wall from where they spread in various directions to the PNS, orbit, palate and cranial cavity. They also arise from the anterior septum, nasal vestibule and nasal floor. Compared with tumours arising from the sinuses, they may present early with nasal obstruction, and hence have a relatively better prognosis. About a tenth of these patients have nodal metastasis at presentation.

Tumours arising from the nasal vestibule are related to skin cancers and behave aggressively, infiltrating nearby cartilage, the upper alveolus and upper lip, making resection and reconstruction more difficult. This situation may lead to radiotherapy being used as the primary modality with surgery being reserved for salvage. Nodal metastasis is common.

Surgery entails a total or partial rhinectomy. Adequate local control is crucial for cure as local recurrence is the most common cause for treatment failure. Partial nasal defects may be repaired using local flaps, such as the forehead or nasolabial flaps. The cosmetic defect due to total rhinectomy is best managed using a prosthodontist-designed artificial nose.

Carcinoma of the PNS

Maxillary sinus

The maxilla is the most common site and accounts for >80% of sinus neoplasms. Squamous cell carcinoma is the most common variety. A male preponderance is evidenced by two-thirds of the patients being men. It affects mostly middle-aged people.

Ethmoid sinuses

Ethmoidal cancers demonstrate a definite aetiological

relationship to exposure to wood dust. There is considerable proportion of adenocarcinomas among ethmoid neoplasms, although squamous cell carcinoma remains the most common histology. They cause nasal obstruction early and so have a greater chance for early detection. Nodal involvement is rare.

Frontal and sphenoid sinuses

Primary neoplasms of these sinuses are exceedingly rare. Their involvement is often secondary to ethmoid neoplasms. Neoplasms in these sinuses constitute <1% each of sinus neoplasms. Sphenoid sinus neoplasms may present with a chronic headache and multiple cranial nerve palsies. Because of their anatomical location, surgical resection of sphenoid sinus neoplasms is technically complex.

Tumour Node Metastasis (TNM) classification

The current American Joint Committee on Cancer (AJCC 7th ed., 2010) classification is applicable to epithelial tumours and not to tumours of lymphoid tissue, soft tissue, bone and cartilage. T4 tumours have been sub-divided into stages T4a and T4b to provide guidelines for unresectability (T4b). Tumours extending to the orbital apex, dura of the anterior cranial fossa, brain, or to the middle cranial fossa, nasopharynx and clivus are considered unresectable.

TNM staging (AJCC 7th ed, 2010)[14]

Primary Tumour (T)
TX Primary tumour cannot be assessed
T0 No evidence of primary tumour
Tis Carcinoma *in situ*

Maxillary Sinus
T1 Tumour limited to maxillary sinus mucosa with no erosion or destruction of bone
T2 Tumour causing bone erosion or destruction including extension into the hard palate and/or middle nasal meatus, except extension to posterior wall of maxillary sinus and pterygoid plates
T3 Tumour invades any of the following: Bone of the posterior wall of maxillary sinus, subcutaneous tissues, floor or medial wall of orbit, pterygoid fossa, ethmoid sinuses
T4a Moderately advanced local disease
Tumour invades anterior orbital contents, skin of cheek, pterygoid plates, infratemporal fossa, cribriform plate, sphenoid or frontal sinuses
T4b Very advanced local disease
Tumour invades any of the following: Orbital apex, dura, brain, middle cranial fossa, cranial nerves other than

maxillary division of trigeminal nerve (V2), nasopharynx, or clivus

Regional Lymph Nodes (N)
NX Regional lymph nodes cannot be assessed
N0 No regional lymph node metastasis
N1 Metastasis in a single ipsilateral lymph node, 3 cm or less in greatest dimension
N2 Metastasis in a single ipsilateral lymph node, more than 3 cm but not more than 6 cm in greatest dimension, or in multiple ipsilateral lymph nodes, none more than 6 cm in greatest dimension, or in bilateral or contralateral lymph nodes, none more than 6 cm in greatest dimension
N2a Metastasis in single ipsilateral lymph node, more than 3 cm but not more than 6 cm in greatest dimension
N2b Metastasis in multiple ipsilateral lymph nodes, none more than 6 cm in greatest dimension
N2c Metastasis in bilateral or contralateral lymph nodes, none more than 6 cm in greatest dimension
N3 Metastasis in lymph node, more than 6 cm in greatest dimension

Distant metastasis (M)
M0 No distant metastasis
M1 Distant metastasis

TREATMENT

Treatment rationale

Treatment decisions regarding the use of surgery or radiation or chemotherapy are based on the tumour histology and the stage of disease. Surgery is usually the initial treatment of choice for tumours of the nasal cavity (both epithelial and non-epithelial) but not for lymphomas, for which radiation therapy and chemotherapy are the initial treatments of choice.

Early presentation is rare, except in the palate or the nasal cavity, and these patients receive single modality treatment by surgery or, occasionally, by radiation. Most sinus malignancies, however, are advanced at presentation (T3/T4) and for these a combined therapy with surgical excision and radiation is the standard treatment. Adequate resection is crucial as local recurrence remains the main cause of treatment failure. Radiation therapy has limited efficacy in situations with bone involvement and so is usually preferred in the post-surgical setting. Further, non-epidermoid cancers (adenocarcinoma and adenoid cystic carcinoma) are not very radiosensitive and, therefore, primary surgery with postoperative radiation is preferred. The added advantage of postoperative radiotherapy is that it is possible to give a higher radiation dose as there are no concerns regarding wound healing being adversely affected.

A situation in which preoperative radiation may be used is for shrinking an unresectable tumour in a medically fit patient in order to render it resectable. However, today induction chemotherapy can achieve the same objective. The practice of limiting the surgical resection following chemotherapy or radiotherapy shrinkage is against general oncological surgical principles.

T4b disease (orbital apex, dura, brain, middle cranial fossa, nasopharynx, clivus extension) indicates unresectability. Base of skull erosion is not a contraindication for surgery and can be tackled by craniofacial resection. Isolated Level II cervical nodes lead to a suspicion of disease extension via the retropharyngeal nodes and are indicative of advanced disease with a limited potential for cure.

Radiation therapy as a sole modality of treatment is used in patients who are poor surgical candidates, for lymphomas, unresectable neoplasms, and when patients are unwilling to undergo surgery. The role of combined chemotherapy and radiotherapy is in patients with positive margins after resection and extracapsular spread in nodal metastasis, as well as in those who do not undergo surgery for various reasons.[15] Chemotherapy can also be used for palliation of unresectable, advanced disease.

Surgical treatment

The main surgical procedures employed in the treatment of malignant neoplasms of the nose and PNS are partial and total maxillectomy, maxillectomy with orbital exenteration and craniofacial resection. Modern imaging allows oncological resections to be tailored to the disease extent in order to minimize needless morbidity resulting from resection of the palate, orbital floor or orbit. With careful case selection this may offer adequacy of resection equivalent to a total maxillectomy.[16]

Figures 1 (a–d) show the soft tissue incisions/approaches to maxillo-ethmoid tumours. The approach to the bony midface is undertaken sub-labially (midfacial degloving) or by a lateral rhinotomy (with or without a lip split), or by a Weber–Fergusson incision (Figs 1a to 1c). A craniofacial resection requires a bicoronal flap (Fig. 1d) or may be undertaken by a 'butterfly incision' extending along and between the eyebrows.

Lateral rhinotomy with medial maxillectomy (Figs 1b and 2a)

The lateral rhinotomy incision, known as the Moure incision (after Moure 1902), was initially described by Michaux in 1848. This is the incision that is most commonly used to carry out a medial maxillectomy, an operation used to resect the

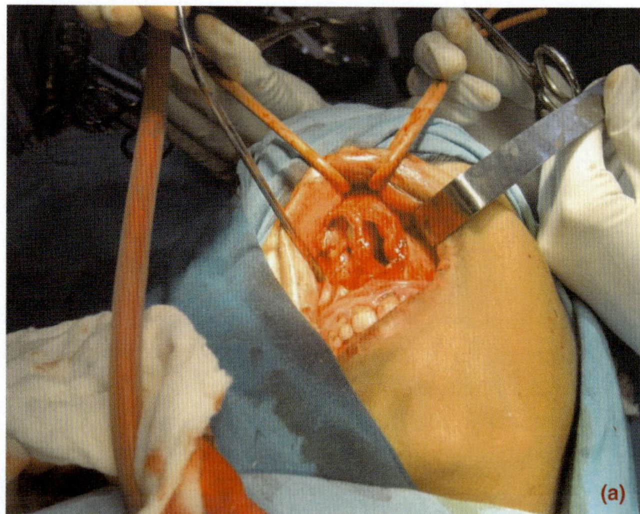

Fig. 1a. Midfacial degloving approach

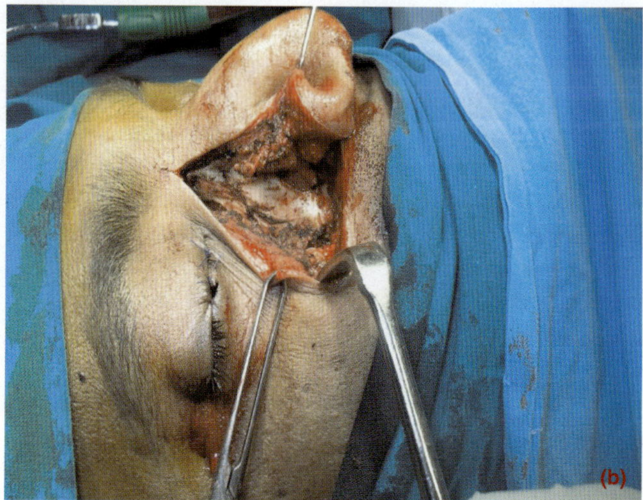

Fig. 1b. Lateral rhinotomy (Moure) incision

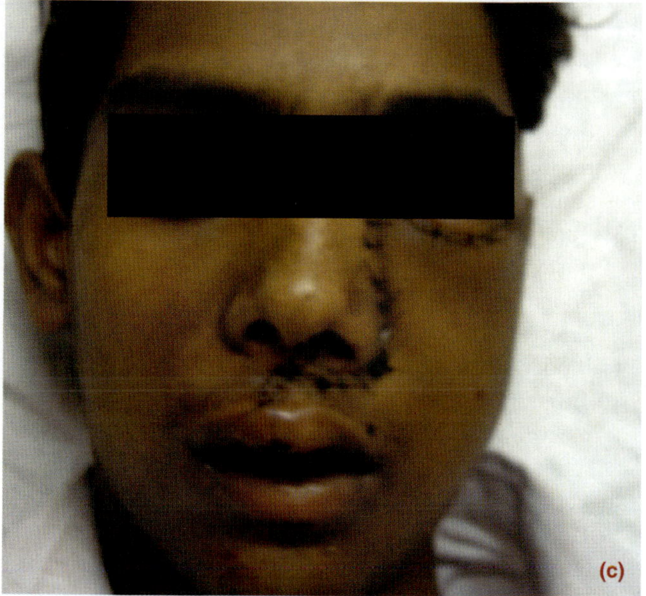

Fig. 1c. Weber–Fergusson incision

medial wall of the maxilla and the ethmoid labyrinth *en bloc*. This operation was initially performed in 1968 by Doyle but the term 'medial maxillectomy' was coined by Sessions and Larson in 1977.[17,18]

The incision starts just inferior to the medial end of the eyebrow and extends inferiorly midway between the nasal dorsum and the medial canthus to the nasofacial groove. It then curves around the nasal ala to the midline or onto the anterior nasal floor across the nasal sill. The incision may be extended superiorly from its upper end to the forehead in the midline in situations necessitating a craniofacial resection. The medial part of the maxilla and the orbit, as well as the nasal fossa, can be exposed widely by elevating the cheek flap laterally, sub-periosteally. The soft tissues over the nasal bony pyramid are elevated medially to expose the nasal bone partly and the frontal process of the maxilla. The soft tissues at the piriform rim are divided to open into the nasal fossa. The medial canthal ligament is detached. The nasolacrimal duct is divided at the lower end of the lacrimal fossa and periosteal elevation is continued over the lamina papyracea posteriorly to expose the fronto-ethmoid suture and the anterior and posterior ethmoid arteries. They are located at the level of the fronto-ethmoid suture approximately 24 mm and 12 mm posterior to the anterior lacrimal crest. The anterior ethmoid artery is cauterized and divided and the posterior one, which is 6 mm away from the optic nerve, is preserved as a landmark. This frees the orbital contents, which can then be retracted laterally taking care to preserve the integrity of the periorbita. Minimal periosteal elevation is done over the medial part of the floor of the orbit to expose it as well.

A bony cut is then made along the inferior part of the lateral nasal wall, across the piriform rim, and carried posteriorly up to the posterior antral wall and just beyond it. Another cut is made vertically across the anterior wall of the maxillary sinus, medial to the level of the infra-orbital foramen, to the medial part of the inferior orbital rim and then posteriorly across the orbital floor to its posterior part. Another osteotomy is made along the superior part of the piriform aperture to the anterior end of the fronto-ethmoid suture, an important landmark that indicates the level of the cribriform plate and the superior extent of the resection. This osteotomy is then carried posteriorly to the level of the posterior ethmoid artery and then curved inferiorly to meet the posterior end of the cut made along the orbital floor. A pair of large curved scissors is introduced through the inferior osteotomy in the lateral wall of the nose and its blades directed superiorly, anterior to the sphenoid face, to divide the posterior attachments of the specimen to deliver it. Haemostasis is secured by diathermy and ligation.

It is important to tackle the nasolacrimal duct suitably in order to prevent post-operative epiphora. This can be done by dividing the lacrimal sac at its junction with the duct at the inferior end of the lacrimal fossa and then everting its cut end with fine 5-0 sutures.

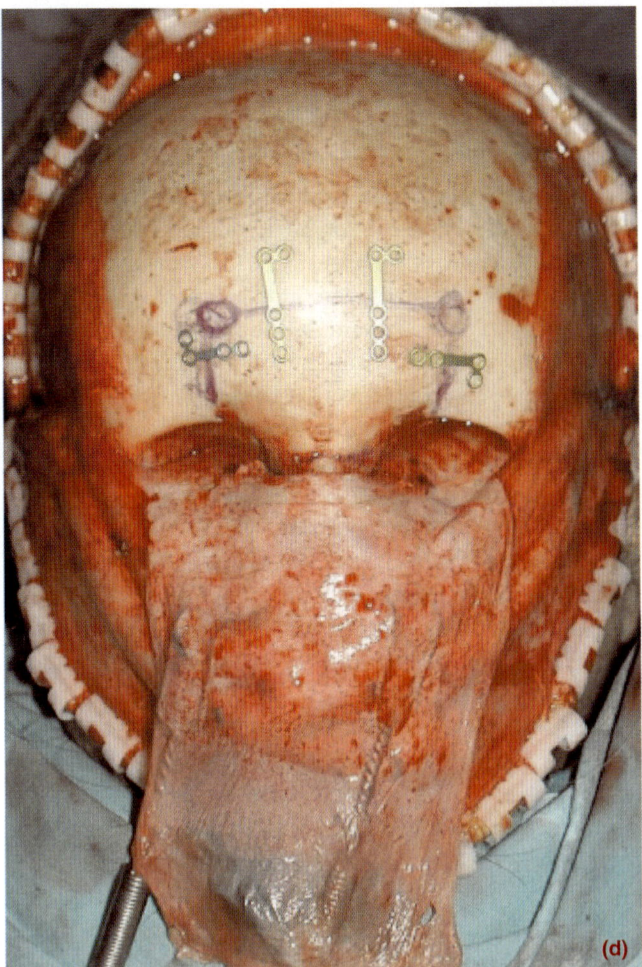

Fig. 1d. Bifrontal craniotomy incision. The pericranial flap has been raised and shall be used for subsequent reconstruction of the dura or for wrapping around the bone flap. The bone flap has been marked. Plates are applied prior to cutting the bone flap so as to allow accurate anatomical positioning of the bone plates and screws. The plates are then removed and the bone flap taken, and then reapplied at the end of the procedure.

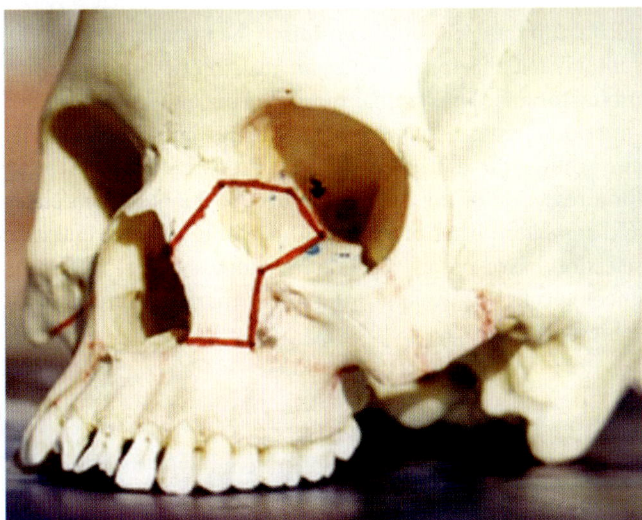

Fig. 2a. Medial maxillectomy

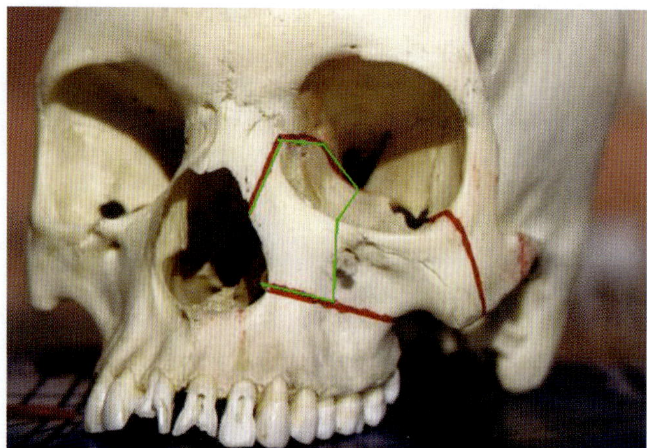

Fig. 2b. Suprastructure maxillectomy

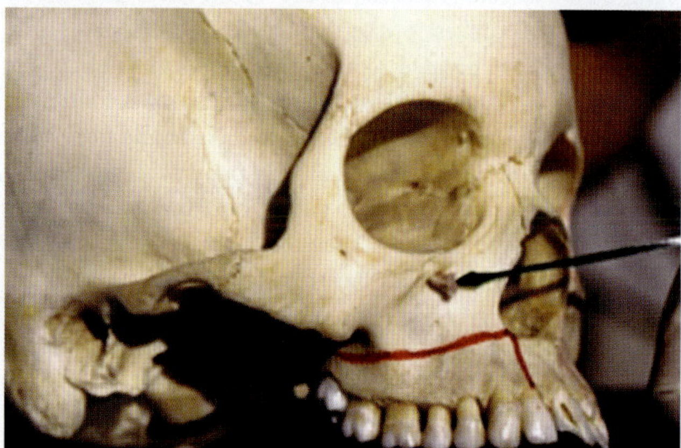

Fig. 2c. Infrastructure maxillectomy

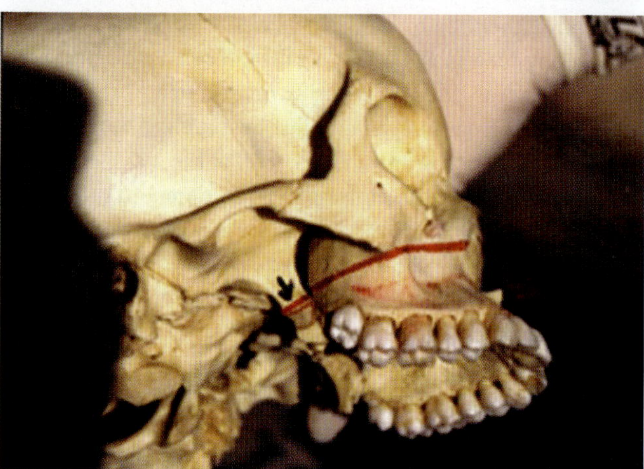

Fig. 2d. Subtotal maxillectomy

Although a bony window can be cut out in the anterior maxillary wall to facilitate exposure of the antral cavity and make posterior cuts under better vision, often this may not be practicable as the antrum contains a neoplasm that obscures view. Following the initial resection, the residual ethmoid cells are cleared of mucosa and the sphenoid opened to examine and clear it of any disease. The medial canthal ligament is sutured to the septal perichondrium or nasal bone periosteum to reduce chances of telecanthus postoperatively. The cavity is packed and the incision closed in layers.

Midfacial degloving approach

This is another means of exposing the midfacial skeleton for a medial maxillectomy. This approach avoids a facial scar but can produce nasal vestibular stenosis. The midfacial degloving approach was first described in the French literature by Georges Portmann and Henri Retrouvey in 1927.

A complete transfixation incision is made across the membranous septum in the columella and joined laterally to an intercartilaginous incision on either side. A circumvestibular incision is made laterally and across the floor of the nose to join the inferior end of the transfixation incision with the lateral ends of the intercartilaginous incisions. This is deepened in the nasal floor to join another superior gingivobuccal sulcus incision made from one maxillary tuberosity to the other. As in a rhinoplasty, scissors are then introduced through the intercartilaginous incision to release the skin and soft tissues from the nasal skeleton and from the maxillae in a subperiosteal plane, thus exposing the midface skeleton (Fig. 1a). With adequate retraction, the frontoethmoid sutures on either side can be exposed. Lateral and superior exposure may be enhanced by sectioning the infra-orbital nerve, but if this is preserved, then exposure in this area is limited.

The approach offers good exposure for work below the level of the infra-orbital foramen. The exposure is better posteriorly than anteriorly. Exposure, however, is inadequate for oncological resections, which involve the anterior ethmoid or the skull base.

Partial maxillectomy

Many variations of the partial maxillectomy exist and are designed to minimize morbidity to the palate or orbit (Figs 2a–2c). The infrastructure maxillectomy (Fig. 2c) is for palatal tumours with no extension to the maxillary sinus. The subtotal maxillectomy (bone cut just inferior to the infra-orbital foramen) has similar morbidity but allows for a greater superior margin of resection; the higher cut in the maxilla also allows for a better posterior exposure, thus allowing for a resection of the inferior portion of the pterygoid plates and a greater posterior margin, if need be. With careful case selection based on appropriate radiology, surgical resections oncologically equivalent to a total maxillectomy can be achieved.[16]

Total maxillectomy

This is the operation most often employed for cases of maxillary sinus cancer. It may have to be combined with an orbital exenteration when the orbit is involved.

The Weber–Fergusson incision is used for a total maxillectomy. It starts as a midline lip-splitting incision turning laterally below the nasal sill and curving round the ala nasi and extending superiorly along the nasofacial crease to the medial canthus, thereafter turning laterally—3–4 mm inferior to the lower lid margin—to end just beyond the lateral canthus. This lateral limb is ideally placed 5–8 mm below the eyelashes. If too close to the lid margin, it may lead to ectropion; if too distal, it may produce lymphoedema of the lower eyelid.

From the lower end of the lip-splitting incision, an extension is made along the superior gingivobuccal sulcus laterally to just beyond the maxillary tuberosity. Another incision is made from the anterior end of the gingivobuccal sulcus incision posteriorly across the alveolus and onto the palate ipsilaterally, just off the midline to the junction of the hard and soft palates. This is then taken laterally along the junction of the hard and soft palates, posterior to the maxillary tuberosity, to meet the posterior end of the superior gingivobuccal sulcus incision.

The facial flap can be elevated just superficial to the bone if the anterior maxillary wall has not been breached by the tumour. If the patient has, however, had a previous sublabial biopsy, it is then presumed that the subcutaneous tissues have been breached and these tissues along with the sublabial incision line should then be included in the specimen. The flap thickness can be adjusted, depending on the extension of the growth anteriorly.

Prior to removal of the maxilla, access can be gained to the infra-temporal fossa by separating the anterior edge of the masseter muscle from the zygoma so as to expose the coronoid process, and then by chipping away the coronoid process (Figs 3a–d). This exposes the maxillary artery, which can be ligated at this point, thus minimizing surgical bleeding and also allowing exposure of the pterygoid plates to permit a good infra-temporal fossa clearance, if required.

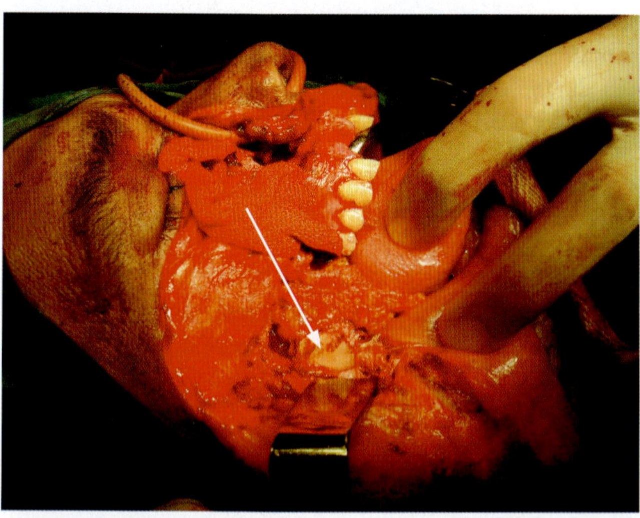

Fig. 3a. Separation of the anterior massetter muscle from the zygoma to expose the coronoid process

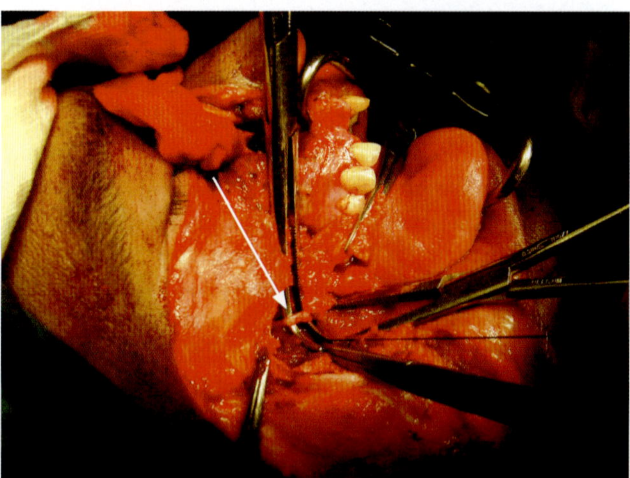

Fig. 3b. Excision of the coronoid process to expose the anterior infra-temporal fossa and the maxillary artery

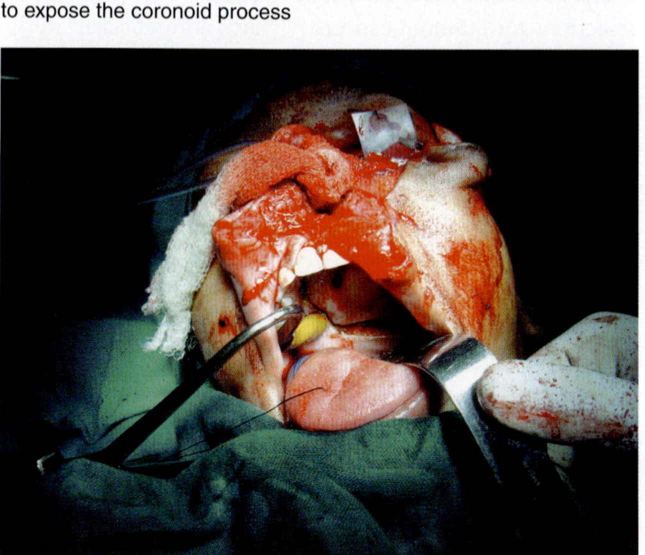

Fig. 3c. Palatal cuts

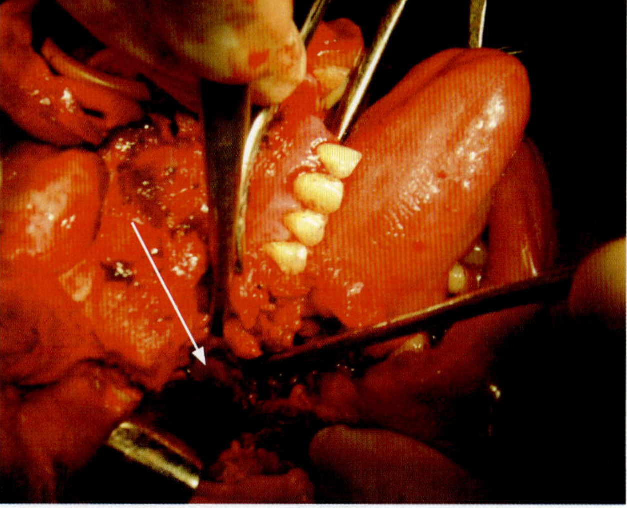

Fig. 3d. The pterygoid plates in the anterior infratemporal fossa prior to resection

The orbital periosteum is elevated off the floor and medial wall. Osteotomies to separate the maxilla are then made in the following manner: (i) along the hard palate in a paramedian line along the incision already described. This incision and osteotomy are usually made simultaneously by using a Gigli saw introduced through the ipsilateral nasal fossa and a perforation at the junction of the hard and soft palates; (ii) along the junction of the nasal bone and frontal process of the maxilla from the piriform rim to the level of the frontoethmoid suture; (iii) along the medial orbital wall, just inferior to the frontoethmoid suture; (iv) from the anterior end of the inferior orbital fissure across the body of the malar (zygomatic) bone. This may be modified to go across the frontal process of the zygomatic bone in the lateral orbital margin, and then another across the anterior part of the zygomatic arch, if the zygomatic bone is invaded by neoplasm; (v) a bony cut is made across the posterior part of the medial orbital wall and the orbital floor to connect the medial osteotomy to the inferior orbital fissure. The maxilla is then detached from the skull by introducing a heavy, curved chisel posteriorly between the maxilla and the pterygoid plates.

Haemostasis is secured. A split thickness skin graft is applied to the cavity and tacked in place with sutures. The lacrimal sac is managed in the same way as after a medial maxillectomy. The orbit may be supported by a temporalis muscle sling which may be swung across the orbital floor like a hammock to the septum after detaching it from the coronoid process, but this often falls short of the septum when attempted. A pre-fabricated palatal obturator, fabricated preoperatively from an impression of the patient's palate, is clipped into place, greatly aided by the presence of maxillary dentition contralaterally. The cavity is packed with an antibiotic-soaked or bismuth subnitrate iodoform paraffin paste (BIPP) tape gauze and the wound is repaired in layers.

In most patients, oral feeds can be resumed by day 2 post-surgery. The pack is removed after about 10 days in the case of a BIPP pack or earlier in the case of antibiotic packs. Impression is taken for an intermediate palatal prosthesis and later, when the cavity is fully healed, a final prosthesis is made. This should be large enough to provide a satisfactory facial contour.

A common complication encountered after total maxillectomy is the breakdown of the incision at the medial canthus, resulting in a fistula between the skin and the maxillectomy cavity. This is best prevented by avoiding a sharp angle as well as thinning of the flap at this vulnerable point. A fistula, if it occurs, may be repaired by a local advancement flap, a rotation flap from the medial canthus, or a midline forehead flap.

Management of the orbit

Obvious clinical involvement with visual loss and ophthalmoplegia or a painful eye may lead to the clinical decision for orbital exenteration. Attempts to avoid orbital exenteration and treat disease extending to the eye by radiation therapy is often inadvisable as radiation is not as efficacious, and further leads to a shrunken and blind eye, which is often complicated by cataract and keratitis and is chronically painful.

Proptosis alone is, today, not necessarily an indication for orbital exenteration as it may be caused by a pushing of the periorbita by the tumour and not by tumour invasion of the orbital contents. Orbital exenteration is undertaken in situations in which the orbital contents (fat/muscle) are invaded. Infiltration of the periorbita too may not necessarily be an indication for orbital exenteration, as there is another inner fascial layer deep to the periorbita, which separates it from the orbital contents; the contents could be spared in such situations.[19]

Preoperative radiology may not always be definitive when deciding on orbital exenteration, which may have to be based on surgical findings. Frozen sections are of limited value because although the fascial layers can be evaluated, it can be difficult to freeze the fat for evaluation. It is important in this situation to discuss these issues with the patients prior to surgery to obtain their views, and if required, their informed consent for orbital exenteration.

Craniofacial resection

Although the concept of craniofacial resection (CFR) for PNS tumours was first described by Smith in 1954,[20] it was Ketcham *et al.* in 1973[21] and Terz *et al.* in 1980[22] who advocated the efficacy of the procedure in dramatically enhancing the cure rate of ethmoid cancers that abut the roof of the ethmoid bone. In 1977, Clifford[23] proposed the single-team approach for craniofacial resection and later Cheesman *et al.* (in 1986) published their experience with anterior craniofacial resections for ethmoid cancers.[24] Shah[25] and Janecka[26] in the 1990s further added data to support the efficacy of CFR for malignant sinonasal neoplasms.

Anterior craniofacial resection involves monobloc resection of the sinonasal malignancy invading the ethmoid roof by means of an osteotomy. This procedure encompasses the roofs of both the ethmoids and the cribriform plate and passes through the frontal sinus anteriorly and sphenoid posteriorly. The structures that are removed in a classical CFR include the entire cribriform plate and the crista galli, foramen caecum and the posterior wall of the frontal sinus, and roof of the ethmoid labyrinth and the jugum of the sphenoid (Fig. 4a), the commonly amenable tumours being esthesioneuroblastomas, sarcomas, carcinomas and salivary gland tumours. The procedure has the potential of doubling the cure rate for these tumours, which abut the anterior skull base.[24–26]

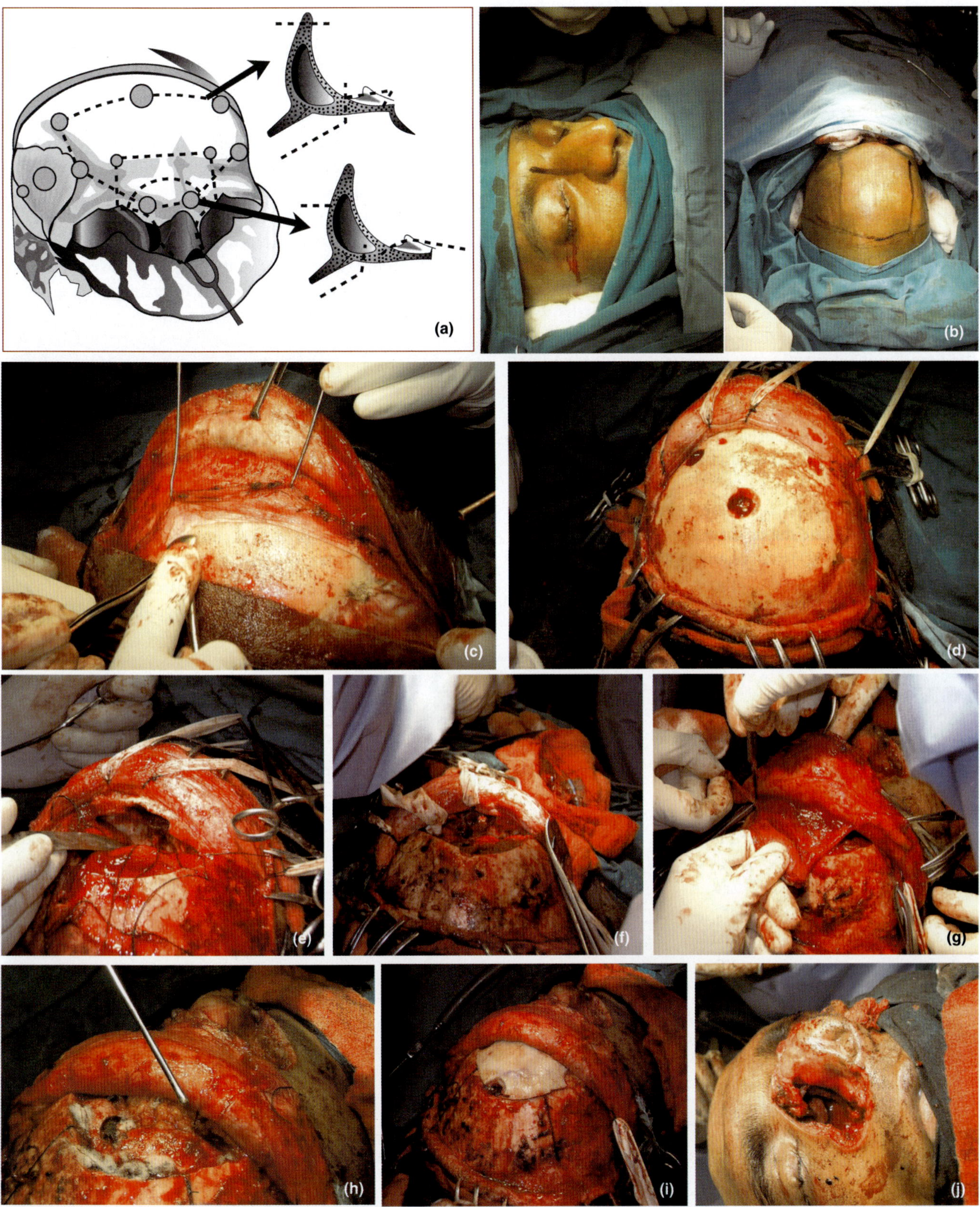

Fig. 4. Single stage craniofacial resection **(a)** Superior bone cuts for a craniofacial resection undertaken by a bifrontal craniotomy or a sub-cranial approach, **(b)** Incisions—lateral rhinotomy (Moure incision) for facial exposure and a bicoronal incision for subcranial and intracranial exposure. The galeo-pericranial flap is also marked, **(c)** Galeopericranial flap being harvested, **(d)** Burr holes for bifrontal craniotomy, **(e)** Exposure of anterior skull base, **(f)** Post-surgical defect, **(g)** Galeopericranial flap of suitable size being fashioned to reconstruct the cranial base defect by the carpeting and quilting technique, **(h)** Abdominal fat to reinforce the dural closure and to obliterate the dead space in the region of the frontal sinus, **(i)** Repositioning of bone flap of bifrontal craniotomy, **(j)** Galeo-pericranial flap as seen through the facial end, ready for split skin grafting.

Contraindications

The general oncological principle regarding tumour resection in the deeper tissues has been to remove an additional layer to the one that is obviously involved. The CFR is, therefore, best applied to tumours restricted to the mucosa of the skull base at the ethmo-fronto-sphenoid. Bone erosion at the fovea or cribriform plate or the posterior wall of the frontal sinus can be oncologically resected by including the frontal lobe dural layers, but this cannot be easily undertaken at the level of the roof of the sphenoid or its lateral wall. Absolute contraindications include extension beyond the dura to involve the optic chiasm or cavernous sinus or the temporal lobe, although early cavernous sinus invasion on the side of the non-dominant carotid may be sometimes resected in an otherwise favourable lesion. Patients who may be medically unfit or of advanced age are unsuitable candidates, and tumours with aggressive behaviour or those tumours with early recurrence after chemo-radiotherapy are contraindicated for resection.

The standard approaches described for the cranial component of CFR are the classical bicoronal incision with a bifrontal craniotomy (Fig. 4), or any of its modifications, and the subcranial approach. These approaches can be combined with orbital resection if required. Selection of an approach depends on the tumour type, extent of lesion, its vascularization, chemo/radiosensitivity, and the reconstructive options available at hand. Shrinkage of the brain during the procedure is achieved by deliberate hyperventilation to produce an end-tidal pCO_2 of 20–25 mm, a head-up tilt of 15–20°, hypotension of 70–90 mmHg systolic pressure, intravenous mannitol and controlled lumbar drainage of cerebrospinal fluid (CSF).

The facial component of the CFR can be undertaken by a classical medial maxillectomy incision (lateral rhinotomy or the Moure incision) or any of the above-mentioned modifications, as are appropriate for the extent and the nature of the tumour.

Reconstruction

After a CFR, the cranial base defects require precise and durable reconstruction to (i) form a watertight dural seal, (ii) provide a barrier between the contaminated sinonasal space and the sterile subdural compartment, (iii) prevent airflow into the intracranial space, (iv) maintain a functional sinonasal system, and (v) provide a good cosmetic outcome.[27–30]

The most challenging part of a CFR is the reconstruction of the cranial base (Fig. 5), which in most cases can be achieved with a pediculed vascularized galeo-pericranial flap (GP)[30] or a

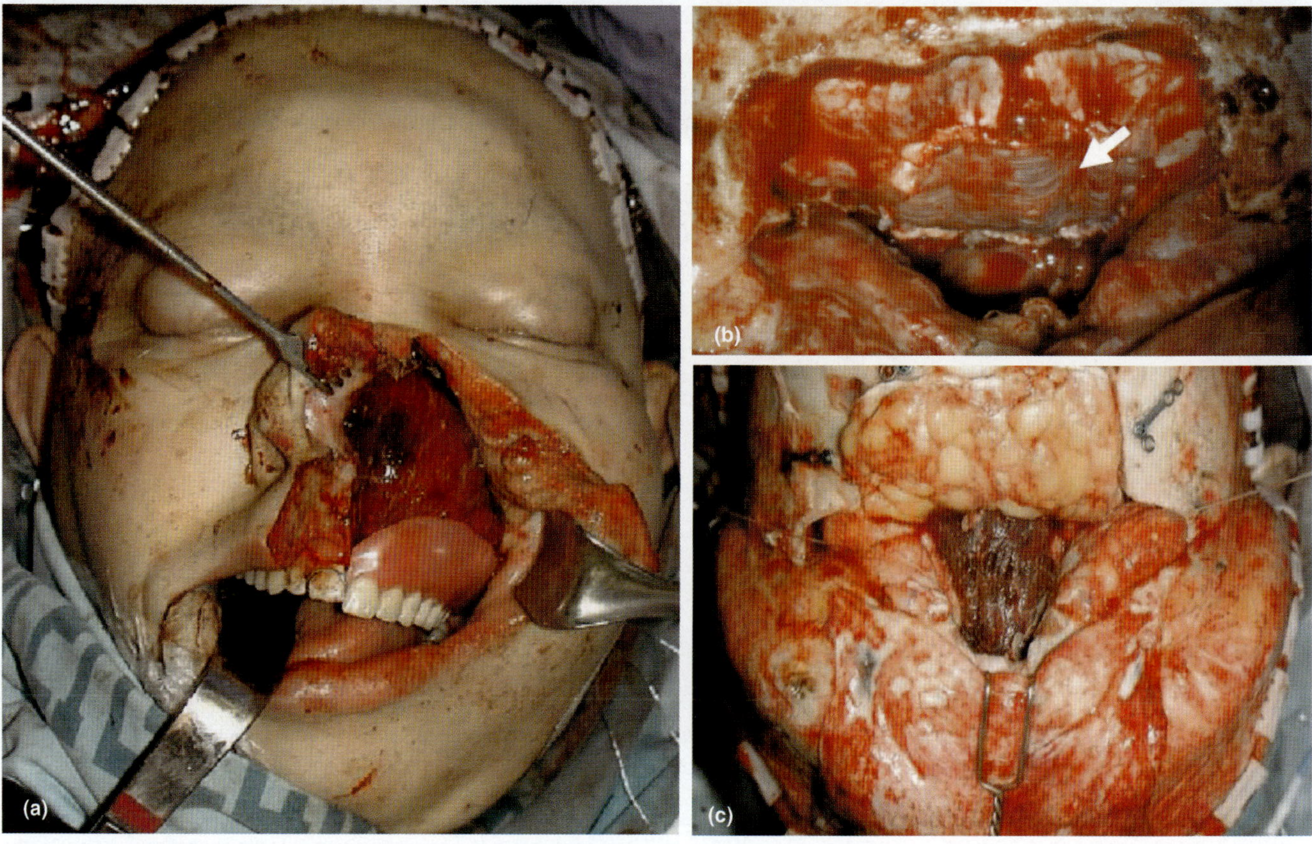

Fig. 5. Reconstruction **(a)** Placement of prefabricated palatal obturator at completion of procedure, **(b)** Small dural defect patched with temporalis fascia, **(c)** Rectus abdominis myocutaneous free flap reconstruction of a large central defect of the skull base. In this picture, the skull base proper has been reconstructed with a generous piece of fascia lata and fat.

Table 2. Reconstruction options following anterior skull base tumour resection proposed by Gil *et al.*[31]

Type of defect	Reconstructive option
Minimal dural tear	Primary closure
Small dural defect	Temporalis fascia
Moderate to large dural defect	Fascia lata
Bony defect: Orbital wall, nasal, and frontal bones	Posterior frontal sinus wall graft, split calvarial bone graft, titanium mesh
Posterior sinus wall, intact	Frontal sinus obliteration with abdominal fat
Posterior sinus wall, involved	Frontal sinus cranialization
Orbital exenteration	Temporalis muscle flap
Orbitomaxillary resection	Rectus abdominus free flap and obturator
Orbital wall resection	Titanium mesh, Fascia lata sling, septal cartilage
Orbital wall resection or medial maxillectomy	Dacryocysto rhinostomy
Perioperative radiotherapy	Pericranial wrapping of all osteotomized bony segments or titanium mesh

Adapted from *Skull Base* 2007;**17**:25–37.

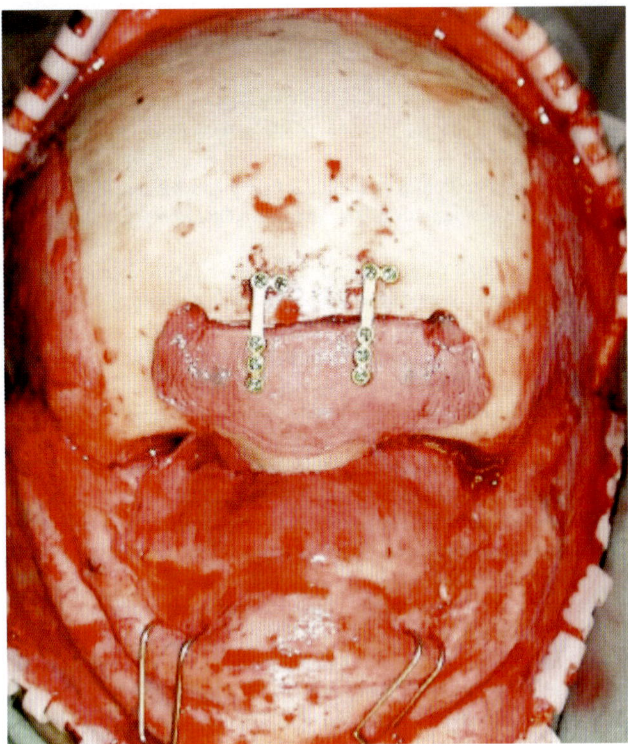

Fig. 5(d). Pericranial wrapping technique

double layered fascia lata graft. Small dural defects need to be patched by temporalis fascia and the larger ones by fascia lata. The GP flap is superior to a pericranial flap as it is better vasularized and will suffice if the dura is not disrupted and can be closed primarily. The flap can be insinuated through the bifrontal craniotomy bone defect and used to carpet the base of the defect in the anterior cranial fossa. It may be quilted to the cranial base. Abdominal fat may be sandwiched between the carpeted floor of cranium and the repaired/preserved dura. The raw nasal surface of the GP flap may be skin grafted if needed, or 'spot welded' with tissue glue. Bone *per se* need not be replaced in the anterior cranial base defect. The nasal cavity is packed for 10 days after which it is inspected for healing.

The reconstructive options[31–35] available for small calvarial and naso-fronto-orbital bone defects are hydroxyapatite paste or 3D titanium mesh, posterior wall of the frontal sinus, or a split calvarial bone graft. For larger defects a biometrical implant may be used. However, all of these options carry the disadvantage of not being able to withstand postoperative radiotherapy. The pedicled pericranial wrapping technique (Fig. 5d) enhances the vascular supply of the free bone and makes it suitable to receive postoperative radiotherapy without the risk of osteoradionecrosis.[32] If the pericranial flap is used for this purpose, a double layered fascia lata graft may be then used instead of a GP flap for reconstructing the skull base. Defects of the orbit that accompany a CFR will require a pedicled temporalis muscle flap reconstruction and those of the orbitomaxillary complex will require a rectus abdominis or an anterolateral thigh flap. An algorithm for skull base reconstruction proposed by Gil *et al.*[31] is shown in Table 2.

Common complications of CFR are CSF leak, meningitis, brain herniation and tension pneumocephalus, all of which result from inadequacies in reconstruction. Other complications include acute brain syndrome due to excessive intra-operative brain retraction, telecanthus, epiphora, wound infection, deep vein thrombosis, ptosis, mucocele, facial nerve paralysis, blindness and serous otitis media.

Neck dissection

Neck dissection is undertaken in cases with nodal metastasis. However, there is no role for elective neck dissection in the clinically N0 neck, as the chance for occult nodal metastasis is insignificant.

References

1. Acheson ED, Cowdell RH, Hadfield E, *et al.* Nasal cancer in woodworkers in the furniture industry. *Br Med J* 1968;**2**:587.
2. Engzell H, Englund A, Westerholm P. Nasal cancer associated with occupational exposure to organic dust. *Acta Otolaryngol* 1978;**86**:437.
3. Barton RT. Nickel carcinogenesis of the respiratory tract. *J Otolaryngol* 1977;**6**:412.
4. Bryan RL, Bovan IS, Crocker J, *et al.* Detection of HPV 6 and 11 in tumours of the upper respiratory tract using the polymerase chain reaction. *Clin Otolaryngol* 1990;**15**:177–80.

5. Respler DS, Jahn A, Pater A, *et al.* Isolation and characterisation of papilloma virus DNA from nasal inverting (Schneiderian) papillomas. *Ann Otol Rhinol Laryngol* 1987;**96**:170–3.

6. Weber RS, Shillitoe EJ, Robbins KT. Prevalence of human papilloma virus in inverted nasal papillomas. *Arch Otolaryngol Head Neck Surg* 1988;**114**:23–6.

7. Hyams VJ. Papillomas of the nasal cavity and paranasal sinuses: A clinicopathologic study of 315 cases. *Ann Otol Rhinol Laryngol* 1971; **80**:192.

8. Stankiewicz JA, Girgis SJ. Endoscopic surgical treatment of nasal and paranasal sinus inverting papilloma. *Otolaryngol Head Neck Surg* 1993;**109**:988–95.

9. Lund VJ. Optimum management of inverted papilloma. *J Laryngol Otol* 2000;**114**:194–7.

10. Kadish S, Goodman M, Wang CC. Olfactory neuroblastoma. A clinical analysis of 17 cases. *Cancer* 1976;**37**:1571–6.

11. Dulguerov P, Calcaterra T. Esthesioneuroblastoma: The UCLA experience 1970–1990. *Laryngoscope* 1992;**102**:843–9.

12. Srigley JR, Dayal JR, Gregor RT, *et al.* Hyponatremia secondary to olfactory neuroblastoma. *Arch Otolaryngol Head Neck Surg* 1983;**109**: 559–62.

13. Lederman M. Cancer of the upper jaw and nasal chambers. *Proc R Soc Med* 1969;**62**:65.

14. Edge SB, Byrd DR, Compton CC (eds). *AJCC Cancer Staging Manual.* 7th ed. New York, NY: Springer; 2010:71–72.

15. Bernier J, Cooper JS, Pajak TF, *et al.* Defining risk levels in locally advanced head and neck cancers: A comparative analysis of concurrent post-operative radiation plus chemotherapy trials of the EORCT (#22931) and RTOG (# 9501). *Head Neck* 2005;**27**:843–50.

16. Roy BC, Bahadur S, Thakar A. Partial maxillectomy for management of neoplasms of paranasal sinuses and hard palate. *Indian J Cancer* 2002;**39**:83–90.

17. Doyle PJ. Approach to tumours of the nose, nasopharynx and paranasal sinuses. *Laryngoscope* 1968;**78**:1756.

18. Sessions RB, Larson DL. *En bloc* ethmoidectomy and medial maxillectomy. *Arch Otolaryngol Head Neck Surg* 1977;**103**:195.

19. Tiwari R, van der Wal J, *et al.* Studies of the anatomy and pathology of the orbit in carcinoma of the maxillary sinus and their impact on preservation of the eye in maxillectomy. *Head Neck* 1998;**20**: 193–6.

20. Smith RR, Klopp CT, Williams JM. Surgical treatment of cancer of the frontal sinus and adjacent areas. *Cancer* 1954;**7**:991–4.

21. Ketcham AS, Wilkins RH, Van Buren JM, *et al.* A combined intracranial approach to the paranasal sinuses. *Am J Surg* 1963;**106**: 698–703.

22. Terz JJ, Young HF, Lawrence W. Combined craniofacial resection for locally advanced carcinoma of the head and neck. *Am J Surg* 1980; **140**:613–24.

23. Clifford P. Transcranial approach for cancer of the antroethmoidal area. *Clin Otalaryngol* 1977;**2**:115–30.

24. Cheesman AD, Lund VJ, Howard DJ. Craniofacial resection for tumors of the nasal cavity and paranasal sinuses. *Head Neck Surg* 1986;**8**:429–35.

25. Shah JP, Kraus DH, Arbit E, *et al.* Craniofacial resection for tumors involving the anterior skull base. *Otolaryngol Head Neck Surg* 1992; **106**:387–93.

26. Janecka IP, Sen C, Sekhar LN, *et al.* Treatment of paranasal sinus cancer with cranial base surgery: Results. *Laryngoscope* 1994;**104**:553–5.

27. Neligan PC, Mulholland S, Irish J, *et al.* Flap selection in cranial base reconstruction. *Plast Reconstr Surg* 1996;**98**:1159–66.

28. Fliss DM, Zucker G, Amir A, *et al.* The subcranial approach for anterior skull base tumors. *Oper Tech Otolaryngol Head Neck Surg* 2000;**11**:238–53.

29. Snyderman CH, Janecka IP, Sekhar LN, *et al.* Anterior cranial base reconstruction: Role of galeal and pericranial flaps. *Laryngoscope* 1990;**100**:607–14.

30. Potparic Z, Fukuta K, Colen LB, *et al.* Galeopericranial flap in the forehead: A study of blood supply andvolumes. *Br J Plast Surg* 1996; **49**:519–28.

31. Gil Z, Abergel A, Leider-Trejo L, *et al.* A comprehensive algorithm for anterior skull base reconstruction after oncological resections. *Skull Base* 2007;**17**:25–37.

32. Fliss DM, Abergel A, Cavel O, *et al.* Combined subcranial approaches for excision of complex anterior skull base tumors. *Arch Otolaryngol Head Neck Surg* 2007;**133**:888–96.

33. Fliss DM, Gil Z, Spektor S, *et al.* Skull base reconstruction after anterior subcranial tumor resection. *Neurosurg Focus* 2002;**12**:e10.

34. Shlomi B, Chaushu S, Gil Z, *et al.* Effects of the subcranial approach on facial growth and development. *Otolaryngol Head Neck Surg* 2007;**136**:27–32.

35. Gil Z, Fliss DM. Pericranial wrapping of the frontal bone after anterior skull base tumor resection. *Plast Reconstr Surg* 2005;**116**:395–8; discussion 399.

15

Cancer of the nasopharynx

CESSAL THOMMACHAN, REJNISH KUMAR, K. RAMADAS, B. RAJAN

Nasopharyngeal cancer (NPC) is a disease with a variable incidence rate across the world. It is endemic in south-east Asia, southern parts of China, Mediterranean basin, and a few parts of north Africa.[1–4] It differs from other head and neck malignancies in the following aspects:

- *Aetiology:* Most of the head and neck tumours are associated with tobacco or tobacco-related products. NPC is associated with Epstein–Barr virus (EBV) infection.[5]
- *Geographical distribution:* NPC is the only tumour in the head and neck region with a defined geographical distribution.[2,4]
- *Nodal involvement:* Early and bilateral nodal involvement[6,7] is common, and the nodal staging is different from other head and neck tumours.
- *Distant metastasis:* NPC is unique from other tumours in the head and neck in that it has maximum potential for systemic spread.
- *Treatment:* NPC shows an excellent response to chemoradiation. The role of surgery is limited.
- *Recurrence:* Systemic relapse is more common in NPC compared with other head and neck tumours.

Aetiological features

The incidence of NPC is attributed to the interaction between three major risk factors, viz. ethnic, geographical and genetic. Their effect is described below:

- *EBV:* This has a universal association with this cancer and exists in a latent form exclusively in the cancer cells. EBV antibody, especially IgA, is seen in patients with NPC.[8]
- *Genetics:* Some individuals have a genetic predisposition to the disease.

- *Environmental factors:* Diet and exposure to high levels of volatile nitrosamines in preserved foods, such as Cantonese-style salted fish.[9,10]

Cancer-related genes in NPC

High frequencies of deletion on chromosomes 3p, 9p, 9q, 11q, 13q, 14q and 16q are associated with an increased incidence of NPC.[11–18]

Pathology

Carcinomas constitute 85% of the malignant tumours in NPC.[5] Lymphomas constitute 10% of the tumours,[5] the majority of which are non-Hodgkin lymphomas, with diffuse, large B-cells being the most common cell types.

WHO classification of NPC is as follows:[5]

- *Type I:* Keratinizing squamous cell carcinoma (SCC), characterized by the formation of keratin pearls or intracellular keratin
- *Type II:* Non-keratinizing carcinoma
  —Differentiated carcinoma (Type 2.1)
  —Undifferentiated carcinoma (Type 2.2)
- *Type III:* Basaloid SCC. Type III is very rare; the frequency of occurrence is <0.2% and it is a less aggressive cancer.[5]

Other rare cancers of the nasopharynx include the following:[5]

- Melanoma
- Minor salivary gland tumours
- Extra medullary plasmacytoma
- Carcinosarcoma
- Rhabdomayosarcoma.

Benign tumours involving the nasopharynx are: (i) Paraganglioma, (ii) Juvenile angiofibroma, (iii) Chordoma.

TNM staging (AJCC 7th ed, 2010)[19]

Primary Tumour (T)

TX   Primary tumour cannot be assessed

T0   No evidence of primary tumour

Tis   Carcinoma *in situ*

T1   Tumour confined to the nasopharynx, or tumour extends to oropharynx and/or nasal cavity without parapharyngeal extension*

T2   Tumour with parapharyngeal extension#

T3   Tumour involves bony structures of skull base and/or paranasal sinuses

T4   Tumour with intracranial extension and/or involvement of cranial nerves, hypopharynx, orbit, or with extension to the infratemporal fossa/masticator space

#*Note:* Parapharyngeal extension denotes posterolateral infiltration of tumour.

*Regional Lymph Nodes (N)**

The distribution and the prognostic impact of regional lymph node spread from nasopharynx cancer, particulary of the undifferentiated type, are different from those of other head and neck mucosal cancers and justify the use of a different N classification scheme.

NX   Regional lymph nodes cannot be assessed

N0   No regional lymph node metastasis

N1   Unilateral metastasis in cervical lymph node(s), 6 cm or less in greatest dimension, above the supraclavicular fossa, and/or unilateral and bilateral, retropharyngeal lymph nodes, 6 cm or less, in greatest dimension*

N2   Bilateral metastasis in cervical lymph nodes(s), 6 cm or less in greatest dimension, above the supraclavicular fossa*

N3   Metastasis in a lymph node(s), more than 6 cm and/or to supraclavicular fossa*

N3a   Greater than 6 cm in dimension

N3b   Extension to the supraclavicular fossa

Note: Midline nodes are considered ipsilateral nodes.

Distant metastasis (M)

M0   No distant metastasis

M1   Distant metastasis

Anatomy (Figs 1–3)

The nasopharynx is cuboidal in shape. Anteriorly, it is continuous with the nasal cavity. The roof is formed by the basisphenoid, basiocciput and anterior arch of atlas.

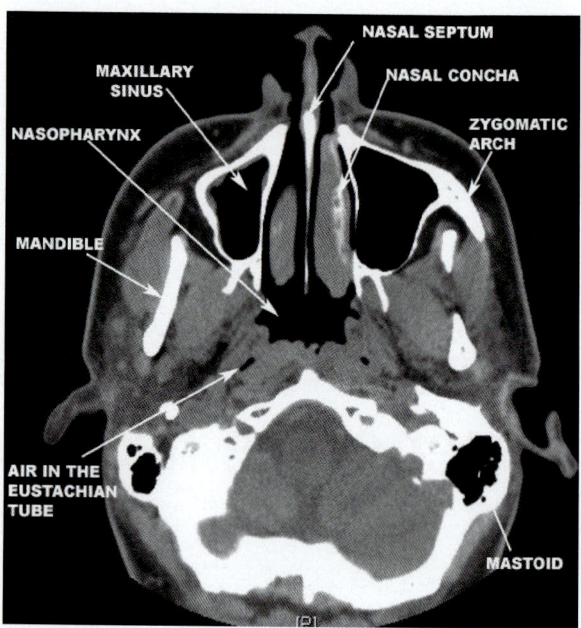

Fig. 1. CT scan showing the normal anatomy of the nasopharynx

Posteriorly, it is bounded by the first and second cervical vertebrae and is continuous with the roof. Laterally, it is bounded by the Eustachian tube orifice, surrounded by the torus tubaris—the recess behind the Eustachian tube—and fossa of Rosenmuller (the most common site for cancer). The floor is formed by the upper surface of the soft palate and communicates with the oropharynx through the pharyngeal isthmus. The posterior wall has four layers, consisting of the mucous membrane of the pharynx, superior constrictor muscle layer, pharyngeal aponeurosis, and buccopharyngeal fascia. The muscular wall in the roof is incomplete at the point of entry of the Eustachian tube.

Lymphatics

Ipsilateral lymph node metastasis occurs in 85%–90% of cases of NPC. Bilateral spread occurs in 50% of cases.[7,20,21]

The submucosal lymphatic capillary plexus is extensive. Lymphatics spread by the following three different pathways:
- The jugular chain
- Spinal accessory chain
- Retropharyngeal pathway.

Local extension

Anterior

Direct extension into the nasal cavity is common. When the lateral wall is invaded, it can lead to destruction of the pterygoid plates. Involvement of the maxilla and post-ethmoid sinus is less common. In very advanced disease, orbital involvement can occur.

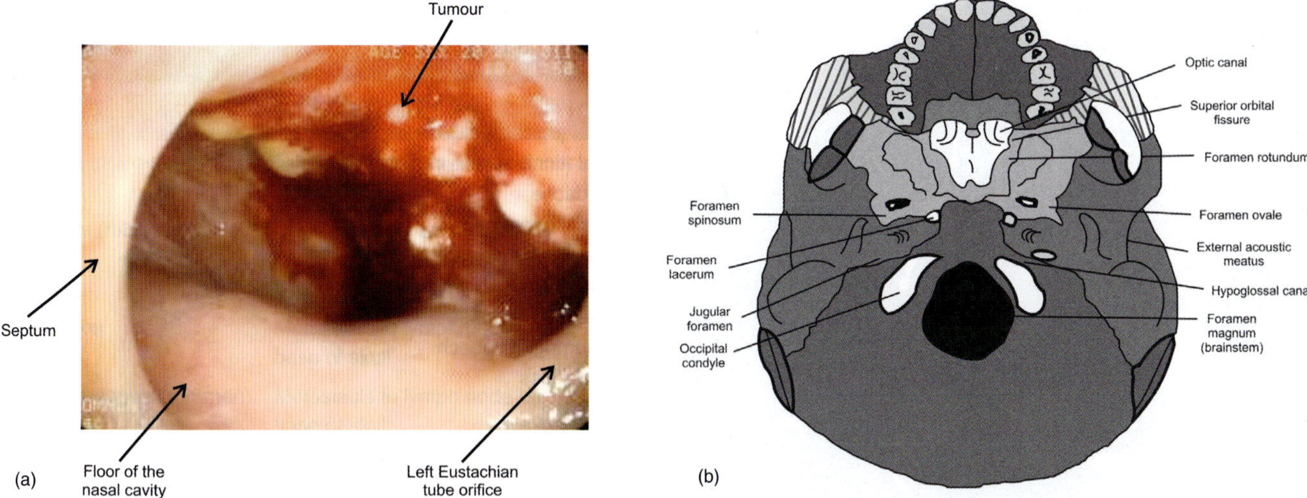

Fig. 2 (a, b). Patterns of spread of NPC. (a) Endoscopic view via left nostril of extensive nasopharynyal carcinoma with involvement of the fossa of Rosenmuller (b) Base of skull showing foramiae.

Table 1. Foramina of base of skull close to the nasopharynx

Foramen/fissure	Cranial nerve
Cribiform plate	Olfactory nerve (I)
Optic foramen	Optic nerve (II)
Superior orbital fissure	Oculomotor (III), trochlear (IV), ophthalmic division of trigeminal (V1) nerve, abducent (VI) nerves
Foramen rotundum	Maxillary division of trigeminal (V2) nerve
Foramen ovale	Mandibular division of trigeminal (V3) nerve
Foramen lacerum	
Foramen spinosum	Recurrent branch of V3 nerve
Stylomastoid foramen	Fascial (VII) nerve
Internal acoustic meatus	Auditory (VIII) nerve
Jugular foramen	Glossopharyngeal (IX), vagus (X), spinal accessory (XI) nerves
Hypoglossal canal	Hypoglossal (XII) nerve
Foramen magnum	Spinal cord

Superior and posterior

Superior and posterior extensions can lead to invasion of the following structures:

- Base of skull
- Sphenoid sinus
- Clivus

The foramen lacerum is located directly above the fossa of Rosenmuller and it is the weakest portion of the base of skull. The tumour can gain direct access to the cavernous sinus and middle cranial fossa. This leads to invasion of cranial nerves II–VI. The most common cranial nerves to be involved are V and VI. Cranial nerves I, VII and VIII are less involved. The tumour can also invade through the foramen ovale into the middle cranial fossa. Posterior extension of the tumour can lead to pre-vertebral muscle invasion.

Inferior

Inferior extension leads to oropharyngeal involvement.

Lateral (Fig. 3)

Lateral extension leads to involvement of the parapharyngeal space and invasion of the levator and tensor veli palati. Invasion of the pterygoid muscle occurs in more advanced disease. Direct tumour extension or lateral retropharyngeal lymph node metastasis can lead to compression of cranial nerve XII as it exits through the hypoglossal canal. It can also compress cranial nerves IX–XI and cervical sympathetic nerves as they emerge through the jugular foramen.

Haematogenous spread

Distant metastasis at presentation is uncommon (6%).[22] The most common site of distant metastasis is bone, followed by the lungs and liver.[23] Hui *et al.*[23] found that lung metastasis was associated with better prognosis compared with other sites. Brain and skin metastases are extremely rare.[24,25]

Clinical presentation

The most common presenting symptom is evidence of a neck mass.[6,7] Twenty per cent of patients present with cranial nerve palsies.[26,27]

40. Hunt Ma, Zelefsky MJ, Wolden S, *et al*. Treatment planning and delivery of intensity-modulated radiation therapy for primary nasopharynx cancer. *Int J Radiat Oncol Biol Phys* 2001;**49**:623–32.

41. Kam MK, Chau RM, Suen J, *et al*. Intensity-modulated radiotherapy in nasopharyngeal carcinoma: Dosimetric advantage over conventional plans and feasibility of dose escalation. *Int J Radiat Oncol Biol Phys* 2003;**56**:145–57.

42. Xia P, Fu KK, Wong GW, *et al*. Comparison of treatment plans involving intensity-modulated radiotherapy for nasopharyngeal carcinoma. *Int J Radiat Oncol Biol Phys* 2000;**48**:329–37.

43. Juncharek M, Kupelnick B. Combined chemoradiation versus radiation therapy alone in locally advanced nasopharyngeal carcinoma: Results of a meta-analysis of 1,528 patients from six randomized traials. *Am J Clin Oncol* 2002;**25**:219–23.

44. Fu KK. Combined radiotherapy and chemotherapy for nasopharyngeal carcinoma. *Semin Radiat Oncol* 1998;**8**:247–53.

45. Preliminary results of a randomized trial comparing neoadjuvant chemotherapy (cisplatin, epirubicin, bleomycin) plus radiotherapy vs radiotherapy alone in stage IV (>or=N2, M0) undifferentiated nasophryngeal carcinoma: A positive effect on progression-free survival. International Nasopharynx Cancer Study Group. VUMCA trial. *Int J Radiat Oncol Phys* 1996;**35**:463–9.

46. Al-Sarraf M, LeBlanc M, Giri PG, *et al*. Chemoradiotherapy versus radiotherapy in patients with advanced nasopharyngeal cancer: Phase III randomized inter group study 0099. *J Clin Oncol* 1998;**16**:1310–17.

47. Chua DT, Ma J, Sham JS, *et al*. Long-term survival after cisplatin-based induction chemotherapy and radiotherapy for nasopharyngeal carcinoma: A pooled data analysis of two phase III trials. *J Clin Oncol* 2005;**23**:1118–24.

48. Langendijk JA, Leemans CR, Buter J, *et al*. The additional value of chemotherapy to radiotherapy in locally advanced nasopharyngeal carcinoma: A meta-analysis of the published literature. *J Clin Oncol* 2004;**22**:4604–12.

49. Posner MR, Hershock DM, Blajman CR, *et al*. Cisplatin and fluorouracil alone or with docetaxel in head and neck cancer. *N Engl J Med* 2007;**357**:1705–15.

50. Vermorken JB, Remenar E, Van Herpen C, *et al*. Cisplatin, fluorouracil, and docetaxel in unresectable head and neck cancer. *N Engl J Med* 2007;**357**:1695–704.

51. Lu TX, Mai WY, The BS, *et al*. Initial experience using intensity-modulated radiotherapy for recurrent nasopharyngeal carcinoma. *Int J Radiat Oncol Biol Phys* 2004;**58**:682–7.

52. Chua DT, Sham JS, Leung LH, *et al*. Re-irradiation of nasopharyngeal carcinoma with intensity-modulated radiotherapy. *Radiother Oncol* 2005;**77**:290–4.

53. Poon D, Yap SP, Wong ZW, *et al*. Concurrent chemoradiotherapy in locoregionally recurrent nasopgaryngeal carcinoma. *Int J Radiat Oncol Biol Phys* 2004;**59**:1312–18.

54. Lee AWM, Lau WH, Tung SY, *et al*. Preliminary results of a randomized study on therapeutic gain by concurrent chemotherapy for regionally-advanced nasopharyngeal carcinoma: NPC-9901. Trial by the Hong Kong Nasopharyngeal Cancer Study Group. *J Clin Oncol* 2005;**23**:6966–75.

55. Lee AWM, Tung SY, Chan AT, *et al*. Preliminary results of a randomized study (NPC-9902 Trial) on therapeutic gain by concurrent chemotherapy and/or accelerated fractionation for locally-advanced nasopharyngeal carcinoma. *Int J Radiat Oncol Biol Phys* 2006;**66**:142–51.

56. Al-Sarraf M, LeBlanc M, Giri PG, *et al*. Chemoradiotherapy versus radiotherapy in patients with advanced nasopharyngeal cancer: Phase III randomized Intergroup study 0099. *J Clin Oncol* 1998;**16**:1310–17.

57. Al-Sarraf M, LeBlanc M, Giri PG, *et al*. Chemoradiotherapy (CT-RT) vs radiotherapy (RT) in patients (PTS) with advanced nasopharyngeal cancer (NPC). Intergroup (0099) (SWOG8892, RTOG8817, ECOG2388) Phase III Study: Progress report. *J Clin Oncol* 1998;**17**:385 (abstr 1483).

58. Lin JC, Jan JS, Hsu CY. Concurrent chemoradiotherapy versus radiotherapy alone for advanced nasopharyngeal carcinoma: Positive effect on overall and progression-free survival. *J Clin Oncol* 2003;**21**:637–7.

59. Kwong DL, Sham JS, Au GK, *et al*. Concurrent and adjuvant chemotherapy for nasopharyngeal carcinoma: A factorial study. *J Clin Oncol* 2004;**22**:2643–53.

60. Wee J, Tan EH, Tai BC. Randomized trial of radiotherapy versus concurrent chemoradiotherapy followed by adjuvant chemotherapy in patients with American Joint Committee on Cancer/International Union Against Cancer Stage III and IV nasopharyngeal cancer of the endemic variety. *J Clin Oncol* 2005;**23**:6730–8.

61. Lee AWM, Tusg SY, Chan AT, *et al*. Preliminary results of a randomized study (NPC-9902 Trial) on therapeutic gain by concurrent chemotherapy and/or accelerated fractionation for locally-advanced nasopharyngeal carcinoma. *Int J Radiat Oncol Biol Phys* 2006;**66**:142–51.

62. Zheng XK, Ma J, Chen LH, *et al*. Dosimetric and clinical results of three dimensional conformal radiotherapy for locally recurrent nasopharyngeal carcinoma. *Radiother Oncol* 2005;**75**:197–203.

63. Pryzant RM, Wendt CD, Delclos L, *et al*. Re-treatment of nasopharyngeal carcinoma in 53 patients. *Int J Radiat Oncol Biol Phys* 1992;**22**:941–7.

16

Cancer of the thyroid and parathyroid glands

MADAN KAPRE

The thyroid is a composite endocrine gland wrapped in deep cervical fascia with the basic connective tissue support. It has two distinct cell populations producing two different hormones. It is intimately connected to a pair of parathyroid glands and a set of laryngeal nerves on either side. The arterial supply is also shared by these endocrine glands.

The pathology often alters the anatomy and as such a thorough knowledge of anatomy of the region and sound philosophy of treatment is the cornerstone in surgical management. Historically, thyroid surgery has been at the helm of innovativeness, bringing together the various disciplines of anatomy, physiology, pathology, biochemistry and imaging. The author frequently comes across huge goitres in the tribal belt of Melghat, Madhya Pradesh, India (Fig. 1). The present chapter discusses diseases of the thyroid gland that are amenable to surgery, and also their treatment options.

Surgical anatomy

Thyroid gland

The thyroid gland consists generally of two lobes connected by an isthmus; it weighs ~25 g in the adult. Occasionally there can be a prominent pyramidal lobe, mostly to the left, or there may be significant thyroid tissue along the descent of thyroid from the foramen caecum to its adult position. It straddles the cervical trachea, with the isthmus at the level of the third and fourth tracheal rings and the superior pole overlying the cricoid cartilage and cricothyroid muscle. It is enveloped by a fine capsule from which septa pass into the gland to separate the lobules. The pretracheal fascia also envelops the gland to form the 'surgical capsule'. Dissection beneath this capsule and on the true capsule comprises the 'capsular dissection'. The gland adheres to the trachea by the surgical capsule, and in addition is suspended to the lateral surfaces of the cricoid cartilage, cricothyroid joint, and upper tracheal rings by a condensation of the fascia known as Berry ligament.

The recurrent laryngeal nerve on each side usually lies in the tracheo-oesophageal (TE) groove but can also be outside the groove, particularly on the right side. Each nerve passes up in loose areolar tissue posteromedial to the lobe and is

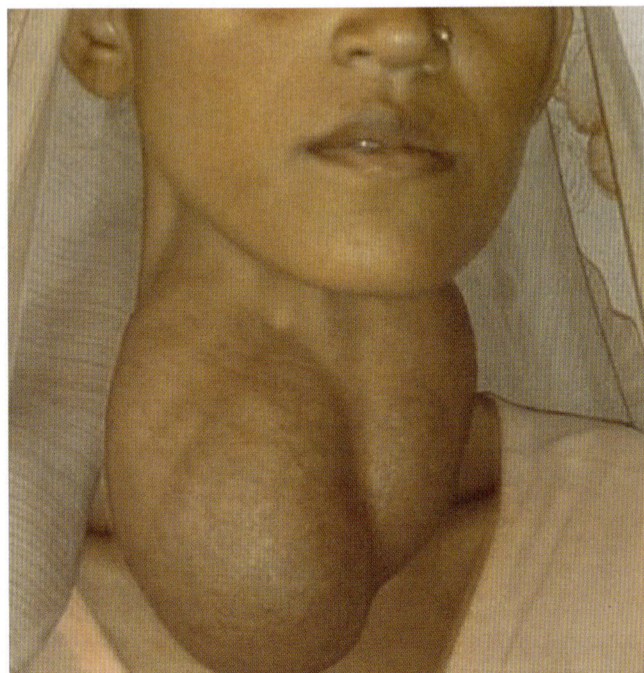

Fig. 1. Endemic thyroid goitre

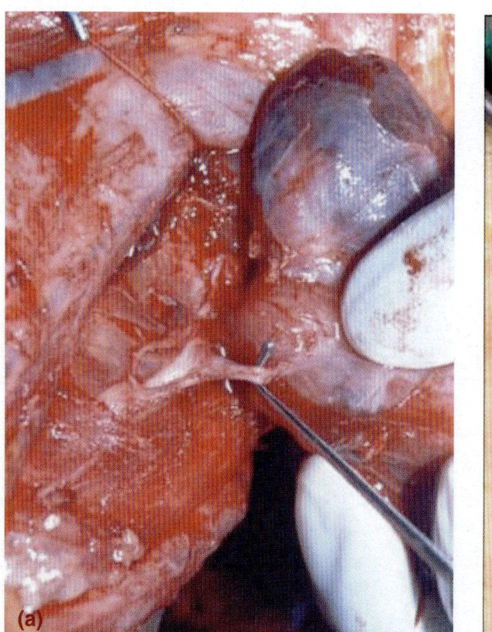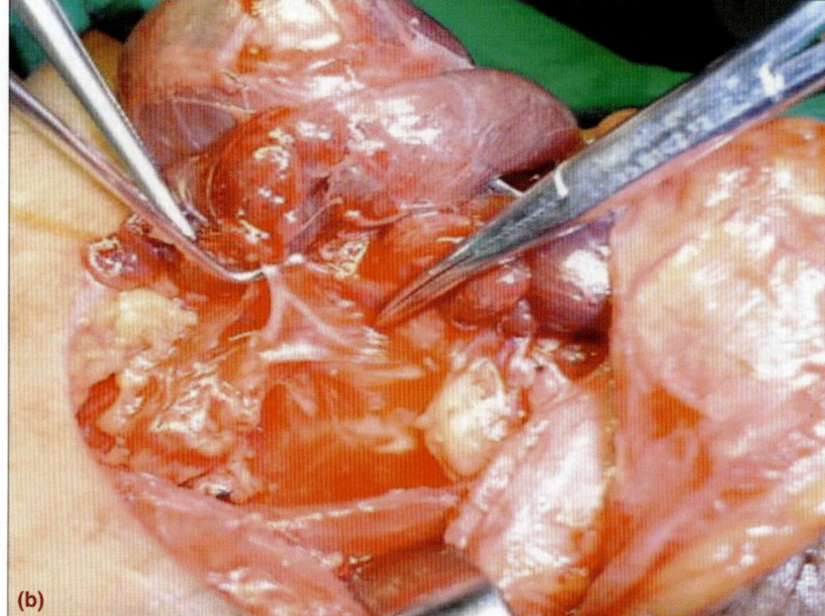

Fig. 2a and b. The recurrent laryngeal nerve—comparative variations

variably but intimately related to the inferior thyroid artery or its branches, which run from lateral to medial when the gland is retracted during surgery. Thereafter, the nerve passes behind, but sometimes between, the fibres of Berry ligament to enter the larynx behind the cricothyroid joint. A small branch of the inferior thyroid artery and small veins invariably course the Berry ligament, which can make dissection of the nerve through the ligament hazardous. In ~1% of cases the right nerve is non-recurrent and is closely related to the superior pole of the thyroid gland as it passes lateral to medial, directly from the vagus nerve to the larynx.

The parathyroid glands

The parathyroid glands are small (1 mm × 3 mm × 6 mm), soft and ovoid, and lie adjacent to the thyroid gland, usually within the surgical capsule. They are most easily recognized by their characteristic caramel colour, but are often camouflaged by associated adipose tissue. The total number of glands varies between two and six, but sometimes there may be more. An upper and a lower gland are usually present on each side. The upper gland is the more constant of the two and usually lies posterior to the nerve on the posterior surface of the superior pole, near the level of the cricothyroid joint. This 'constancy' arises because the thyroid and superior parathyroids have a common embryological origin from the fourth pharyngeal pouch. The inferior gland usually lies on the posterior surface of the inferior pole and anterior to the recurrent laryngeal nerve, although it is not uncommon for it to be in the thymus and out of the surgical field. This is because of its embryological origin from the third pharyngeal pouch, the other structure of similar origin being the thymus, which normally rests in the superior mediastinum.

Inferior thyroid artery and recurrent laryngeal nerve (Figs 2a and b)

Surgical techniques have evolved around protecting the recurrent laryngeal nerve. The variable relationship this nerve has with the thyroid gland is mostly due to the variable branching pattern of the inferior thyroid artery and the pathology in the gland. Different statistics are quoted for how often the nerve passes below, above, or between the branches of the inferior thyroid artery. In the author's experience, the most constant point of identification of the nerve is at its entry into the larynx at the cricoarytenoid joint, which aids in preserving the parathyroids.

Right recurrent laryngeal nerve (Fig. 3)

- Loops around subclavian artery
- Rather lateral in root of neck
- Rises medially at 45° angle in TE groove.

Left recurrent laryngeal nerve (Fig. 4)

- Loops around ligamentum arteriosus
- Rather early in TE groove
- Close to oesophagus at the point where oesophagus slants to the left.

The external branch of superior laryngeal nerves

These are often called 'children of the lesser God', as they have not received adequate attention in the past. They also have a variable relation with the superior thyroid vascular pedicle, passing either medially and out of harm's way, or they may

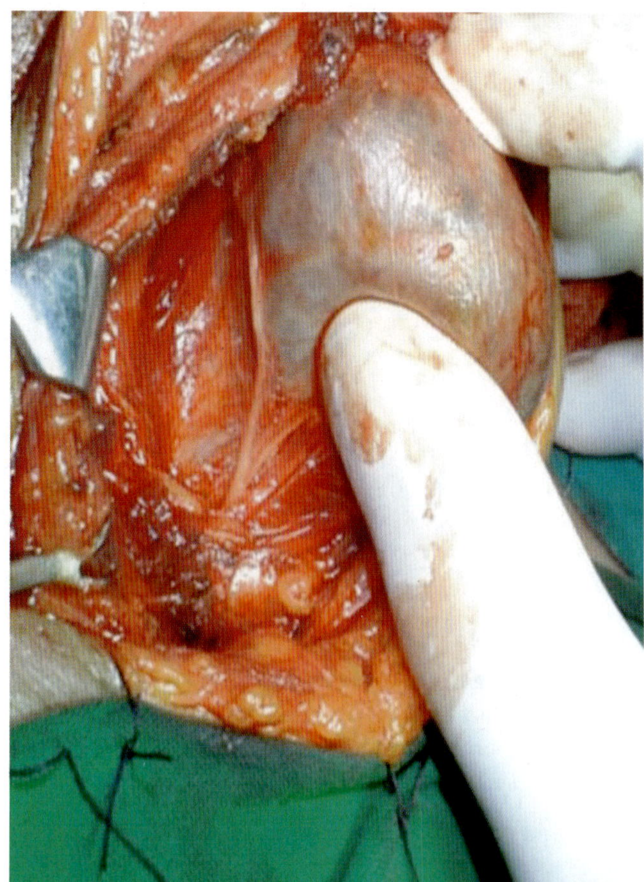

Fig. 3. Anteriorly placed right recurrent laryngeal nerve

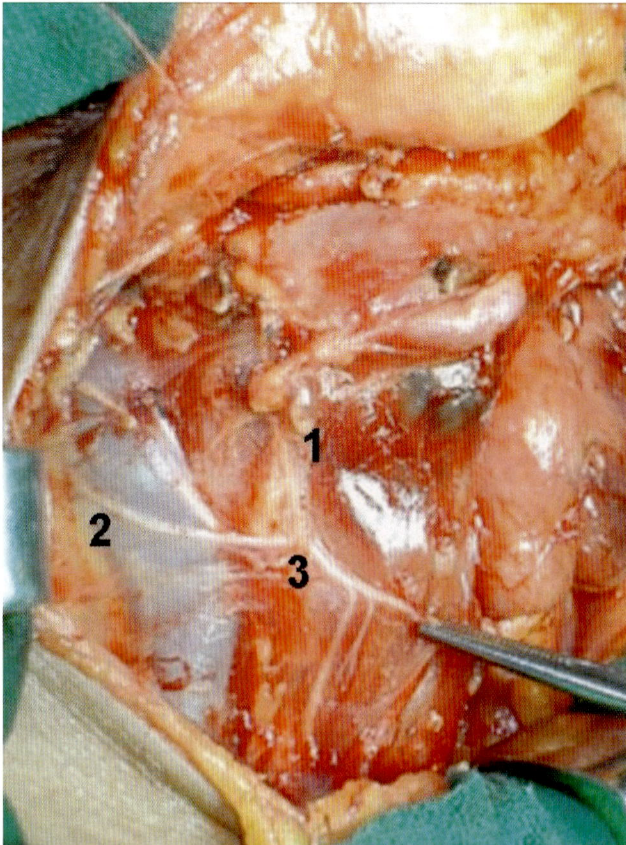

Fig. 5. Ansa cervicalis supplying the strap muscle: **(1)** descendens hypoglossi; **(2)** cervical contribution; **(3)** ansa cervicalis

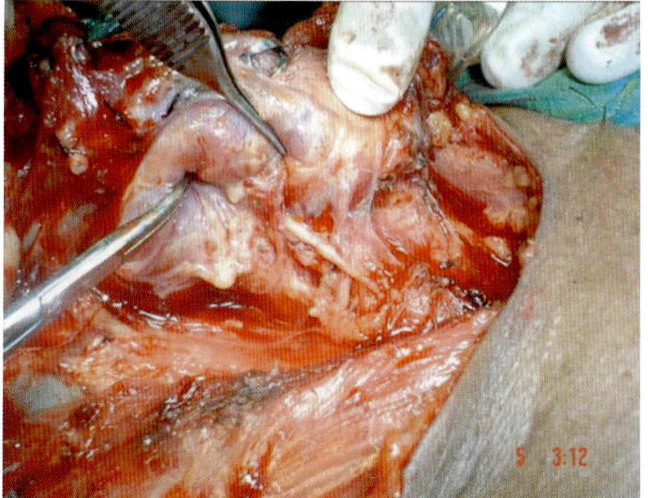

Fig. 4. Left recurrent laryngeal nerve

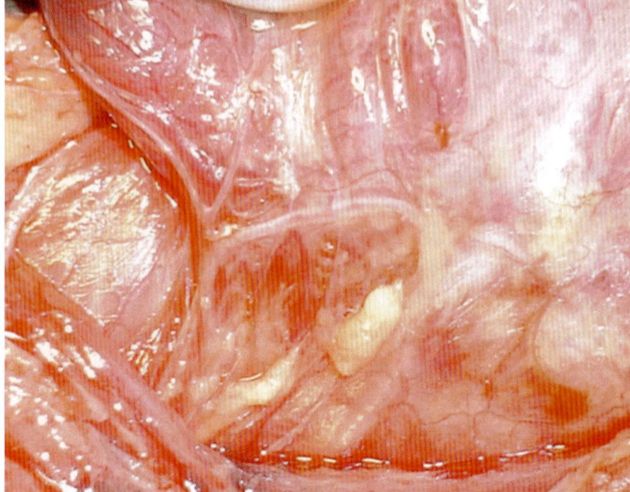

Fig. 6. Arterial supply to the thyroid

cross from lateral to medial posteriorly, which makes them vulnerable to damage.

Ansa cervicalis (Fig. 5)

This nerve is formed by the union of descendens hypoglossi and cervical 2, 3 contribution, supplying the strap muscles in the lower half. When these muscles need to be transected for approach, it is best to do so in the upper third (Fig. 2)

The vascular loop of the parathyroid (Fig. 6)

The main arterial supply is from the superior thyroid artery; the inferior thyroid artery's supply is insignificant as it is by its

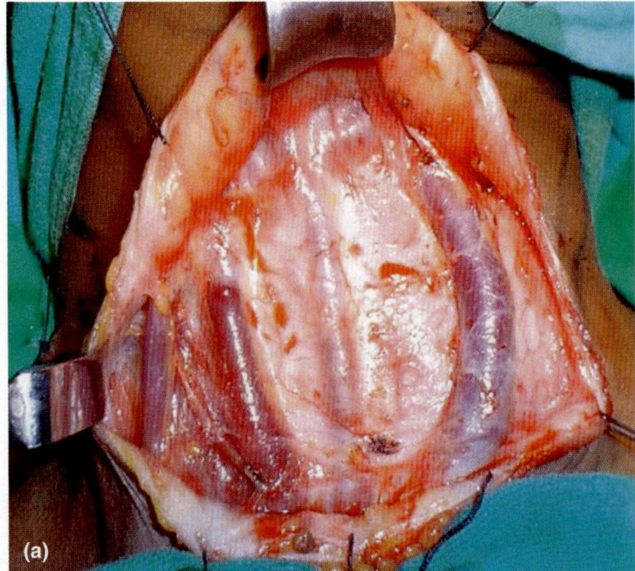

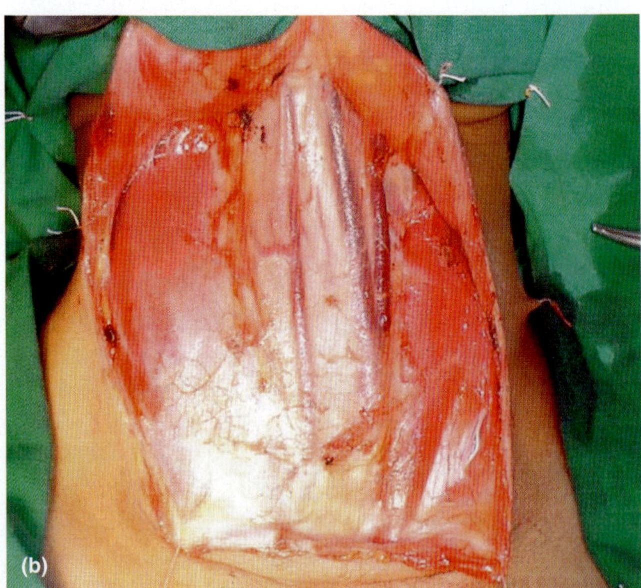

Figs 7a and b. The venous drainage

terminal branches. An arterial loop constitutes the vascular supply of the parathyroids; it is located between the posterior branch of the superior thyroid artery and the terminal branch of the inferior thyroid artery. The thyroidea ima artery is rarely present and enters just to the right of the isthmus; it arises from the arch of the aorta in the superior mediastinum. The variability of the terminal branches of the inferior thyroid artery is the main cause of concern during surgery, as it influences the dissection of the recurrent laryngeal nerve.

Inferior thyroid vein with usual variations

The thyroid gland is drained by the superior thyroid vein, the middle thyroid vein and the inferior thyroid veins. However, their number and location can be inconsistent. The middle thyroid vein is rather short and is easily torn by injudicious finger dissection. The tear can extend into the jugular vein with consequent bleeding. Capsular veins are devoid of the muscular coat and bleeding needs to be controlled by special surgical techniques. When present, the fourth vein of Kocher needs special attention as it normally drains into the internal jugular vein ~1 cm below the middle thyroid vein.

Anterior jugular veins

These are usually paired on either side and offer excellent landmarks for midline. However, they may be present in multiples (Figs 7a and 7b)

The lymphatic drainage of the thyroid gland

The major lymphatic drainage is in the middle and lower deep jugular nodes. Through these routes it may drain into the lateral compartment of the neck, i.e. level V. More significantly, the thyroid lymphatics drain into the pre- and para-tracheal nodes and thence into the superior mediastinum. Literature exists about intraglandular and subcapsular lymphatics within the gland which leads to the advocacy for more radical surgery for malignant thyroid diseases.

Clinical features

A solitary thyroid nodule is evident to the clinician by virtue of its position in front of the neck. The task of deciding whether it needs excision and with what urgency and to what extent is a clinical challenge (Fig. 1). In a head extended position, the ability to insinuate finger below the inferior border of thyroid indicates an easy cervical approach for excision (Fig. 8). Pain and increase in size indicates that there could either be bleeding in the cyst, or more ominously, a malignant change. Posteriorly placed nodules may cause discomfort on swallowing by their movement in the TE groove. However, dysphagia usually points to a malignant invasion. A change

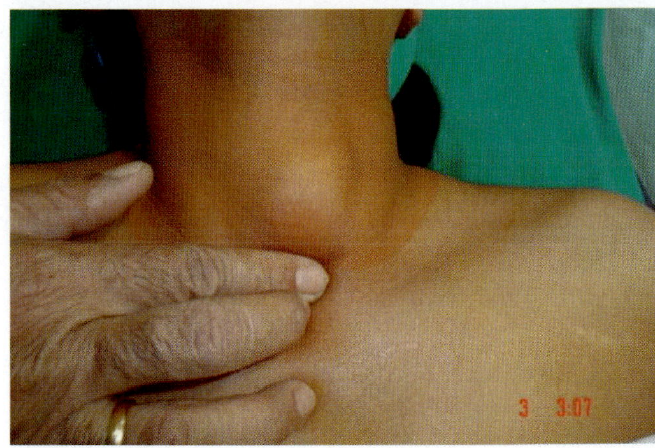

Fig. 8. Assessing the tetrosternal extent

in voice and difficulty in breathing indicate malignancy. The breathlessness associated with retrosternal goitre is usually postural, lying supine, or can be demonstrated with Pemberton manoeuvre, wherein the neck also has vascular congestion, indicating mediastinal compression.

The presence of palpable neck nodes (indicators of papillary or medullary carcinoma of the thyroid), sometimes without a palpable thyroid swelling, requires confirmation by fine-needle aspiration cytology (FNAC). It is also imperative to enquire into the functional aspect of the gland which may or may not help to decide the pathological nature of the tumour in the thyroid, but would certainly keep the clinician well ahead in anticipation of post-operative complications and their management. It is pertinent to note that more and more thyroid diseases, particularly malignancies, are now diagnosed in laboratories rather than in the surgical setting.

Surgical pathology

Although tumours of the thyroid gland are common, the incidence of malignancy is quite low. Tribal populations of India (e.g. Melghat tribe) apparently show a lower incidence of malignancy compared with European goitrous areas, which report a higher incidence of malignancy (unpublished data). The incidence of thyroid nodules varies in relation to the diagnostic criterion applied. Clinical palpation suggests a prevalence of 1%–7%.[1] A British study indicates 3.2%,[2] whereas a study from the United States of America reports a prevalence of 4.2%.[3] However, if ultrasonography is added to the screening techniques, the incidence rises to 19%, and even to 46% in some studies.[4] Mortensen's well recognized study of the autopsy specimen has almost 49.5% malignancy in an otherwise normal thyroid specimen.[5] Much interest is generated from the changing pattern of follicular carcinomas to papillary carcinomas in goitrous areas, which are no more iodine deprived.

Aetiology and pathophysiology

As with most endocrine systems, the thyroid gland is controlled by a feedback mechanism. Regulation of the thyroid gland is primarily via the hypothalamic–pituitary–thyroid axis. High levels of serum thyroxine (T4) and triodothyronine (T3) provide a negative feedback to the anterior pituitary gland, which consequently secretes thyroid stimulating hormone (TSH), and to the hypothalamus, which secretes thyrotropin-releasing hormone (TRH), which in turn stimulates the anterior pituitary to release TSH. Thus, increased levels of plasma TRH or decreased levels of plasma T4/T3 stimulate the release of TSH, which is the major regulator of the thyroid. The gland has TSH receptors, which when activated by its ligand, initiate the production of thyroid hormones by the organification process that attaches iodine to portions of the stored thyroglobulin (TG). Processing of the iodinized TG ultimately releases T4 and T3. In addition, most of the serum T3 is formed from conversion of T4 peripherally.

In iodine-deficient regions, hypothyroidism is endemic and contributes to the aetiology of multinodular goitre (MNG). Through the feedback mechanism, hypothyroidism increases TSH, which stimulates the growth of the thyroid gland. In iodine-replete areas, however, patients are generally euthyroid, with a normal TSH level, providing evidence that other factors, such as genetics, play a role. More recently, a gene located on chromosome 14q, dubbed 'MNG-1', has been associated with familial non-toxic MNG.[5] In addition, polymorphism of codon 727 has been associated with toxic MNG. Individual follicular cells, furthermore, demonstrate variable activity, morphology, and growth potential, and nodular formation occurs through an ill-defined mechanism. Areas of growing follicular cells create nodules whose increasing sizes begin to outgrow their blood supply, leading to localized haemorrhage and reparative fibrosis.

Multinodular goitre (Fig. 9)

The natural history of MNG encompasses an increase in

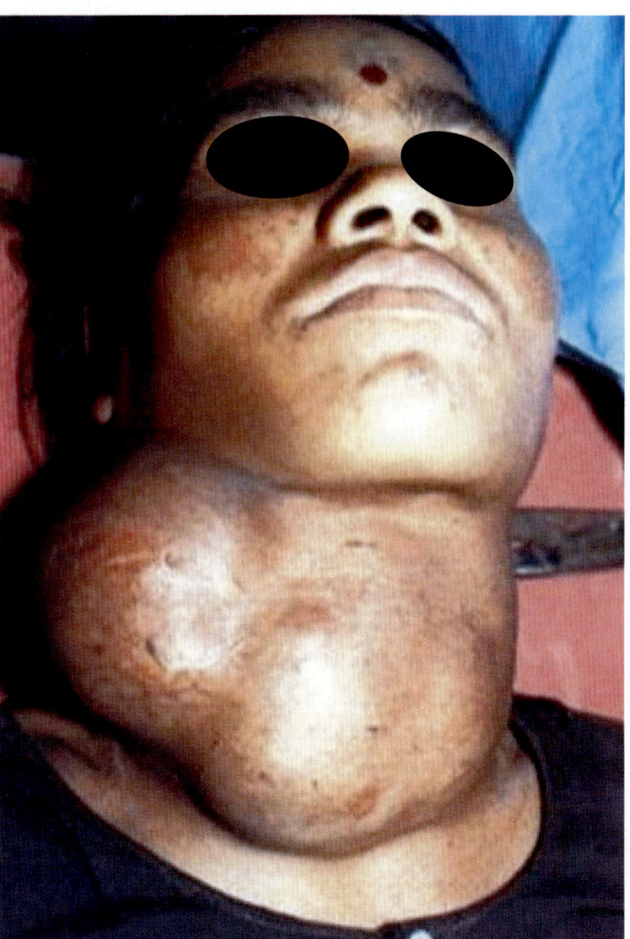

Fig. 9. Multinodular goitres and their malignant potential

tissue with an annual growth potential of up to 20%. Areas of the thyroid with increased functioning may progress to hyperthyroidism or toxic MNG (Plummer disease), which occurs in 5%–10% of MNG cases in a 5-year period. These conditions may occur slowly as an autonomous, adenomatous form or they may occur more acutely following an excessive source of iodine such as radiographic contrast material, or medications such as amiodarone. Although not corroborated by controlled trials, patients with these conditions may be placed on prophylactic antithyroid drug therapy.

It is well established that MNG may harbour occult malignancy, although the true incidence is disputed. Formerly, it was thought that solitary nodules had an increased risk of malignancy (7.5%–24%) compared with MNG (4%–12%).[6–9] However, more recent studies have demonstrated similar frequencies of malignancy in solitary and multinodular conditions of approximately 4%.[10–13] This could be reflected by the improved detection of multinodular disease with radiographic imaging.

Malignancies of thyroid

The incidence of thyroid cancer is reported to be rising in the western world, probably because of more aggressive screening and more advanced diagnostic tools. However, the development and availability of imaging modalities as primary investigatory tools for early diagnosis has not made any impact on survival statistics and disease-related deaths.

Pathology of well differentiated carcinoma

Papillary carcinoma of the thyroid

The most common histological type of thyroid cancer is papillary carcinoma, which represents 80%–90% of all newly diagnosed thyroid cancers. Papillary carcinoma has the best prognosis of the thyroid malignancies. Women are more commonly affected than men, and the average age at diagnosis is around 40 years. Papillary carcinoma is probably much more prevalent than is clinically evident. Papillary 'microcarcinoma' is a term applied to an incidentally identified papillary cancer, which measures <1.0 cm in diameter. It is often identified at the time of thyroid surgery for benign disease or at autopsy, with an incidence ranging from 1% to 35% in autopsy specimens.[14] Papillary microcarcinoma theoretically harbours some malignant potential, including the potential for recurrence and regional or distant metastasis. This possibility is minute, however, and these microcarcinomas are generally considered to be of little clinical significance. Further treatment is typically not warranted other than increased vigilance and routine follow up with, possibly, the addition of thyroid hormone suppression therapy.

Papillary carcinoma arises from the follicular cells of the normal thyroid gland. It is characterized by a papillary growth pattern of tumour cells that exhibit distinctive nuclear features, which can usually be diagnosed by fine-needle aspiration biopsy (FNAB), and include: (i) Nuclear membrane irregularities that manifest as indentations, pseudonuclear inclusions, or nuclear grooves; (ii) overlapping and enlarged nuclei; and (iii) an empty appearance of the nuclei that look pale, optically clear, and resemble 'orphan Annie eyes'.

Other variants of papillary carcinoma also exist, and include the follicular-type papillary carcinoma, tall cell variant, and columnar cell variant. Follicular-type papillary cancer exhibits a follicular growth pattern but the nuclear characteristics resemble those of papillary carcinoma. The prognosis is believed to be roughly the same as traditional papillary carcinoma and treatment algorithms do not differ.

Follicular carcinoma of the thyroid

Follicular carcinoma exhibits a pattern of growth that resembles normal thyroid follicles. In fact, the follicles of a hyperplastic thyroid adenoma are indistinguishable from those of follicular carcinoma. Rather, it is the presence or absence of invasiveness that distinguishes it from the malignant potential of a follicular neoplasm. This fact limits the usefulness of fine-needle aspiration cytology (FNAC) and frozen section pathological analysis in establishing a diagnosis of follicular carcinoma. The two principal histological features of invasiveness that confirm the diagnosis of carcinoma in a follicular neoplasm are invasion of the capsule or of the vascular channels of the lesion. Complete histological sections of formalin-fixed, paraffin-embedded surgical specimens of the thyroid gland are best used to confirm capsular and vascular invasion.

In contrast to papillary carcinoma, follicular carcinoma of the thyroid spreads more commonly by haematogenous dissemination. This fact reiterates the diagnostic criterion and its clinical tolerance of vascular invasion. Intra-glandular, multicentric disease is much less common than papillary carcinoma, as is nodal spread, which again reflects the strong lymphotropic tendency of papillary thyroid cancer. However, when nodal spread is present it clearly has a negative influence on recurrence and survival in patients with follicular carcinoma of the thyroid.

Hurthle cell carcinoma

Hurthle cell carcinoma is also referred to as oncocytic carcinoma. Hurthle cells (oncocytes) are large, polygonal cells that contain abundant cytoplasm with pink granularity. Ultrastructurally, these cytoplasmic granules are predominantly abnormal mitochondria. Hurthle cells can be seen in benign and malignant thyroid pathology. Hurthle cell carcinoma has long been considered to be a variant of follicular carcinoma. Recently, the Hurthle cell variant has been assigned more autonomy and is now considered by most investigators to be a distinct, clinical entity.[15] The behaviour of Hurthle cell carcinoma is highly variable, and depends largely on the histopathological features of the tumour. Aggressive features, such as large size, invasiveness, and regional or distant metastases indicate a more guarded prognosis. The treatment of Hurthle cell carcinoma mirrors that of the other well differentiated varieties, especially follicular carcinoma. Like follicular carcinoma, the diagnosis of Hurthle cell carcinoma can be difficult to distinguish from benign adenoma.

Medullary thyroid carcinoma

Medullary carcinoma accounts for ~5% of all cases of thyroid malignancy. It may occur as part of the multiple endocrine neoplasia (MEN) syndrome, as familial non-MEN disease, or it can be sporadic. In patients with MEN, medullary thyroid carcinoma is frequently bilateral (90%) and multifocal. In sporadic cases, medullary carcinoma is likely to be unifocal. The cervical node metastasis varies from 25% to 50%. Medullary cancers arise from the parafollicular or C cells. Parafollicular cells secrete calcitonin, which is therefore a valuable tumour marker.

Macroscopically, the tumour is grey or white with a gritty texture and areas of haemorrhage, necrosis, fibrosis and calcification. Histologically, it consists of uniform spindle-shaped cells within a variable fibrous stroma that may contain amyloid.

Lymphoma

Primary thyroid lymphomas are uncommon, accounting for <5% of all cases of lymphoma. They usually present as rapidly increasing swellings of the neck; elderly women are most at risk. This clinical presentation can be very similar to that of anaplastic thyroid carcinoma and so histological confirmation of the diagnosis is necessary. On purely morphological grounds, lymphoma can sometimes resemble anaplastic carcinoma, so appropriate immunocytochemistry is essential to differentiate these two diseases. Accurate diagnosis is important as the treatment of the two conditions is different. The response to treatment and prognosis of lymphoma is much better than that of anaplastic cancer.

Grossly, most thyroid lymphomas appear as large, grey, fleshy masses, often extending outside the capsule. Infiltration of the residual thyroid tissue may be seen. Lymphoma usually arises on a background of chronic autoimmune thyroiditis, and the non-tumour thyroid tissue may show the gross appearance of lymphocytic thyroiditis. Histologically, the majority of lymphomas are high-grade B-cell non-Hodgkin lymphomas. Rarely, low-grade mucoid-associated lymphoid tissue (MALT) lymphomas may be encountered. Most often,

primary thyroid lymphomas are localized stage I or II disease. The thyroid may occasionally be involved in patients with widespread systemic lymphoma. The response to steroids to alleviate stridor is strikingly dramatic and is also diagnostic of a lymphoma.

Anaplastic cancers

Anaplastic tumours are more common in elderly people and in women, and many of them are superimposed on a long standing enlargement of the thyroid gland, which then begins to increase in size rapidly and is accompanied with referred pain to the ear and hoarseness. These tumours are aggressively malignant and have a high metastatic potential. They rapidly invade surrounding structures, such as the larynx, pharynx and oesophagus, and carry a uniformly bleak prognosis. Treatment is often ineffective and the overwhelming majority of patients are dead within 1 year of presentation.

Histologically, anaplastic or undifferentiated thyroid cancers have no characteristic architecture and resemble normal thyroid cells. Traditionally, they have been divided into the following two categories, depending on the predominant cell morphology: (i) The uncommon small cell carcinoma, and (ii) the spindle and giant cell carcinoma. The more common, latter category has a wide variety of histological patterns. The differential diagnosis includes lymphoma, sarcoma, spindle cell medullary cancer and metastatic cancer. The kidney and the breasts are the most common sites for neoplasms metastatizing to the thyroid.

Evaluation of thyroid nodule

While evaluating a thyroid nodule, one needs to consider several factors such as age, sex, onset, rapidity of growth, pain, thyroid dysfunction, etc. Summarily giving any algorithm would expose situational inadequacies and demand mature experienced individualized decision-making. However, the judicious application of imaging modalities and FNAC, coupled with astute clinical examination and history, is the best method of diagnosis. Radioisotope scanning is generally regarded as a surveillance tool and as an adjunct to diagnosing a solid follicular neoplasia with a 'high-risk' clinical status. Analytical biochemistry and assays also have little diagnostic application, yet they are useful for post-operative management. Although ultrasonography (USG), computed tomography (CT) and magnetic resonance imaging (MRI) have immense diagnostic applications, the scope and objective of these techniques must be understood. These techniques are used essentially to determine the physical character of the nodule and the surrounding architecture, be it within the thyroid gland itself or in its adjoining soft tissues, i.e. muscle, trachea, larynx, vessels, nerve and pharyngo-oesophagus. FNAB, on the other hand, highlights the biology of the pathology. A

The lateral release

This procedure entails unwrapping the gland and mobilizing it from the carotid fascia. The middle thyroid vein and the fourth vein of Kocher are divided, but should this not be feasible, it is best to perform this step by the operator standing on the opposite side of the lobe to be excised.

Managing the upper pole

Here the crucial skills are to leave no thyroid tissue behind and save the external branch of the superior laryngeal nerve. This is best achieved by skeletonizing the vessels, superior thyroid artery and vein. This will also save the branch that supplies the superior parathyroid gland.

Managing the recurrent laryngeal nerve

Whereas it is mandatory to demonstrate the recurrent laryngeal nerve in all thyroid surgeries, caution should be exercised to avoid unnecessary dissection. The overlying fascia contains the microvasculature of the parathyroids and should not be violated. The recurrent laryngeal nerve can be identified by a below–upwards or lateral to medial approach by identifying the inferior thyroid artery as a leading landmark. However, the medial to lateral approach is more desirable, as the recurrent laryngeal nerve is identified at its entry into the larynx at the cricoarytenoid joint; it is minimally exposed to facilitate the surgery.

Managing the inferior thyroid artery

It is often ligated very close to the gland just before it enters the gland. It is our experience that with due care the terminal branch of the inferior thyroid artery can be seen anastomosing with its counterpart from the superior thyroid artery. Together they supply the parathyroids and must be saved.

Managing the inferior thyroid veins

These veins are numerous and should be saved until the last minute to minimize congestion of the gland. Rarely, one of the inferior thyroid veins may run parallel to the recurrent laryngeal nerve and cause concern. However, this problem can be resolved quickly, as the veins empty on stretch.

Managing the ligament of Berry

The ligament of Berry is a posterior condensation of the deep cervical fascia and needs to be divided. Rarely, the recurrent laryngeal nerve may pass through it and needs to be dissected carefully.

Division of the isthmus

The author removes the pyramidal lobe and the isthmus routinely in all cases of a hemi-thyroidectomy to avoid the unsightly hypertrophy of this thyroid tissue after this procedure. It is best to release the isthmus of its tracheal attachment so that the opposite lobe retracts in the lateral neck postoperatively.

References

1. Cusick EL, Krukowski ZH, MacIntosh CA, *et al.* Risk of neoplasia and malignancy in 'dormant' thyroid swellings. *BMJ* 1991;**303:** 20–2.
2. Witterick IJ, Abel SM, Noyek AM, *et al.* Non-palpable occult and metastatic papillary thyroid carcinoma. *Laryngoscope* 1993;**103:** 149–55.
3. Cerise EJ, Randall S, Ochsner A. Carcinoma of the thyroid and non-toxic nodular goiter. *Surgery* 1952;**31:**552–61.
4. Neumann S, Willgerodt H, Ackermann F, *et al.* Linkage of familial euthyroid goiter to the multinodular goiter-1 locus and exclusion of the candidate genes thyroglobulin, thyroperoxidase, and Na+/I-symporter. *J Clin Endocrinol Metab* 1999;**84:**3750–6.
5. Perez LA, Gupta PK, Mandel SJ, *et al.* Thyroid papillary microcarcinoma. Is it really a pitfall of fine needle aspiration cytology? *Acta Cytol* 2001;**45:**341–6.
6. Belfiore A, La Rosa GL, La Porta GA, *et al.* Cancer risk in patients with cold thyroid nodules: Relevance of iodine intake, sex, age, and multinodularity. *Am J Med* 1992;**93:**363–9.
7. Cusick EL, MacIntosh CA, Krukowski ZH, *et al.* Management of isolated thyroid swellings: A perspective six year study of the fine needle aspiration cytology in diagnosis. *BMJ* 1990;**301:**318–21.
8. Sugino K, Ito K Jr, Ozakio O, *et al.* Papillary microcarcinoma of the thyroid. *J Endocrinol Invest* 1998;**21:**445–8.
9. Mazzaferri EL, Jhiang SM. Long-term impact of initial surgical and medical therapy on papillary and follicular thyroid cancer. *Am J Med* 1994;**97:**418–28.
10. Vander JB, Gaston EA, Dawber TR. The significance of nontoxic thyroid nodules: Final report of a 15-year old study of the incidence of thyroid malignancy. *Ann Intern Med* 1968;**68:**537.
11. Bramley MD, Harrison BJ. Papillary microcarcinoma of the thyroid gland. *Br J Surg* 1996;**83:**1674–83.
12. Shah J. *Head and neck surgery and oncology.* 3rd ed. New York: Elsevier; 2003:395–429.
13. Koh KB, Chang KW. Carcinoma in multinodular goiter. *Br J Surg* 1992;**79:**266–7.
14. Castro MR, Gharib E. Thyroid nodules and cancer: When to wait and watch, when to refer. *Postgrad Med* 2000;**107:**113–24.
15. Turnbridge WMG, Evered DC, Hall R, *et al.* The spectrum of thyroid disease in a community: The Wickham survey. *Clin Endocrinol* 1977; 7:481–93.

17

Cancer of the major salivary glands

MADAN KAPRE

Parotid surgery involves dissection around the facial nerve which poses a challenge to a head and neck surgeon. Also, because the majority of parotid tumours are benign, inadvertent facial nerve injury during surgical resection of a tumour, with the resulting morbidity inflicted upon the patient, could cause much embarrassment to the surgeon and the patient alike.

Approximately 3%–6% of tumours in the head and neck region occur in salivary glands, approximately 70% of which occur in the parotid gland; 22% occur in minor salivary glands and only 8% in the submandibular salivary gland (Fig. 1).[1] It is pertinent to note that 75% of parotid tumours are benign, whereas 80% of the tumours of the minor salivary glands are malignant (Fig. 2). In a review of the Memorial Sloan Kettering experience with salivary neoplasms over a 35-year period, benign tumours accounted for 54% and malignant tumours for 46% of all salivary gland tumours. Pleomorphic adenoma was the most common benign tumour, while mucoepidermoid carcinoma was the most common malignant tumour.[1] The biology of the tumour is such that the larger the salivary gland the more benign the tumour, and the smaller the salivary gland the more malignant the tumour.

Anatomy of the parotid gland

The parotid gland is described as having a superficial lobe and a deep lobe with an isthmus in between. These lobes are separated by the facial nerve, which runs through the gland. The facial nerve is surrounded by parotid tissue and intimately attached on all sides to glandular tissue. A sizable number of anatomists categorically deny the existence of the deep and superficial lobes as two distinct entities, suggesting

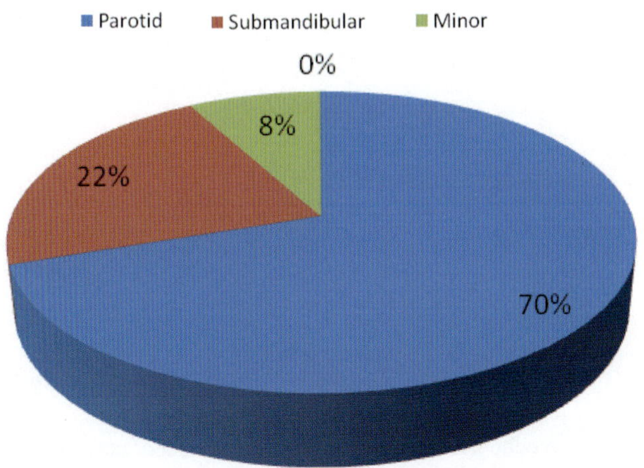

Fig. 1. Site of origin of salivary gland tumours

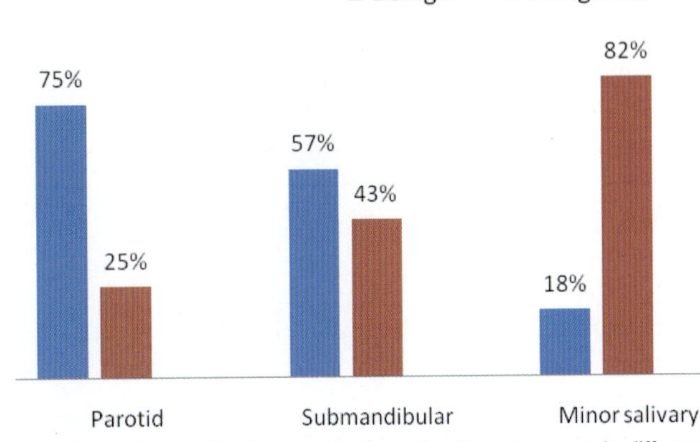

Fig. 2. Incidence of benign and malignant salivary tumours in different sites of origin

that division into two lobes is a myth created by surgeons.

The parotid gland extends from the zygoma superiorly to the oblique line of the sternocleidomastoid inferiorly and anteriorly to the midpoint of the masseter muscle. The parotid duct (Stensen duct) runs over the anterior border of the masseter muscle to enter the mouth opposite the second molar tooth in the interdental line. The gland is covered by the investing fascia of the neck. There are 6–8 lymph nodes outside this fascia and 10–12 lymph nodes embedded in the glandular tissue, largely in the superficial lobe. Very few nodes are present in the deep lobe.

The deep lobe of the parotid gland—the retromandibular portion—lies in the parapharyngeal space anterior to the carotid sheath and styloid process, and posterior to the infratemporal fossa. Medial to the deep lobe is the superior constrictor muscle, separating it from the tonsil and oropharynx. Tumours may extend deeply into the lateral parapharyngeal space either by passing through the narrow space between the mandible and stylomandibular ligament or by passing behind the ligament.

The key to conservative parotid surgery is total preservation of the facial nerve and its branches, making a detailed knowledge of the anatomy of this region mandatory (Fig. 3). The commonest method of identification is to locate the nerve at the point where it emerges from the skull base at the stylomastoid foramen. The following markers may be used:

- The most reliable landmark is the tympanomastoid groove, formed by the anterior part of the mastoid and the edge of the bony external auditory meatus (EAM). The facial nerve bisects the apex of this groove 5 mm below the bony meatal edge. It then passes forwards, downwards and laterally, where it occurs immediately above the upper border of the posterior belly of the digastric muscle, and lateral and slightly posterior to the base of the styloid process.
- The main trunk of the facial nerve lies 1–1.5 cm inferior and deep to the tragal 'pointer', which is the antero-inferior edge of the tragal cartilage.
- Branches of the nerve can be found peripherally and traced proximally. Usually, the marginal mandibular branch is identified where it crosses the posterior facial vein at the tail of the gland; it can then be traced proximally to the lower division.

This, in the author's opinion, is labour-intensive. Where difficulty arises in nerve identification (such as in large malignant tumours), the best way to find the facial nerve is by opening the mastoid.

The presence of a tumour dictates the location of the facial nerve. A deep lobe tumour would force the nerve more superficially and *vice versa*. Imaging modalities may help to resolve the issue and assist the surgeon pre-operatively. The greater auricular nerve lies on the deep cervical fascia, which invests the sternomastoid muscle and inclines upwards to cross the superficial aspect of the parotid gland. It can be used in collaboration with other branches of the cervical plexus for free cable grafts in facial-nerve reconstruction.

Vasculature of the parotid

The posterior facial vein traverses the deep lobe of the gland from above downwards, lying immediately medial or deep to the branches of the facial nerve. Maintenance of the deep parotid vein as well as avoiding early ligation of the external jugular vein avoids congestion of the parotid, and thereby reduces embarrassing bleeding during dissection (Fig. 4).

Clinical features

Parotid swellings of inflammatory aetiology occur as a uniform enlargement obliterating the post-aural sulcus and lifting the pinna. These swellings may be tender or bilateral, depending on the causative pathology. They do not require surgical intervention except occasionally, fine needle aspiration cytology (FNAC) or open biopsy. An abscess of the parotid gland may not produce fluctuance due to the firmness of the enveloping fascia; nevertheless, drainage via a standard parotidectomy incision is mandatory if it does not respond to antibiotics within 48 hours.

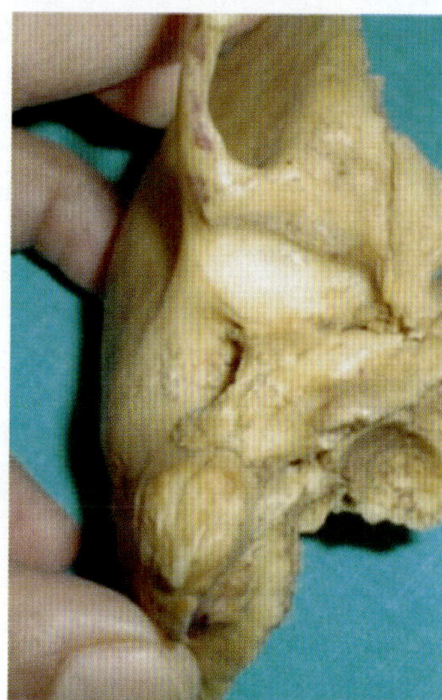

Fig. 3. Relevance of tympanomastoid suture and stylomastoid foramen

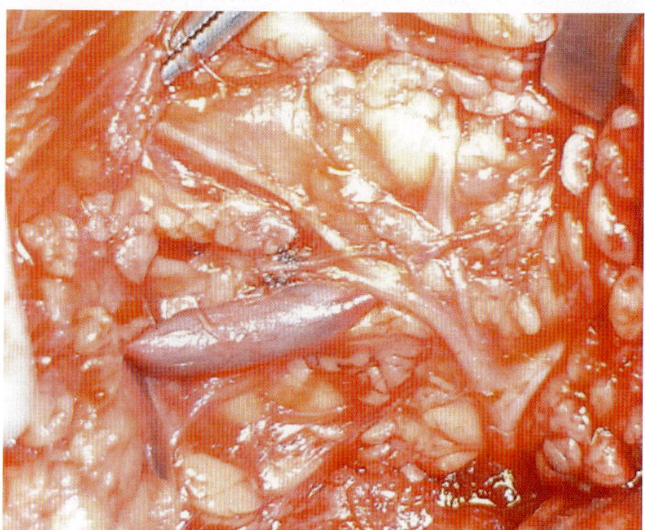

Fig. 4. The deep parotid vein lies always at a deeper plane than the facial nerve

The usual clinical presentation of a tumour of salivary gland origin is the presence of a mass. The majorities of parotid tumours arise in the superficial lobe and present as a rubbery nodular mass. Most benign mixed tumours are asymptomatic. Involvement of the facial nerve or its peripheral branches needs full pre-operative assessment, as it has much relevance to pathology of the tumour and also to the treatment outcome. Facial paralysis does not occur with benign mixed tumours, regardless of the size of the tumour. Enlarged ipsilateral cervical lymph nodes or the presence of facial nerve dysfunction or invasions of the overlying skin are almost invariably suggestive of a malignant tumour. Tumours in the deep lobe of the parotid gland usually present with diffuse enlargement and fullness in the retromandibular portion of the gland. At times, these may present as an oropharyngeal bulge. Radiographic studies are essential to delineate accurately the location of the deep lobe tumour. Swelling of the soft palate associated with a parotid mass is diagnostic of a tumour originating in the deep lobe of the parotid gland. Occasionally, a tumour may arise in accessory parotid tissue along the course of the Stensen duct and may present as a mass in the soft tissues of the mid-portion of the cheek.

Metastatic tumours to the parotid gland are usually from primary cutaneous malignant lesions of the scalp and forehead, such as squamous carcinomas and melanomas; and rarely haematogenous metastases from lung, kidney, or breast. These constitute important differential diagnostic entities.

Aetiopathology of parotid tumours

According to the multicellular theory,[2] each type of salivary gland tumour arises from a distinctive cell type. Thus, Warthin tumour, oncocytic tumour, mucoepidermoid or squamous cell carcinomas (SCCs) arise from the striated ductal cells, acinic tumour from the acinar cells, and pleomorphic adenomas and myoepithelial carcinomas from the intercalated duct cells. On the other hand, the bicellular theory assumes that the various types of salivary gland tumours arise from the basal cells of either the excretory or the intercalated duct.[3] Evidence is accumulating that Epstein–Barr virus (EBV) may be associated with parotid tumours, particularly lymphoepithelial carcinoma.[4,5]

Radiographic evaluation

Diagnostic imaging studies are seldom necessary in the evaluation of salivary gland neoplasms, unless the patient presents with a deep-seated or a fixed lesion, whence invasion into adjacent structures becomes a matter of concern. The goals of imaging studies are to delineate accurately the location and extent of the tumour and to identify whether the lesion is intraglandular or has extraglandular extension. Plain X-rays, sialography, nuclear scans and ultrasonography

(USG) add very little to the diagnostic information and are seldom indicated. A better utility for ultrasound is in guiding FNAC. On the other hand, computerized tomography (CT) and magnetic resonance imaging (MRI) permit better visualization of masses within the salivary glands. CT and MRI are equally satisfactory in differentiating cystic from solid lesions and allow evaluation of the relationship of the mass to the major salivary gland or adjacent structures, including soft tissues and bones. Both can be used to assess perineural spread. CT scan is cheaper, widely available and better for assessment of bone destruction and skull base. MRI, though more expensive, is superior to CT scan in assessment of early perineural spread, deep lobe tumours, parapharyngeal space extension or intracranial extension. Deep lobe tumours lie in the prestyloid compartment and characteristically displace the parapharyngeal fat medially.

Fine-needle aspiration cytology

The overall sensitivity of FNAC ranges from 85.5% to 99%, and the overall specificity ranges from 96.3% to 100%.[6–8] Accuracy is greater for benign rather than malignant pathologies. FNAC diagnosis may be very useful in pre-operative counselling of the patient about the nature of the tumour and explaining the treatment aspects such as the extent of surgery, the management of the facial nerve or the need for a neck dissection. Certain disadvantages of FNAC in parotid tumours are: Difficulty in differentiating a low-grade malignancy and benign tumour, false-negative diagnosis and inflammation or fibrosis at the site making the dissection more difficult.

Benign tumours of the parotid

Although several benign tumours occur in the parotid gland, such as pleomorphic adenoma, Warthin tumour, oncocytoma, cysts, vascular malformation and tumours of other tissues (nerves, collagen, etc.), only the commoner ones are discussed in this chapter.

Pleomorphic adenoma

This is the most common tumour of the major salivary glands. Around 84% of benign parotid tumours are pleomorphic adenomas.[1] The ratio of men to women is 1:1 with an average age of 40 years at presentation. A few bilateral tumours have been described.

Mixed-cell tumours arise from intercalated duct cells and myoepithelial cells.

Warthin tumour

This is also known as 'adenolymphoma'; its incidence is 6%–8% of salivary gland tumours. It arises in heterotopic parotid tissue occurring within parotid lymph nodes, usually in the parotid tail. These tumours are never malignant. The male to female incidence is 7:1 and the average age at presentation is 70 years. Approximately 10% of these tumours are bilateral. Clinically, the tumour appears as a fluctuant, slow-growing, smooth, not bosselated, soft and compressible swelling. Cystic ones contain mucoid fluid whereas the solid ones have a lymphoid component. The solid white areas seen occasionally are because of lymphoid tissue.

Oncocytoma

Oncocytoma comprises only 1% of all salivary gland tumours; it is also known as 'oxyphil cell adenoma'. It arises from striated duct cells and the malignant variants are exceedingly rare. The incidence is equal in males and females and its occurrence is rare before 50 years of age. Clinically, it appears as a painless, slow-growing lump.

Malignant tumours of the parotid

Primary malignant tumours occur rarely in the parotid gland. Facial nerve paralysis spells the diagnosis on clinical examination. The tumours could be mucoepidermoid carcinoma, acinic cell carcinoma, adenoid cystic carcinoma, adenocarcinoma, and carcinoma ex-pleomorphic adenoma. SCCs, lymphoma, lymphoepithelial carcinoma and sarcomas are rarely seen.

Pathology of malignant tumours

Mucoepidermoid tumour

Mucoepidermoid carcinoma is the commonest salivary gland malignancy accounting for 34%–36% of malignant tumours. It is also the commonest salivary gland malignancy in children. These are most commonly encountered in the parotid gland (70%), followed by the minor salivary glands (25%) and submandibular gland (5%). It comprises 4%–9% of salivary tumours; the male to female ratio is 1:1. It usually presents in the fifth decade of life. It may be solid or cystic and is usually not encapsulated.

Mucoepidermoid carcinoma may be classified into low grade, intermediate grade and high grade tumours. High-grade tumours have a higher incidence of nodal involvement, loco-regional recurrence, distant metastasis and a worse prognosis than low-grade tumour. Forty per cent of cases present with lymphadenopathy, and if the tumour is high grade, the 5-year survival rate is about 40%.[9]

Acinic cell tumour

This tumour comprises 2.5%–4% of all parotid tumours, and is sometimes bilateral. It arises from the terminal tubular intercalated duct cells and is often encapsulated. The male to female ratio is 1:1 with a peak in the fifth decade of life. It is

also the second most common salivary tumour in children. Most of these tumours behave like pleomorphic adenomas. However, some of them have an aggressive malignant course. The 5-year survival rate is 85%, and the 15-year survival rate is 65%.[10] It has a propensity for late recurrence, even 30 years after excision. Nearly 15% of recurrences have regional lymphadenopathy, and 15% have distant metastases.

Adenoid cystic carcinoma

Adenoid cystic carcinoma is the second most common salivary gland tumour. This tumour is slightly more common in females than in males with a median age at presentation in the sixth decade. It comprises approximately 40% of malignant tumours at all salivary sites. The minor salivary glands are the more common site, with adenoid cystic carcinomas making up 71% of tumours arising in the minor salivary glands.[11] The most probable source of origin is the intercalated ducts. Four main pathological patterns are recognized: cribriform, tubuloglandular, solid cellular and cylindromatous. The cribriform pattern has a glandular architecture and is reported to have the best prognosis.[12] The solid pattern is more epithelial in nature and is associated with a poorer prognosis. The tubular pattern has a clinical prognosis of intermediate nature between the other two patterns. Eight per cent of cases present with lymphadenopathy, whereas 7% have a late node appearance. The tumour is unencapsulated but appears circumscribed. It is moist and grey–pink on section, with an infiltrative growth pattern. It also has a marked tendency to invade nerves, and is associated with a high frequency of pain. The characteristics of adenoid cystic carcinoma are slow growth, neurotropism, late local recurrence and distant metastases. Neurotropic spread may lead to recurrences at the skull base.

Adenocarcinoma

This tumour comprises around 3% of parotid tumours. The gender incidence is equal and it can occur at any age. It may present as an asymptomatic mass or with typical malignant features. In the parotid, most adenocarcinomas occur in the deep lobe or extend beyond the gland when first seen. They are highly metastatic and the 5-year survival is only 10%.

Carcinoma ex-pleomorphic adenoma

The majority of these tumours arise from a pre-existing pleomorphic adenoma; only 1% arise *ab initio*. The malignancy takes about 10 years to develop into an adenoma. About 1%–5% of pleomorphic adenomas that are present for more than 10 years may become malignant. However, the tumour may still be grossly encapsulated. The suspicious features are pain, its rapid growth spurt, excessive bosselation and infiltration at the periphery. The rate of metastasis to the regional lymph nodes is 25%, and distant metastases occur in 30% of cases. The 5-year survival is around 40%, and 15-year survival is 19%.

Squamous cell carcinoma (SCC)

SCC is extremely rare in the parotid, and comprises only about 1% of tumours. The male-to-female ratio is 2:1 with average age of presentation being in the seventh decade. It is an aggressive tumour with no tendency for encapsulation. It grows rapidly, causing pain, facial nerve paralysis, skin fixation and ulceration. Approximately 50% of patients have metastatic neck nodes at presentation. SCC has a very poor prognosis, irrespective of the treatment modality used.

Histological assessment

Though an accurate pre-operative histological assessment is helpful in patient counselling and treatment planning, it should not dictate the surgeon's decision about the extent of resection or the sacrifice of critical structures. It is true that an experienced cytologist will give histological diagnosis in almost 95% of cases. Rarely, an open biopsy is indicated, either externally or intra-orally. It is obvious that such an open biopsy site will need to be included in future excisions.

Staging of primary salivary gland tumours (AJCC 7ed, 2010)[13]

Primary Tumour (T)

Tx Primary tumour cannot be assessed

T0 No evidence of primary tumour

T1 Tumour 2 cm or less in greatest dimension without extraparenchymal extension*

T2 Tumour more than 2 cm but not more than 4 cm in greatest dimension without extraparenchymal extension*

T3 Tumour more than 4 cm and/or tumour having extraparenchymal extension*

T4a Moderately advanced disease
Tumour invades skin, mandible, ear canal, and/or facial nerve

T4b Very advanced disease
Tumour invades skull base and/or pterygoid plates and/or encases carotid artery.

*Note: Extraparenchymal extension is clinical or macroscopic evidence of invasion of soft tissues. Microscopic evidence alone does not constitute extraparenchymal extension for classification purposes.

Regional Lymph Nodes (N)

Nx Regional lymph nodes cannot be assessed

N0 No regional lymph node metastasis

N1 Metastasis in a single ipsilateral lymph node, 3 cm or less in greatest dimension

N2 Metastasis in a single ipsilateral lymph node, more than 3 cm but not more than 6 cm in greatest dimension, or in multiple ipsilateral lymph nodes, none more than 6 cm in greatest dimension, or in bilateral or contra lateral lymph nodes, none more than 6 cm in greatest dimension

N2a Metastasis in a single ipsilateral lymph nodes, more than 3 cm but not more than 6 cm in greatest dimension

N2b Metastasis in multiple ipsilateral lymph nodes, none more than 6 cm in greatest dimension

N2c Metastasis in bilateral or contralateral lymph nodes, none more than 6 cm in greatest dimension

N3 Metastasis in a lymph node, more than 6 cm in greatest dimension.

Distant Metastasis (M)

M0 No distant metastasis

M1 Distant metastasis

(Used with the permission of the American Joint Committee on Cancer (AJCC), Chicago, Illinois. The original source for this material is the *AJCC Cancer Staging Manual*, Seventh Edition (2010) published by Springer Science and Business Media LLC, www.springer.com.)

Treatment strategy of parotid tumours

The following factors need to be considered while deciding the optimum surgical procedure for parotid tumours:

- Histology and grading of the tumour
- Tumour's propensity to disseminate, particularly along nerves, as in adenoid cystic tumours
- Location of the tumour within gland
- Involvement of facial nerve
- Involvement of adjoining soft tissues
- Presence of metastatic neck nodes.

Choice of surgical procedure

Since most of the parotid tumours are located in the tail of the parotid in the superficial lobe and are benign or low stage and low grade, a simple superficial parotidectomy would be adequate. It is customary to perform a very wide excision sacrificing all the involved tissue, along with a total parotidectomy, for extremely advanced lesions, in which adjoining bone, skin, muscles and nerves are involved. In high grade, high stage malignancies, very wide excision sacrificing all the involved tissue along with total parotidectomy would be the order.

The dilemma occurs when malignancies do not involve the facial nerve. In such cases the uninvolved facial nerve should not be sacrificed except when the diagnosis is adenoid cystic carcinoma and/or when perineural spread is evident on MRI. In these situations every attempt should be made to cable graft the nerve with the adjoining great auricular nerve, or perform any similar procedure, according to the availability of resources.

Management of neck nodes

It is not common for a parotid malignant tumour to present with neck node metastasis. However, it is good practice to sample the level II nodes as a preliminary surgical step, even in the N0 neck, and plan a suitable neck dissection for a given case. In a patient with high grade mucoepidermoid carcinoma or squamous cell carcinoma, elective neck dissection has been advocated by several authors.[14,15] Adenocarcinoma is best treated surgically and hence primary elective neck dissection is well recommended. Occasionally, and for practical reasons, if the lower neck is to be exposed (such as for a reconstructive procedure), it is correct to carry out a modified or conservative neck dissection. Thus, the indications for elective neck dissection would be:

- Tumours >4 cm in size
- High-grade tumours (SCC, undifferentiated carcinoma, adenocarcinoma, high-grade mucoepidermoid carcinoma)
- Large tail of parotid tumours in which a neck dissection would facilitate exposure.

Radiation therapy

Most of the parotid tumours are conventionally thought to be radio-resistant, and hence radiation therapy as a primary choice of treatment is not the standard of care. Exceptions are made. of course, for very advanced, inaccessible disease. Disease involving base of skull, lateral pharyngeal wall or base of tongue would require an extensive procedure with unacceptable morbidity. However, in advanced cases post-operative radiation therapy is practised with good results in several centres.[16,17] For adenoid cystic carcinoma, neutron beam radiotherapy is strongly advocated by some authors.[18]

Traditionally, external beam therapy is practised in most centres, but availability of intensity-modulated radiation therapy (IMRT) has considerably reduced radiation-induced morbidity. The indications of post-operative radiotherapy in salivary gland malignancy would include:

- High-grade tumours
- Close or positive margins
- Facial nerve involvement
- Perineural spread
- Bone involvement
- Lymph node metastasis
- Extranodal spread
- Recurrent disease

Treatment outcome

For benign parotid tumours, successful surgical excision is performed with almost 95% success rate. Only 5% show local recurrence, which can be adequately excised at a revision surgery, albeit with increased risk of facial nerve injury. In selected cases, neutron beam on IMRT could be considered.

However, there is a genuine incidence of malignant transformation; hence injudicious post-operative radiation therapy for adequately excised benign tumour should be avoided.

For the outcome of malignant tumours, clinical stage of the disease is the single most prognostic determinant for all histological subtypes of parotid tumours.[19] Acinic cell tumours carry the best prognosis, whereas squamous cell carcinoma and adenoid cystic carcinoma are among the poor performers. Long-term survival is determined by histological grading of adenocarcinoma or mucoepidermoid carcinoma.

Clinical staging is the real determinant of outcome in adenoid cystic carcinoma. Although the first recurrence may be delayed for several years, subsequent recurrences are rapid and quickly become surgically unresectable.

Pearls in surgery of parotid

Because of the variations in surgical techniques dictated by the disease itself and the surgeon's own preferences, a detailed discussion on surgery on parotid tumours is beyond the scope of this chapter. However, the routine steps that are recommended, and the author's personal preference on surgical technique, are described briefly.

Recommended incision for large parotid tumour

The incision is made from the tragus, running parallel and occasionally dipping in the external auditory meatus and gently curving around the pinna while staying well behind the angle of the mandible, and then running parallel to it for a variable length (Fig. 5). This incision has three components—cartilaginous, fibrous and muscular. Flaps are raised deep to skin in the face and deep to platysma in the neck. Anteriorly, the flaps are raised until the anterior border of the parotid

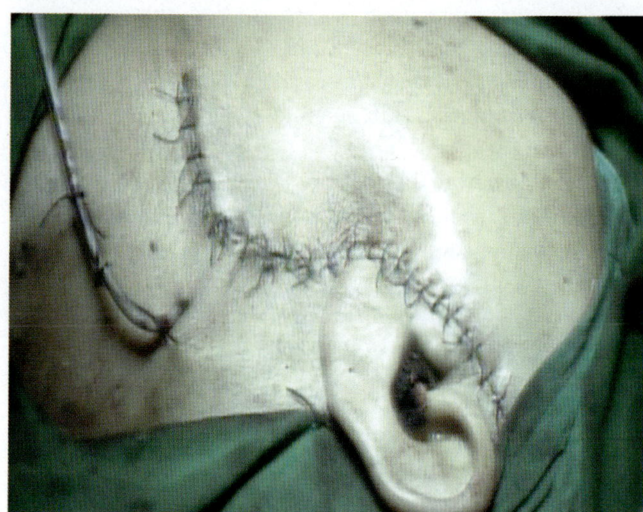

Fig. 5. Incision and initial exposure

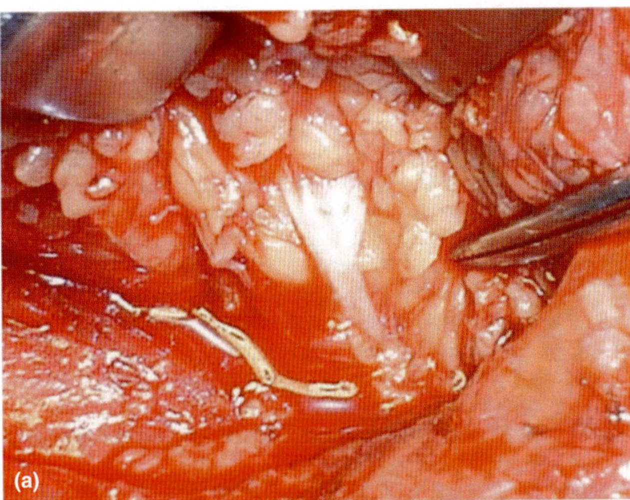

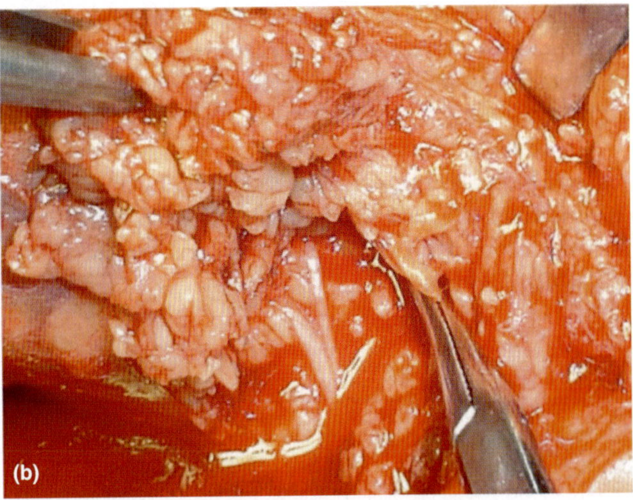

Fig. 6. Identifying the facial nerve

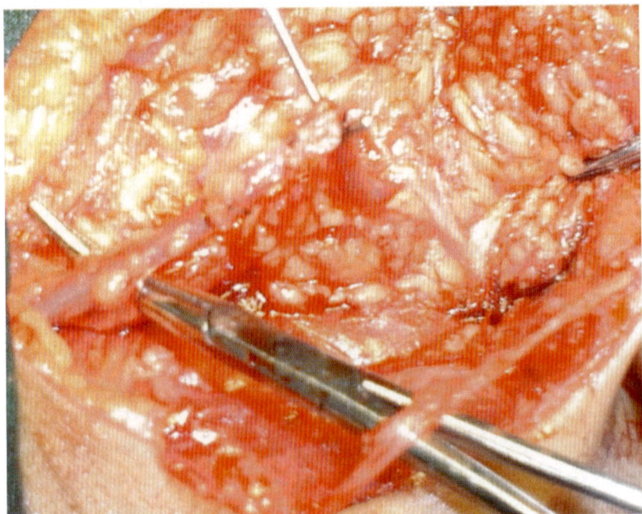

Fig. 7. Superficial parotidectomy completed with deep parotid vein auricle nerve and facial nerve

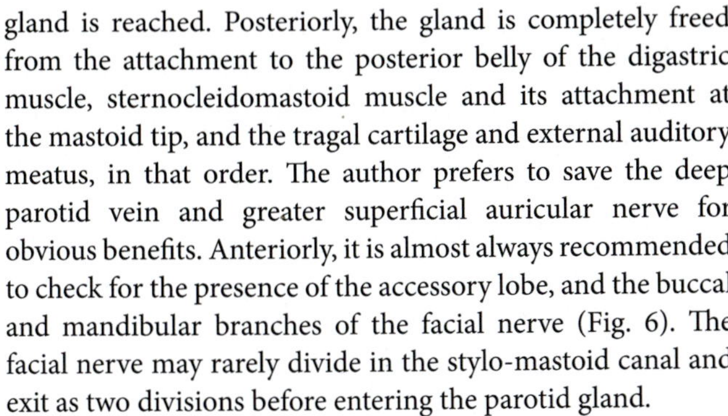

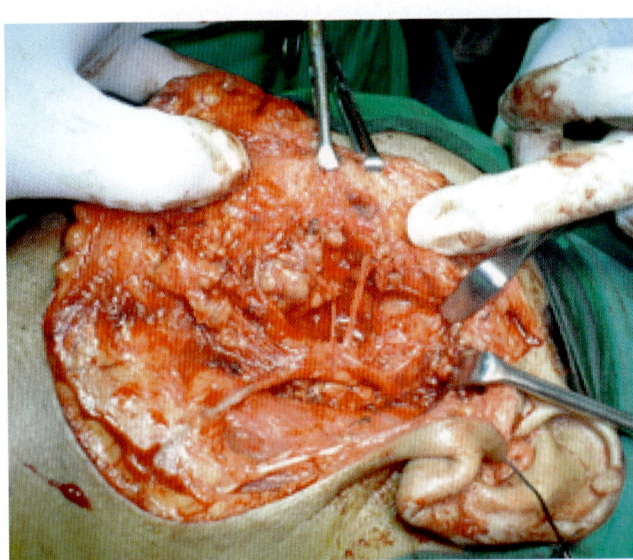

Fig. 8. Dissecting the deep lobe tumour

gland is reached. Posteriorly, the gland is completely freed from the attachment to the posterior belly of the digastric muscle, sternocleidomastoid muscle and its attachment at the mastoid tip, and the tragal cartilage and external auditory meatus, in that order. The author prefers to save the deep parotid vein and greater superficial auricular nerve for obvious benefits. Anteriorly, it is almost always recommended to check for the presence of the accessory lobe, and the buccal and mandibular branches of the facial nerve (Fig. 6). The facial nerve may rarely divide in the stylo-mastoid canal and exit as two divisions before entering the parotid gland.

One cannot overemphasize the old saying: 'Look for the facial nerve outside the parotid gland'. Hence, the cornerstone of the surgical procedure is to completely release the gland posteriorly of all its attachments. Various surgical landmarks have been described earlier in this text. The author's own recommended surgical landmarks are the tympanomastoid

suture and the attachment of the posterior belly of the digastric muscle. The nerve emerges within 5 mm of this bisection and moves forwards and superficially to bisect the parotid gland (Fig. 7). Modern imaging techniques will come to the surgeons' aid in locating the tumour in relation to the facial nerve; their use preoperatively is strongly recommended.

Managing deep lobe parotid tumours

If the pathology of the parotid tumour is ascertained as benign, it is appropriate to complete a superficial parotidectomy and then deliver the deep lobe tumour between the branches of the facial nerve (Fig. 8). In cases where the pathology is known to be malignant, the recommended procedure is total parotidectomy, but the facial nerve poses a special concern. The author recommends that all the functioning facial nerves be saved and only those that are paralysed preoperatively should be sacrificed. Because of the propensity of adenoidcystic carcinoma for perineural spread, it is best to excise the nerve for long-term safety, with prior consultation with the patient.

In all cases of facial nerve excision, the nerve should be replaced by a greater auricular nerve graft in a suitable manner. The insertion of a gold weight in the upper lid immediately post-operatively achieves good cosmetic rehabilitation and is advisable.

References

1. Spiro RH. Salivary neoplasms: Overview of a 35-year experience with 2,807 patients. *Head Neck Surg* 1986;**8**:177–84.
2. Dardick I. Mounting evidence against current histogenetic concepts for salivary gland tumorigenesis. *Eur J Morphol* 1998;**36**:257–61.
3. Batsakis JG, Regezi JA. The pathology of head and neck tumors: Salivary glands, part 1. *Head Neck Surg* 1978;**1**:59–68.
4. Tsai CC, Chen CL, Hsu HC. Expression of Epstein–Barr virus in carcinomas of major salivary glands: A strong association with lymphoepithelioma-like carcinoma. *Hum Pathol* 1996;**27**:258–62.
5. Leung SY, Chung LP, Yuen ST, *et al.* Lymphoepithelial carcinoma of the salivary gland: *In situ* detection of Epstein–Barr virus. *J Clin Pathol* 1995;**48**:1022–7.
6. Al-Khafaji BM, Afify AM. Salivary gland fine needle aspiration using the ThinPrep technique: Diagnostic accuracy, cytologic artifacts and pitfalls. *Acta Cytologica* 2001;**45**:567–74.
7. Stewart CJ, MacKenzieK, McGarry GW. Fine-needle aspiration cytology of salivary gland: A review of 341 cases. *Diagn Cytopathol* 2000;**22**:139–46.
8. Michael CW, Hunter B. Interpretation of fine-needle aspirates processed by the ThinPrep technique: Cytologic artifacts and diagnostic pitfalls. *Diagn Cytopathol* 2000;**23**:6–13.
9. Clode AL, FonsecaI, Santos JR, *et al.* Mucoepidermoid carcinoma of the salivary glands: A reappraisal of the influence of tumor differentiation on prognosis. *J Surg Oncol* 1991;**46**:100–6.
10. Spiro RH, Huvos AG, Strong EW. Acinic cell carcinoma of salivary origin: A clinicopathologic study of 67 cases. *Cancer* 1978;**41**:924.
11. Spiro RH. Distant metastasis in adenoid cystic carcinoma of salivary origin. *Am J Surg* 1997;**174**:495.
12. Fordice J, Kershaw C, El-Naggar A. Adenoid cystic carcinoma of the head and neck. Predictors of morbidity and mortality. *Arch Otolaryngol Head Neck Surg* 1999;**125**:149.
13. Edge SB, Byrd DR, Compton CC (eds). *AJCC Cancer Staging Manual.* 7th ed. New York, NY: Springer; 2010:80.
14. Kelly DJ, Spiro RH. Management of the neck in parotid carcinoma. *Am J Surg* 1996;**172**:695.
15. Armstrong JG, Harrison LB, Thaler HT. The indications for elective treatment of the neck in cancer of the major salivary glands. *Cancer* 1992;**69**:615.
16. Armstrong JG, Harrison LB, Spiro RH. Malignant tumors of major salivary origin: A matched-pair analysis of the role of combined surgery and postoperative radiotherapy. *Arch Otolaryngol Head Neck Surg* 1990;**116**:290.
17. Spiro RH, Armstrong J, Harrison L. Carcinoma of major salivary glands: Recent trends. *Arch Otolaryngol Head Neck Surg* 1989;**115**:316.
18. Laramore GE, Krall JM, Griffin TW. Neutron versus photon irradiation for unresectable salivary gland tumors: Final report of an RTOG-MRC randomized clinical trial. *Int J Radiat Oncol Biol Phys* 1993;**27**:235.
19. Frankenthaler RA. Prognostic variables in parotid gland cancer. *Arch Otolaryngol Head Neck Surg* 1991;**117**:1251–6.

18

Cancer of the skull base

C. RAYAPPA, K. KUMARESH

Tumours that arise from the skull base or from various neighbouring structures were, in the past, considered inoperable and therefore incurable. Although a wide variety of tumours arise in this region, they share common problems, namely, their inaccessibility because of the difficulty of accurately defining the extent of the lesion radiologically, complex regional anatomy, proximity to adjacent neurovascular structures, and the fear of causing life-threatening complications.

The skull base was the watershed, which separated the areas of work of neurosurgeons and ENT surgeons. Today, the collaborative work of ENT surgeons, neurosurgeons and plastic surgeons has given rise to many innovative approaches to the skull base for resecting these tumours, as well as for reconstruction of the complex defects created at the skull base.

In the past 2 decades, considerable progress has been made in the management of skull base tumours, both in terms of diagnosis and treatment. With the introduction of CT in the 1970s and the later introduction of MRI, surgeons are now able to determine the size and extent of the tumour and its relationship to the neurovascular structures. This helps the surgeon to determine the operability and the possible risks involved in the planned resection. Significant progress in neuroanaesthetic techniques, and the ability to intra-operatively monitor cranial nerve and brain functions, have all played a big role in the development of skull base surgery. Microvascular free tissue transfer has made it possible to reconstruct large defects in the skull base after tumour resection.

The skull base is closely related to the cranial as well as facial structures. To reach a desired section of the skull base, one or both of these compartments have to be displaced. Operative displacement produces oedema of the affected structures. Facial swelling is self-limiting with minimal long-term consequences. Excessive and prolonged brain retraction causes oedema and contusion of the brain. This neurovascular injury can lead to loss of consciousness and seizure. Therefore, in skull base surgery, the amount of brain retraction is reduced by temporarily or permanently removing the facial structures to expose these tumours.

Craniofacial resection was first described by Smith and colleagues[1] in 1954. During the same period, Parsons and colleagues[2] described en bloc resection of tumours of the temporal bone. Almost a decade later, in 1963, Ketcham and colleagues[3] performed craniofacial resection on a series of 29 patients with sinonasal tumours involving the anterior cranial base, with good results.

Successful skull base surgery depends not only on the coordination of the skull base team but also on expert nursing care. Surgery has become the optimal treatment modality for most of the tumours of the skull base because of the coordinated efforts of various members of the team.

Advances in radiotherapy, including proton therapy, neutron therapy, intensity-modulated radiation therapy (IMRT), and stereotactic radiosurgery are important adjuncts for the curative therapy of patients with malignant tumours of the skull base, and/or palliative treatment of inoperable patients. These advanced approaches have a reduced incidence of complications compared with conventional radiation therapy.

Surgical anatomy

Skull base anatomy is complex, and for effective surgical treatment the performing surgeon should understand the

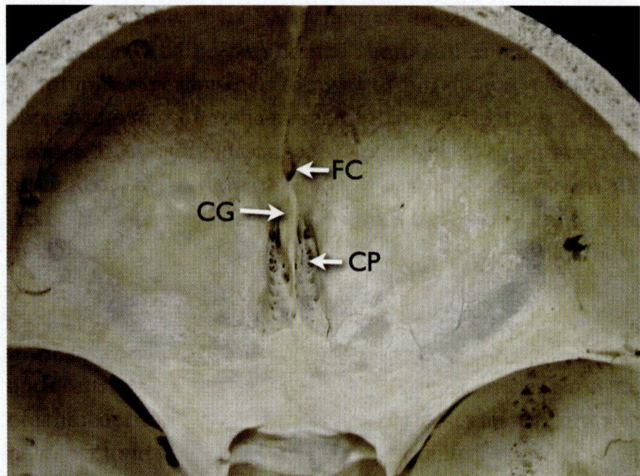

Fig. 1. Floor of anterior cranial fossa
FC foramen caecum   CG crista galli   CP cribriform plate of ethmoid

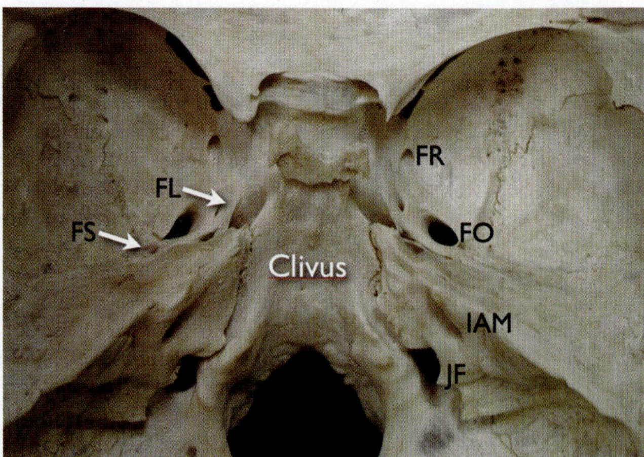

Fig. 2. Floor of middle and posterior cranial fossa
FR foramen rotundum   FO foramen ovale   FL foramen lacerum
FS foramen spinosum   IAM internal auditory meatus   JF jugular foramen

three-dimensional topography and anatomy of the region in both the normal and diseased conditions. The skull base that forms the floor of the cranial cavity and separates the brain from facial structures is composed of five bones, viz. the ethmoid, sphenoid, occipital, paired temporal and paired frontal bones. It can be divided into three compartments, viz. anterior, middle, and posterior cranial fossae.

Anterior cranial base

The anterior cranial base is bound anteriorly by the frontal bone, which contains two surgically important structures, viz. the frontal sinus and the supraorbital foramina. The frontal sinus is extremely variable in size and extent. This must be taken into account in most anterior skull base operations. The supraorbital foramina, which may be incomplete in some individuals, transmit the supraorbital nerves and vessels. These vessels must be preserved if the galea and pericranium are to be used in the reconstruction of anterior cranial base defects.

Intracranially, the anterior cranial base is formed by the frontal, ethmoid, and sphenoid bones. There are several landmarks in the intracranial side (Fig. 1). The most anterior of these is the foramen caecum, which usually ends blindly. When it is patent, it can be a site of developmental anomalies, such as nasal dermoid cysts, nasal gliomas, encephaloceles, and meningoencephaloceles. The next anatomical landmark is the crista galli, which protrudes upward from the midline to provide attachment for the falx cerebri. On either side of the crista are the many openings in the cribriform plate, which transmit the olfactory nerves inferiorly. Just posterior to the last of these olfactory foramina is a smooth-surfaced area known as the planum sphenoidale. It forms the roof of the sphenoid sinus. The anterior clinoid processes and lesser sphenoid wings delineate the most posterior limit of the anterior cranial base.

Extracranially, the anterior cranial base is related to the nasal cavity, the ethmoid and sphenoid sinuses, and the orbits. The anterior and posterior ethmoid foramina transmit the anterior and posterior ethmoid arteries. These ethmoid foramina mark the position of the frontoethmoid suture line, a guide to the level of junction of the ethmoid roof and anterior fossa floor. In the majority of individuals the optic nerve will be found 4–7 mm posterior to the posterior ethmoid foramen.

Middle cranial base

Intracranially, the middle cranial base begins anteriorly at the posterior edge of the lesser wing of sphenoid; posteriorly, it ends at the posterosuperior edge of the petrous part of the temporal bone. The greater wing and body of the sphenoid bone, as well as the petrous and squamous portions of the temporal bone, form the intracranial surface of the middle cranial base. It forms the roof of the infratemporal fossa, middle ear, mastoid, and condylar fossa, as well as the lateral wall of the sphenoid sinus.

The floor of the middle fossa has a series of important foramina (Fig. 2). There are the superior orbital fissure (which transmits the oculomotor, trochlear, ophthalmic and abducent cranial nerves, as well as the ophthalmic vein), optic canal (which transmits the optic nerve), foramen rotundum (which transmits maxillary nerve V2), the foramen ovale (which delivers the mandibular nerve [V3] to the infratemporal fossa below) and the foramen spinosum (which transmits the middle meningeal artery). The superior petrosal sinus, which runs along the rim of the petrous bone, separates the middle from the posterior cranial fossa. The anteromedial petrous tip houses the trigeminal or gasserian ganglion in a region known as Meckel cave. This area is superior to the point at which the internal carotid artery (ICA) enters the cavernous sinus just above the foramen lacerum.

Along the superomedial surface of the petrous part of the temporal bone, the roof of the carotid canal is frequently dehiscent, revealing the horizontal petrous ICA and the foramen lacerum. This foramen receives the greater superficial petrosal nerve (GSPN) after its exit from the facial hiatus a few millimetres posterolaterally and conducts it to the pterygopalatine fossa inferiorly. This relationship between the GSPN, the foramen lacerum, and the carotid canal is often helpful in surgery, because the GSPN, which is readily identifiable, can be followed medially to the distal petrous ICA.

Extracranially, it extends from the posterolateral walls of the maxillary sinuses anteriorly to the petro-occipital sutures posteriorly, and is formed by the greater wing and body of the sphenoid bone and by the temporal bone. Like its intracranial surface, this region also contains numerous openings for major nerves and blood vessels, including the previously mentioned foramina ovale, spinosum, and lacerum, as well as the stylomastoid foramen (cranial nerve VII), the jugular foramen (internal jugular vein [IJV], cranial nerves IX, X, XI), and the carotid canal (entrance of ICA into the temporal bone).

The muscles of mastication, including the temporalis, and medial and lateral pterygoids, are present in the infratemporal fossa. The pterygoid muscles originate, in part, from the lateral pterygoid plate of the sphenoid bone. It is palpable during surgery and can be exposed easily by dissecting medially along the greater wing of sphenoid. The root of this lateral pterygoid plate is situated immediately posterior to the foramen rotundum and anterior to the foramen ovale. It can thus be used as an index to the positions of the maxillary (V2) and mandibular (V3) divisions of the trigeminal nerve. Once the foramen ovale is identified, the foramen spinosum (transmitting the middle meningeal artery) will be found just posterior to it. Knowing the close relationship between these foramina, Eustachian tube and the horizontal petrous ICA is extremely important to resect skull base tumours without injuring the ICA. This can be understood easily by three imaginary parallel lines drawn at an angle of 45° to the midsagittal plane. The outer line incorporates the lateral pterygoid plate, foramen ovale, foramen spinosum and spine of sphenoid, the middle line incorporates the Eustachian tube, and the innermost line incorporates the horizontal petrous ICA.[4] While approaching from the lateral to medial direction, methodical dissection and identification of the structures described would prevent accidental injury to the ICA.

Posterior cranial base

The posterior skull base is composed of the clivus anteriorly, the petrous and mastoid portions of the temporal bone anterolaterally, and the occipital bone laterally and posteriorly. The clivus receives contributions from the sphenoid and occipital bones. It is separated from the petrous apex of the temporal bone by the petro-occipital (petroclival) fissure. At this junction lies the groove for the inferior petrosal sinus, which connects the cavernous sinus to the jugular bulb. Several important foramina of the posterior skull base are present, which include the foramen magnum, internal auditory canals, hypoglossal canals, and jugular foramina. The facial (cranial nerve VII) and vestibulocochlear (cranial nerve VIII) nerves exit the cranium through the internal auditory canals, and cranial nerve XII exits the posterior fossa through the anterior and obliquely oriented paired hypoglossal canals. The paired jugular foramina are actually focal widening of the posterior petro-occipital fissure consisting of two parts: the anteriorly located pars nervosa, which transmits the glossopharyngeal nerve (cranial nerve IX), and the pars vascularis, transmitting the jugular vein, and the vagus and spinal accessory nerves (cranial nerves X and XI, respectively). Ventrally, the posterior cranial base is situated over the nasopharynx.

Clinical features

Symptoms of skull base tumours are related to compression or invasion of neurovascular structures in the area of growth. The dysfunction may be related to cranial nerve deficits, nasal function, vision and hearing. Headache is a non-specific symptom found in most of the skull base tumours. The site of skull base lesions can often be localized by the cranial nerve deficits. Nasal obstruction, epistaxis and anosmia (CN I) suggest a tumour of the anterior cranial base. Proptosis, diplopia (CN III, IV, VI) or visual loss (CN II) indicates involvement of the orbit, optic chiasm, or cavernous sinus. Sensory loss in the face (CNV) may suggest a tumour in the middle cranial base, or infratemporal fossa, or the pterygopalatine fossa. Hearing loss (CN VIII), facial palsy (CN VII), voice change or swallowing difficulty (CN IX, X) may indicate a tumour in the posterior cranial base.

Pathology

A wide variety of neoplasms and infectious diseases can affect the cranial base because of the presence of different kinds of tissues in that region. They can arise from the extracranial tissues or the skull base or an intracranial lesion eroding the skull base. The lesions arising from the anterior skull base can be divided broadly into the following four categories: (i) Aggressive sinonasal diseases that extend intracranially (most common), (ii) lesions arising from the bone of the skull base, (iii) uncommon intracranial lesions that extend inferiorly into the paranasal sinuses and nasal cavity, and (iv) developmental lesions.[5]

Tumour spread to the skull base may occur by the following three methods: (i) Direct extension, (ii) perineural spread along the nerve sheaths of cranial nerves, and (iii) haematogenous spread.

The tumour can spread intracranially from the primary site along tissue planes of the cranial nerves.[6] Although adenoid cystic carcinoma is notorious for spreading in this fashion, squamous cell carcinoma also spreads in this way. Perineural spread may occur in any head and neck malignancy, including salivary gland tumours, mucosal lesions and skin carcinoma. Infrequently, infections such as rhinocerebral mucormycosis may extend to cranial nerves in a perineural fashion.[7] The second and third divisions of the trigeminal nerve and the descending facial nerve are most commonly affected by perineural spread.

Rare tumours

Chordoma

Chordoma is a malignant bone tumour derived from notochordal remnants. It is slow growing, and the average age at presentation is 40 years. Chordomas occurring in the skull base represent approximately one-third of all chordomas, and the majority of the rest occur in the caudal end of the spine. Within the cranial area, the sites in which chordomas occur most frequently are the clivus and parasellar areas. The most common symptoms associated with cranial chordomas are headache and visual disturbances, including diplopia and nerve palsies, which occur particularly in cranial nerve VI because of its proximity to the major site of tumour origin, namely the clivus. Bone is destroyed in an irregular manner, as is evident on the CT scan. The chordomas have two patterns: (i) conventional and (ii) chondroid. Chordomas are characteristically gelatinous with semi-translucent grey and blue areas and focal haemorrhage. Conventional chordomas are highly mucinous in nature and semi-fluid. Chordomas with chondroid differentiation (chondroid chordoma) are semisolid. The chondroid types have a hyaline-type chondroid or cartilaginous tissue within the chordoma tumour. These cause the most difficulty in accurate histological distinction between chondrosarcoma and chondroid chordoma.[8,9] Immunohistochemically, tumour cells for conventional and chondroid areas of chordomas express vimentin, S100, and epithelial markers (cytokeratin and epithelial membrane antigen [EMA]). Chondrosarcomas express positivity for vimentin and S100, but typically do not express epithelial markers, such as cytokeratin or EMA.[9] They are extradural in origin and tend to displace the dura. Large tumours invade and penetrate the dura and surround important arteries and cranial nerves. Chordomas are relatively radio resistant, and aggressive surgical resection is the treatment of choice. As the local recurrence is high, postoperative radiotherapy is given. Metastasis occurs in 10%–40% of cases.

Chondroma

Chondromas are slow-growing tumours. Their occurrence in the skull base region is rare. These tumours arise from well-differentiated cartilage cells and are locally invasive. Surgery is the treatment of choice, as these tumours are radio-resistant.

Paragangliomas

Paragangliomas are benign, slow growing, hypervascular tumours. They arise from paraganglionic tissue (of neural crest origin) found along major blood vessels of the head and neck and superior mediastinum.[10] In addition, they are found in the orbit, larynx and along the course of the vagus nerve. The average age at the time of presentation is 45 years, and women are affected more frequently. These tumours are divided into adrenal paragangliomas (pheochromocytomas) and extra-adrenal paragangliomas. In the past, these tumours were known as glomus tumours, chemodectoma and non-chromaffin tumours. Currently, the correct terminology is paraganglioma, based on the anatomical location (e.g. carotid paraganglioma and jugulotympanic paraganglioma). Of this group, the glomus jugulare, tympanicum and vagale arise in the region of the skull base. In approximately 10% of patients, these paraganglia can develop at multiple sites. The incidence goes up to 50% in familial cases. The most common presenting symptom is pulsatile tinnitus, followed by hearing loss. Paragangliomas are locally invasive, and hence lower cranial nerve dysfunction is common. Facial nerve paralysis signals advanced disease, and is an indication of poor facial nerve prognosis. A majority of these tumours are non-functional and surgery is the treatment of choice. Their response to radiation is variable. Radiation is given for residual/recurrent tumours. The incidence of malignancy in these tumours is 2%–6%, and they are indistinguishable histologically from benign tumours. Metastases to lymph nodes and distant sites are indicative of malignancy.

Other benign skull tumours

Other benign lesions that affect bone and sometimes involve the skull include aneurysmal bone cysts, osteoid osteoma, ossifying and non-ossifying fibromas, and some variants of giant cell tumours. Bony involvement is best demonstrated on CT scan with bone windows. MRI can demonstrate intracranial extension.

Chondrosarcoma

These are slow-growing malignant tumours that originate from primitive mesenchymal cell rests in the cartilagenous matrix at the skull base. They are most common in men in the fourth decade of life. The gross appearance and biological behaviour of chondrosarcomas are similar to the chordoma. Their most common location is the parasellar region. Chondrosarcomas are separated into conventional, clear cell, mesenchymal, and dedifferentiated variants on the basis of cellularity, nuclear pleomorphism and mitotic activity.[9] Conventional chondrosarcomas have been further subdivided into histological grades I–III. The lower-grade tumours are less aggressive and have minimal malignant potential. These tumours do not stain for epithelial markers or oncofetal antigens, distinguishing them from chordomas. In contrast to conventional chondrosarcomas, mesenchymal and dedifferentiated chondrosarcomas exhibit aggressive behaviour and have a poor prognosis. These are primarily extradural with dural invasion occurring at a later stage. Radical excision is the treatment of choice. Local recurrence rate is high and is usually the ultimate cause of the patient's death.

Metastatic tumours

These tumours enter the brain from another cancerous location in the body. The most common metastatic brain tumours are caused by cancers of the lung, breast, renal cell (kidney), colon or a melanoma (skin cancer). These tumours can be single or multiple. The involvement of the skull base is a serious complication of cancer. Skull base metastatic lesions may present with signs and symptoms, depending on tumour location and the dysfunction of cranial nerves affected by the tumour, which is typically sudden in onset. Although skull base metastases are often painless, localized cranial or facial pain at the site of tumour invasion may be a symptom, especially with those arising because of direct extension. CT scan and MRI are complementary modalities of investigating these lesions. These lesions are generally soft and rarely invade vascular structures. Surgery, where feasible, remains the main modality of treatment.

Olfactory neuroblastomas

Esthesioneuroblastoma, also known as an olfactory neuroblastoma, is a rare neoplasm originating from olfactory neuroepithelium. The incidence has two peaks—at 30 and 60 years of age, respectively. It usually presents as a nasal polypoidal mass within the superior one-third of the nasal cavity. The average delay between the appearance of the initial symptom and the diagnosis is 6 months. However, diagnosis is delayed for years in some cases, because initial symptoms tend to be subtle and are frequently banal, occurring also in common nasal diseases, including long-term rhinosinusitis or allergic polypoid sinus disease. Therefore, sending all the tissue removed during sinus surgery for pathological examination is important for diagnosis of esthesioneuroblastoma, as is the vigilance of the pathologist in examining the tissue. It is slow growing and has a 20%–40% metastatic potential to the regional lymph nodes, bone and lungs. Surgery involves *en bloc* removal of the tumour and the surrounding tissues, including

the bone of the cranial base, the dura and the olfactory tracts. These tumours respond favourably to radiation, so surgery is followed by external beam irradiation.

Adenoid cystic carcinomas

This slow-growing, neurotropic, widely infiltrative malignant tumour affects the major and minor salivary glands, lacrimal gland, and ceruminous glands. It has a protracted, relentless clinical course, delayed onset of distant metastasis (lung, bone, or brain), and a tendency for late death—10–20 years after definitive treatment.[11] A poor prognosis could be attributable to the anatomical location of the minor salivary glands, the tumour's tendency for widespread submucosal dissemination, and its distinctive propensity for perineural invasion. Lymphatic spread of adenoid cystic carcinoma is uncommon. The location of the intraoral minor salivary gland could give the tumour ready access to a neural network leading to the skull base, cranial nerves, and brain. It occurs most often in the fifth decade of life and affects women slightly more than men. The three histological subtypes are based on architectural growth patterns: (i) Cribriform (most common), (ii) tubular, and (iii) solid. Of the histological variants, tumours containing 30% solid growth patterns appear to have the worst prognosis. The status of surgical margins, perineural invasion of major nerves, and solid histological pattern are three components frequently correlated with patient outcome.[11,12] The treatment of choice for adenoid cystic carcinoma is wide local surgical excision with negative margins. Although adenoid cystic carcinomas do not respond well to irradiation, postoperative radiotherapy is used often as adjunctive therapy to take care of the microscopic, residual disease. Recurrence rates are high and relate to the difficulty in obtaining a negative surgical margin. Despite incomplete excision, long periods of survival are not uncommon. Multiple treatments for recurrent disease are justified to provide symptomatic relief.

Meningioma

Meningiomas are benign neoplasms arising from arachnoid cells of the arachnoid villi. Roughly 3% of all meningiomas secondarily involve the sinonasal tract.[13] Meningiomas can arise outside the central nervous system (CNS) and are divided into primary (no identifiable connection to the CNS) and secondary (communication to the CNS). The most common sites of these infrequent ectopic meningiomas in the head and neck area include the middle ear, temporal bone (internal auditory canal, jugular foramen, geniculate ganglion, roof of the Eustachian tube, sulcus of the greater petrosal nerve), sinonasal cavity, orbit, oral cavity, and parotid gland. The tumours tend to grow by direct extension, invading adjacent structures such as bone, and causing compression of adjacent structures. Meningiomas that extend to the neck have an

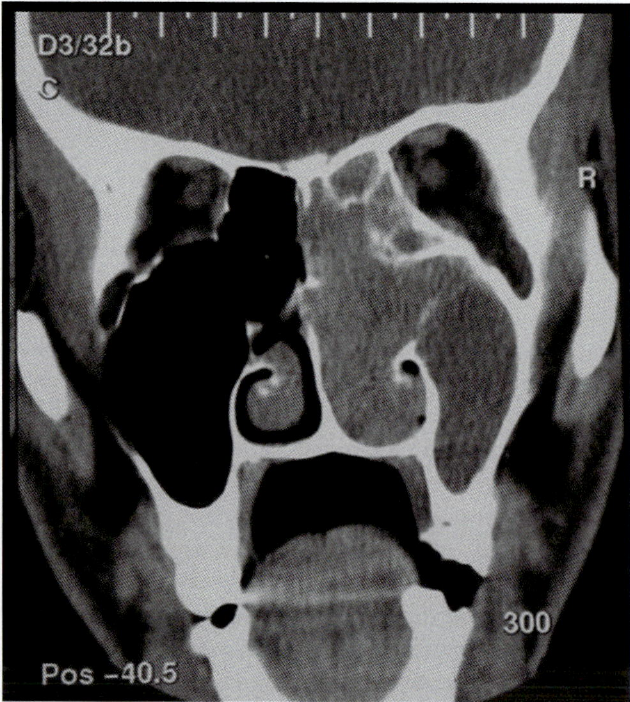

Fig. 3a. CT image shows the tumour involving the entire nasal cavity, maxillary antrum and ethmoid sinus reaching the skull base

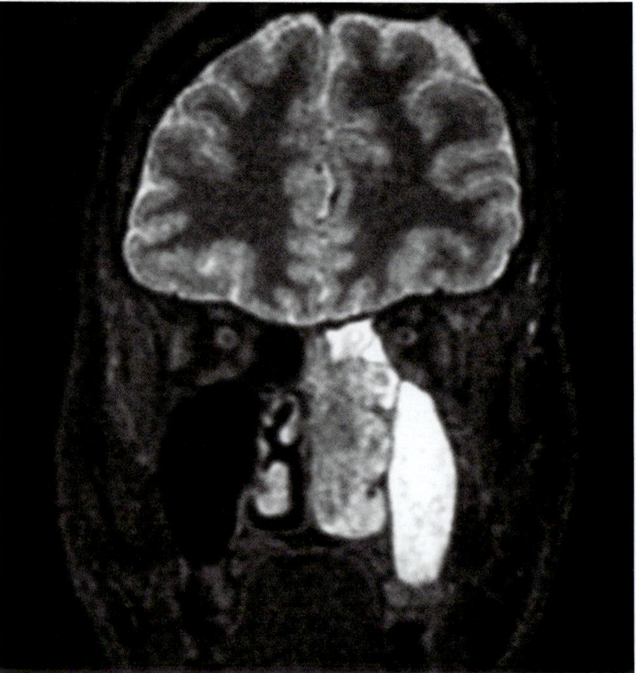

Fig. 3b. MR image of the same patient reveals the true extent of the tumour, maxillary antrum and ethmoid sinus are filled with retained secretion

infiltrative growth pattern into soft tissue that may result in a higher incidence of local recurrences. Meningiomas of the cranial base area are often associated with hyperostosis of the cranium. This can be due to direct invasion of the tumour into the bone or it can occur as a reaction to the tumour resulting from increased vascularity. Complete surgical excision is the treatment of choice. The complex anatomy of the skull base, however, may preclude complete excision, making recurrence likely. Although meningiomas do not respond well to irradiation, this treatment modality is used in inoperable lesions.

Imaging

Diagnostic imaging of cranial base lesions has improved dramatically in the last decade because of refinements in CT and MRI techniques. These developments have made it possible to accurately map cranial base lesions, to define involvement of critical structures and to plan optimal surgical approaches—all in a non-invasive way.

CT scans define the bony boundaries better than MRI. Intravenous contrast increases the sensitivity of detecting neoplasms. The effect of the mass on the adjacent bone may be suggestive of the type of pathological condition.[5] For example, squamous cell carcinoma, the most common of the sinonasal neoplasms, characteristically destroys bone aggressively. Conversely, lesions that cause expansion of the paranasal sinuses and smooth remodelling of adjacent bone are more likely to be benign entities, such as mucocoeles or sinonasal polyposis. A combination of bony destruction and remodelling is associated with aggressive chronic infection or fungal sinusitis. These lesions are usually associated with reactive sclerosis and bony thickening.

In general, MRI is the primary imaging modality for any skull base process that is suspected to involve the brain or meninges, or which may interface between the brain and extracranial head or neck structures. Compared with CT, MRI easily can image the skull base in any plane and is more sensitive in detecting leptomeningeal, dural, or cranial nerve involvement (perineural spread), marrow space processes and intracranial spread. It is also better suited to differentiate retained secretions from a tumour in processes involving the paranasal sinuses and mastoid air cells (Fig. 3). Pulse sequences, such as fat saturation techniques, are useful in suppressing high signal from fat, maximizing tissue–tumour contrast. This is particularly useful in distinguishing bone marrow or orbital fat from the tumour. The intravenous administration of gadolinium helps to maximize the contrast between normal and pathological tissues and is used almost universally in skull base studies. Multiplanar, post-gadolinium T_1-weighted images with a small field of view and fat saturation are used routinely in skull-base imaging.[14] It should be noted that meningeal enhancement in itself does not necessarily indicate neoplastic invasion, because reactive dural enhancement may occur as a result of fibrovascular changes. The following criteria are suggestive of dural invasion: (i) Nodular, irregular enhancement, (ii) dura of >5 mm thickness, (iii) pial enhancement, and (iv) parenchymal

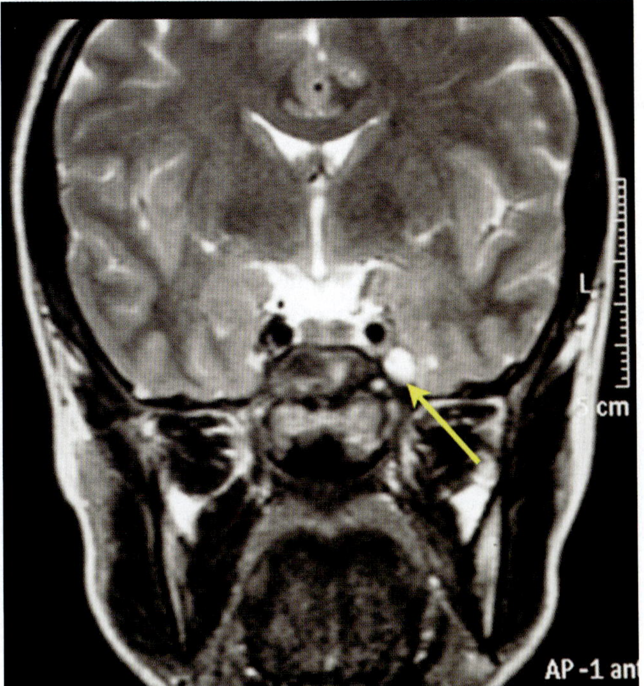

Fig. 4. MR image of an asymptomatic patient who underwent surgery of a patent adenoid cystic carcinoma of palate. Perineural spread resulted in thickening of the maxillary division of trigeminal nerve (yellow arrow).

enhancement or vasogenic brain oedema.[15]

Perineural spread is associated with decreased survival. Identification of this process may indicate either the need for a wider resection or non-resectability, thereby necessitating radiotherapy. Imaging evidence of perineural spread includes the following: (i) Widening or destruction of and excessive enhancement within neural foramina, (ii) replacement of fat density on CT scan or signal intensity on MRI and abnormal enhancement or widening of the pterygopalatine fossa or pterygomaxillary fissure, and (iii) expansion or abnormal enhancement of Meckel cave or the cavernous sinuses.[7] Post-gadolinium axial and coronal T_1-weighted MRIs with fat suppression identify perineural spread well (Fig. 4). Although CT scan frequently demonstrates this entity, CT scanning is better at detecting cortical bone destruction associated with perineural spread.

PET is particularly useful in postoperative patients in differentiating between a residual or recurrent tumour versus post-treatment changes, which may have an identical appearance on CT scanning or MRI. Fluorodeoxyglucose is the most commonly used agent and is taken up by metabolically active tumours that use glucose as a substrate, whereas post-treatment scar or granulation tissue does not.[16] A current limitation of PET is its limited sensitivity in detecting small lesions.

MR angiography (MRA) or CT angiography (CTA) is adequate for delineating the vascular anatomy of the affected area. Angiography is preferred over MRA and CTA when preoperative embolization of the tumour is indicated. Paragangliomas and juvenile nasopharyngeal angiofibromas are hypervascular lesions that have a near pathognomonic appearance on arteriography. The diagnosis of these lesions can usually be made from the arteriogram, obviating the need for biopsy. Angiography can delineate the vascularity of the tumour and its relationship to the ICA, and demonstrates the cerebral circulation and its collateral vasculature. These tests, however, do not predict the adequacy of the intracranial collateral blood supply after sacrificing the ICA.

Cerebral blood flow evaluation

In the surgical management of aggressive skull base tumours encasing the ICA or, more rarely, the vertebral artery, the tumour can be removed only when the encased artery is sacrificed. *En bloc* resection or ligation of the ICA without reconstruction for head and neck tumours is associated with a high rate of neurovascular morbidity and mortality. In a study of 156 patients undergoing carotid artery ligation for head and neck malignancy, Konno *et al.*[17] reported a 30% rate of permanent plegia, coma and death. Trial balloon occlusion (TBO) is first recommended to determine whether the patient will safely tolerate permanent occlusion or whether an arterial bypass procedure is needed. Six-vessel cerebral angiography is necessary to evaluate the collateral circulation via the anterior and posterior communicating arteries.

The TBO procedure is performed via a transfemoral approach in an awake, sedated, heparinized patient. The balloon is placed in the proximal ICA and inflated slowly to occlude the ICA under fluoroscopic control. The patient is assessed neurologically every 2–3 minutes at first, and then every 5 minutes over a period of 30 minutes. If the patient experiences a neurological deficit the balloon is deflated immediately. During the period of balloon inflation, contralateral internal carotid angiography (via the other femoral artery) may be performed to demonstrate cross-flow across the anterior communicating artery and, more importantly, assessment of the ipsilateral venous phase. A delay in the appearance of the cerebral veins on the occluded side is evidence of inadequate collateral cross-filling.

TBO is itself associated with a 0.4% incidence of permanent neurological deficit and no mortality. This complication rate is similar to that in diagnostic cerebral angiography.[18,19] Up to 20% of patients, who tolerate temporary occlusion, will develop infarction after permanent occlusion.[20,21] In 20% of these, the onset could be after 48 hours but is sometimes up to 2 weeks later.[22] This is due to clot propagation or embolic phenomena from static blood in the distal ligated stump of the ICA.[17,23] Methods combining balloon occlusion with simultaneous measurements of cerebral blood flow using xenon-enhanced CT,[24] single photon CT,[25] or transcranial doppler,[26] have been

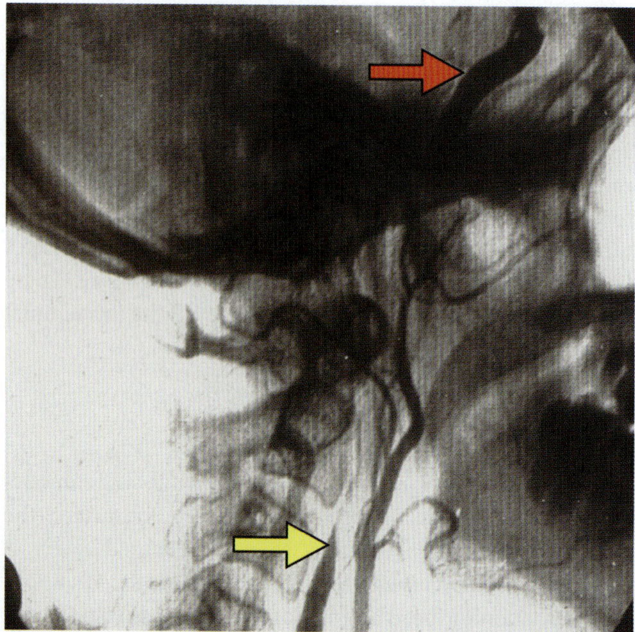

Fig. 5. Permanent balloon occlusion. Red arrow points to the contrast filled balloon in the intracavernous portion of ICA. Yellow arrow points to the absence of blood flow through the ICA.

used successfully to identify patients who pass a standard balloon occlusion test but are at risk because of low-flow reserves. Despite this enhanced ability to detect patients at risk, there is no single fail-safe test to predict postoperative neurological complications in patients undergoing carotid resection without reconstruction. Although these tests have reduced the delayed stroke rate to 3%–8%, they cannot predict embolic stroke.[27]

Preoperative embolization

After a successful TBO, and should it be decided preoperatively that the carotid artery will have to be sacrificed, the patient may go on to permanent ICA occlusion using detachable intra-arterial permanent balloons (Fig. 5). Preoperative embolization may be done to minimize intra-operative bleeding during the resection of such vascular lesions as juvenile nasopharyngeal angiofibromas, paragangliomas, or skull base meningiomas.

General considerations of skull base surgery

A wide variety of approaches have been developed for exposure of tumours in the anterior, middle and posterior cranial base regions. Some of the approaches are purely intracranial and some are purely extracranial. Most of the current approaches for dealing with lesions of the skull base employ combined intracranial and extracranial methods.

For anterior cranial base lesions, the most commonly used approaches combine frontal craniotomy with some form of transfacial (transnasal, transmaxillary, or transorbital) exposure. For middle cranial base lesions that combine temporal or frontotemporal craniotomy with infratemporal fossa dissection, transfacial exposure or transtemporal techniques most often provide good access. In both anterior and middle cranial base approaches, craniofacial disassembly techniques are increasingly being applied. For the posterior cranial fossa, the translabyrinthine, retrosigmoid, suboccipital and extreme lateral approaches are employed. Petrosectomy is done to resect malignant tumours. For larger tumours, combined and staged procedures have also been proposed.[28] All these approaches may have to be modified, extended or combined, depending on the pathology, site of tumour and the structures involved.

Planning the operative approach

The planned approach must provide a wide exposure to allow complete removal of the tumour. To preserve the nearby cranial nerves, the ICA, orbital contents, or brain, the exposure is extended beyond the limits of the lesion; it is a major factor in reducing postoperative morbidity. After resection of the tumour, the barrier between the brain and the aerodigestive tract must be restored to reduce the potential for such consequences as cerebrospinal fluid (CSF) fistula and meningitis. All attempts should be made to preserve the vascularity of adjacent tissues, such as the temporalis muscle, galea, and pericranium, which can then be used for the reconstruction. Preservation of function and cosmesis should be considered while choosing the approach. Whenever possible, the facial skeleton should be mobilized temporarily. Even in cases in which aesthetically important segments must be removed for oncological reasons, acceptable cosmesis can usually be accomplished through judicious use of bone grafts and soft tissue flaps.

Preoperative considerations

Skull base surgery is a clean–contaminated procedure. A wide-spectrum perioperative antibiotic with good penetration of the blood–brain barrier is recommended.[29] Neuroanaesthetic measures to prevent brain oedema (intravenous mannitol, controlled hyperventilation, lumbar subarachnoid drainage) and intra-operative neurophysiological monitoring of cranial nerve and brain function reduces the morbidity. Tracheostomy is performed when the patient has permanent trismus, or a bulky free flap is narrowing the airway, or when prolonged mechanical ventilation is anticipated. A nasogastric feeding tube for postoperative enteral feeding and Foley catheter for monitoring of urinary output are routinely used during these procedures. Antiembolic sequential compression stockings are used to prevent deep venous thrombosis.

Approaches to anterior skull base

The majority of malignant cranial base tumours involving the anterior or anterolateral skull base originate in the paranasal sinuses, or nasal cavity, or orbit. In addition, anterior cranial base dura, brain, cavernous sinus and their neurovascular components are often involved.[30]

Craniofacial approach

The craniofacial approach has gradually evolved over the past 5 decades into a safe and reliable technique for resecting both benign and malignant tumours involving the anterior cranial base. In 1963 Ketcham *et al.*[3] presented a satisfactory success rate with low morbidity in a large series in which this procedure was used for treating paranasal sinus cancer. The tumours most commonly requiring combined anterior craniofacial surgery usually begin in the nose or sinuses. The technique can be extended and incorporated as a part of a more complex resection involving the infratemporal fossa and anterolateral cranial base, as well as the middle cranial fossa, cavernous sinus, etc. Tumours with a primary intracranial origin, such as meningioma, chordoma or chondrosarcoma require combined resection when they clearly violate the anterior fossa floor.

Technique

The procedure is performed under general anaesthesia. A lumbar drain is routinely placed and patients are given prophylactic peroperative antibiotic. The patient is then placed in a Mayfield head holder or in a head ring to stabilize the head and positioned to optimize both the neurosurgical and facial approaches. The leg is prepared to obtain a skin graft and fascia lata if needed. The anterior craniofacial approach incorporates a combination of transfacial and transcranial procedures. The sequence of steps may vary from patient to patient. The nature of the tumour and its primary location determine whether the intracranial or extracranial part of the operation is performed first. Author (CR) prefers to do the transfacial part first.

Facial approach

The facial approach depends on the extent of the tumour. Modifications of a lateral rhinotomy incision that may or may not transect the upper lip is used (Fig. 6). This depends on whether a total maxillectomy is done in conjunction with the resection. The periosteum is elevated from the nasal bone as well as from the medial and inferior surfaces of the orbit. The nasolacrimal duct is identified and transected distally. The anterior and posterior ethmoidal arteries are then identified and cauterized or clipped. In most cases it is necessary

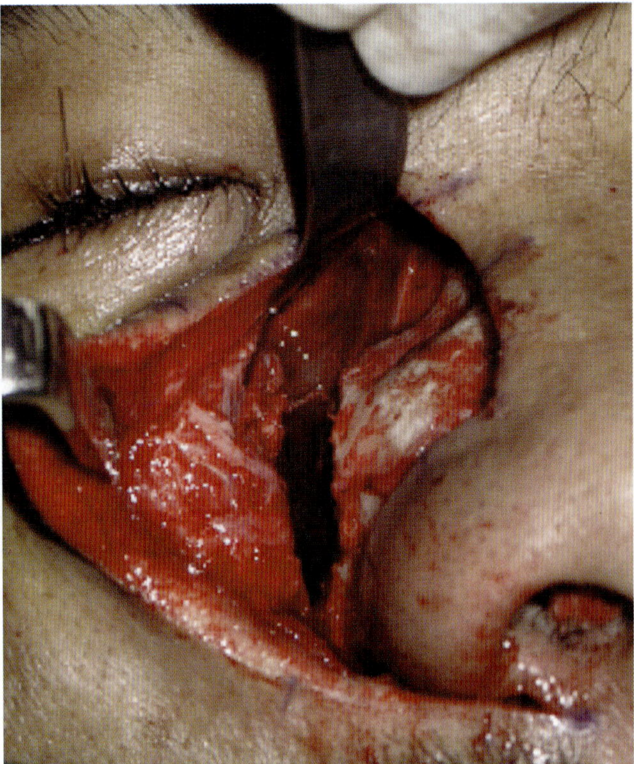

Fig. 6. Lateral rhinotomy incision. Medial maxillectomy is being done

to perform a complete *en bloc* ethmoidectomy. For this purpose a contralateral Lynch incision is made to elevate the contralateral periorbita, cauterize the anterior and posterior ethmoidal vessels, and make the appropriate osteotomies. The septum is cut at the oncologically suitable site.

If preoperative imaging studies confirm the presence of a tumour in the soft tissues of the orbit, then extending the incision laterally to include a portion of the eyelids may facilitate orbital exenteration.

Craniotomy

The craniotomy is tailored according to the extent of involvement of the anterior fossa floor, the sub cranial tumour location and the degree of dural or frontal lobe invasion. A bicoronal scalp incision is made running 2–3 cm behind the hairline. The flap is elevated in the subgaleal plane down to the eyebrows, then to the lateral orbital walls laterally and just below the nasal glabella medially. A large flap of vascularized pericranial tissue is raised that will be used for later reconstruction (Fig. 7). As the dissection proceeds, the supratrochlear and supraorbital neurovascular bundles are exposed and preserved.

Removing a segment of frontal bone, which may be pedicled on the temporalis muscle or completely separated, exposes the anterior cranial fossa. The lower horizontal bone cut should be kept low to lessen the need for subsequent

lesions, which were previously deemed unresectable. These approaches are classified as types Fisch A, B and C.

Type A approach

This approach is used for removal of tumours of the temporal bone involving the jugular foramen and vertical segment of the petrous ICA, primarily glomus temporal tumours. It involves control of lower cranial nerves, ICA and IJV in the neck, subtotal petrosectomy and a permanent anterior rerouting of the facial nerve. This exposes the jugular and the vertical part of petrous ICA. The glomus jugulare tumour is excised with the jugular bulb it is invading after ligating the IJV and sigmoid sinus (Fig. 13). Bleeding from the inferior petrosal sinus is controlled by plugging with surgicel. A dural defect, if present, is closed and the Eustachian tube is plugged to prevent infection. The external auditory canal (EAC) is closed blindly.

Type B approach

This approach is designed to expose more anteriorly located tumours in the petrous apex and clivus. After blind closure of the EAC and subtotal petrosectomy, the zygomatic arch and the temporalis muscle are reflected inferiorly. The temperomandibular joint is then disarticulated, and the bone of the glenoid fossa and the root of the zygoma are removed completely. Complete exposure of the vertical as well as horizontal petrous ICA and its mobilization permits free access to the petrous tip and clivus. It is applicable to glomus tumours involving the horizontal petrous carotid artery, clival chordoma, and congenital cholesteatoma of the petrous apex.

Type C approach

This is an anterior extension of the type B approach and allows for exposure of the parasellar region, nasopharynx, pterygomaxillary fossa and Eustachian tube. It has been used primarily for extensive juvenile nasopharyngeal angiofibroma and nasopharyngeal malignancies. In this approach, the dissection extends further anteriorly and both medial and lateral pterygoid plates are drilled away, exposing the lateral wall of the nasopharynx, which can be resected *en bloc* (Fig. 14). Entire temporalis muscle can be rotated to fill the dead space. Vascularized free flaps are often necessary to provide adequate closure.

Petrosectomy

Malignancies of the ear and temporal bone are rare. These tumours spread mainly by direct invasion into the temporal bone and neighbouring structures (parotid, infratemporal fossa, dura, brain).[54] Lymphatic metastases are uncommon

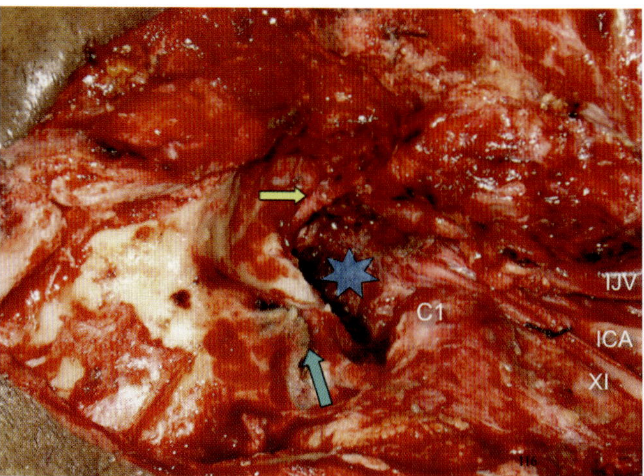

Fig. 13. Dissected lower cranial nerves, ICA and IJV are marked. Yellow arrow—anteriorly rerouted facial nerve. Green arrow—site of occlusion of sigmoid sinus. Blue star—site of jugular bulb (after excision)

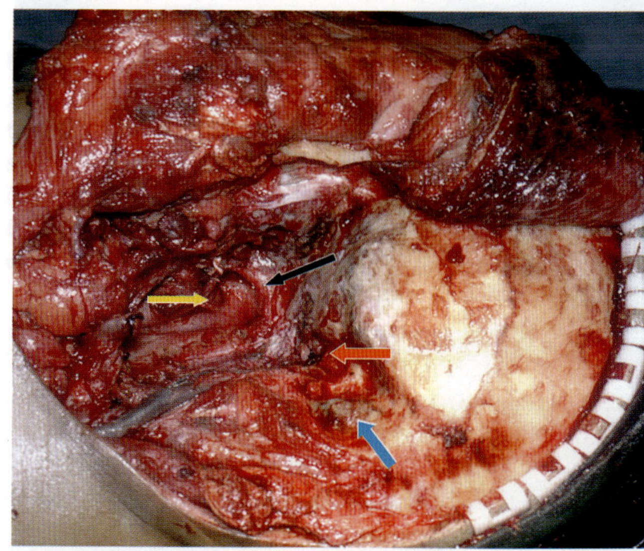

Fig. 14. Nasopharyngectomy had been done using modified ITF type C approach. Subtotal petrosectomy is done. Blue arrow—sigmoid sinus. Involved ICA is sacrificed. Red arrow—cut distal end of ICA. Black arrow—posterior end of nasal septum. Yellow arrow—contralateral Eustachian tube

and distant spread extremely rare. Surgical treatment of malignant tumours of the ear and temporal bone is not universally agreed upon. In general, lesions localized to the EAC (T1 lesions) are treated with a limited resection (i.e. local resection, radical mastoidectomy), whereas more advanced lesions (T2–T4) are treated by partial temporal bone resection, subtotal petrosectomy, or total petrosectomy.[55–58]

A temporal craniectomy is performed initially and the dura is elevated from the temporal bone. If the dura is involved, it is also resected. Thereafter, the craniectomy is extended into the posterior cranial fossa, allowing the sigmoid sinus and the jugular bulb to be mobilized from their attachment to bone.

Total parotidectomy with facial nerve dissection is done for tumour clearance as well as to remove preauricular nodes. The mandibular condyle is resected for exposure of the ICA and jugular vein.

Through the temperomandibular joint, the intratemporal carotid is identified and, using a drill, mobilized from its attachment to the temporal bone. A partial or subtotal resection of the temporal bone may now be accomplished by creating a controlled fracture across the axis of the petrous bone with a chisel. Depending on the location of the tumour, the temporal bone may be resected medial to the ear drum, medial to the cochlea, or medial to the internal auditory meatus.

Approaches to posterior skull base

Posterior cranial base lesions are complex and occur in different locations. Surgery of the petroclival, foramen magnum, cerebello pontine angle (CPA), jugular foramen lesions, and complex vertebral and basilar aneurysms require a skull base approach.

Transtemporal approaches

These are lateral, primarily extradural techniques that traverse the mastoid and petrous portions of the temporal bone to provide exposure of lesions at the petrous apex, clivus and CPA (for lesions such as acoustic neuroma, petroclival meningioma and aggressive cholesteatoma). They include the transcochlear,[59] translabyrinthine[60] and combined techniques.

Complications

As skull base resections have increased in complexity and magnitude, so have the complications associated with the procedures. Many methods have evolved not only to completely extirpate the cancer but also to avoid complications. The major complications of skull base surgery include CSF leak, bleeding, stroke, meningitis, cranial nerve deficits and recurrent disease. The most common medical complications are pneumonia, electrolyte disturbance and cardiac complications.

Cerebrospinal fluid leak: After extirpation of the tumour and separation of the intracranial cavity from the upper aerodigestive tract, creating a watertight closure is the keystone to preventing CSF leakage and consequent central complications. Dural closure is best accomplished by autografts of fascia lata or temporalis fascia. The best closure is by direct suturing, but in difficult areas, such as the planum sphenoidale and over the clivus under the pons, the use of fibrin glue helps to fix dural grafts in place. After dural closure, a second layer of well vascularized tissue enhances dural healing and aids in the prevention of CSF leakage. For defects in the anterior cranial fossa, the pericranial flap, which is a richly vascularized tissue, is used to aid in closure. In the middle fossa, after dural closure, either a pedicled temporalis muscle flap or a vascularized free flap is used as a second layer.[61] A watertight closure of the dura after skull base resection may not be possible in all cases, especially around nerves and blood vessels. Most of these leaks can be managed by reducing the CSF pressure with a spinal drain. Surgical repair of the dural defect is done if the leak does not resolve within a week because of the risk of meningitis. Sometimes, profuse ipsilateral rhinorrhoea is seen after dissection of the petrous ICA and is probably due to loss of sympathetic fibres that travel along the ICA en route to the nasal mucosa.[62]

Tension pneumocephalus: Whenever the CSF leak is present, air can enter into the cranial cavity. The forcing of air into the intracranial compartment by grunting respirations in a semi comatose patient will result in a tension pneumocephalus if a ball-valve type of situation is established through an incompletely closed dura. This can happen in a non-compliant patient by blowing the nose in the postoperative period. The patient will have a deepening of unconsciousness with a deterioration of his or her score on the Glasgow coma scale. Aspiration of the air through the burr hole is the initial treatment. If the tension pneumocephalus recurs, bypassing the airway with a tracheostomy or surgical exploration to close the defect is required.

Cerebral oedema/contusion: Excessive retraction of the brain causes cerebral oedema and contusion. Further injury to the brain, because of increased intracranial pressure due to parenchymal oedema, can be avoided with corticosteroids, stabilization of the haemodynamic problems, and correction of electrolyte imbalance. Medical prophylaxis of seizures is recommended.

Trismus: Postoperative pain and scarring of the pterygoid musculature causes trismus. Performing stretching exercises for the jaw using stacked up ice-cream sticks or a Therabite® (Atos Medical AB: Sweden) appliance helps to relieve the trismus. In select cases coronoidotomy and/or releasing the scar band are needed.

Eustachian tube dysfunction: This can result from surgical resection of tumours in the infratemporal fossa. Inserting a ventilation tube can correct the resulting conductive hearing loss.

Cranial neuropathies: Surgical resection of tumours of the middle cranial fossa can result in paralysis of the lower cranial nerves.[63] Intraoperative electrodes to monitor brain, spinal cord, and cranial nerve function help to prevent neurological compromise. If vagus nerve injury or sacrifice occurs, paralysis of the pharynx, palate and the vocal cord will ensue. In most cases, the initial breathiness and aspiration of liquids gradually resolve when the contralateral vocal cord compensates. However, if this compensation is inadequate, complete glottic closure can be re-established by surgically medializing the paralysed vocal cord. This does not improve the sensory deficits produced by denervation of the afferent pathways. Thus, patients with lower cranial neuropathies remain at risk of aspiration, even after the glottic insufficiency has been corrected. An experienced speech-language pathologist can assist with the monitoring of the patient, recommend diet modifications, and provide intensive swallowing therapy.[64,65] Additionally, velopharyngeal insufficiency may result from paralysis of the palatal branch of the vagus nerve. Palatopexy (nasopharyngeal surface of the palate is sutured to the posterior pharyngeal wall) helps to stop the nasal regurgitation.[66]

Spinal accessory nerve injury results in shoulder pain and restricted range of motion because of the paralysis of the sternomastoid and trapezius muscles. Aggressive postoperative physical therapy can prevent the development of adhesive capsulitis and scapular 'winging', although normal shoulder range of motion and strength are not possible.[67]

Surgical interruption of the facial nerve can result in either partial or total paralysis of the facial musculature. The resulting corneal exposure, oral incompetence, and cosmetic deformity are formidable rehabilitation challenges. A variety of surgical procedures are available for providing either static or dynamic facial reanimation, including nerve crossovers, muscle transfers, and skin tightening procedures. Placement of a gold weight in the supratarsal plane of the upper eyelid re-establishes complete eye closure and prevents exposure keratopathy. This can be reversed when the facial nerve function returns, in those instances in which the anatomical integrity of the nerve has been maintained.

References

1. Smith RR, Klopp CT, Williams JM. Surgical treatment of cancer of the frontal sinus and adjacent areas. *Cancer* 1954;**7**:991–4.
2. Parsons H, Lewis JS. Subtotal resection of the temporal bone for cancer of the ear. *Cancer* 1954;**7**:995–1000.
3. Ketcham AS, Wilkins RH, van Buren JM, *et al*. A combined intracranial facial approach to the paranasal sinuses. *Am J Surg* 1963;**106**:698–703.
4. Lyons BM. Surgical anatomy of the skull base. In: Donald PJ (ed). *Surgery of the skull base*. Philadelphia: Lippincott-Raven Publishers; 1998:15–30.
5. Som PM, Shugar JM, Parisier SC. A clinical-radiographic classification of skull base lesions. *Laryngoscope* 1979;**89**:1066–76.
6. Ginsberg LE. Imaging of perineural tumor spread in head and neck cancer. *Semin Ultrasound CT MR* 1999;**20**:175–86.
7. McLean FM, Ginsberg LE, Stanton CA. Perineural spread of rhinocerebral mucormycosis. *Am J Neuroradiol* 1996;**17**:114–16.
8. O'Connell JX, Renard LG, Liebsch NJ, *et al*. Base of skull chordoma: A correlative study of histologic and clinical features of 62 cases. *Cancer* 1994;**74**:2261–7.
9. Rosenberg AE, Nielsen GP, Keel SB, *et al*. Chondrosarcoma of the base of the skull: A clinicopathologic study of 200 cases with emphasis on its distinction from chordoma. *Am J Surg* 1999;**23**:1370–8.
10. Grimley PM, Glemmer GG. Histology and ultrastructure of carotid body paragangliomas: Comparison with normal gland. *Cancer* 1967;**20**:1473–88.
11. Fordice J, Kershaw C, El-Naggar A, *et al*. Adenoid cystic carcinoma of the head and neck. *Arch Otolaryngol Head Neck Surg* 1999;**125**:149–52.
12. Pitman KT, Prokopakis EP, Aydogan B, *et al*. The role of skull base surgery for the treatment of adenoid cystic carcinoma of the sinonasal tract. *Head Neck* 1999;**12**:402–7.
13. Perez-Ordonez B, Huvos AG. Non-squamous lesions of nasal cavity, paranasal sinuses, and nasopharynx. In: Gnepp DR (ed). *Diagnostic surgical pathology of the head and neck*. Philadelphia: WB Saunders; 2001:115–26.
14. Durden D, Williams D. Radiology of skull base neoplasms. *Otolaryngologic Clin North Am* 2001;**34**:1043–64.
15. Eisen MD, Yousem DM, Montone KT, *et al*. Use of preoperative MR to predict dural, perineural, and venous sinus invasion of skull base tumors. *Am J Neuroradiol* 1996;**17**:1937–45.
16. Keyes JW, Watson NE, Williams DW. FDG PET in head and neck cancer. *Am J Radiol* 1997;**169**:1663–9.
17. Konno A, Togawa K, Iizuka K. Analysis of factors affecting complications of carotid ligation. *Ann Otol Rhinol Laryngol* 1981;**90**:222–6.
18. Dion JE, Gates PC, Fox AJ, *et al*. Clinical events following neuroangiography: A prospective study. *Stroke* 1987;**18**:997–1004.
19. Ernst F, Forbes G, Sandok BA, *et al*. Complications of cerebral angiography: Prospective assessment of risk. *AJR* 1984;**142**:247–53.
20. de Vries EJ, Sekhar LN, Horton JA, *et al*. A new method to predict safe resection of the internal carotid artery. *Laryngoscope* 1990;**100**:85–8.
21. Gonzalez CF, Moret J. Balloon occlusion of the carotid artery prior to surgery for neck tumours. *AJNR* 1990;**11**:649–52.
22. Larson JL, Tew JM, Tomsick TA, *et al*. Treatment of aneurysms of the internal carotid artery by intravascular balloon occlusion: Long-term follow-up of 58 patients. *Neurosurgery* 1995;**36**:23–30.
23. Ehrenfeld WK, Stoney RJ, Wylie EJ. Relation of carotid stump pressure to safety of carotid artery ligation. *Surgery* 1983;**93**:299–305.
24. Erba SM, Horton JA, Latchaw RE, *et al*. Balloon test occlusion of the internal carotid artery with stable xenon/CT cerebral blood flow imaging. *AJNR* 1988;**9**:533–8.
25. Eckard DA, Purdy PD, Bonte FJ. Temporary balloon occlusion of the carotid artery combined with brain blood flow imaging as a test to predict tolerance prior to permanent carotid sacrifice. *AJNR* 1992;**13**:1565–9.
26. Takeuchi Y, Numata T, Konno A, *et al*. Evaluation of brain collateral circulation by the transcranial color doppler-guided Matas' test. *Ann Otol Rhinol Laryngol* 1993;**102**:35–41.
27. Linksey ME, Jungreis CA, Yonas H, *et al*. Stroke risk after abrupt internal carotid artery sacrifice: Accuracy of preoperative assessment with balloon test occlusion and stable xenon-enhanced CT. *AJNR* 1994;**15**:829–43.
28. Tamaki N, Nagashima T, Ehara K, *et al*. Surgical approaches and strategies for skull base chordomas. *Neurosurg Focus* 2001;**10**:E9.
29. Carrau RL, Snyderman CH. Antibiotic prophylaxis in cranial base surgery. *Infect Dis Dig* 1992;**3**:22–3.
30. Shah JP, Bilsky MH, Patel SG. Malignant tumors of the skull base. *Neurosurg Focus* 2002;**13**:Article 6.
31. Donald PJ. Extended transfacial subcranial approach. In: Donald PJ (ed). *Surgery of the skull base*. Philadelphia: Lippincott-Raven Publishers; 1998:287–308.
32. Har-El G. Anterior craniofacial resection without facial skin incisions. *Otolaryngol Head Neck Surg* 2004;**130**:780–7.
33. Yuen APW, Fung CT, Hung KN. Endoscopic craniofacial resection of anterior skull base tumor. *Am J Otolaryngol* 1997;**18**:431–3.
34. Thaler ER, Kotapka M, Lanza DC, *et al*. Endoscopically assisted anterior cranial skull base resection of sinonasal tumors. *Am J Rhinol* 1999;**13**:303–10.

35. Carrau RL, Snyderman CH, Kassam AB, *et al.* Endoscopic and endoscopic-assisted surgery for juvenile angiofibroma. *Laryngoscope* 2001;**111**:483–7.

36. Devaiah AK, Larson C, Tawfik O, *et al.* Esthesioneuroblastoma: Endoscopic nasal and anterior craniotomy resection. *Laryngoscope* 2003;**113**:2086–90.

37. Casiano RR, Numa WA, Falquez AM. Endoscopic resection of esthesioneuroblastoma. *Am J Rhinol* 2001;**15**:271–9.

38. Casiano RR. Anterior skull base resection. In: *Endoscopic sinus surgery dissection manual.* New York: Marcel Dekker; 2002:99–101.

39. Har-El G. Anterior craniofacial resection without facial skin incisions. *Otolaryngol Head Neck Surg* 2004;**130**:780–1.

40. Har-El, Todor R. Anterior craniofacial resection without facial skin incisions. *Skull Base* 2003;**13** (Suppl 1):22.

41. Carrau RL, Kassam AB, Snyderman CH, *et al.* Endoscopic transnasal anterior skull base resection for the treatment of sinonasal malignancies. *Operative Techniques in Otolaryngology* 2006;**17**:102–10.

42. Har-El, Casiano RR. Endoscopic management of anterior skull base tumors. *Otolaryngol Clin North Am* 2005;**38**:133–44.

43. Hadad G, Bassagasteguy L, Carrau RL, *et al.* A novel reconstructive technique after endoscopic expanded endonasal approaches: Vascular pedicle nasoseptal flap. *Laryngoscope* 2006;**116**:1882–6.

44. Fairbanks-Barbosa J. Surgery of extensive cancer of paranasal sinuses. Presentation of a new technique. *Arch Otolaryngol* 1961;**73**:129–38.

45. Fisch U. The infratemporal fossa approach for the lateral skull base. *Otolaryngol Clin North Am.* Symposium of Skull Base Surgery. Philadelphia: WB Saunders; 1984:513–52.

46. Sekhar LN, Schramm VL, Jones NF. Subtemporal–preauricular infratemporal fossa approach to large lateral and posterior cranial neoplasms. *J Neurosurg* 1987;**67**:499.

47. Janecka IP, Sen CN, Sekhar LN. Facial translocation: A new approach to the cranial base. *Otolaryngol Head Neck Surg* 1990;**103**:413–19.

48. Catalano PJ, Biller HF. Extended osteoplastic maxillotomy. A versatile new procedure for wide access to the central skull base and infratemporal fossa. *Arch Otolaryngol Head Neck Surg* 1993;**119**:394–400.

49. Janecka IP. Facial translocation approach. In: Janecka IP, Tiedemann K (eds). *Skull base surgery: Anatomy, biology and technology.* Philadelphia: Lippincott-Raven Publishers; 1997:183–22.

50. Wei WI, Larn KH, Sham JS. New approach to the nasopharynx: The maxillary swing approach. *Head Neck* 1991;**13**:200–7.

51. Nuss DW, Janecka IP, Sekhar LN, *et al.* Craniofacial disassembly in the management of skull base tumours. *Otolaryngol Clin North Am* 1991a;**24**:1465–97.

52. Fisch U. Infratemporal fossa approach to tumours of the temporal bone and base of skull. *J Laryngol Otol* 1978;**92**:949–67.

53. Fisch U. Infratemporal fossa approach for extensive tumours of the temporal bone and base of skull. In: Silverstein H (ed). *Neurological surgery of the ear.* Birmingham, AL: Aesculapius Publishing; 1977: 34–53.

54. Michaels L, Wells M. Squamous carcinoma of the middle ear. *Clin Otolaryngol* 1980;**5**:235–48.

55. Nyrop M, Grontved A. Cancer of the external auditory canal. *Arch Otolaryngol Head Neck Surg* 2002;**128**:834–7.

56. Gillespie MB, Francis HW, Chee N, *et al.* Squamous cell carcinoma of the temporal bone: A radiographic–pathologic correlation. *Arch Otolaryngol Head Neck Surg* 2001;**127**:803–7.

57. Austin JR, Stewart KL, Fawzi N. Squamous cell carcinoma of the external auditory canal: Therapeutic prognosis based on a proposed staging system. *Arch Otolaryngol Head Neck Surg* 1994;**120**:1228–32.

58. Moffat DA, Grey P, Ballagh RH, *et al.* Extended temporal bone resection for squamous cell carcinoma. *Otolaryngol Head Neck Surg* 1997;**116**:617–23.

59. House WF, Hitselberger WE. The transcochlear approach to the skull base. *Arch Otolaryngol Head Neck Surg* 1976;**102**:334–42.

60. House WF. Translabyrinthine approach. In: House WF, Luetje CM (eds). *Acoustic tumours.* Baltimore: University Park Davis; 1979: 438–87.

61. Donald PJ. Complications in skull base surgery for malignancy. *Laryngoscope* 1999;**109**:1959–66.

62. Carrau RL, Snyderman CH, Nuss DW. Surgery of the anterior and lateral skull base. In: Myers EN, Suen JY, Myers J, Hanna E (eds). *Cancer of the head and neck.* Philadelphia: WB Saunders; 2003: 207–28.

63. Netterville JL, Civantos FJ. Rehabilitation of cranial nerve deficits after neurotologic skull base surgery. *Laryngoscope* 1993;**103** (Suppl 60):45–54.

64. Murry R, Carrau RL. *Clinical manual for swallowing disorders.* San Diego, California: Singular Publishing; 2001.

65. Carrau RL, Murry T (eds). *Comprehensive management of swallowing disorders.* San Diego, California: Singular Publishing; 1998.

66. Roberts WL. Rehabilitation of the head and neck cancer patient. In: McGarvey CL (ed). *Physical therapy for the cancer patient.* New York: Churchill Livingstone; 1990:47–65.

67. Tucker HM. Postoperative management and rehabilitation of cranial nerve deficits. In: Jackson CG (ed). *Surgery of skull base tumours.* New York: Churchill Livingstone; 1991:273–86.

19

Cancer of the skin and ear

B.E. MOSTAFA, P. ARUN, BIPIN T. VARGHESE

SKIN TUMOURS

The skin is the interface between human beings and their environment. It is the largest organ in the body weighing an average of 4 kg and covering an area of 2 m². The skin of the head and neck represents approximately 9% of this surface and is the most exposed to environmental factors. Skin has two layers—the outer epithelial layer named the epidermis, and the underlying layer, the dermis, which is firmly attached to the epidermis and supported by connective tissues. Beneath the dermis is the loose connective tissue, the subcutis or the hypodermis. The epidermis is avascular and it is composed of many cell types, the most important being the keratinocytes, melanocytes, Langerhans cells and Merkel cells. In addition, the skin also contains appendages derived from epithelial remnants during embryogenesis that lie in the dermis. They are the hair, sweat glands and sebaceous glands. The commonest skin tumours are squamous cell carcinoma (SCC), basal cell carcinoma (BCC) and malignant melanoma (Table 1).[1,2]

Epidemiology

General risk factors associated with the development of

Table 1. Tumours of the skin

Skin component	Benign	Premalignant / carcinoma *in situ*	Malignant
Epidermis and appendages	Viral wart Squamous cell papilloma Seborrheic keratosis Linear epidermal naevus Milium Melanocytic naevus Sebaceous cyst	Keratoacanthoma Intraepidermal carcinoma Actinic keratosis Sebaceous naevus	Squamous cell carcinoma Basal cell carcinoma Malignant melanoma
Dermis	Haemangioma Lymphangioma Neurofibroma Neuroma Glomus tumour Pyogenic granuloma Dermatofibroma Keloid Lipoma Lymphocytoma cutis Mastocytosis		Kaposi sarcoma Lymphoma Dermatofibrosarcoma protuberans Metastases

malignant skin tumours include the following:[2–5] (i) Age more than 50 years; (ii) male sex; (iii) light skin; (iv) blonde or light brown hair; (v) green, blue, or gray eyes; (vi) skin that sunburns easily (Fitzpatrick skin types I and II); (vii) geographical location (closer to the equator); (viii) history of prior non-melanoma skin cancer; (ix) exposure to ultraviolet light (high cumulative dose of sunshine, tanning beds, or medical UV treatments); (x) exposure to chemical carcinogens (e.g. arsenic, tar) or ionizing radiation (medical treatments, occupational or accidental radiation exposure); (xi) chronic immunosuppression; (xii) chronic inflammatory and scarring conditions (burn scar or thermal injury); (xiii) chronic infections; and (xiv) genetic syndromes and chromosomal abnormalities (oculocutaneous albinism, KID [keratitis, ichthyosis and deafness] syndrome, CDKN2A gene and p16 chromosomal mutation [associated with melanoma], patched gene inactivation/altered hedgehog intracellular signalling pathway [in sporadic BCCs and in nevoid BCC syndrome or Gorlin syndrome] presence of activated *BCL2* [an anti-apoptosis proto-oncogene commonly found in BCCs] and chromosome 1 abnormalities [in Merkel cell carcinoma]).

Malignant melanoma

Melanoma[1,2,5,6] is a malignant neoplasm originating from skin or mucosal melanocytes. It represents 1% of all malignancies, 3% of skin malignancies and 65% of skin cancer deaths. Melanoma is primarily found among the white population and is infrequent in black and oriental people. A majority of patients with melanoma have a pre-existing pigmented lesion, such as a melanocytic nevus. The changes in a benign mole that should alert the clinician towards the possibility of the onset of cutaneous melanoma are itch, enlargement, increased or decreased pigmentation, altered shape or contour, inflammation, or ulceration and bleeding.

The traditional ABCD of malignant melanoma is:
* Asymmetry
* Border irregularity
* Colour variegation
* Diameter >0.6 cm

To this list, E (Evolving lesions) has been added recently.[7]

Types of cutaneous malignant melanoma

The main types of malignant melanoma in the head and neck are described below.[7,8]
* *Lentigo maligna (LM) melanoma* occurs on the exposed skin of the elderly. Approximately 20% of head and neck melanomas are of the LM type. These are flat melanomas with a long radial growth phase. LMs are regarded as the least invasive form of melanoma.
* *Desmoplastic melanomas (DMs)* are a rare subtype of melanoma. Although they account for only 1% of all cutaneous lesions, more than 75% of them are found within the head and neck region. DM tumours tend to be locally aggressive and highly infiltrative. Consequently, they are frequently associated with involvement of the cranial nerves and skull base. Approximately half of these lesions recur.
* *Superficial spreading melanoma* is the most common type in Caucasoids. Its radial growth phase shows varied colours and is often palpable. A nodule coming up within such a plaque signifies deep dermal invasion and a poor prognosis. Superficial spreading melanomas account for approximately 50% of all head and neck melanomas. The growth of a superficial spreading melanoma is biphasic, with an initial radial growth phase, when growth is confined to the epidermis, followed by a vertical phase, when melanocytes invade deeply into the papillary and reticular dermis.
* *Nodular melanoma* appears as a pigmented nodule with no preceding *in situ* phase. It is the most rapidly growing and aggressive type of melanoma. Nodular melanomas are aggressive lesions that have only a vertical growth phase. These lesions make up 15%–30% of head and neck melanomas.
* *Mucosal melanomas* originate from dendritic melanocytes. They account for approximately 1%–4% of cases of head and neck melanoma; most (55%–75%) arise in the nasal cavity, followed by the oral cavity (40%). Although the growth patterns of mucosal melanoma tend to mirror the nodular pattern of their cutaneous counterparts, they differ in that thickness of the tumour is not well correlated with the prognosis. The average tumour thickness at presentation is 3.72 mm, and the most frequent symptom is bleeding or a mass swelling. Approximately 40% of patients have regional metastatic spread at the time of the primary diagnosis. The biological aggressiveness may be related to a greater propensity of mucosal melanomas for not only lymphatic but for haematogenous spread as well.

Although most patients present with clinically localized disease, over 50% experience local recurrence after treatment. Prognosis is dismal, regardless of the thickness of the primary lesion.[9,10]

Histology

Numerous atypical melanocytes, many in groups, are seen initially along the basal layer extending downwards in the walls of hair follicles. Later, dermal invasion occurs, with a breach of the basement membrane region. *In situ* changes are seen in the adjacent epidermis.[1,8]

Microstaging

Histology can be used to assess prognosis. The Breslow

method is to use an ocular micrometer to measure the vertical distance from the granular cell layer to the deepest part of the tumour. The Clark method is to assess the depth of penetration of the melanoma in relation to the different layers of the dermis.[1] The thicker and more penetrating a lesion, the worse is its prognosis.

Stages

- Stages I and II—Localized primary melanoma
- Stage III—Metastasis to single regional lymph node basin (with or without in-transit metastases)
- Stage IV—Distant metastatic disease.

Prognostic factors

Overall, the two most important prognostic factors for cutaneous melanoma of the head and neck are the thickness of the tumour and the status of the regional lymph-node basin. The presence of ulceration has also been found to be an important predictor of outcome. The most important indicator for patients with nodal metastasis is the number of positive lymph nodes (macroscopic disease) and the tumour burden within the lymph nodes (microscopic disease).[6,8,11]

Management

Owing to the dismal prognosis in general, treatment strategies have to be carefully charted out on the basis of the principles described below.[12–15]

Surgery: The lesion should be excised with a wide safety margin. The safety margin increases incrementally with the depth of the tumour (10 times as wide as the deepest penetration of the tumour). However, in aesthetically important areas in the face, a margin as narrow as 5 mm may be enough. The management of lymph nodes is controversial. In the node-positive neck, a selective or comprehensive radical neck dissection is warranted. In the clinically negative neck, sentinel lymph node mapping may be useful in planning further management. With intermediate thickness lesions (1–4 mm) an elective neck dissection may be planned. It should be noted that the lymph node status significantly influences the prognosis. If one node is involved the 5-year survival is 40%, if two or three nodes are involved the 5-year survival drops to 30%, and if >3 nodes are involved the 5-year survival drops to 18%.

Chemotherapy: Malignant melanoma is known to be a relatively chemoresistant tumour. Dacarbazine (DTIC) has been the only chemotherapeutic agent to demonstrate significant activity against melanoma. Adjuvant radiotherapy (RT) may improve regional control in patients with two or more involved nodes.

RT: High dose, post-operative RT may be used to improve survival in mucosal melanomas.

Alternative therapies: Those that have been tried to improve survival and prognosis include high-dose interferon alpha-2b (IFN alpha-2b), polyvalent or ganglioside peptide vaccines, or gene therapy.

Mucosal melanoma of the head and neck

Mucosal melanomas are rare but well recognized and reviewed.[16,17] Their aetiology, however, is unknown. They constitute approximately 2% of all melanomas and 4%–5% of all head and neck cancers. In contrast to their counterparts, they are more common in Japanese people. Common sites of involvement are the oral cavity, nasal cavity and paranasal sinuses, alveolus and tongue. Oropharynx, larynx and nasopharynx are rare sites for this tumour. The man to women ratio is 2:1, unlike cutaneous melanomas, which show an equal predisposition. The mean age of occurrence is 56 years, being 51–60 years for men and 61–70 years for women.

Staging

Commonly used clinical prognostic staging is the Ballantyne staging, in which stage I represents those melanomas that are confined to the primary site, irrespective of their extent. Stage II melanomas show lymph node metastasis, and stage III melanomas represent melanomas with distant metastasis. Eighty per cent patients present with local disease and 5%–10% with enlarged lymph nodes.

The Clarke grading and Breslow thickness obtained after histopathological examination of the excised specimen are less reliable because of the absence of the basement membrane, and papillary and reticular dermis. Largely macular, sometimes nodular or even pedunculated lentigomaligna and nodular melanomas carry poor prognosis, whereas the superficial spreading type carries a better overall prognosis. Therefore, tumour thickness (those that are <0.75 mm thick rarely metastasize) and lymph node metastasis are reliable prognostic indicators.

Investigations

Management: The dictum of management of oral melanotic lesions is that, unless otherwise proven, all of them need to be biopsied because the chance of a melanotic mucosal lesion (black or blue) being a melanoma is much higher than that of a similar pigmented lesion in the skin. A long standing melanosis can undergo sudden malignant change characterized by an increase in thickness or bleeding from the site.

Lesions of <3 mm can be excised with a 1–2 mm margin and those that are >3 mm need an incisional biopsy. Once the tissue diagnosis is obtained, a chest X-ray, an ultrasound scan of the abdomen and a bone scan need to be done to rule

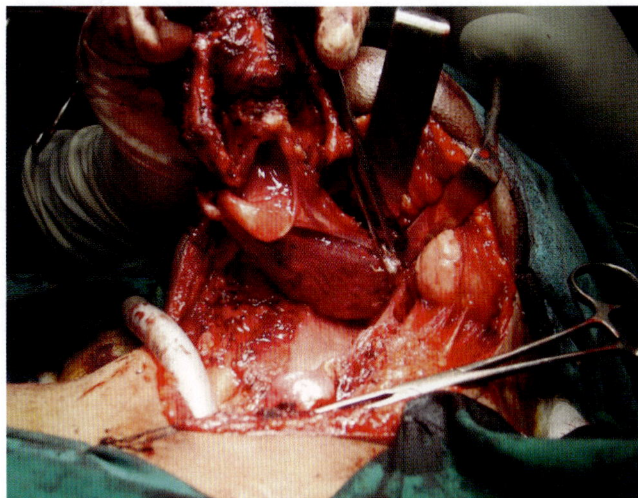

Fig. 1. An extensive mucosal melanoma of the supraglottis vallecula tonsils and tongue being radically resected

out distant metastasis. Endoscopy of the upper aerodigestive tract is done to rule out similar lesions and to delineate the tumour extent when the lesion is beyond the lower pole of the tonsil. Contrast-enhanced CT and MRI help to gauge the deep extent of disease and lymph node status.

Treatment: The mainstay of treatment of mucosal melanoma (Fig. 1) is surgical excision with adequate margins, which ideally would be 2 cm all around. However, this may not be feasible in all locations, especially the oropharynx, larynx and hypopharynx, where a margin of 1 cm can be considered satisfactory. Elective neck dissection for the N0 neck is not warranted and a comprehensive neck dissection needs to be done when the neck is clinically or radiologically positive for nodes.

Although not radiosensitive, melanomas, especially those that are inoperable or those that have metastasized to a distant site, are treated upfront by RT either with a curative or a palliative intent. There are very occasional reports of a radio response of these tumours. Radiotherapy, however, is used as adjuvant treatment after radical surgical excision, with or without neck dissection, to enhance the loco-regional control (hyperfractionated RT).

Immunotherapy in the form of interferon, interleukin and adoptive cell therapy are the recent adjuvants that are being tried, with limited success. When other forms of treatment are not feasible, immunotherapy is occasionally given as the primary treatment. Apart from their direct action on the mediators of immunity, interferons (INF–A) alfa-2b act on the receptors in the tumour cells and make the tumour susceptible to the innate immunity of the host. Interleukin (IL-2) enhances the action of natural killer cells and acts on the hypothalamus releasing immunomodulators and pyrogens. Adoptive cell therapy is a technique by which highly tumour avid lymphocytes are cultured *ex vivo* to be transferred after a lymphocyte-depleting chemotherapy to

the host.[18] However, the role of immunotherapy has not been evaluated clearly in mucosal sites.

Unlike cutaneous melanomas, mucosal melanomas do not benefit from sentinel node biopsy because of their complex drainage patterns. Chemotherapy with dacarbazine is of questionable value.

Differential diagnoses, besides benign conditions, includes poorly differentiated carcinoma and anaplastic large cell lymphoma. Histopathological confirmation is by immuno-histochemistry, which shows positivity for S–100 protein, HMB45 (homatropine methylbromide), and vimentin with micropthalmic transcription factor. Tyrosinase and melan immunostains are also positive.

Prognosis

The 5-year survival rate is 10%–25%. Death in one-third of the cases occurs due to metastasis, one-third is due to recurrence, and one-third due to both relapse and metastasis; these events could possibly occur even after 5 years.

Basal cell carcinoma (BCC)

BCCs arise from pleuripotent cells in the basal layer of the epidermis or follicular structures. This is the most common form of skin cancer. Patients often present with a non-healing sore of varying duration. The lesions are typically seen on the face, ears, scalp, neck, or upper trunk. Mild trauma, such as face washing or drying with a towel, may initially cause bleeding from the lesions. Lesions invade locally but, for practical purposes, never metastasize.[1,2,4]

Clinical presentation

BCCs present in various forms as follows.[1,2,19,20]

Nodulo-ulcerative: This is the most common type. An early lesion is a small glistening translucent skin coloured papule that slowly enlarges. Central necrosis, although not invariable, leaves an ulcer with an adherent crust and a rolled pearly edge. Fine telangiectatic vessels often run across the tumour's surface. Without treatment, such lesions may reach 1–2 cm in diameter in 5–10 years.

Cystic: The lesion is at first like the nodular type, but later cystic changes predominate and the nodule becomes tense and more translucent, with marked telangiectasia.

Cicatricial (morphoeic): These are slowly expanding yellow or white waxy plaques with an ill-defined edge. Ulceration and crusting, followed by fibrosis, are common, and the lesion may look like an enlarging scar.

Superficial (multicentric): These arise most often on the trunk. Several lesions may be present, each expanding slowly as a pink or brown scaly plaque with a fine 'whipcord' edge. Such lesions can grow to >10 cm in diameter.

Pigmented: Pigment may be present in all types of BCC, causing all or part of the tumour to be brown or have specks of brown or black within it.

Histology

Several authors[1,5,20] have described BCC as characteristically consisting of small, dark blue staining basal cells that grow in well defined aggregates which invade the dermis. The outer layer of cells is arranged in a palisade. Numerous mitoses and apoptotic bodies are seen. In the cicatricial type of BCC, the islands of tumour are surrounded by fibrous tissue. Tumour cells of nodular BCC have large, hyperchromatic, oval nuclei and little cytoplasm with few mitotic figures. Tumour cells tend to align more densely in a palisade pattern at the periphery of these nests. The more aggressive morpheaform and infiltrating BCCs have growth patterns resulting in strands of cells rather than round nests. Basosquamous carcinoma, which exhibits features of both BCC and SCC, is also considered an aggressive skin cancer.

Management[2,21–24]

Management policies vary according to the size of the lesion and its site. For lesions <2 cm, complete surgical excision with a 4 mm safety margin is usually adequate with 98% cure rate. Mohs micrographic surgery with immediate histopathological analysis is usually reserved for cosmetically critical regions (lids, nose, lips). In selected cases, this gives a 5-year cure rate of 99%. Topical imiquimod, an immunomodulatory agent with antineoplastic activity, has been used successfully in areas where surgery is not feasible or desirable. Phototherapy has been attempted with variable degrees of success. Radiation therapy is seldom used for primary cases but may be used in recurrences and for salvage.

Squamous cell carcinoma (SCC)

This is a malignant proliferation of epidermal keratinocytes. SCC may manifest as a variety of primary morphologies with or without associated symptoms. Tumours may arise as thickenings in an actinic keratosis or, *de novo* as small scaling nodules; rapidly growing anaplastic lesions may start as ulcers with a granulating base and an indurated edge.

Clinical presentation

SCCs are common on the lower lip and in the mouth. SCC of the lip usually arises on the vermillion border of the lower lip. It is sometimes predated by a precursor lesion, actinic cheilitis, which manifests as xerosis, fissuring, atrophy and dyspigmentation. SCC on the lip manifests as a new papule, erosion, or focus of erythema/induration. Intra-oral SCC typically manifests as a white plaque (leukoplakia) with or without reddish reticulation (erythroplakia). Common locations include the anterior floor of the mouth, the lateral tongue and the buccal vestibule. SCC arising in sun-exposed areas and in actinic keratoses seldom metastasize. Tumours >2 cm in diameter are twice as likely to recur and metastasize compared with smaller tumours. Metastatic potential is also high in tumours >4 mm in depth or invading the subcutaneous tissue, in poorly differentiated tumours, in tumours with perineural involvement and in those arising in immunosuppressed patients.[1,2,5]

Histology

SCC *in situ* is characterized by an intra-epidermal proliferation of atypical keratinocytes. Hyperkeratosis, acanthosis, and confluent parakeratosis are seen within the epidermis, and the keratinocytes lie in complete disorder, resulting in the classic 'windblown' appearance. Cellular atypia, including pleomorphism, hyperchromatic nuclei, and mitoses, is prominent. Atypical keratinocytes may be found in the basal layer and often extend deeply down hair follicles, but they do not invade the dermis. Squamous eddies or keratin pearls arise from keratinization. The neoplastic cells may show varying degrees of squamous differentiation and atypia. Immunohistochemical staining with antibodies to cytokeratins and epithelial membrane antigen is used to confirm the epithelial (i.e. keratinocyte) origin of the tumour.[2,4,5]

Staging

SCC is staged according to American Joint Committee on Cancer guidelines, which use the TNM (tumour, node, metastasis) classification system. Most cutaneous SCCs are not metastatic at the time of presentation; therefore, the tumour stage in such cases is based solely on the characteristics of the primary lesion. Staging of metastatic disease takes into account the presence or absence of regional lymph node and distant metastasis.[1,4,5] Tx denotes those tumours which cannot be assessed due to previous intervention; in T0 stage there is no clinical evidence of a primary tumour; T1s is carcinoma *in situ;* T1 is tumour <2 cm in its greatest diameter; T2 between 2 and 5 cm in its greatest diameter; T3 >5 cm in its greatest diameter; and T4 tumours invade the cartilage muscle or bone.

Spread

Spread occurs by local invasion along tissue plains, between muscles, over the periosteum, and along nerves, lymphatics and blood vessels. Distant metastases by blood-borne dissemination occur towards the later stages.

Management

Management is by wide excision with margins of 2–10 mm or by Moh micrographic surgery. Other methods are curretage and cautery, cryotherapy, lasers, photodynamic therapy, retinoids and radiation therapy, of which radiation alone has stood the test of time. Management of the neck nodes will be required in node-positive disease, the preferred option being neck dissection. Irradiation of the neck is an alternative when surgery is not feasible.[2,23,25]

Follow-up

Most recurrences occur within 5 years (95%). Follow-up should be every 3 months for 2 years and then twice yearly. Close examination of the scar site and draining lymph node areas is recommended.

Merkel cell carcinoma

Merkel cell carcinoma (neuroendocrine carcinoma of the skin, cutaneous APUDoma [amine precursor uptake and deamination] or primary small cell carcinoma) of the skin with endocrine differentiation, is an uncommon, aggressive, cutaneous neoplasm. It is the deadliest skin malignancy. Merkel cell carcinoma is located principally on the head and neck. It occurs primarily in caucasians.

Most patients are in their sixties and seventies at the time of diagnosis. Merkel cell carcinoma presents most often as a solitary, painless, pink to reddish-blue or brown dome-shaped nodule or plaque on sun-exposed skin of elderly individuals. The lesion may sometimes ulcerate, and can range in size from 0.2 to 5.0 cm.[2,26]

Histology

Merkel cell carcinoma is composed of small, monomorphic, basophilic tumour cells with round to oval-shaped nuclei and scanty cytoplasm. The definitive diagnosis of Merkel cell carcinoma requires the use of immunohistochemistry. Antibodies to low molecular weight cytokeratins are the most sensitive markers.

Staging

- Stage I—a local disease without lymph node or systemic involvement
- Stage II—refers to regional lymph node disease without evidence of systemic spread
- Stage III—refers to metastatic disease.

Management

Multimodality treatment is thought to offer the best results.

Surgical excision includes using a wide local excision with 2–3 cm margins, and dissecting up to the fascia. Excision may be followed by elective lymph node dissection or lymphoscintigraphy and sentinel node biopsy. Postoperative radiation may also be considered in higher stages. Stage III disease most often requires systemic chemotherapy.

TUMOURS OF THE EAR

Tumours are unusual in the ear. Tumours in the external ear arise from the skin, ceruminous glands, or bone. Tumours of the middle ear may arise from the lining cuboidal epithelium as adenomas or adenocarcinomas, from minor salivary glands or from glial tissue (choristomas). SCC may arise from metaplastic epithelium in chronically discharging middle ears.[27,28] The commonest tumours of the temporal bone are those arising from Schwann cells, such as vestibular or facial schwannomas. Tumours may also arise from paraganglia (glomus tumours) or from the endolymphatic sac.

The WHO classification of tumours of the ear is as follows:[29]

Tumours of the external ear
- Benign tumours of ceruminous glands
  —Adenoma
  —Chondroid syringoma
  —Syringocystadenoma papilliferum
- Cylindroma
- Malignant tumours of ceruminous glands
  —Adenocarcinoma
  —Adenoid cystic carcinoma
  —Mucoepidermoid carcinoma
- Squamous cell carcinoma
- Embryonal rhabdomyosarcoma
- Osteoma and exostosis
- Angiolymphoid hyperplasia with eosinophilia

Tumours of the middle ear
- Adenoma of the middle ear
- Papillary tumours
  —Aggressive papillary tumour
  —Schneiderian papilloma
  —Inverted papilloma
- Squamous cell carcinoma
- Meningioma

Tumours of the inner ear
- Vestibular schwannoma
- Lipoma of the internal auditory canal
- Haemangioma
- Endolymphatic sac tumour

Haematolymphoid tumours
- B-cell chronic lymphocytic leukaemia/small lymphocytic lymphoma
- Langerhans cell histiocytosis

Secondary tumours

Tumours of the external ear

The most common tumours of the auricle are SCC or BCC. They behave like their cutaneous counterparts anywhere in the body. The external auditory meatus may also give rise to ceruminoma or adenocarcinoma.

Ceruminoma

These are rare benign tumours of the ceruminous glands of the external meatus. The tumour usually manifests as a non-ulcerating superficial mass causing conductive hearing loss and occasional discharge.

Histology

The neoplasm lacks a capsule. It is composed of regular oxyphil glands with intra-luminal projections. The glandular epithelium is bilayered.

Management

Local excision.

Malignant tumours of the ceruminous glands

These infiltrating neoplasms from the ceruminous glands arise from the superficial part of the external canal. They may be confused with adenoid cystic carcinoma or mucoepidermoid tumours. Extension from primary parotid tumours should be excluded. Recurrences, local and distal extension may complicate high-grade lesions. Treatment is by wide primary surgical excision. Postoperative RT may improve the prognosis, especially in adenoid cystic carcinoma.

SCC of the external meatus

This malignant tumour arises from the stratified squamous epithelium covering the external canal and pinna. Lesions of the pinna show a male preponderance whereas tumours of the external canal show a female preponderance.[27,30]

Aetiology

Lesions of the pinna show the same aetiological factors as other skin tumours, especially actinic overexposure. Lesions of the external canal are mostly secondary to prolonged chronic inflammation.

Clinical presentation

Most of the lesions of the canal present late because of the minimal symptoms they generate. Pain, hearing loss and discharge which may be purulent or blood-stained are the major presenting symptoms. A plaque-like lesion or a polypoid mass may occlude the canal. The lesion may invade through the drum into the middle ear, or into the parotid region, or the sternomastoid muscle. Increasing pain and facial paralysis may occur later. Metastases are usually late but may occur in up to 20% of cases to the jugulodigastric parotid or group IIb nodes.[31]

Staging

The University of Pittsburgh staging proposed by Arriaga *et al.*[32] is the most popular. According to this, T1 tumours are confined solely to the external auditory canal (EAC); T2 tumours show limited bone erosion or soft tissue (<0.5 cm) extension; T3 tumours show extensive (full thickness) involvement of bony EAC and limited (<0.5 cm) soft tissue involvement or show middle ear or mastoid involvement or the involvement of both; T4 tumours erode the cochlea, petrous apex, medial wall of middle ear, carotid canal, jugular foramen or dura or show extensive (>0.5 cm) soft tissue involvement. The N status significantly affects the prognosis and places the patient in an advanced stage, i.e. T1N1 is stage III and any T >2 with N1 makes it stage IV.

Treatment

Radical surgical excision with lymph node dissection in N+ lesions.[33–35]

Osteomas and exostosis

These are benign bony lesions of the deeper portion of the external meatus. An osteoma is a single unilateral spherical mass on a distinct pedicle. They usually arise in the region of the tympanomastoid or tympanosquamous sutures. They have been reported in the middle ear, mastoid, and other regions. Exostoses are commoner broad-based lesions—often bilateral and symmetrical. They usually arise deeper in the canal and are related to repeated trauma, especially exposure to cold water in swimmers.

Clinical presentation

Hearing loss and occlusion of the canal are the usual presenting symptoms. Repeated wax impaction or inflammation of the skin of the meatus deep to the lesion may also occur. In some patients an external canal cholesteatoma or keratosis obturans may develop deep to the lesion leading to localized bone destruction.

Treatment

Surgical excision. Osteomas are pedunculated and can be easily excised. Attempts at chiselling off the lesion may cause a radiating fissure with the potential for facial nerve damage, ossicular disruption or even labyrinthine damage. Exostoses may be shaved off with a drill after elevating skin flaps to line the refashioned meatus.[27,28]

Tumours of the middle ear

Masses in the middle ear may be primary or secondary extensions from surrounding areas.[33,34,36] Primary lesions include benign and malignant tumours and mass like-lesions.

Benign:
- Cholesteatoma
- Cholesterol granuloma
- Choristomas
- Benign adenoma

Malignant:
- SCC
- Adenocarcinoma
- Rhabdomyosarcoma

Adenoma

These are benign glandular neoplasms with variable neuro-endocrine or mucin-secreting pathways. These lesions usually appear in middle-aged persons with progressive unilateral hearing loss and a reddish-brown, non-pulsating mass behind an intact drum.

Histology

The tumour is formed of closely apposed small glands. In some places a solid or trabecular pattern may be seen. Periodic acid–Schiff and alcian blue stains may be positive for mucin, and immunohistochemical markers for neuroendocrine activity are positive in most of these lesions.

Management: Surgical excision is done, with possible ossiculoplasty for repair of a damaged ossicular chain.

Adenocarcinoma (papillary tumours)

These are rare tumours which may arise in any part of the middle ear and mastoid air cell system or from the endolymphatic sac. They are aggressive tumours that may lead to extensive destruction and spread beyond the confines of the middle ear cleft. Most are treated by extensive surgery followed by RT.

SCC

These are malignant tumours arising from the cuboidal or pseudostratified epithelium of the middle ear.[27,28,34,36] Most cases arise secondary to squamous metaplasia in long standing chronic suppurative otitis media.

Clinical presentation

The usual scenario is a patient with long standing chronic suppurative otitis media with increasing persistent discharge, blood-stained discharge, pain and a fleshy polypoid mass arising from the middle ear and extending into the external meatus. Hearing usually worsens.

The tumour can infiltrate the surrounding areas intra-cranially with dural invasion, anteriorly along the Eustachian tube and into the nasopharynx and posteriorly with mastoid destruction. Facial paralysis is a common presentation and may be the first suspicious sign of malignant transformation in a chronically discharging ear. The inner ear resists invasion for a long time but erosion of the promontory may lead to sensorineural hearing loss and vertigo. Lymphatic spread to the retropharyngeal nodes may occur by lymphatics along the Eustachian tube.

Stages

- T1—Tumour limited to the site of origin with no facial paralysis or bone destruction
- T2—Facial paralysis or bone destruction. No extrapetrous extension
- T3—Extension to the dura, skull base, parotid, etc.

Management

The best results are achieved by radical surgery followed by RT. Some patients present late without any feasibility of any effective treatment other than pain-relief.

Rhabdomyosarcoma

This is a primitive malignant tumour arising from embryonal skeletal muscle elements. It is a rare tumour with a distinct subgroup arising in very young children, with a predilection for the palate, middle ear and orbit. Most tumours arise in the middle ear and extend into the external meatus as a fleshy polyp.

The tumour must be suspected in any young child presenting with an aural polyp. Later, there is otorrhoea, facial paralysis and swelling, and destruction of the mastoid region. Extensive destruction of the skull base may complicate these lesions. The mainstay of management is a combination of surgery, RT and chemotherapy.[28]

Management of tumours of the ear and temporal bone

Introduction

Tumours of the ear and temporal bone are rare and usually present with signs and symptoms of inflammatory ear disease. Suspicion of malignancy is aroused by the presence of blood-stained ear discharge, onset of facial paralysis and, in the event of local spread, by the presence of cranial nerve involvement and intractable pain. Usually, these tumours are detected when they are in a fairly advanced stage, which contributes to poor treatment outcomes. Owing to the rarity of these tumours and varied histology, no consensus on staging and prognostication has been arrived at. However, from the experience of most centres, surgery is the mainstay of treatment. The complex anatomy of the ear and temporal bone, where a plethora of vital structures are packed into a small area, makes surgery a formidable challenge. Usually, treatment requires a multidisciplinary team comprising of head and neck surgeons/skull base surgeons, neurosurgeons, plastic reconstructive surgeons, and speech and swallowing therapists.

General considerations

Age and sex

This is a disease of the elderly, even though middle ear cancer may present in younger individuals. The possibility of sarcoma must be considered in the paediatric population. No significant differences in predilection have been reported between the sexes.[37]

Incidence

The age-adjusted incidence for a SCC is 1 per 1 million women and 0.8 per 1 million men annually.[38]

Aetiology

No definite aetiological factors have been identified. UV exposure from sunlight may be attributed to lesions arising from the pinna or the outer EAC. Chronic inflammation has been suggested as a causative factor for those arising deep in the meatus.[39] Radiotherapy to the nasopharynx has also been documented as a predisposing factor.[40]

Pathology

SCC is the commonest histological type encountered. Other types include BCC and primary adenocarcinomas, of which the papillary subtype is the commonest. Other less commonly encountered pathologies include adenoid cystic carcinoma, melanoma, sarcoma, metastasis and rhabdomyosarcoma, especially in younger individuals.

Clinical presentation

The disease presents insidiously as a chronic external otitis. The presence of pain, bloody otorrhoea or facial weakness alerts the clinician to the possibility of underlying malignancy.[41] In a review by Pensak, the symptoms of patients ranged from ear pain (74%), through hearing loss (62%) and bleeding (28%) to facial numbness (12%) and vertigo (10%). The clinical signs included ear canal lesion (88%), aural discharge (84%), preauricular swelling (25%), facial paralysis (18%) and abnormal neck nodes (8%). It is uncommon to find cervical lymphadenopathy in these patients. It is usually present in very advanced stages and has a very poor prognosis.[42,43]

Spread and natural history

The temporal bone is endowed with numerous vascular and neural foramina and preformed channels through which tumours may traverse. The complexity of extensions through the labyrinth of critical structures makes surgery particularly challenging and hinders complete excision, leading to a high chance of local recurrence.

Laterally, the tumour may track along the skin of the EAC, leading to oedema and granulations in the external canal, or it may present as an aural polyp. A high index of suspicion is needed to detect the lesion at this time (Fig. 2a). Over a period of time, the lesion may spread into the conchal bowl and pinna with destruction of cartilage (Fig. 2b). Anterior extension occurs into the parotid, temporomandibular joint and the infra-temporal fossa through the fissures of Santorini, the petrosquamous and petrotympanic fissures and preformed defects in the external canal (foramen of Huschke). Inferiorly, it may involve the jugular foramen and give rise to lower cranial nerve palsies. Medial extension through the tympanic membrane provides access to the middle ear cleft and the pneumatized spaces of the mastoid, eventually involving the facial nerve, the internal carotid artery and the Eustachian tube. The otic capsule resists invasion and features of its invasion occur late in the course of the disease with the patient presenting with sensorineural hearing loss or vertigo. Superior spread occurs into the epitympanic space and extension to the middle cranial fossa dura. Posteriorly, the tumour may extend through the air cells to invade the posterior fossa dura.

Distant metastasis is rare. Reports indicate the lung

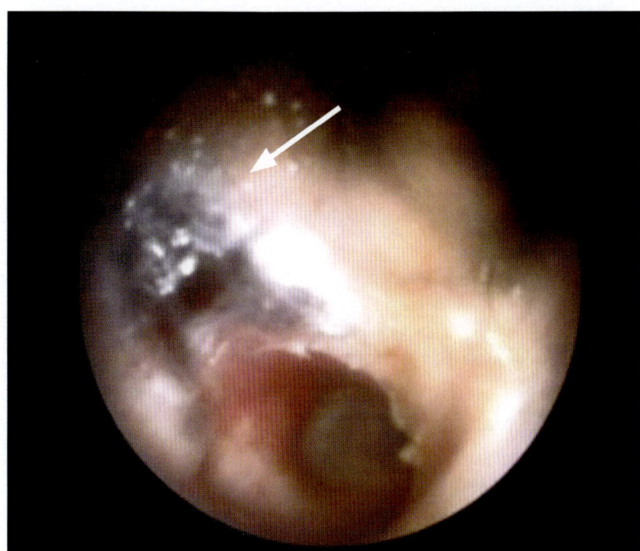

Fig. 2a. Otomicroscopy shows a haemorrhagic proliferative area at the junction of the bony and cartilaginous external auditory meatus (arrow). Histology was consistent with squamous cell carcinoma.

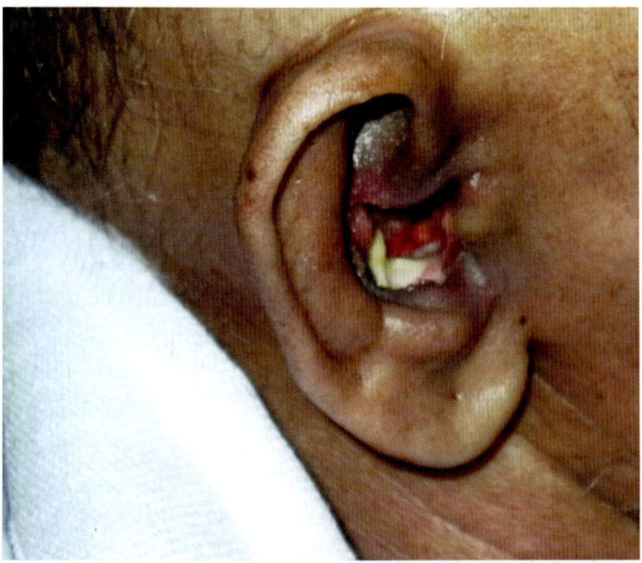

Fig. 2b. Advanced squamous cell of the external auditory meatus with involvement of the pinna and exposure of conchal cartilage

and bone as the most common sites and may occur with squamous cancer, adenoid cystic carcinoma, adenocarcinoma, and sarcoma. Perineural spread has been reported most commonly with adenoidcystic carcinoma, but may also occur in SCCs and BCCs. The temporal bone may also be a site for distant metastasis for primaries arising in the breast, lung, prostate, kidney, salivary glands, pharynx or nasopharynx, gastrointestinal tract, or from an occult primary.[44]

Evaluation of patients

History and examination of patients with ear and temporal

bone cancers is done with intent to confirm diagnosis, assess extent of disease and, accordingly, formulate a treatment plan. Malignancy is suspected in recalcitrant otorrhoea of long duration or in the presence of facial nerve weakness. More extensive lesions may present with other cranial nerve involvement. Deep-seated headache may suggest dural involvement. It is essential to conduct a detailed otomicroscopy and to obtain a biopsy from granulations in the EAC. In case a vascular lesion is suspected, it is better to wait for radiological examination to be complete before biopsy.

Imaging studies include a coronal and axial computed tomogram [CT] and an MRI. According to Hugh and Curtin, both these modalities are 'complementary and not competitive in the initial evaluation of skull base tumours'. Whereas CT offers excellent detail of bone involvement, MRI contributes by providing excellent tissue demarcation, visualization of perineural extension and dural and intracranial extension, especially when enhanced by gadolinium contrast. Sub-millimetric resolution, 3-D reformatting and multiplanar imaging capabilities have generated a strong case for high resolution CT as a first line imaging, with MRI supplemented for additional detail.[42]

Four-vessel angiography, including the venous phase, is considered in a surgical candidate with internal carotid artery involvement. Pre-operative cerebral blood flow studies done after a 15-minute carotid balloon occlusion study with neurological monitoring would indicate whether it would be feasible to safely resect the internal carotid on one side or employ revascularization using a graft.[45]

Staging

Owing to the extreme rarity of these tumours, no centre has sufficient data to generate meaningful staging or prognostication guidelines. Staging systems have been suggested by Stell and McCormick,[46] which was later revised by Clark *et al.*[47] The Pittsburgh university staging system is the most popular and has been extensively adopted in studies on temporal bone cancer.[32]

Treatment

Even though the histology and biological behaviour of ear and temporal bone tumours are varied, broad guidelines in their management may be adopted. Surgery remains the mainstay of treatment and RT is used sometimes in the adjuvant setting. The CT and MRI scans must be studied and carefully read to plan the surgical approach. Attempts must be made to remove the tumour *en bloc* with negative margins. Some skull base surgeons prefer to perform a step-wise removal of disease starting with an *en bloc* resection with a gross estimate of the extent and, using a drill to clear out remaining disease, offer adjuvant RT thereafter.[48] Very small tumours whose borders

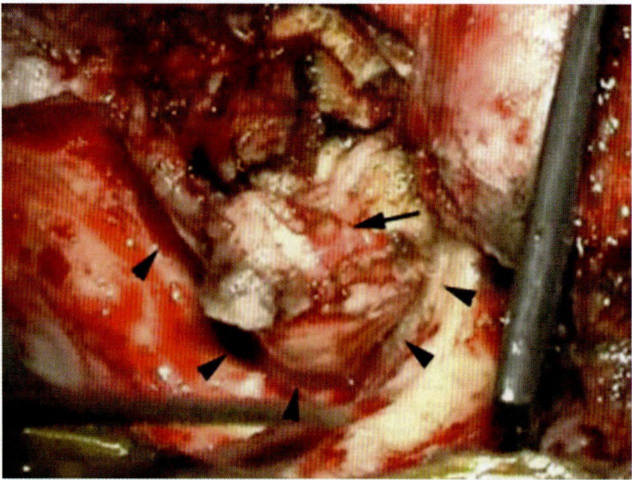

Fig. 3. Lateral temporal bone resection. Arrow shows transected external auditory canal containing the tumour. The extended facial recess extending all the way from the mastiod tip to the temporomadibular joint is shown by the arrowheads.

are visible completely in the EAC may be approached per meatally.

Sleeve resection

This is used for very small lesions limited to the cartilaginous external auditory meatus with limited extension to the bony part where the ear canal may be excised as a cuff of skin. Once the tumour encroaches into the bony canal, a lateral temporal bone resection is to be considered as the skin in this area is extremely thin and there is a high possibility of microscopic invasion of underlying bone.

Lateral temporal bone resection

This is indicated for lesions in the EAC involving the bony meatus but not extending into the mesotympanum. This operation entails excising the entire bony and cartilaginous meatus with the tympanic membrane. A circular incision is placed in the conchal bowl, including the tragus, and the sleeve is closed. A post-aural incision is placed and a mastoidectomy is performed, leaving the canal wall intact. This is followed by an extended facial recess approach, and the facial nerve is preserved along its entire length. The incudostapedial joint is dislocated and the bony canal fractured using an osteotome. The lateral temporal bone resection may be extended to involve the head of the mandible or the parotid gland (Fig. 3).

Subtotal temporal bone resection

The vertical part of the internal carotid artery is identified and the resection includes the glenoid fossa and the Eustachian tube orifice. The sigmoid sinus may also have to be ligated.

Total temporal bone resection

While total temporal bone resections have been performed, the morbidity arising from palsies of the VII, VIII, IX, X, XI and XII cranial nerves and the risk of compromise of vascularity to the brainstem must be weighed against the limited survival following these extensive surgeries.

RT in ear and temporal bone tumours

The role of RT in the primary treatment of ear and temporal bone tumours is limited. In Zhang's series, radiation alone offered a 5-year survival rate of only 28.7%.[49] The intimate relation of the tumour to the bone, skull base and cartilage of the pinna makes it difficult to deliver a high dose effectively. RT, however, may be used for palliation of symptoms in a small group of patients. Various studies have demonstrated effectiveness of RT in the adjuvant setting after primary surgical resection.[50,51]

Reconstruction

Temporal bone resections leave a bony defect sometimes with extension to skin, parotid and pinna. Minimal defects may be allowed to epithelialize over a temporal fascia graft. The temporalis muscle may be turned in to cover a larger defect. For larger defects, local flaps of choice are the latissimus dorsi and trapezius flap. In our group's experience, free flaps offer the best reconstructive option. Radial forearm free flaps offer thin pliable skin for superficial defects. For larger defects, especially where there is dural breach or exposure, it is ideal to use a muscle containing flap, such as the rectus abdominis, or anterolateral thigh flap with vastus lateralis muscle, which forms an effective seal.

Prognosis and outcomes following treatment

The rarity of the disease and the variety in terms of histopathology make it difficult to arrive at meaningful tools for staging and prognostication, but certain large series reported in the literature allow us to obtain a broad overview of the behaviour of these tumours and their outcome. The local extent of the tumour is a good indicator of survival. In most studies, treatment outcomes are good when the disease is localized.[52] Studies show overall survival, for all stages together, to vary from 37% to 75.6% with radical surgery and post-operative RT.[51,53] A dramatic difference in survival was noted between early and advanced stages in a study conducted by Kunst *et al.*,[54] in which the Kaplan–Meier survival curves showed survival rates at 5 years of 83% and 25% for the stages pT1 and pT4, respectively. Similar disparity in survival between early and late stages was noted by Moffat *et al.*[36] in whose series the overall disease-free survival was 43.2% across all stages. Disease-free survival for stages II and III disease was 100%, whereas for stage IV tumours it dropped to 34.3%. In the same study, node-positive disease, poorly differentiated squamous cell histological findings, brain involvement, and salvage surgery were associated with a poorer outcome. Failure of treatment is most commonly caused by local failure (83%) followed by loco-regional failure (9%), regional failure (5.5%), and distant metastasis (2%).[55]

Rehabilitation

Surgery for temporal bone tumours results in problems that would require rehabilitative measures that range from deficits of cranial nerves to cosmetic defects. The facial nerve, if resected, should be reconstructed using a nerve graft. A gold weight may be placed in the upper lid at the same time while waiting for function to recover. Lower cranial nerve deficits result in dysphagia and dysphonia which may settle in due course with active assistance from a speech and swallowing therapist. Medialization of the vocal cord may be considered for vocal cord paralysis. Prosthetic ear, either as adhesive borne or as an osseointegrated implant may be provided for defects of the pinna.

References

1. Hunter J, Savin J, Dhal M. *Clinical dermatology.* 3rd ed. Oxford, England: Blackwell Scientific; 2002.
2. Morgan MB, Smoller BR, Somach SC. *Deadly dermatologic diseases.* 1st ed. Malaysia, Springer Science +Business Media, LLC, 2007.
3. Bale AE, Yu KP. The hedgehog pathway and basal cell carcinomas. *Hum Mol Genet* 2001;**10**:757–62.
4. Ponten F, Lundeberg J. Principles of tumour biology and pathogenesis of BCCs and SCCs. In: Bolognia JL, Jorizzo JL, Rapini RP (eds). *Dermatology.* Vol. 2. China: Mosby; 2004;107:1020–35.
5. Kirkham N. Tumors and cysts of the epidermis. In: Elder D, Elenitas R, Jaworsky C, *et al.* (eds). *Lever's histopathology of the skin.* 8th ed. Philadelphia, Pa: Lippincott-Raven; 1997:719–46.
6. Garbe C, Büttner P, Bertz J, *et al.* Primary cutaneous melanoma. Prognostic classification of anatomic location. *Cancer* 1995;**75**:2492–98.
7. Abbasi NR, Shaw HM, Rigel DS. Early diagnosis of cutaneous melanoma, revisiting the ABCD criteria. *JAMA* 2004;**292**:2771.
8. Balch CM, Buzaid AC, Soong SJ, *et al.* Final version of the AJCC staging system for cutaneous melanoma. *J Clin Oncol* 2001;**19**:3635–48.
9. Paytrick RJ, Fenske NA, Messina JL. Primary mucosal melanoma. *J Am Acad Dermatol* 2007;**56**:828–34.
10. Penel N, Mallet Y, Mirabel X, *et al.* Primary mucosal melanoma of head and neck: Prognostic value of clear margins. *Laryngoscope* 2006;**116**:993–5.
11. Golger A, Young DS, Ghazaria D, *et al.* Epidemiological features and prognostic factors of cutaneous head and neck melanoma: A population based study. *Arch Otolaryngol Head Neck Surg* 2007;**133**:442–7.
12. Balch CM, Urist MM, Karakousis CP, *et al.* Efficacy of 2-cm surgical margins for intermediate thickness melanomas (1 to 4 mm). Results of a multi-institutional randomized surgical trial. *Ann Surg* 1993;**218**:262–7; discussion 267–69.
13. Bricca GM, Brodland DG, Ren D, *et al.* Cutaneous head and neck melanoma treated with Mohs micrographic surgery. *J Am Acad Dermatol* 2005;**52**:92–100.
14. Kirkwood JM, Manola J, Ibrahim J, *et al.* A pooled analysis of eastern cooperative oncology group and intergroup trials of adjuvant high dose interferon for melanoma. *Clin Cancer Res* 2004;**10**:1670–77.
15. Schmalbach CE, Johnson TM, Bradford CR. The management of head and neck melanoma. *Curr Probl Surg* 2006;**43**:781–835.
16. Hicks MJ, Flaitz CM. Oral mucosal melanoma: Epidemiology and pathobiology. *Oral Oncol* 2000;**36**:152–69. Review.
17. Mendenhall WM, Amdur RJ, Hinerman RW, *et al.* Head and neck mucosal melanoma. *Am J Clin Oncol* 2005;**28**:626–30. Review.
18. Dudley ME, Wunderlich JR, Yang JC, et al. Adoptive cell transfer therapy following non-myeloablative but lymphodepleting chemotherapy for treatment of patients with refractory metastatic melanoma. *J Clin Oncol* 2005;**23**:2346–57.
19. Maloney ME, Miller SJ. Aggressive versus non-aggressive subtypes: Basal cell carcinoma. In: Maloney ME, Miller SJ (eds). *Cutaneous Oncology.* Oxford, England: Blackwell Science; 1998:609–13.
20. Lowe L. Histology: Basal cell carcinoma. In: Maloney ME, Miller SJ (eds). *Cutaneous Oncology.* Oxford, England: Blackwell Science; 1998.
21. Lang PG, Maize JC. Basal cell carcinoma. In: Friedman RJ, Kopf AW, Harris MN, *et al.* (eds). *Cancer of the skin.* Philadelphia, Pa: WB Saunders; 1991.
22. Ratner D, Skouge JW. Surgical management of local disease: Basal cell carcinoma. In: Maloney ME, Miller SJ (eds). *Cutaneous oncology.* Oxford, England: Blackwell Science; 1998.
23. Robinson JK. What are adequate treatment and follow-up care for non-melanoma cutaneous cancer? *Arch Dermatol* 1987;**123**:331–3.
24. Silverman MK, Kopf AW, Grin CM, *et al.* Recurrence rates of treated basal cell carcinomas. Part 1: Overview. *J Dermatol Surg Oncol* 1991;**17**:713–18.
25. Preston DS, Stern RS. Nonmelanoma cancers of the skin. *N Engl J Med* 1992;**327**:1649–62.
26. Gollard R, Weber R, Kosty M, *et al.* Merkel cell carcinoma: Review of 22 cases with surgical, pathologic, and therapeutic considerations. *Cancer* 2000;**88**:1842–51.
27. Michaels L, Hellquist HB. *Ear nose and throat histopathology.* 2nd ed. Springer Verlag 2001.
28. Barnes L, Eveson JW, Reichhart P, *et al. Pathology and genetics of head and neck tumours.* 2nd ed. IARC, Lyon: France; 2005.
29. Thompson LDR. Pathology and genetics of head and neck tumours. In: Barnes L, Eveson JW, Reichart P, *et al.* World Health Organization Classification of Tumours; 2005:330.
30. Lim LH, Goh YH, Chan YM, *et al.* Malignancy of the temporal bone and external auditory canal. *Otolaryngol Head Neck Surg* 2000;**122**:882–6.
31. Moody SA, Hirsch BE, Myers EN. Squamous cell carcinoma of the external auditory canal: An evaluation of a staging system. *Am J Otol* 2000;**21**:582–8.
32. Arriaga M, Curtin H, Takahashi H, *et al.* Staging proposal for external auditory meatus carcinoma based on preoperative clinical examination and computed tomography findings. *Ann Otol Rhinol Laryngol* 1990;**99**:714–21.
33. Nakagawa T, Kumamoto Y, Natori Y, *et al.* Squamous cell carcinoma of the external auditory canal and middle ear: An operation combined with preoperative chemoradiotherapy and a free surgical margin. *Otol Neurotol* 2006;**27**:242–8.
34. Pemberton LS, Swindell R, Sykes AJ. Primary radical radiotherapy for squamous cell carcinoma of the middle ear and external auditory canal—a historical series. *Clin Oncol (R Coll Radiol)* 2006;**18**:390–4.

35. Nyrop M, Grontved A. Cancer of the external auditory canal. *Arch Otolaryngol Head Neck Surg* 2002;**128**:834–7.

36. Moffat DA, Wagstaff SA, Hardy DG. The outcome of radical surgery and post-operative radiotherapy for squamous carcinoma of the temporal bone. *Laryngoscope* 2005;**115**:341–7.

37. Michaels L, Wells M. Squamous cell carcinoma of the middle ear. *Clin Otolaryngol Allied Sci* 1980;**5**:235–48.

38. Morton RP, Stell PM, Derrick PP. Epidemiology of cancer of the middle ear cleft. *Cancer* 1984;**53**:1612–17.

39. Austin JR, Stewart KL, Fawzi N. Squamous cell carcinoma of the external auditory canal. Therapeutic prognosis based on a proposed staging system. *Arch Otolaryngol Head Neck Surg* 1994;**120**: 1228–32.

40. Lim LH, Goh YH, Chan YM, *et al*. Malignancy of the temporal bone and external auditory canal. *Otolaryngol Head Neck Surg* 2000;**122**:882–6.

41. Sekhar LN, Pomeranz S, Janecka IP, *et al*. Temporal bone neoplasms: A report on 20 surgically treated cases. *J Neurosurg* 1992;**76**: 578–87.

42. Arriaga M, Curtin HD, Takahashi H, *et al*. The role of preoperative CT scans in staging external auditory meatus carcinoma: Radiologic–pathologic correlation study. *Otolaryngol Head Neck Surg* 1991;**105**:6–11.

43. Hahn SS, Kim JA, Goodchild N, *et al*. Carcinoma of the middle ear and external auditory canal. *Int J Radiat Oncol Biol Phys* 1983;**9**:1003–7.

44. Imamura S, Murakami Y. Secondary malignant tumors of the temporal bone. A histopathologic study and review of the world literature. *Nippon Jibiinkoka Gakkai Kaiho* 1991;**94**:924–37.

45. Sen C, Sekhar LN. Direct vein graft reconstruction of the cavernous, petrous, and upper cervical internal carotid artery: Lessons learned from 30 cases. *Neurosurgery* 1992;**30**:732–42; discussion 742–3.

46. Stell PM, McCormick MS. Carcinoma of the external auditory meatus and middle ear. Prognostic factors and a suggested staging system. *J Laryngol Otol* 1985;**99**:847–50.

47. Clark LJ, Narula AA, Morgan DA, *et al*. Squamous carcinoma of the temporal bone: A revised staging. *J Laryngol Otol* 1991;**105**:346–8.

48. Kinney SE, Wood BG. Malignancies of the external ear canal and temporal bone: Surgical techniques and results. *Laryngoscope* 1987;**97**:158–64.

49. Zhang B, Tu G, Xu G, *et al*. Squamous cell carcinoma of temporal bone: Reported on 33 patients. *Head Neck* 1999;**21**:461–6.

50. Bibas AG, Ward V, Gleeson MJ. Squamous cell carcinoma of the temporal bone. *J Laryngol Otol* 2008;**122**:1156–61.

51. Cristalli G, Manciocco V, Pichi B, *et al*. Treatment and outcome of advanced external auditory canal and middle ear squamous cell carcinoma. *J Craniofac Surg* 2009;**20**:816–21.

52. Chang CH, Shu MT, Lee JC, *et al*. Treatments and outcomes of malignant tumors of external auditory canal. *Am J Otolaryngol* 2009;**30**:44–8.

53. Lobo D, Llorente JL, Suarez C. Squamous cell carcinoma of the external auditory canal. *Skull Base* 2008;**18**:167–72.

54. Kunst H, Lavieille JP, Marres H. Squamous cell carcinoma of the temporal bone: Results and management. *Otol Neurotol* 2008;**29**: 549–52.

55. Prasad S, Janecka IP. Malignancies of the temporal bone—radical temporal bone resection. In: Prasad S, Janecka IP (eds). *Otologic surgery*. Philadelphia: WB Saunders; 1994:49–62.

20

Swallowing rehabilitation following head and neck cancer

KAPILA MANIKANTAN, RAGHAV C. DWIVEDI, REHAN KAZI

Introduction

Dysphagia is a term derived from the Greek term 'phage in', meaning 'to eat'. Dysphagia is essentially a symptom that 'translates' as a delay in the passage of solids or liquids from the oral cavity to the stomach. Head and neck cancer (HNC) patients may complain of dysphagia, which is caused either by the disease itself or as a consequence of the treatment modality used. The various organ preservation modalities, which have been on the increase in recent years, do not necessarily mean 'functional' preservation.

Dysphagia and aspiration are recognized as potentially devastating complications arising from the treatment of HNC. Anything that restricts the opening of the upper oesophageal sphincter and results in residuals of swallow may cause spillage into the airway. Aspiration is thus a consequence of dysphagia.[1] Aspiration can be prevented by an intact cough reflex. Patients with a suppressed cough reflex tend to aspirate and this silent nature of aspiration has been corroborated by videofluroscopic studies. The incidence of this 'silent aspiration' is not known. Aspiration can be caused broadly by factors such as those causing aspiration before the swallow, during the swallow, and after the swallow. Aspiration before the swallow is caused by reduced oromotor control and delayed or absent reflex. During the swallow it is caused by reduced laryngeal closure, decreased epiglottic inversion, or decreased laryngeal elevation. After the swallow aspiration is caused by reduced pharyngeal peristalsis, cricopharyngeal sphincter dysfunction, reduced laryngeal elevation and structural abnormalities.[2] Patients who undergo chemoradiation are considered to have a higher risk of aspiration and they may lack laryngeal sensation, which makes it difficult to detect the aspiration.[3]

In this review we look at the normal swallowing mechanism (Fig. 1), the effects of various treatment modalities on this mechanism, and the swallowing rehabilitation methods employed in HNC.

Normal swallowing mechanism

The process of swallowing includes the conscious effort

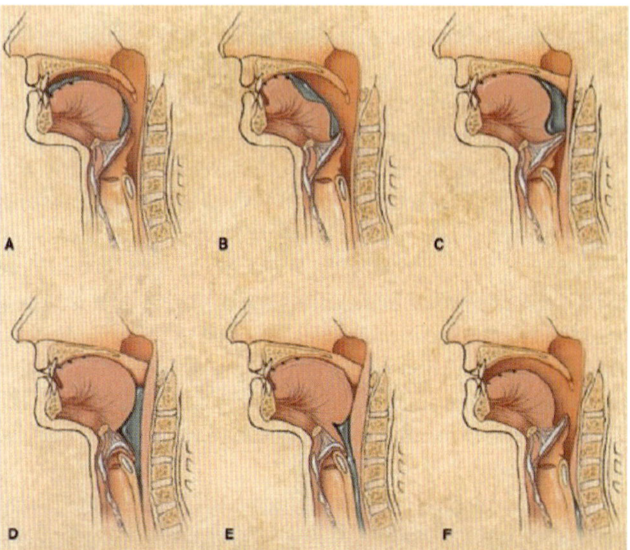

Fig. 1. Sequence of normal swallowing mechanism
A and B Oral phase of swallowing; C and D Oropharyngeal phase of swallowing; E and F Pharyngeal phase of swallowing

to ingest food and the subconscious or reflex act of bolus preparation. The preparation of the bolus is referred to as the preparatory phase, its transport from the oral cavity and pharynx to the oesophagus as the transport phase, and its passage through the oesophagus as the oesophageal transport phase. The rhythm and pattern of the swallowing mechanism is controlled by a central pattern generator located in the medulla.[4]

In the oral preparatory phase, food is chewed and prepared for swallowing. The tongue plays an important role in this phase by mixing the food and moving it towards the occlusal surface of the teeth. Sensory innervation across the oral mucosa and the tone of the facial muscles help to keep the bolus within the oral cavity and in its manipulation. The soft palate approximates to the tongue to create a glossopalatal seal, which prevents premature spillage into the pharynx, while the various movements of the mandible create adequate grinding of the bolus. The bolus is mixed with saliva, and when it is ready for the oral phase of swallowing, the tongue forms a trough containing the bolus with the lateral edges curved upwards. The tongue then contracts anterioposteriorly, pushing the bolus back into the pharynx. The entire process takes approximately one second. This phase involves cranial nerves V, VII and XII.[4–6]

The pharyngeal phase, which usually lasts one second, is involuntary, with sensations travelling through cranial nerves IX and X. In this phase, five physiological actions take place simultaneously—the soft palate closes the nasopharynx to prevent nasal regurgitation, the larynx is elevated and closed, the pharyngeal constrictors contract, and the cricopharynx relaxes. The true cords, the false cords, the epiglottis and the aryepiglottic folds constrict to form a barrier of several layers to protect the airway and prevent aspiration. Elevation of the larynx occurs by the contraction of the suprahyoid musculature.[6] The pharyngeal stage generally occurs during a brief phase of apnoea, which occurs during the expiratory phase of respiration during which time post-swallow continues, thus providing a degree of inherent airway protection.[7]

When the larynx is elevated superiorly and anteriorly, the cricopharyngeus relaxes by inhibition of its normal resting tone. This relaxation creates a negative pressure in the upper oesophagus, which helps in the bolus movement. In addition to true and false vocal fold closure, the laryngeal inlet is closed through epiglottic deflection by the action of the aryepiglottic muscles, the elevation of the larynx, pressure exerted by the base of the tongue and the pressure exerted by the bolus itself.[6] This phase lasts for one second but may vary, depending on size of the bolus.[8]

The oesophageal phase is characterized by a single primary peristaltic wave travelling at 3–4 cm/sec. Several secondary peristaltic waves occur spontaneously within one hour, thus helping to clear residue and any gastric reflux. Oesophageal transit time increases with age.[5]

HNC and swallowing

HNC is the sixth most common cancer worldwide, accounting for 2.8% of all malignancies. The main treatment modalities for HNC are surgery and radiotherapy, with an increasing role for chemotherapy. The choice of modality is dependent on patient variables, the primary site, clinical stage and resectability of the tumour. Patients presenting with early-stage disease can be managed by curative surgery or radiotherapy. Patients presenting with loco regionally advanced disease may be treated with complete surgical excision followed by postoperative (chemo)radiotherapy or with concomitant chemoradiotherapy. In spite of using an aggressive bimodality treatment approach, patients have a poor prognosis, with 5-year survival rates of 30%–40%.[9] The presence of the tumour itself, as well as the treatment, can result in neuromuscular damage affecting any stage of the swallow.[10]

Dysphagia following surgery for HNC

Surgical interventions for HNCs result in specific anatomical or neurological insults with site-specific patterns of dysphagia and aspiration.[5]

Oral and oropharyngeal surgery

Sessions *et al.*[11] showed that for oral surgery the size of the lesion excised was less predictive of subsequent dysphagia than the area excised. Logemann *et al.*[12] found that swallowing was worse in patients with tumours in the tongue base rather than in the anterior floor of the mouth. The swallowing deficits that occur after oral resections vary with the site of resection and type of reconstruction. The various reconstruction types for oral and pharyngeal defects are primary closure, skin graft, tissue flap, or microvascular free flap. McConnell *et al.*[13] found that skin grafts gave better results than reconstruction done with a distal flap. A multi-centre prospective study was undertaken to compare the swallowing function before and after oral and oropharyngeal surgery and to compare primary closure, distal myocutaneous flap and microvascular free flap reconstruction.[14] Measurements made were the oral transit time, pharyngeal transit time, pharyngeal delay time, duration of laryngeal closure, duration of cricopharyngeal opening and oropharyngeal swallowing efficiency (OPSE), which is calculated by dividing the approximate percentage of bolus swallowed by the total transit time. The normal numerical value for OPSE is 50, which indicates that 100% bolus is swallowed in 2 minutes. Patients with distal flap reconstruction (50.9±8.7) had significantly lower OPSE scores compared with patients with primary closure (79.9±8.2) for liquid boluses (p=0.01). The distal flap patients, however, had significantly faster oral transit times on paste boluses, but significantly more pharyngeal residue. Patients with free flaps had significantly lower OPSE scores and more pharyngeal residue when compared with patients with primary closure. The distal flap group had significantly more pharyngeal residue in comparison to the free flap group. The study showed that resections of the tongue (<30%) and tongue base (<60%) had better swallowing efficiency with primary closure on liquid boluses. The authors felt that a flap may be acting as an adynamic segment reducing the swallow efficiency by impairing the driving force of the tongue.[14]

A pilot study[14] for surgical variables affecting swallowing efficiency showed that as the percentage of the resected tongue and tongue base increased, the efficiency of the swallow decreased. Hence, it is better to replace oral and pharyngeal tissue with a flap so that the functional tongue is not affected. In a case–control study of 30 patients, Logemann and Bytell[12] showed better swallowing in patients without use of tongue-flap for closure of oral cavity defects than in patients with a tongue-flap closure. A study of 278 consecutive patients with oral cancer assessed using the University of Washington Quality of Life questionnaire concluded that primary closure results in a better swallowing outcome than reconstruction with a distal or free flap.[15] The radial forearm free flap is a fasciocutaneous flap with a wide use in HNC reconstruction. A bilobed sensate design of the flap was introduced by Urken and Biller[16] to preserve tongue mobility. The main disadvantage of this flap has been donor site morbidity. This has led authors to advocate the anterolateral thigh flap. The anterolateral thigh flap was first advocated by Song *et al.*[17] in 1984 and is a popular reconstructive method after head and neck surgery. In a study of 20 patients who underwent hemiglossectomy, 10 had primary reconstruction with a forearm free flap and 10 with an anterolateral thigh flap. Eight patients in each group received postoperative radiotherapy. The patients' functional outcome was assessed after 6 months and no significant difference was seen in the mean scores for deglutition (p>0.05) between the two groups. The donor site was closed primarily in all cases for the anterolateral thigh flaps, and by skin graft and immobilization for 1 week in all cases for the forearm free flaps. No complications were noted in the anterolateral thigh flap group, but they were evident in 4 cases in the forearm free flap group. The authors concluded that the anterolateral thigh flap is ideal for reconstruction of surgical defects after hemiglossectomy.[18]

A videofluoroscopic study of 15 patients who underwent total, subtotal (10% of base tongue is preserved) or partial glossectomy showed stasis in all areas of the oropharyngeal tract after subtotal and total glossectomies.[19] The oral transit times were greater for food of all consistencies. Moderate aspiration after deglutition was noted in 2 patients. Patients who underwent partial glossectomy showed increased oral transit times and required a greater number of swallows to clear the valleculae. Total glossectomy has been associated with the risk of aspiration, for which simultaneous total

laryngectomy used to be carried out prophylactically.[5] Laryngeal preservation with total glossectomy was proposed in 1973.[20] The postoperative swallowing outcome was compared in patients on the basis of the postoperative MRI appearance of the tongue, in a study of 30 patients who underwent total or subtotal glossectomy with reconstruction and with preservation of the larynx.[21] Deglutition was significantly poorer in patients with flat or depressed tongues compared with patients with protuberant or semi-protuberant tongues (p<0.003). The authors suggested that wider and thicker flaps, such as rectus abdominis musculocutaneous flaps, be used for reconstruction of the tongue and that the flaps be designed to be 30% wider than the defect; laryngeal suspension was also advocated to prevent prolapse of the flap.[21]

Some tumours may infiltrate the mandible and require resection. Mandibular defects that are not reconstructed and are not pure lateral defects give a poor functional and aesthetic outcome.[22] Urken and co-workers[23] compared functional parameters between 10 patients with reconstruction of mandibular defects and 10 patients without mandibular reconstruction. A clear advantage in function was seen in the reconstructed patients.[23] This highlights the importance of maintaining the 3-dimensional anatomical relationship during oro-mandibular reconstruction, after composite resection of oral neoplasms, for preserving physiological function.[24] Use of non-vascularized bone grafts often resulted in complications of bone graft resorption and wound healing.[23] The free fibular flap for reconstruction of composite head and neck defects has distinct advantages in terms of the combination of tissue match and favourable attributes of pedicle length, no repositioning, and the remote distance from the defect, making it a popular choice.[25] A retrospective study of 163 patients who underwent mandibular reconstruction, compared a osseo-cutaneous radial forearm free flap with free fibular and scapular flaps, and showed a similar swallowing outcome between the flap types.[24] In this study the maximum length of bone harvested from the radial forearm was 12 cm. The authors felt that for larger defects, the fibula graft can offer up to 25 cm of bone. Seikaly *et al.*[26] performed a prospective study of free fibular reconstruction of mandibular defects and compared the swallowing outcome across treatment times preoperatively, and pre- and post-radiation; no significant difference in swallowing was seen. They concluded that free fibular grafts are an excellent option for reconstruction of mandibular defects.[26]

Tumours involving the palate and maxillary sinus that are treated by surgical extirpation often require the creation of large oronasal and oromaxillary fistulae, and loss of tooth bearing segments that impair oral alimentation.[27] These defects can be managed by skin for lining the defect, and a prosthesis for swallowing. The prosthesis requires regular cleaning.[28] The oral and nasal cavities can be sealed by local flaps or by microvasular-free tissue transfer. In a retrospective study of

56 patients who underwent partial or total maxillectomy with free flap reconstruction, 37 patients returned to a normal diet and 19 were able to consume a soft diet.[29]

Tracheostomy

Tracheostomy may be used as a short- or long-term solution when the tumour occludes the airway, for postoperative oedema, or where supraglottic and glottic oedema may occur during chemoradiation. It may also be indicated in cases of significant laryngeal incompetence and aspiration risk. The presence of an inflated cuff may have an impact on the range of laryngeal motion and thus, on airway protection and cricopharyngeal opening.[30]

Material collecting above the cuff has already passed the true cords and is considered aspirated; micro-aspiration can occur with an inflated cuff. Manometers are essential for cuff pressure management and deflation trials are needed to prevent blunting of the cough reflex. A retrospective study using videofluoroscopy in 623 tracheostomized patients with inflated and deflated cuffs showed a higher incidence of silent aspiration and reduction in laryngeal elevation in the cuff-inflated condition.[30] The authors also concluded that patients should undergo instrumental evaluation in both a cuff-inflated and -deflated condition, thus returning patients with adequate swallow function to oral intake at the earliest.[30]

Mechanical and neurophysiological factors broadly account for the causes of aspiration after a tracheostomy.[31] The mechanical factors constitute local compressive forces exerted by the inflated cuff, which cause a decreased laryngeal elevation from suturing the trachea to the skin, and stasis of secretions in the upper airway and cervical oesophagus. The patient may experience pain and discomfort due to the presence of an inflated cuff, which impinges on the oesophagus.[12] The neurophysiological factors include desensitization of the protective cough reflex and a loss of coordination of laryngeal closure. An inflated cuff is not protective against aspiration in tracheostomized patients. High volume, low pressure cuffs significantly decrease this risk of aspiration.[32] It is crucial that the supraglottic airway be evaluated to ensure successful removal of the tube prior to decannulation of the postsurgical patient.

Dysphagia following laryngeal surgery

Endoscopic laser surgery on the larynx

In a study of 117 patients who underwent transoral laser microsurgery for stage III and stage IV glottic and supraglottic carcinoma of the larynx, swallowing was assessed by the functional outcome of the swallowing scale (FOSS).[33] Of the 68 patients who were alive on the latest follow up, 7% were on tube-dependent feeding, and 44% were assessable by the FOSS system, which revealed an overall median post-treatment FOSS stage 1, which reflects normal function with episodic or daily symptoms of dysphagia. The authors used a definition of FOSS stage 2 or better as the functional endpoint, and found that 22 of the 28 patients for whom follow up data were available were able to achieve the endpoint.

Partial laryngectomy

Partial laryngectomy procedures were introduced to decrease the functional impact of total laryngectomy on swallowing and speech. The degree of impairment of swallowing depends on the extent of the resection. The conventional vertical hemilaryngectomy gives relatively the best results. However, symptoms worsen when the resection includes the arytenoids or large portions of the endolaryngeal soft tissues.[34] A study comparing the dysphagia outcome in 25 total laryngectomy and 11 frontolateral laryngectomy patients found a statistically significant difference between the two groups (p<0.027). Of the total 36 patients experiencing difficulties, 12 had undergone total laryngectomy and one a frontolateral laryngectomy.[35] A speech language pathologist interviewed the patients, using a semi-structured questionnaire. In a study of functional outcome of 29 male patients variously undergoing cricohyoidopexy, frontolateral laryngectomy and laryngofissure cordectomy, the time taken to resume oral feeding was found to be significantly longer (p=0.036) in patients who underwent cricohyoidopexy (day 20) and frontolateral laryngectomy (day 6), compared with cordectomy (day 0).[36] No statistically significant difference (p>0.05) was seen on the swallowing outcome when these procedures were combined with arytenoidectomy. In a study comparing 17 patients treated by cricohyoidoepiglottopexy (CHEP) with 21 patients with near total laryngectomy with epiglottic reconstruction (NTLER), nasogastric tubes were removed at a mean of 23.0 (SD 13.6) days in the CHEP group and 17.0 (SD 11.4) days in the NTLER group.[37] The difference was not significant (p>0.05) and the swallow function was good on long-term follow up in both groups. All the patients selected for the study had T1b glottic cancer.[37]

Supraglottic laryngectomy

Supraglottic laryngectomy involves the removal of the epiglottis, aryepiglottic folds, false cords, upper third of the thyroid cartilage, and one or both superior laryngeal nerves, while at the same time preserving the most important laryngeal sphincter—the true vocal cords. Aspiration can occur during swallow after supraglottic laryngectomy because of incomplete airway closure, secondary to pharyngeal residue spilling into the airway, inadequate laryngeal elevation, or weak propulsive forces.[38] When the supraglottic laryngectomy is extended to involve the tongue base or arytenoids and adjacent valleculae or the pyriform fosse, aspiration is more likely. In a study of 55 patients undergoing partial laryngectomy, those who underwent extended supraglottic laryngectomy took significantly longer to achieve swallowing rehabilitation.[39]

Supracricoid laryngectomy

Supracricoid laryngectomy includes removing the true and false cords of both sides, the paraglottic space, the thyroid cartilage and, occasionally, the epiglottis and one arytenoid. Supracricoid partial laryngectomy in 27 patients, who were evaluated by modified barium swallow, resulted in initial aspiration and impaired base of tongue and laryngeal movements.[40] The median tube removal was 9.4 weeks and 81% of the patients returned to a normal diet. Pneumonia and subcutaneous emphysema were reported to be the most common complications.[40]

Near total laryngectomy

Near total laryngectomy involves removing three-fourths of the larynx, while preserving the strip of larynx. The arytenoid cartilage, one vocal fold and one false vocal fold are preserved to form a myomucosal shunt from the trachea to the pharynx. If the opening or inlet of the tracheopharyngeal shunt is too wide, aspiration is inevitable during swallowing. This is true particularly in cases of endolaryngeal lesions in which laryngeal augmentation is carried out.[41] Near total laryngectomy falls midway between total laryngectomy and partial laryngectomy. As in total laryngectomy, nasal breathing is sacrificed and as in partial laryngectomy, speech is preserved. Although the patient has a permanent tracheotomy, verbal communication is preserved, as one of the vocal cords is retained. A study on 137 near total laryngectomies found that only 2 cases with major aspiration required conversion to a total laryngectomy. However, most patients were seen to be on a regular diet within 2–3 weeks.[42]

Total laryngectomy

Dysphagia is a predominant, negative sequel after total laryngectomy. The occurrence of dysphagia ranges from 10% to 60%.[41] It can result from tumour recurrence, a benign stricture, a second primary, radiation, pseudo-epiglottis formation,[12] or loss of coordination of the pharyngeal constrictors. A spatial distortion may occur in the hypopharynx and cervical oesophagus due to the tethering of the tracheostomy.[44] After a total laryngectomy, clearance of the bolus from the pharynx takes longer.[45] In an evaluation of lifestyle changes post-total laryngectomy, Ackerstaff *et al.*[46] reported that 25% patients had a change in diet, consistency of the food, and style of eating. Successful swallowing has been described in various ways by different authors, such as

maintenance of nutrition without tube feeding, and the ability to swallow modified consistencies of the food as the optimal outcome. Hillman *et al.*[47] reported 76% of laryngectomy patients resuming a normal diet by 2 years post-surgery. In a study of 55 patients[48] who underwent total laryngectomy and 37 who underwent laryngopharyngectomy with jejunal reconstruction, 27% of the laryngectomy group and 65% of the laryngopharyngectomy group developed statistically significant (p<0.001) swallowing-related complications in the one month post-surgery. All patients were on postoperative nasogastric (NG) tube feeding, with the mean duration of 10.7±2.0 days to oral feeding in the total laryngectomy group. Late complications requiring non-oral nutrition on follow up were seen in 27% of the laryngectomy group. Percutaneous endoscopic gastrostomy (PEG) feeding for a mean duration of 23.3±17.9 days was required in 5% of the laryngectomy patients. Upon being discharged, one laryngectomy patient was on a normal diet and 98% were unable to consume a diet of normal consistency. On long-term follow up, 58% of patients continued to have dysphagia. Dysphagia was defined by these authors as an inability to achieve normal dietary status, stating that this may be the reason for the higher incidence of dysphagia seen. Following laryngectomy, the drop in hypopharyngeal pressure, which results from laryngeal elevation during the pharyngeal phase of the swallow, is lost.[44] The pseudo-epiglottis is a mucosal fold at the junction of the tongue base and the reconstructed pharynx.[12] Lateral radiographic visualization gives the appearance of the contour of an epiglottis, hence the term 'pseudo-epiglottis'. On clinical examination the pseudo-epiglottis tends to collapse against the tongue base in the resting state, giving the false impression of adequate space. However, as a result of pharyngeal contraction, this pseudo-epiglottis forms a pocket during a swallow, accumulating food and causing dysphagia[44] (Fig. 1).

Hypopharyngeal surgery

The multiple goals of hypopharyngeal surgery have been to minimize morbidity and mortality with a single stage reconstruction, a short hospital stay, and early restoration of swallowing. Ogura *et al.*[49] advocated partial pharyngolaryngectomy in patients whose tumour did not involve the true cords and arytenoids and the apex of the pyriform sinus, and which did not invade the thyroid cartilage. The defect can be closed by a hinge flap or local mucosal flap when the resection does not involve the lateral wall of the pyriform sinus.[49] In a study of 55 patients who underwent transoral laser surgery for pharyngeal and pharyngolaryngeal tumours of stages T1, T2 and T3, 67% of the patients required a feeding tube, which was removed at a median period of 7 days.[50] Of the 32 patients followed up, 16 had returned to a normal diet.[50]

Myocutaneous flaps, visceral transpositions and free flaps have been used for circumferential reconstruction of the hypopharynx. Myocutaneous flaps have the problem of developing local complications, such as fistulae and dysphagia, which are difficult to treat because of the thickness of the flaps. Proximal lesions of the pharynx and hypopharynx are reconstructed by free jejunal transfer, whereas gastric transposition is used for reconstruction when the resection extends beyond the thoracic inlet. In an analysis of 209 patients who underwent total laryngopharyngectomy between 1982 and 1999,[51] 61% of patients underwent total oesophagectomy with pharyngogastric anastomosis, 37% underwent cervical oesophagectomy with free jejunal transfer, and 2% underwent pharyngocolic anastomosis. The average time for resumption of feeding was 19.7 days, with 98.4% of patients achieving swallowing. The survival rate without dysphagia was higher for gastric anastomosis (89%) than for jejunal grafts (76%). Swallowing is better with gastric transposition because of the low rate of fistula and stricture formation. In a study of 29 patients who underwent hypopharyngeal resection with jejunal free transfer, the nasogastric tube was removed at a mean of 15 days (9–150 days); in 25 patients it was removed before day 15. Patients who received adjuvant radiotherapy (15 patients) did not show any swallowing impairment.[52]

Skull base surgery

Surgery involving the skull base poses a problem because of the presence of vital structures in its vicinity. In a retrospective study of 19 patients with nerve sheath tumours of the skull base,[53] 57.8% patients presented with a soft tissue lump, and dysphagia was a presenting symptom in 3 patients with a neck lump. Patients with extensive tumours usually do not present with significant dysphagia, as the swallowing mechanism adapts to the slow onset of the cranial nerve paresis. However, postoperative dysphagia can be acute on account of injuries to the adjoining cranial nerves.[54] The various approaches used for accessing the skull base may affect the swallowing mechanism in different ways. The anterior approach involving maxillectomies may cause palatal defects and nasal reflux. The lateral approach through the zygoma and mandible may injure cranial nerves V, VII, IX, X, XI and XII. Temporal bone resections and temporal bone approaches may injure cranial nerve VII with subsequent difficulties.[55] In fact, not just the nerves, but the pharynx itself may be injured in a skull base surgery.[54]

Radiotherapy

The conventional effective radiotherapy dosage in HNC is daily fractions of 1.8–2.0 Gray (Gy), up to total doses of 66.0–70.0 Gy over 6 or 7 weeks. Present evidence suggests that alterations in the fractionation schedule, as well as concomitant chemotherapy, may significantly improve tumour responses.[1] However, these aggressive treatment regimens have also contributed to significant dysphagia.[1] Radiotherapy to the head and neck results in appreciable dose delivery to critical structures necessary for normal deglutition, such as the tongue, larynx and pharyngeal muscles. Acute side-effects of radiotherapy are mucositis, dysphagia, hoarseness, erythema and desquamation of the skin. The potential late sequelae of this high radiation dose include osteonecrosis, dental decay, trismus, hypogeusia, subcutaneous fibrosis, thyroid dysfunction, oesophageal stenosis hoarseness and damage to the middle or inner ear.[56]

The various structures of the head and neck have their inherent response to the radiation. Mucocutaneous tissues subjected to irradiation develop increased vascular permeability leading to fibrin deposition, collagen formation and eventually fibrosis.[57] The type and severity of the effects are related directly to radiation dosimetry, including total dose, fraction size, and duration of treatment.[58] The oral sequelae were evaluated in 100 patients with HNC at a mean post-radiotherapy time of 28 months. Thirty per cent of the patients were found to have dysgeusia, 38% had dysphagia, and 68% had xerostomia.[59] The authors concluded that the post-radiotherapy sequelae are dependent on radiation dose, the radiation field, use of xerostomic medication, and the time post-radiotherapy.[59] European organisation for research and treatment of cancer (EORTC) protocol 22791 compared daily fractionation to pure fractionation of 80.5 Gy in 70 fractions in 7 weeks using 3 fractions of 1.15 Gy per day in advanced oropharyngeal carcinoma.[60] An improved locoregional control was noted in the hyperfractionation schedule and no difference was seen in the late normal tissue damage between the modalities.[58] In an analysis of 39 patients undergoing rapid hyperfractionated radiotherapy, the common late complications included cervical fibrosis, mucosal necrosis, bone necrosis, trismus, and laryngeal oedema.[61] Late complications were seen in 70% of the patients, 54% of whom had severe complications. No relationship was seen between the field sizes, dosimetric data and frequency of late effects. The authors concluded that the interval between the daily sessions is of critical importance in multi-fractionation schedules.[61] An analysis of 784 patients of squamous cell carcinoma of the pharynx and larynx treated by external beam radiotherapy, compared site and size of the tumour, total dose, fraction size and treatment time.[62] A weak relationship was noted between the late effects and patient and fractionation schedules. The size of the primary had a significant influence on the complication rate, independent of the fractionation schedule. In recent years, favourable results have been reported with the introduction of conformal 3-dimensional radiotherapy techniques and, in particular, intensity-modulated radiation therapy (IMRT), which allows for radiation to be delivered to the tumour while sparing surrounding healthy tissues.[63]

Studies relating to swallowing in IMRT suggest a potential for improved functional outcomes with targeted therapy that avoid key structures.[64] In particular, the superior and middle constrictor muscles have been implicated as key swallowing structures to be avoided.[65] The functional and anatomical changes were studied in 31 dysphagic nasopharyngeal carcinoma patients treated by radiotherapy alone, with a mean follow up of 8.5 years.[66] Pharyngeal retention and an incidence of 77.4% post-swallow aspiration were seen in 93.5% patients. Also noted were atrophy of the tongue (54.8%), vocal cord palsy (29%), velopharyngeal insufficiency (58%), premature leakage (41.9%), delay or absence of the swallow reflex (87.1%), poor pharyngeal constriction (80.6%) and silent aspiration (41.9%). A significant role of poor pharyngeal constriction and abnormal upper oesophageal sphincter function in post-swallow aspiration were also observed. In a study of 40 patients receiving radiotherapy for advanced laryngeal carcinoma,[67] aspiration was identified in 84% of patients and 44% aspirated silently. Impaired hyolaryngeal motion, incomplete epiglottic inversion and reduced base of tongue retraction to the posterior pharyngeal wall were the most prevalent abnormalities. Only 15% of the total number of patients required a feeding tube prior to radiotherapy. During the course of treatment 78% of the patients had a feeding tube at some point in time, and 52% of these were removed eventually. Of the disease-free patients, 72% returned to oral nutrition. Patients who were on tube-dependent feeding in the pre-treatment stage remained so on assessment post-radiotherapy. Fibrosis and functional deterioration of the swallow can be avoided by encouraging patients to swallow during therapy.[1] However, the ability to maintain a normal diet or swallow does not indicate a normal swallow mechanism, and safe limits of aspiration have not been quantified. In a retrospective study of 158 patients[68] treated for HNC, 16 of 50 patients undergoing radiotherapy needed tube placement, whereas 75 of 108 patients undergoing chemoradiotherapy underwent tube placement (p<0.001). The authors also concluded that a PEG was required for longer periods of time and was associated with more dysphagia and required more pharyngo-oesophageal dilatation in comparison to NG tubes. In a multi-centre cross-sectional study for the clinical factors influencing the placement of an enteral feeding tube in HNC patients, 28% of patients receiving chemoradiation were found to require tube feeding.[69] According to the European Society for Clinical Nutrition and Metabolism guidelines on enteral nutrition for non-surgical oncology,[70] patients with obstructive HNC lesions interfering with swallowing should be started on tube-delivered enteral feeding. Tube feeding is also indicated for severe oral and oesophageal mucositis with dysphagia, and a PEG is preferred to an NG tube. In a recent randomized study of 33 patients undergoing chemoradiation for HNC, no evidence was found to support the use of PEG over NG tubes for enteral nutrition.[71]

Xerostomia is a common side-effect of radiotherapy. Due to the challenges of bolus formation in the absence of saliva, patients may have to make permanent changes to their diet.[9] Research has shown that whereas patients with xerostomia perceive that their swallowing is impaired from a sensory and comfort perspective, swallowing physiology and bolus transport were unaffected.[72] Transforming growth factor $\beta 1$ (TGFβ1) expression can be activated after high-dose radiation and this is known to be involved in collagen deposition and degradation. As a result, swallowing can be affected several years after treatment with a fixation of the hyolaryngeal complex, reduced range of tongue motion, reduced glottic closure and cricopharyngeal relaxation, resulting in the potential for aspiration.[58] Irradiated patients have longer oral transit times, increased pharyngeal residue, and reduced cricopharyngeal opening times.[9]

Chemotherapy

Chemotherapeutic agents can impact the ability to swallow and affect nutrition in HNC patients. Various side-effects, such as nausea, vomiting, neutropenia, generalized weakness and fatigue can occur. Nutritional supplementation by routes other than oral may be required when the pain from mucositis prevents adequate nutritional intake. Approximately 40% of patients undergoing chemotherapy are reported to have mucositis.[73] On the other hand, almost 100% of patients receiving chemoradiation report mucositis.[73] Symptoms of mucositis include odynophagia, dysphagia, dehydration, heartburn, vomiting, nausea, and sensitivity to salty, spicy, and hot/cold foods. Stomatitis may result in eating difficulty. Anti-metabolites such as methotrexate and 5-fluorouracil are the cytotoxic agents most commonly associated with oral, pharyngeal and oesophageal symptoms of dysphagia.[74,75]

Concurrent chemoradiation was introduced to improve the prognosis by increasing the killing of tumour cells with chemotherapy, which also acts as a radiosensitizer.[76] Inoperable tumours showed good control rates, but the toxicity of the two modalities was significant with severe mucositis.[77] Videofluoroscopic swallowing studies performed after chemoradiation showed a severe dysfunction of the base of the tongue, larynx and pharyngeal muscles, leading to stasis of the bolus, vallecular residue, epiglottic dysmotility and, in severe cases, aspiration.[58] The combination of aspiration with neutropenia arising from chemotherapy may lead to aspiration pneumonia, sepsis and respiratory failure.[58] It is also believed that aspiration is under-reported by chemoradiation patients, because it is often silent.[78] In a cross-sectional study comparing the swallowing outcome (as assessed by the MD Anderson Dysphagia Inventory [MDADI]) after treatment with chemoradiation or surgery followed by radiation in stage III and stage IV patients with oropharynx, larynx and hypopharynx cancers, the swallowing outcome was better in patients with chemoradiation for oropharyngeal primaries.[79] Of a total of 40 subjects, 22 underwent surgery followed by radiation and 18 underwent chemoradiation. The MDADI scores for patients treated by chemoradiation for oropharyngeal tumours was significantly better than patients treated by surgery followed by radiation. No difference in scores was seen for the laryngeal and hypopharyngeal tumours, and between the oropharyngeal and laryngeal/hypopharyngeal tumours.[79] Another cross-sectional study on patients with advanced oropharyngeal cancer compared the laryngeal penetration and aspiration between patients treated by chemoradiation (CRT) and surgery followed by radiation (SRT).[80] Of a total of 21 subjects studied, 11 were in the SRT group and 10 in the CRT group. All patients were seen 12 months after completion of their treatment. The patients were assessed using the validated penetration–aspiration scale and the MDADI. Significantly fewer patients in the SRT group (2/11) were able to consume a complex diet of all solids and liquids after treatment, compared with patients in the CRT group (8/10). Patients in the CRT group demonstrated better airway protection during swallowing and swallow-related quality-of-life when their scores were compared. Hanna *et al.*[81] conducted a retrospective study in 127 patients of advanced squamous cell carcinoma of the head and neck treated by intensive chemoradiotherapy, to evaluate the efficacy and toxic effects of this therapy. The toxic effect data collected included the rate and grade of treatment-related complications and the rate of unscheduled hospital admissions for the management of treatment-related toxic effects. Primary tumour sites in the patients were as follows: 46% in the oropharynx, 28% in the larynx, 16% in the hypopharynx, 8% in the oral cavity, and 3% were oesophageal and sinonasal. Neutropenia was seen in 50% of the patients, of which 50% had grade 3–4 neutropenia. Mucositis was seen in 64% of the patients, 33% of whom had severe mucositis. Nausea was seen in 44% of patients, severe nausea in 15%, and vomiting in 11%. Gastrostomy tubes were placed in 73% of the patients. Dysphagia was the most common long-term complication and 40% of the patients required a change from their pretreatment diet. The authors felt that early or pretreatment placement of a gastrostomy tube resulted in 'defunctioning' of the swallowing mechanism, which may have a detrimental effect on the long-term outcome of swallowing function. They also felt that active swallowing rehabilitation should be continued even when a gastrostomy tube is placed. They surmised that the cause of dysphagia may be due to stricture formation as a consequence of ulcerative mucositis. Therefore, in cases of dysphagia it may be better to use a NG tube than a gastrostomy tube for nutritional support, as it helps to maintain a patent lumen. Generalized weakness and lack of coordination in deglutition, caused by fibrosis of the musculature or toxic effects on the neuromuscular junctions, could be more likely causes of dysphagia after chemoradiotherapy. Pharyngeal dysmotility and aspiration could result from the weakness and the lack of sensation.[82]

Swallowing rehabilitation

It is important that patients who are at risk of swallowing difficulty should receive preoperative/treatment counselling from a speech/swallowing therapist. The counselling should include the likely impact of the treatment on both swallowing function and rehabilitation planning. Counselling the patient prior to the planned treatment helps prevent frustration and uncertainty in the post-treatment period, and should form an integral part of the informed consent of the treatment process.

Swallowing disorders arising from HNC impairs the quality of life of the patient. All available biochemical, technical and physical measures need to be used to improve the swallowing function of the patient. The multidisciplinary team attending to the patients should be vigilant towards those who have had treatment for HNC and who report swallowing difficulty. Patients should undergo a comprehensive clinical assessment for optimal rehabilitation planning; the choice of instrument will be on the basis of the recommendation of the speech language pathologist. Recurrence is a possibility that has to be considered when post-treatment patients present with recent onset of dysphagia, or any worsening of the existing dysphagia.

Radiation mucositis shows similarities to the mucosal toxicity of chemotherapy. However, radiation mucositis is more difficult to prevent and treat. The Consensus Development Panel of the National Institutes of Health, United States stated that no drug is able to prevent mucositis.[83] The oral care programmes aim to remove mucosal irritating factors, cleanse the oral mucosa, maintain the moisture of the lips and oral cavity, relieve mucosal inflammation, and prevent and treat the inflammation.[84,85] Sharp teeth and fillings need to be smoothened or polished to reduce the chances of trauma. Irritating factors, such as spices, alcohol, tobacco and 'pungent' foods need to be avoided.[84] Aqueous chlorhexidine rinses have been shown to benefit chemotherapy-induced mucositis, but not radiotherapy-induced mucositis.[84] Sutherland and Browman[86] rated several anaesthetics, analgesics and mucosal coating agents as cytoprotective but not therapeutic. They also showed that narrow-spectrum antibiotic lozenges are prophylactic for radiation mucositis. The results with the administration of growth factors and free radical scavengers are promising but need further evaluation.[84]

Dysgeusia results from the effect of radiation on taste buds and changes the physiological nature of the saliva. The condition usually reverts to normal within a year in most cases.[87,88] Taste loss can be prevented by the use of shields and by repositioning the fields. Zinc supplements have been shown to be helpful in reducing dysgeusia after radiotherapy.[89]

The best way to avoid salivary gland hypofunction post-radiotherapy is to arrange the radiation beam to avoid the salivary glands altogether.[57] IMRT has been shown to reduce the radiation-induced salivary gland impairment and improve the xerostomia-related quality of life, compared with conventional radiotherapy.[90] Post-radiotherapy salivary loss can be prevented by the use of sialogogues, of which pilocarpine has been extensively studied.[91] The effect of pilocarpine can be attributed to the stimulation of the minor salivary glands, which are more resistant to the effects of radiation than the parotid glands. Systemic administration of amifostine (a free radical scavenger) has been shown to reduce xerostomia pre- and post-radiation.[92] The drug has also been shown to have the undesirable effect of tumour protection.[93] If the amount of saliva produced after stimulation is insufficient then stored autologous saliva collected prior to radiotherapy or donor saliva is an option; however most patients find this gruesome.[94] A variety of rinsing solutions are available which moisten the mucosa. Other options are frequent moistening of the mouth with water, tea, saline, sodium bicarbonate solution, and diluted milk of magnesia.[95] Viscous glycerine-containing mouthwashes require less frequent mouth rinses. Complex saliva substitutes that moisten the mucosa, maintain viscosity and retard enamel solubility have also been developed. These are based on carboxymethylcellulose or mucin.[96] Other substitutes are xanthan gum-based and polyglycerylmethacrylate-based substitutes.[97] Each of these substitutes has its own advantages and disadvantages. Several authors believe that the effectiveness of artificial saliva can be judged by indices such as the degree of night-time discomfort and difficulty in talking.[96] The effectiveness is also dependent on adequate instructions for usage of saliva substitutes and maintenance of oral hygiene by the speech language pathologist.[95]

Rehabilitation can be broadly divided into the following three main areas: (i) Preventative, (ii) compensatory, and (iii) therapeutic exercises and manoeuvres.[82] From the preventative perspective, there is a growing body of evidence to suggest that patients should commence prophylactic swallowing exercises prior to starting radiotherapy.[98,99] However, it is recognized that patients receiving chemoradiotherapy may find it difficult to continue the exercises during treatment due to the side-effects of the therapy.[100] Amifostine decreases the mucositis and xerostomia associated with chemotherapy.[92] However, objective data on the effectiveness of this therapy in reducing swallowing disorders are absent. The range of compensatory approaches include postural changes, such as a chin tuck posture, to increase airway protection, or manoeuvres, such as the supraglottic swallow that requires the patient to consciously protect the airway by holding the breath during the swallow, and coughing immediately post-swallow to expectorate penetrated or aspirated material from the airway. In addition, changes to consistency and temperature of food and taste may also be introduced. Postural changes and manoeuvres may be used in isolation or in combination, including adaptation to solids and liquids. Strategies should be implemented only after evaluation of the nature and extent of the oropharyngeal dysphagia under video fluoroscopy, or functional endoscopic evaluation of swallowing (FEES), especially when it is known that silent aspiration is a risk factor in HNC patients, as it occurs after chemoradiation.[78] Compensatory approaches can yield immediate benefit and may facilitate some oral intake. Instrumental evaluation allows for the speech language pathologist to evaluate the most appropriate rehabilitative strategies. These could include strengthening and a range of motion exercises,[101] such as those that improve base of tongue strength.[102] Some strategies have a dual compensation-exercise role, such as the Mendelsohn manoeuvre, which involves voluntary elevation of the larynx and prolonged opening of the cricopharyngeal sphincter. In the postoperative period and after adequate healing, exercises can be introduced after the assessment. A detailed specific review of preventative and rehabilitative strategies for HNC patients undergoing radiotherapy, chemotherapy and surgery has been published in 2003.[82]

Postsurgical patients may have a decreased sensory feedback from the oral cavity and pharynx. Sensory feedback can be increased by changing the size and temperature of the bolus, and pressure on the tongue. Instruments, such as a cold spoon, ice-cream sticks and chop-sticks can be used to apply pressure on the back of the tongue to increase the sensory feedback in the patient. Encouraging the patient to feed themselves also increases sensory feedback.[100] Postoperative patients can be taught a range of motion exercises for strengthening musculature of the head and neck.[103] These exercises specifically address musculature of sites such as jaws, lips, tongue, and closure of the airway, and for laryngeal elevation. FEES and videofluoroscopy can be used to study the success of therapy.[100]

Prosthetic devices can be used to improve the efficiency of the swallowing mechanism. Palatal defects can be closed by prosthetics for the oral phase of swallowing and, at the same time, they also prevent nasal leakage of the food.[104] The prosthetic device should be designed to provide maximum functional rehabilitation. It is advantageous to have a prosthodontist working with the speech pathologist for the design of the prosthetic device.[100]

Apart from functional rehabilitation, malnutrition associated with the treatment of the cancer is also a matter for concern. Factors influencing the development of malnutrition and its severity include the pre-treatment nutritional status of the patient, the site of the primary tumour, and the type of treatment delivered.[105]

Dysphagia arising from the treatment of HNC also affects the psychosocial behaviour of the patient.[106] The patient may

introduction of the first useful, reliable voice prosthesis by Singer and Blom in 1980,[1] a number of different prostheses were developed, and the success rate of vocal rehabilitation after total laryngectomy improved considerably.

TE voice using voice prostheses

TEP with prostheses has revolutionized the rehabilitation of the laryngectomized patient over the past 2 decades. This was due to a major conceptual development in the late 1970s by Eric Blom and Mark Singer.[1] Their technique involved creating a simple TEP between the posterior wall of the tracheostome and the upper oesophagus into which was inserted a one-way silicone valve. The basis of TE speech is that during expiration tracheal air is shunted into the pharynx through a small, silicone-valved prosthesis in a fistulous tract. Sound is produced by vibrating the mucosa of the pharyngo-oesophageal sphincter (PES). Speech is then produced by articulation of this sound in the oral cavity using the remaining anatomical resonators, including the tongue, teeth and lips. The prosthesis also serves as a one-way valve to prevent salivary soiling of the airway. In the early years the puncture technique was used as a secondary procedure in post-laryngectomy patients who failed to achieve oesophageal speech. Consistently good results and the superior quality of voice of secondary puncture prompted Hamaker *et al.*[2] in 1985 to incorporate the TEP at the time of laryngectomy as a primary procedure. The first voice prostheses (Blom–Singer®, Panje) were designed as non-indwelling devices, to be taken care of by the patient.[1-5] In Europe, as early as the early 1980s, indwelling voice prostheses (Groningen, Traissac) were developed and preferred, as they required less dexterity from the patient.[6,7] A number of indwelling devices are available today, namely the Blom–Singer®, Provox® 1 and 2, Groningen, VoiceMaster, Nijdam and Bordeaux voice prostheses. In the last 2 decades the valve has been improved and modified by manufacturers the world over with the introduction of hands-free, low pressure, indwelling and fungal-resistant valves. The Provox® voice prosthesis, developed in The Netherlands Cancer Institute (1988), is currently one of the more widely used devices.[8,9] The many advantages of TE voice include the following:

- It can be achieved after a laryngectomy, neck dissection, and/or radiotherapy.
- The fistula is a convenient route for oesophagogastric feeding in the immediate postoperative period.
- Easily reversible if desired by the patient
- More quickly attained than oesophageal speech
- High success rate for prosthetic vocal rehabilitation (approximating 95% in long-term users)
- Fair-to-excellent voice quality in close to 88% cases
- Similar to laryngeal speech on a range of voice parameters, such as fundamental frequency, jitter, shimmer, words per minute and maximum phonation time (compared with oesophageal speech)
- More intelligible, natural sounding, with improved intensity and duration of speech.

The disadvantages of TE speech include the following:
- Need to manually cover the stoma when voicing; although, in many devices, this has been relieved by the creation of hands-free valves.
- An adequate pulmonary reserve is necessary.

Disadvantages unique to secondary TEP include the following:
- Additional surgery needed for secondary punctures
- Violation of the posterior oesophageal wall
- Passage of the catheter through a false passage, and oesophageal perforation.

Primary speech restoration

Selection of patients

Primary voice restoration is today a standard practice for patients undergoing total laryngectomy. However, a few but rare contraindications to primary puncture are prevalent, and are related to the potentially increased risk of developing a postoperative fistula or wound breakdown. These contraindications are:

- Extensive pharyngolaryngeal surgery and separation of the party wall (absolute contraindication)
- Inadequate psychological preparation of the patient
- Doubtful ability of the patient to cope physically
- Suspected difficulty with post-operative radiotherapy.

Insertion of voice prostheses

Approximately a week after the primary voice restoration procedure, an appropriately sized voice prosthesis is fitted. It is generally advisable to wait a few more days before voice rehabilitation is begun in non-irradiated patients, or about a week in irradiated patients. After a secondary puncture, the prosthesis may be fitted after 2–3 days unless a myotomy has been performed, in which case fitting is best delayed for a week.

Immediate insertion of the indwelling voice prostheses: In this case, the indwelling voice prosthesis is inserted immediately at the time of the primary TEP, with no need for temporary stenting of the fistula tract with a feeding tube.[8-10] Numerous advantages of this technique have been claimed, provided a device of sufficient length is used. The advantages include:
- Diminished risk of separation of the TE wall due to the retrograde insertion technique, using a special trocar and cannula for the TEP and a disposable guidewire (Provox®)
- Stabilization of the TE wall by the voice prosthesis to some degree

- Optimal protection against leakage of saliva and gastric reflux provided by flanges of prosthesis
- Less irritation of the stoma and the fistula tract than a feeding tube
- No post-operative interference with a cannula or an HME.
- Familiarization with maintenance of voice prosthesis soon after operation by patients
- Obviates the need for early postoperative prosthesis fitting at a time when the stoma is not yet healed completely and when the patient's mental and physical status is not yet optimal
- Postoperative radiotherapy not a contraindication
- The first replacement is usually months later, when wound healing is completed.

The only disadvantages are the presence of a feeding tube in the nose and throat for 10 days, and temporary deterioration of the voice during postoperative radiotherapy. Giving reassurance to the patient during this period is important, as most of them eventually regain a useful voice.

Secondary speech restoration

Assessment and selection criteria

The first and the most important step is an assessment of the tonicity of the pharyngoesophageal (PE) segment. The most reliable and accurate way of assessing PE segment physiology is video fluoroscopy, which has three important components: A modified barium swallow, attempted phonation, and an oesophageal insufflation test (Taub test). Selection criteria for secondary voice restoration are:

- Good motivation
- Mental stability of patient
- Adequate understanding by patient of post-surgical anatomy and TEP voice prosthesis. No alcohol or other substance dependency
- Adequate manual dexterity
- Adequate visual acuity
- Positive oesophageal air insufflation test
- No significant pharyngeal stenosis or stricture
- Adequate pulmonary reserve
- Stoma of adequate depth and diameter
- Intact TE party wall.

PE segment tonicity

The PE segment needs to be tonic to allow a steady stream of air through it for good voice production. Hypertonicity or spasm has been considered to be a cause of failure in 10%–12% of patients.[11] Treatment options for PE spasm include pharyngeal constrictor myotomy, unilateral pharyngeal plexus neurectomy and, more recently, chemical denervation of the PE segment through the use of clostridium botulinum toxin.

Replacement technique

Indwelling voice prosthesis replacement is carried out by either a speech therapist, or nurse, or an otolaryngologist in an outpatient clinical setting. The technique of insertion varies for each prosthesis. The original Provox® device is replaced in a retrograde manner with a special disposable guidewire, but this technique is somewhat uncomfortable for the patient and the pharyngeal route can be difficult if stenosis of the PE segment is present.[11] For this reason the Provox® 2 voice prosthesis was developed, which can be easily inserted with a simple loading tube in an anterograde fashion, with the retrograde method still available as a backup procedure.[12] The Blom–Singer® voice prostheses also have a similar anterograde method of insertion using the dissolvable gel cap.

Common problems

Leakage through the prostheses

Leakage of fluids through the valve is the most common problem related to maintenance of the TEP, and is also the commonest indication for replacing any voice prostheses. Leakage through the prostheses has several causes, for which careful observation of the prostheses in situ and after removal should be made. The condition and positioning of the flap valve in situ should be checked for the following:

- The presence of deformities that may have occurred during the insertion process, including inversion of the flap valve.
- The presence of a partial remnant of the gel cap, which interferes with proper closure of the flap valve.
- Movement of the flap valve in conjunction with the patient's swallowing or respiratory pattern, which is usually indicative of negative pressure in the oesophagus that acts to suck the flap valve open, resulting in leakage through the prosthesis. Recently, magnets have been used to maintain closure of the valve mechanism and prevent leakage through the prosthesis in order to manage this problem of negative pressure (Provox Acti-valve).[13]

A prosthesis that is too old may present with a curled or deformed appearance of the valves and should be replaced. After removal, attention should be paid to the colour and overall condition of the device. The presence of microbial colonization of the valve mechanism commonly interferes with proper seating of the valve and leakage through the device, and subsequent shortened prosthesis life. Valve incompetence is generally caused by candida deposits on the silicon material and is the most important factor determining the life of voice prostheses.

Leakage around the prostheses

Leakage around the prosthesis the second commonest reason for replacement and is most frequently caused by too long a prosthesis, which in turn causes pistoning in the TE fistula. This is solved easily in most cases by downsizing the device. If this does not help, a possible solution is temporary removal of the prostheses to allow the fistula to shrink. Other causes can be lack of wound healing due to tissue necrosis caused by radiation and hypothyroidism. Assessment for recurrent cancer or metastatic disease must also be made. If the leakage occurs around a 16F diameter prosthesis, then the patient can be inserted with a 20F diameter prosthesis of the same length. Another option is first to remove the prosthesis and insert a smaller diameter rubber catheter (e.g. an 18F for a 20F prosthesis and a 14F for a 16F prosthesis) in an attempt to reduce systematically the diameter of the puncture and then reinsert a new prosthesis of the original diameter and length. Long-term success with type I collagen injections into/around the posterior tracheal wall at the puncture site has been reported by Remacle and Declaye.[14] More recently, success was reported by Luff *et al.*[15] with Hylaform (Collagen [UK] Limted, Thame, Oxon, United Kingdom) and Perie *et al.*[16] with autologous fat injection in the management of intractable leakage around the TEP site. Surgical closure of the TE fistula is rarely performed nowadays.

Other common associated problems are immediate or delayed aphonia or dysphonia, PES hypertonicity problems, puncture tract problems, small or large tracheostoma, granuloma, excessive tracheostoma mucous discharge, and hypotonic voice.

Indwelling versus non-indwelling voice prostheses

Brown *et al.*[10] demonstrated that on acoustic analysis of the voice produced, the frequency range or maximal phonation time between indwelling and non-indwelling devices were not significantly different. A patient satisfaction survey revealed that the quality of voice was perceived to be the same or slightly better with the indwelling prosthesis and that maintenance of the indwelling prosthesis was considered easier.[10]

Primary versus secondary post-laryngectomy voice restoration with TEP

Brown *et al.*[10] demonstrated that no significant difference apparently exists in patient satisfaction or subjective and objective assessments of voice quality in patients undergoing primary or secondary TEP.

Hands-free speech

Excellent results have been reported with the use of voice prostheses for the rehabilitation of laryngectomees. Many patients consider it a disadvantage that the tracheostoma must be closed manually for speech production. It is also difficult or impossible for them to simultaneously communicate through gesture, or to work with both hands. An automatic tracheostoma valve helps patients overcome this problem. For this reason, different types of tracheostoma valves have been developed in recent years and offer the advantage of hands-free speech. The Blom–Singer® tracheostoma valve and the Provox Handsfree Heat and Moisture Exchanger® are common examples. The majority of patients have no major difficulties in producing hands-free speech with theses valves. Little has appeared in the literature concerning automatic speaking valves.

In all studies, the results are similar, indicating the greatest problem as being fixation of the valve to the peristomal skin. Overproduction of mucus, excessive coughing, or a high speaking pressure can be additional unfavourable conditions. Breathing is described as harder with an automatic speaking valve than with a digital system. Automatic speaking valves are easy to use and useful devices in speech rehabilitation; attempts should be made to develop further options, especially for better securing the valve to the tracheostoma, such as the use of different types of adhesives and base plates, cannulas and/or tracheostoma buttons (Barton-Mayo or LaryButton).

Biofilms on voice prostheses

Microbial colonization of voice prostheses has been a major factor in limiting the lifetime of all voice prostheses. Antimicrobials have been used with success to solve this problem. However, long-term medication induces the risk of development of resistant strains. Therefore, recent research has focused on development of other means of preventing biofilm formation on voice prostheses. Numerous techniques have been devised with varied results. Approaches that have been tried include modification of the physicochemical properties of the biomaterial surface, and achieving an antifouling improvement for the silicone rubber material by developing new biomaterials and alternative prophylactic and therapeutic agents, including probiotics and biosurfactants, especially in view of the growing resistance of antimicrobial agents.[17]

Non-surgical restoration of speech after laryngectomy

Non-surgical restoration of speech following total laryngectomy can be broadly divided into two methods— electrolarynx and oesophageal speech.

Electrolarynx

The electrolarynx produces a fundamental sound that can then be shaped into words with the tongue, jaws, lips, and teeth. It uses a battery-powered electronic circuit that causes an electromagnetic plunger to strike a hard membrane or drum, thereby generating a vibrating tone. The tone is designed to have a frequency range close to that of the average human speaking voice, and is adjustable to suit individual preferences. The tone moves through the neck or into the mouth where it is articulated. Electronic artificial larynges fall into two subtypes on the basis of where the generated sound is transmitted to the user—neck placement devices and intraoral placement devices.

Neck placement devices

In neck placement devices, a metal or plastic head on the device transmits the sound vibration to the tissues of the neck. The fundamental sound is transmitted through the tissues in the pharynx, hypopharynx and the oral cavity, and is then articulated into speech, similar to the manner in which speech was generated before surgical intervention. Pitch and loudness can be modulated by adjusting the electronic device. Each patient has to learn the proper placement of the vibratory surface on the neck by trying the device in multiple areas and analysing which location allows the best quality of voice. Placement options vary, with no single correct location for all individuals and even in the same patient; the optimal position may change over time.

Intraoral placement devices

Most of the neck placement devices can be converted also to an intraoral device by using an adapter. A cap with a plastic tube is placed over the vibrating head of the electrolarynx. The sound then enters the mouth through the tube. Sometimes patients using this device complain of a sense of fullness in their mouths, but dysphagia has not been reported. Intraoral devices are also available separately.

Advantages

All electrolarynges are relatively easy to master, especially compared with oesophageal speech.[18] Speech therapy training with the artificial larynx can begin pre-operatively and within a few days postoperatively. Practice is required to achieve fluent speech; the laryngectomee can regain functional oral communication almost immediately.[18] Most of the newer digital devices have pitch and loudness controls that facilitate communication in environments with varying degrees of background noise, with hearing-impaired listeners, or while having telephonic conversation. Newer digital devices also offer a greater pitch range. Because of their relative ease of use and easy availability, electrolarynges are often attractive back-up means of communication. They can be used while learning oesophageal or TEP speech, when healing after extensive oral-pharyngeal-oesophageal surgery, and when access to a speech pathologist for training is limited.

Problems with electrolarynx

The commonest complaint from users of the electrolarynx is the mechanical sound quality and the attention it attracts in public.[19] Another disadvantage is that these devices are not hands-free, although they can be made hands-free with use of a suitable collar, but the positioning and the optimal placement of the device is not always simple. Because they require the use of hands, some daily activities become more challenging while speaking, such as driving, cooking, or holding the telephone. The older generation electrolarynges were relatively big and heavy. With today's advances in technology, some devices are very lightweight and are only a few centimetres in size. Another disadvantage is the need to charge or replace the batteries frequently.

Problems with the intraoral devices

They interfere with articulation because of the need for a plastic tube to be placed in the oral cavity, which gets blocked by saliva, thus impeding the transmission of sound. Although learning to use an artificial larynx for basic function is relatively easy, some training is required for more efficient usage.

Oesophageal speech

Oesophageal speech can be described as producing voice and speech through burping. Air can be trapped in the cervical oesophagus and voluntarily released back through the mouth. The resulting vibration of muscles and mucosa in the cervical oesophagus and hypopharynx produces sound. There are two methods of oesophageal speech—the injection method and the inhalation method. Most successful oesophageal speakers use both types while speaking. The physiology for the two methods is the same. The relative pressure of air within the oral cavity and oesophagus is altered to allow the passage of air into the oesophagus. While inhaling, the expanded chest cavity creates negative air pressure in the lungs and oesophagus. Air consequently rushes into the lungs. Upon exhaling, the chest cavity contracts, which creates positive air pressure and air flows out. Positive or negative pressure can also be created within the oral cavity. By closing the mouth, we can trap air in the oral cavity above the PES, allowing the potential to create a positive pressure relative to that in the oesophagus. By controlling this dynamic system, oesophageal speakers can achieve remarkably fluent speech.

Injection method

The injection method of oesophageal speech requires the

speaker to build up positive pressure in the oral cavity that forces air into the cervical oesophagus. Sufficient positive pressure has to be produced by pressing the tongue against the hard palate and then forcing the tongue back into the oropharynx. This can force air into the oral cavity past the PE segment and into the cervical oesophagus. Some users of oesophageal speech can inject air into the oesophagus by voluntarily swallowing it. In either case, a 'clunk' or 'thump' sound typically is produced as the air enters the upper oesophagus. This method of injecting is also referred to as tongue pumping, glossopharyngeal press, and glossopharyngeal closure.

Inhalation method

The inhalation method utilizes the negative pressure used in normal breathing to allow air to enter the oesophagus. The air in the oesophagus below the PE segment is subjected to the same pressure as the air in the intrathoracic cavity. During inspiration, this pressure falls below that of the atmosphere. Laryngectomees can learn to relax the PE segment during inspiration, thereby allowing air to enter the cervical oesophagus. Regardless of the method used, it is important for the laryngectomee to limit the amount of air that enters the oesophagus. Too much air can fill the stomach, which is inefficient and can cause considerable discomfort.

Advantages of oesophageal speech

The major advantage of oesophageal speech is that it is hands-free speech. Also, it requires no equipment, thus obliterating costs for any new equipment and repairs. Once a patient has mastered oesophageal speech, he/she can change the pitch, intensity, and rate of speech. Bennett and Weinberg[20] found that listeners preferred hearing oesophageal speech rather than the mechanical sound produced by the electrolarynx.

Problems associated with oesophageal speech

The major problem is the amount of speech therapy training required to become a proficient speaker. Forty per cent to 74% of laryngectomees fail to acquire functional oesophageal speech.[18] Improper training can also lead to failure.[21] Considerable amounts of time and practice are required to refine articulatory precision, increase duration of utterances, and develop good rate and phrasing. Controlling pitch, loudness, and rate of speech can be difficult for oesophageal speakers. The fundamental frequency for oesophageal speech, regardless of gender, is approximately 65 Hz, one half that of the normal adult male laryngeal speaker and two octaves lower than the speech frequency of a normal adult female laryngeal speaker.[22] Intensity levels can be 6 dB–10 dB lower than laryngeal speech, which can make noisy environments problematic for oesophageal speakers.[22] Laryngeal speakers'

average rate of speaking is 150–165 words per minute.[23] Approximately 100–110 words per minute is a reasonable goal for oesophageal speakers, according to Shanks.[23] PE segment dysfunction and achalasia can impede learning of oesophageal speech. A video swallow study, insufflation test, or electromyogram testing can help diagnose problems with the PE segment. A surgical myotomy or botulinum toxin injection may be beneficial if this is the case.

Pulmonary rehabilitation after total laryngectomy

Pulmonary rehabilitation is of vital importance to every patient undergoing voice rehabilitation. Some of the lost nasal functions of normal conditioning, i.e. heating, moisturizing and filtering of the air, can be restored by application of a heat and moisture exchanger (HME). HMEs collect heat and moisture during expiration and subsequently ensure that the inhaled air is filtered, warmed and humidified. In addition, HMEs increase the airflow resistance of the stoma, so pulmonary physiology is also improved. Their consistent use appears to have a positive effect on pulmonary function and problems and on the related quality of life dimensions, including voice quality; not only of TE, but of oesophageal speech as well.[25,26]

Olfactory rehabilitation after total laryngectomy

Total laryngectomy results in a permanent disconnection of the upper and lower airways with a wide range of adverse effects. This change in anatomy also leads to loss of the normal senses of smell and taste. The patient's ability to smell severely deteriorates as the normal passive nasal airflow, and thereby the odour stimulation to the olfactory epithelium, is lacking.[27] This may have serious consequences on daily life, as the patients are unable to detect spoiled food, smoke, or leaking gas. Also, since most tastes (such as chocolate, coffee, tea, meat, etc.) are dependent on retronasal stimulation of the olfactory receptors, the perception of such tastes will also be negatively influenced.[28,29] It is evident that these adverse effects on taste and smell have an impact on patients' quality of life.[29] A number of studies have been done in recent years to assess the olfactory ability of laryngectomized patients, leading to the conclusion that the sense of olfaction is affected significantly in these patients.[30] To overcome this, few manoeuvres and devices have been described in the literature, each having some limitations.

Anatomical and physiological changes after total laryngectomy

After total laryngectomy, the gross anatomy of the nose

remains unchanged. The hyposmia occurring after the procedure is primarily caused by the nasal cavity being bypassed during respiration, as the patient breathes through the permanent stoma in the neck. Olfaction is a passive procedure, which goes on continuously and unnoticed during passive respiration. Olfactory neuroepithelium, which remains in the upper part of the nasal cavity, receives only about 15% of inhaled air.[30] So, even a minute change in nasal air-flow, which may not cause any effect on normal respiration, may have a significant impact on the sense of olfaction. As a result, a laryngectomized patient almost always suffers from hyposmia or anosmia. Although the gross nasal anatomy remains unchanged after total laryngectomy, all studies have confirmed that some histological changes definitely occur in the olfactory neuroepithelium after the surgery. In a study based on endoscopic examination, Fujii *et al.*[31] have suggested that although the nasal respiratory mucosa shows atrophic changes in most of the patients after total laryngectomy, the olfactory mucosa appears normal in all patients, irrespective of the time gap after the procedure. However, on histological examination, the olfactory neuroepithelium showed definite degenerative changes, culminating in a complete topical loss; degenerative changes were also seen in Bowman glands.[32] Scanning electron microscopy showed a more densely ciliated nasal epithelium in the laryngectomees compared with the pre-operative controls, and nasal mucociliary transport, measured by saccharine clearance, was significantly faster in laryngectomees.[33] This was further supported by electron microscopic study of olfactory neuroepithelium of 4 laryngectomized patients, which showed apoptic changes. So, the loss of nasal airflow, in combination with degenerative changes of the olfactory epithelium, is responsible for the olfactory deficit after total laryngectomy.[34]

Assessment of olfactory function after total laryngectomy

A number of studies have been conducted to assess olfaction after total laryngectomy, and all of them have suggested that the patients suffer from a significant loss of the sensation of smell. In a normal person, olfaction can be passive (i.e. occurring spontaneously during breathing) or active (i.e. sniffing). Total laryngectomy inevitably results in the loss of passive smelling, whereas only a minority of the patients are still able to smell actively.[35] In their study of 63 laryngectomized patients, Hilgers *et al.*[35] observed that approximately two-thirds were anosmic and the rest had difficulty in smelling. A study aimed at an objective evaluation of the sense of olfaction after total laryngectomy was carried out by Nagamachi *et al.*[36] According to them, as olfactory information is transmitted to the cerebral olfactory cortex, alteration of regional cerebral blood flow (rCBF) in these areas, in conjunction with olfactory stimulation, is likely to be one of the objective methods to assess olfactory function. To test this, the authors performed HMPAO SPECT in both the test and control groups, under baseline and under olfactory stimulation. In the baseline condition, no significant difference was evident in rCBF between the two groups, but under a stimulated condition, a significant increase in rCBF was found in the cerebral olfactory region in the control group, whereas the test group showed no significant rCBF change in the cerebral olfactory region. The sense of taste is also impaired in laryngectomized patients, given the close association of the sense of smell with taste. However, impairment of the taste sensation has been shown to be much less than impairment of the smell sensation.[37,39]

Different techniques for olfactory rehabilitattion

A number of techniques have been described in the literature for olfactory rehabilitation of laryngectomized patients. Some of these are described briefly in the following sections.

Prosthetic device to improve the olfaction

The first prosthetic device to improve olfaction after total laryngectomy was a simple device named 'nipple tube', described by Bosone.[39] Then an 'oral tracheal breathing' tube was introduced by Knudson *et al.*[40], which was similar to the 'larynx bypass'. The larynx bypass consists of a plastic tube that connects the tracheostoma to the mouth with a mouthpiece. The person breathes through the nose, keeping both lips and tracheostoma air-sealed, and the inhaled air reaches the lungs through the larynx bypass tube. The efficacy of larynx bypass was studied by Goktas *et al.*[41] They performed an odour test on 20 laryngectomized patients, and concluded that olfactory ability was significantly better with the larynx bypass than without it. However, they also observed that the first application of the larynx bypass was cumbersome. The authors concluded that although the patients had a better sense of smell with the larynx bypass, it does not seem to be suitable for daily use because of its rather moderate practicability.[41] So, it can be concluded that, although the use of different prosthetic devices definitely improves the sense of smell after total laryngectomy, they are inconvenient for use in daily life and hence their role is limited.

Different manoeuvres

A number of manoeuvres have been described to establish nasal air flow in laryngectomized patients. Examples of this are the glossopharyngeal press,[42] buccopharyngeal sniffing,[33] and the buccopharyngeal manoeuvre.[43] The underlying principle of these manoeuvres is to create an inflow of air through the nose by changing the volume of the oral cavity and the oropharynx, while the lips are closed. These methods have not been described in detail and their effectiveness has not been proven in scientific studies. Hence, they have not been used in general practice and remain fairly unknown.[44] A study has suggested that an early TE fistula for voice reconstruction causes significant improvement in olfaction of laryngectomized patients, and further improvement is possible with the association of the closed mouth nasal outward airflow manoeuvre.[34]

Nasal airflow inducing manoeuvre (NAIM)

The NAIM is the simplest, easiest and most effective technique for olfactory rehabilitation in laryngectomized patients. It was discovered by some authors that laryngectomized patients who are able to smell are more active in using facial muscles and muscles of the neck than those unable to smell.[33,43,45] Based on the observations of the techniques that such patients taught themselves in order to be able to smell, the NAIM, or the so-called 'polite yawning technique', was developed by Hilgers and co-workers.[46] Polite yawning describes the basis of this technique. A negative pressure is created in the oral cavity and oropharynx by lowering the lower jaw with closed lip. Now air comes to the oral cavity and the oropharynx through the nose, at it remains the only entry passage to those areas. This air carries the odour molecule to the olfactory epithelium, leading to olfaction. In their manual, Hilgers et al.[47] described the procedure as follows:

- The mandible, and thus the floor of mouth, is lowered. The mandibular joint rotates, but should not shift.
- Simultaneously, the tongue moves from the hard palate downwards.
- The lips remain closed
- The movement must be repeated quickly a couple of times.
- While performing the movements, relaxed breathing should continue and the breathing rhythm should be independent of the movements of the mandible and tongue.
- The movements must be performed eutonically, not hypokinetically, and certainly not hyperkinetically.

They have also advised that, after adequate practice, the patient should try to make the movements smaller to make it less obvious, and coined a name 'refined polite yawning technique' to describe it. This can be done by repetitive movements of the base of the tongue only, instead of moving the entire tongue.[47] This will make the procedure more acceptable to the patients.

Validation of the NAIM

A number of studies have been done to check the efficacy of this technique, leading to the conclusion that it is indeed the most simple, easy and effective method for olfactory rehabilitation in laryngectomized patients. The first intervention study, performed on 33 laryngectomized patients categorized as non-smellers, showed a success rate of 46% after a single 30 minute NAIM therapy session.[46] Risberg-Berlin et al.[48] observed that 72% of laryngectomized patients with an impaired sense of olfaction became normosmic after rehabilitation with NAIM. The results of long-term follow up of this technique are also encouraging.[35,47,49] Long-term olfactory rehabilitation was achieved in approximately 50% of the patients in the study of Hilgers et al.[35] In a study by Risberg-Berlin et al.[49] 70% of non-smellers became smellers in a 6-month follow-up after NAIM intervention, which increased to 78% after 36 months.

To conclude, loss of a sense of smell is inevitable after total laryngectomy. It definitely creates some restrictions in lifestyle. A number of rehabilitation methods have been described in the literature. Among them the NAIM or 'polite yawning technique' is the most acceptable, convenient, easy to learn and effective method. Both the short- and long-term follow-up results of this manoeuvre are encouraging. Its routine incorporation in the rehabilitation protocol of laryngectomized patients is strongly recommended.

Conclusion

Alaryngeal speech has come a long way since the first laryngectomy was performed in 1873. The 21st century holds further promise for the advancement of communication options following treatment for laryngeal cancer. It will continue to be the responsibility of the physician and speech pathologist to help the patient make an informed decision regarding which speech option to choose. TE speech using voice prostheses has revolutionized vocal rehabilitation after total laryngectomy and, in many centres, has now replaced oesophageal speech as the gold standard for voice rehabilitation. The advantages of these devices are numerous and include immediate voice production, high success rates compared with oesophageal speech, relatively low complication rates, and sustained speech with a more fluent quality than with oesophageal speech. TE speech has clearly improved the quality of life of laryngectomized patients. But it is not without its associated common problems, such as obstruction of the prostheses and leakage through the devices; troubleshooting of these problems should be anticipated. With the development of automatic tracheostomy valves, even hands-free speech is now possible. Biofilm formation on voice prostheses has been a major problem limiting the lifetime of all voice prostheses and the development of novel alternative prophylactic and therapeutic agents, including probiotics and other surface-active compounds, such as biosurfactants, are expected to gain prominence in the future in preventing biofilm formation. Today, the focus is not only on optimal voice rehabilitation but also on adequate pulmonary and olfactory rehabilitation.

References

1. Singer MI, Blom ED. An endoscopic technique for restoration of voice after laryngectomy. *Ann Otol Rhinol Laryngol* 1980;**89:** 529–33.

2. Hamaker RC, Singer MI, Blom ED, *et al.* Primary voice restoration at laryngectomy. *Arch Otolaryngol* 1985;**111:**182–6.

3. Serafini I. Reconstructive laryngectomy. In: Shedd DP, Weinberg B (eds). *Surgical and prosthetic approach to speech rehabilitation.* Boston G.K. Hall; 1980:67–76.

4. Guttman MR. Rehabilitation of voice in laryngectomized patients. *Arch Otolaryngol* 1932;**15:**478–9.

5. Panje WR. Prosthetic vocal rehabilitation following laryngectomy. *Ann Otol Rhinol Laryngol* 1981;**90:**116–20.

6. Nijdam HF, Annyas AA, Schutte HK, *et al.* A new prosthesis for voice rehabilitation after laryngectomy. *Arch Otorhinolaryngol* 1982; **237:**27–9.

7. Jebria AB, Henry C, Petit J, *et al.* Physical and aerodynamic features of the Bordeaux voice prosthesis. *Artif Organs* 1987;**11:**383–9.

8. Hilgers FJM, Schouwenburg PF. A new low-resistance, self-retaining prosthesis (Provox®) for voice rehabilitation after total laryngectomy. *Laryngoscope* 1990;**100:**1202–5.

9. Hilgers FJM, Cornelissen MW, Balm AJM. Aerodynamic characteristics of the low-resistance, indwelling Provox® voice prosthesis. *Eur Arch Otorhinolaryngol* 1993;**250:**375–80.

10. Brown DH, Hilgers FJM, Irish JC, *et al.* Postlaryngectomy voice rehabilitation: State-of-the-art at the millennium. *World J Surg* 2003; **27:**824–31.

11. Hilgers FJM, Balm AJM. Long-term results of vocal rehabilitation after total laryngectomy with the low-resistance, indwelling Provox® voice prosthesis system. *Clin Otolaryngol* 1993;**18:**517–19.

12. Hilgers FJM, Ackerstaff AH, Balm AJM, *et al.* Development and clinical evaluation of a second-generation voice prosthesis (Provox®2), designed for anterograde and retrograde insertion. *Acta Otolaryngol* 1997;**117:**889–95.

13. Hilgers FJM, Ackerstaff AH, Balm AJM, *et al.* A new problem-solving indwelling voice prosthesis, eliminating the need for frequent Candida and 'underpressure'-related replacements: Provox ActiValve. *Acta Otolaryngol* 2003;**123:**972–9.

14. Remacle MJM, Declaye XJ. Gax-collagen injection to correct an enlarged tracheoesophageal fistula for a vocal prosthesis. *Laryngoscope* 1988;**98:**1350–2.

15. Luff DA, Izzat S, Farrington WT. Viscoaugmentation as a treatment for leakage around the Provox 2 voice rehabilitation system. *J Laryngol Otol* 1999;**113:**847–8.

16. Perie S, Ming X, Dewolf E, *et al.* Autologous fat injection to treat leakage around tracheoesophageal puncture. *Am J Otolaryngol* 2002; **23:**345–50.

17. Rodrigues L, Banat IM, Teixeira J, *et al.* Strategies for the prevention of microbial biofilm formation on silicone rubber voice prostheses. *Journal of Biomedical Materials Research Part B: Applied Biomaterials;* 2007;**81B:**367.

18. Graham MS. *Clinician's guide to alaryngeal speech therapy.* Boston: Butterworth-Heinemann; 1997.

19. Casper JK, Colton RH. *Clinical manual for laryngectomy and head and neck cancer rehabilitation.* San Diego (California): Singular Publishing; 1993.

20. Bennett S, Weinberg B. Acceptability ratings of normal, esophageal, and artificial larynx speech. *J Speech Hear Res* 1973;**16:**608.

21. Gilmore SI. Failure in acquiring esophageal speech. In: Salmon SJ, Mounts KH (eds). *Alaryngeal speech rehabilitation for clinicians by clinicians.* Austin (Texas): PRO-ED; 1991:194.

22. Robbins J, Fisher HB, Blom ED, *et al.* A comparative acoustic study of normal, esophageal, and tracheoesophageal speech production. *J Speech Hear Disord* 1984;**49:**202.

23. Shanks JC. Developing esophageal communication. In: Keith RL, Darley FL (eds). *Laryngectomee rehabilitation.* 3rd ed. Austin (Texas): PRO-ED; 1994:211.

24. Hilgers FJM, Aaronson NK, Ackerstaff AH, *et al.* The influence of a heat and moisture exchanger (HME) on the respiratory symptoms after total laryngectomy. *Clin Otolaryngol* 1991;**16:**152–60.

25. Ackerstaff AH, Hilgers FJM, Aaronson NK, *et al.* Improvements in respiratory and psychosocial functioning following total laryngectomy by the use of a heat and moisture exchanger. *Ann Otol Rhinol Laryngol* 1993;**102:**878–82.

26. van Dam FS, Hilgers FJM, Emsbroek G, *et al.* Deterioration of olfaction and gustation as a consequence of total laryngectomy. *Laryngoscope* 1999;**109:**1150–5.

27. Hilgers FJM, Ackerstaff AH, Aaronson NK, *et al.* Physical and psychosocial consequences of total laryngectomy. *Clin Otolaryngol* 1990;**15:**421–5.

28. Ackerstaff AH, Hilgers FJM, Aaronson NK, *et al.* Communication, functional disorders and lifestyle changes after total laryngectomy. *Clin Otolaryngol* 1994;**19:**295–300.

29. Hilgers FJM, van Dam FS, Keyzers S, *et al.* Rehabilitation of olfaction after laryngectomy by means of a nasal airflow-inducing maneuver: The 'polite yawning' technique. *Arch Otolaryngol Head Neck Surg* 2000;**126:**726–32.

30. Scherer PW, Hahn II, Mozell MM. The biophysics of nasal airflow. *Otolaryngol Clin North Am* 1989;**22:**265.

31. Fujii M, Fukazawa K, Hatta C, *et al.* Olfactory acuity after total laryngectomy. *Chem Senses* 2002;**27:**117–21.

32. Miani C, Ortolani F, Bracale AMB, *et al.* Olfactory mucosa histological findings in laryngectomees. *Europian Archives of Oto Rhino Laryngology* 2003;**260:**529–35.

33. Moore-Gillon V. The nose after laryngectomy. *JR Soc Med* 1985;**78:** 435–9.

34. Jin GW, Wei XD, Chen J, *et al.* Olfactory acuity and improvement of olfaction after total laryngectomy. *Zhonghua Er Bi Yan Hou Tou Jing Wai Ke Za Zhi* 2005;**40:**536–40.

35. Hilgers FJM, Jansen HA, Van As CJ, *et al.* Long-term results of olfaction rehabilitation using the nasal airflow-inducing ('polite yawning') maneuver after total laryngectomy. *Arch Otolaryngol Head Neck Surg* 2002;**128:**648–54.

36. Nagamachi S, Wakamatsu H, Fujita S, *et al.* Deficit of olfactory sensation in patients after total laryngectomy – Evaluation of regional cerebral blood flow alteration by Tc-99m HMPAO SPECT and SPM2 analysis. *J Nucl Med* 2006;**47** (Suppl 1):306P.

37. Ackerstaff AH, Hilgers FJ, Aaronson NK, *et al.* Communication, functional disorders and lifestyle changes after total laryngectomy. *Clin Otolaryngol* 1994;**19:**295–300.

38. Finizia C, Hammerlid E, Westin T, *et al.* Quality of life and voice in patients with laryngeal carcinoma: A post-treatment comparison of laryngectomy (salvage surgery) versus radiotherapy. *Laryngoscope* 1998;**108:**1566–73.

39. Bosone ZT. The nipple tube: A simple device for olfaction and nose blowing after laryngectomy. *J Speech Hear Disord* 1984;**49:**106–7.

40. Knudson RC, Williams EO. Olfaction through oral tracheal breathing tube. *J Prosthetic Dentistry* 1989;**61:**471–2.

41. Goktas O, Lammert I, Berl J, *et al.* Rehabilitation of the olfactory sense after laryngectomy—the larynx bypass [in German]. *Laryngorhinootologie* 2005;**84:**829–32.

42. Damsté PH. Extras in rehabilitation: Smelling, swimming, and compensating for changes after laryngectomy. In: Keith RL (ed). *Laryngectomee rehabilitation.* Houston: College-Hill Press; 1979:513–20.

43. Swartz DN, Mozell MM, Youngentob SL, *et al.* Improvement of olfaction in laryngectomized patients with the larynx bypass. *Laryngoscope* 1987;**97**:1280–6.

44. Tatchell RH, Lerman JW, Watt J. Olfactory ability as a function of nasal air flow volume in laryngectomees. *Am J Otolaryngol* 1985;**6**:426–32.

45. Van Dam F, Hilgers F, Emsbroek G, *et al.* Deterioration of olfaction and gustation as a consequence of total laryngectomy. *Laryngoscope* 1999;**109**:1150–5.

46. Hilgers F, van Dam F, Keyzers S, *et al.* Rehabilitation of olfaction after laryngectomy by means of a nasal airflow-inducing maneuver. *Arch Otolaryngol Head Neck Surg* 2000;**126**:726–32.

47. Polak R, van As C, van Dam F, Hilgers F. *Olfaction regained, using the polite yawning technique: A brochure for laryngectomees.* In: Hilgers F (ed). Swets en Zeitlinger, Lisse; 2003.

48. Risberg-Berlin B, Ylitalo R, Finizia C. Screening and rehabilitation of olfaction after total laryngectomy in Swedish patients. *Arch Otolaryngol Head Neck Surg* 2006;**132**:301–6.

49. Risberg-Berlin B, Ryden A, Moller RY, *et al.* Effects of total laryngectomy on olfactory function, health-related quality of life, and communication: A 3-year follow-up study Export. *BMC Ear, Nose and Throat Disorders* 2009;**9**:8.

22

Quality of life (QOL) outcomes in head and neck cancer

SUHAIL SAYED, RAGHAV C. DWIVEDI, ALOK PATHAK, REHAN KAZI

Introduction

The field of head and neck oncology has seen dramatic improvements in cancer detection and therapeutics. In spite of this, cancer continues to ravage the lives of patients, with physical, psychological and social consequences. The structural and functional integrity of the head and neck region holds pivotal importance in a patient's social and emotional life. Hence, when a person is afflicted with a head and neck cancer (HNC), the disease becomes an intrinsic part of his or her personal and social life. Although it is possible to extend the patient's life in a 'disease free' state, it is important to evaluate the patients' quality of life (QOL), so that one 'not only adds years to life but life to years.'[1] In this regard, QOL evaluation and performance outcomes in cancer is critical for optimal patient care, comprehensive evaluation of treatment alternatives, and the development of informed rehabilitative services and patient education.[2–5]

What is QOL?

QOL is subjective to the patients' perceptions of their state of well-being and there is no universally accepted definition. Although this perceptual entity may have myriad definitions, it is important to evaluate QOL from the patient's rather than the clinician's perspective.

- Joyce and McGee defined QOL as: *'How good or bad you feel your life to be.'*[1]
- The World Health Organization (WHO) defines QOL as: *'An individual's perception of their position in life, in the context of the culture and value systems in their life,* *and in relation to their goals, expectations, standards, and concerns.'*[6,7]
- Revicki and colleagues define QOL as: *'A broad range of human experiences related to one's overall well-being'* that minimally includes the broadly defined assessments of the physical, psychological and social domains of functioning.[1]
- Morton and Izzard define QOL as: *'… the perceived discrepancy between the reality of what a person has and the concept of what the person wants, needs or expects'.*[3]

Evaluation of QOL must incorporate the following variables, viz. biological/physical, symptoms and functions, general health perceptions and health-related QOL (HRQOL).[8] The intricate interrelationship of these independent variables need to be understood to get a comprehensive scenario of the patient's 'total health related experience'.

Importance of QOL outcome measures

Including QOL outcome measures in the management armamentarium for a HNC patient will not just help in improving the survival of the patient but also guide in gauging the effectiveness of the treatment imparted. This has been schematically depicted in Fig. 1.[2–5,9]

The QOL outcome measures help clinicians to focus on patients' core problems and issues.[2,3] The QOL assessment also provides additional data on issues that might explain disease severity or coping strategies (response shift – change in internal standards over time), thereby identifying the patient's preferred treatment expectations, and monitoring changes/responses to treatment.[4] Failure to meet these expectations

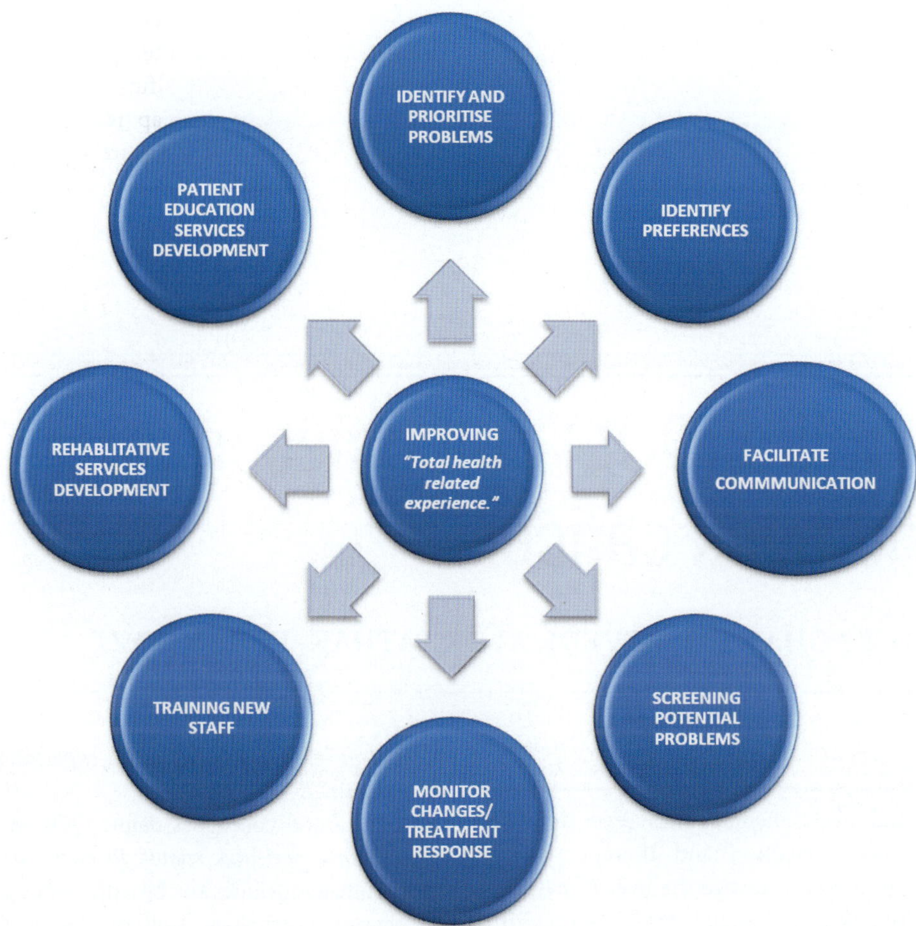

Fig. 1. Diagram depicting the importance of QOL outcome measures in aiding routine clinical practice and governance

may, unfortunately, lead to patients defaulting their treatment. Additionally, QOL data can be constructive in training the staff in patient governance and in auditing the information on patients obtained through the QOL measures, thus making the staff more responsive to the pressing issues.[3–5]

QOL outcome measures can be instrumental in guiding the government and public agencies in formulating policies prioritizing the assets to domains of utmost importance.[5,6] Given the importance of QOL in patient care, QOL measures have been duly incorporated into the strategic and research initiatives of numerous cancer bodies, such as the NCI (National Cancer Institute), NIH (National Institute of Health), ACS (American Cancer Society), NICE (National Institute for Clinical and Health Excellence), ASCO (American Society of Clinical Oncology) and the US FDA.[6,10]

Available QOL outcome measures

To date, overall 24 QOL outcome measures catering to the various domains that influence QOL have been formulated for HNC patients. Although it is challenging to quantify patients' perceptions, a methodological approach can help in devising an outcome measure that caters to all the available domains,

which unfortunately is not the case presently. Of the available 24 outcome measures described in the literature, only 12 are currently employed.[3–6,11–27] The QOL outcome measures are questionnaires/scales that incorporate several questions/ items catering to the various domains that influence QOL. In formulating an outcome measure the questionnaire should be:[5,11]

- *Valid*—appropriateness, meaningfulness and usefulness of a measure for a specific purpose
- *Reliable*—stability and reproducibility of a measure over time
- *Interpretable*—clinically relevant
- *Sensitive*—responsive to change
- *Short*—minimal time-burden
- *Easy to score*
- *Have an overall global score and domain scores*
- *Multidimensional*—covering a broad range of items in multiple domains
- *Self-administered*
- *No floor and ceiling effect*—ability to detect changes at the two extremes of QOL
- QOL scales should undergo rigorous back-translation (to be used in different languages).

To date there is no 'gold standard' questionnaire available and therefore there is a need to individualize it as per the scope of the outcome research.[5]

The commonly employed QOL scales have been broadly classified into two categories: (i) Generic (covers the majority of the aspects of the patient's health); and (ii) specific (caters to the attributes affected by the disease and its treatment). Some examples are: Generic (e.g. the Medical Outcomes Study [MOS] Short Form-36, Sickness Impact Profile [SIP]), disease-specific (e.g. the European Organization for Research into the Treatment of Cancer [EORTC] QLQ-C30, Functional Assessment of Cancer Therapy-General [FACT-G]), site-specific (University of Washington QOL questionnaire [UWQOL], EORTC HN QLQ), domain-specific (e.g. the voice-related QOL [VRQOL], MD Anderson Dysphagia Inventory [MDADI]), treatment-specific (e.g. the UWQOL for surgical patients, QOL-RTI/H&N for radiotherapy patients), and symptom-specific (e.g. the Brief Pain Inventory [BPI] and the Brief Fatigue Inventory [BFI]).[3–6,11–27] These have been depicted schematically and described briefly in Fig. 2 and Table 1, respectively.[5]

Difficulties, limitations and pitfalls of QOL research in HNC

QOL outcome work has grown by leaps and bounds in the recent years. However, it is imperative that, while maintaining the relentless efforts in this evolving discipline of cancer care, a pragmatic approach be employed in the evaluation and interpretation of QOL outcomes. This is because QOL is a multidimensional construct which is complex and highly individualized and any attempt to generalize the outcome results are bound to prove futile. QOL measure is like a rose whose beauty can only be appreciated by the individual, and no number of precise measurements can ever capture its beauty to the fullest.[1]

The practical and methodological constraints faced by a researcher whilst embarking on QOL studies are listed in Table 2.

Self-administered questionnaires are preferable for use in QOL studies, as the patient's self-rating is a more sensitive and reliable indicator than that made by a clinician.[2,3] In situations where the patient is incapable of filling a QOL questionnaire because of cognitive/communication deficits, a proxy (family member) can be considered. However, this can yield biased results because of the carer's own experiences of and feelings for the patient.[30] Furthermore, results generated from outcome measures cannot always be clinically relevant. Results showing different scores by the same patient are difficult to interpret because QOL experienced by a patient is not a static perception but is derived from experiences over a long period. Also, occasionally patients do not demonstrate a logical variation in overall QOL scores. To explain this, the phenomenon of adaptation has been propounded.[4,6] QOL scales must be considered as an adjunct in patient care and the clinician should refrain from using them as an alternative to effective patient communication.[5] QOL studies based on inadequate sample size and retrospective data analysis are bound to yield skewed data, thus failing to draw a broad picture of the patient's problems.[4]

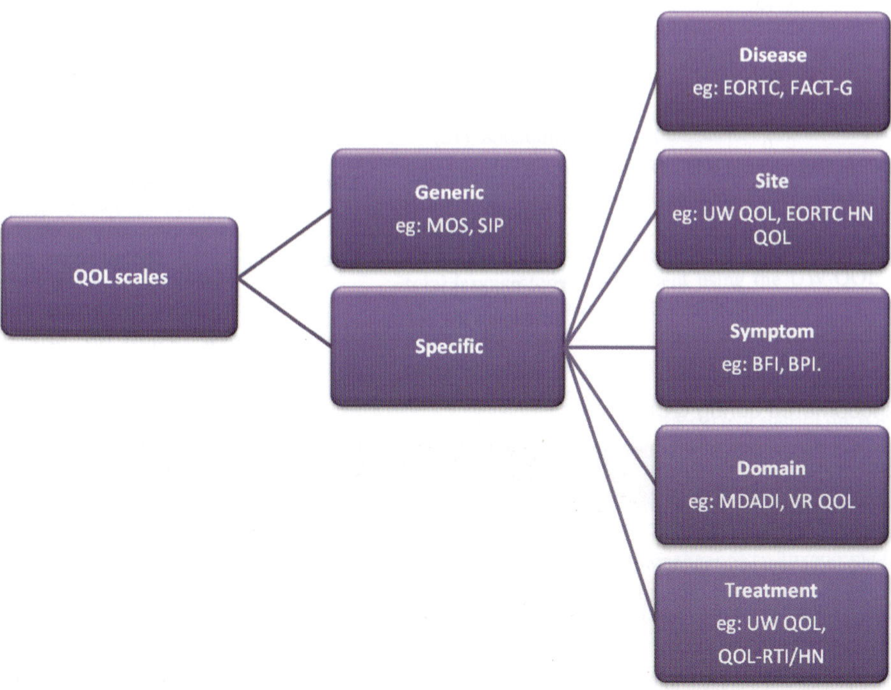

Fig. 2. Types of QOL scales with selected examples (adapted with permission from Sayed *et al.*[5])

8. Wilson IB, Clearly PD. Health-related outcomes. *JAMA* 1995;**273:** 59–63.

9. Higginson IJ, Carr AJ. Measuring quality of life: Using quality of life measures in the clinical setting. *BJM* 2001;**322:**1297–1300.

10. Lipscomb J, Gotay CC, Snyder CF. A Review of recent research and policy initiatives of patient-reported outcomes in cancer. *CA Cancer J Clin* 2007;**57:**278–30.

11. Pusic A, Liu JC, Chen CM, *et al.* A systematic review of patient-reported outcome measures in head and neck cancer surgery. *Otolaryngology-Head and Neck Surgery* 2007;**136:**525–35.

12. Sayed SI, Kazi RA. Need for a paradigm for application of outcome measure (QOL scales) in head and neck cancer patients in India. *J Cancer Res Ther* 2008;**4:**192–4.

13. Ware JE, Sherbourne C. The MOS 36-Item short-form health survey (SF-36). *Med Care* 1992;**30:**473–83.

14. Berbner M, Bobbit RA, Carter WB, *et al.* The sickness impact profile: Development and final revision of a health status measure. *Med Care* 1981;**19:**787–805.

15. Cella D, Tulsky D, Gray G, *et al.* The functional assessment of cancer therapy (FACT) scale: Development and validation of a general measure. *J Clin Oncol* 1993;**11:**570–9.

16. Aaronson NK, Ahmedzai S, Bergman B, *et al.* The European Organization for Research and Treatment of Cancer QLQ-C30: A quality-of-life instrument for use international clinical trials in oncology. *J Natl Cancer Inst* 1993;**85:**365–76.

17. Sherman AC, Simmonton S, Adams DC, *et al.* Assessing quality of life in patients with head and neck cancer: Cross-validation of the European Organization for Research and Treatment of Cancer (EORTC) Quality of Life Head and Neck Module (QLQ-H&N35). *Arch Otolaryngol Head Neck Surg* 2000;**126:**459–67.

18. Bjordal K, de Graeff A, Fayers PM, *et al.* A 12 country field study of the EORTC QLQ-C30 (version3.0) and the head and neck cancer specific module (EORTC QLQ-H&N35) in head and neck patients. *Eur J Cancer* 2000;**36:**1796–1807.

19. Hassan SJ, Weymuller EA. Assessment of quality of life in head and neck cancer patients. *Head Neck* 1993;**15:**485–96.

20. List MA, Ritter-Sterr C, Lansky S. A performance status scale for head and neck cancer patients. *Cancer* 1990;**66:**564–9.

21. Daut R, Cleeland C, Flanery R. Development of the Wisconsin brief pain questionnaire to assess pain in cancer and other patients. *Pain* 1983;**17:**197–210.

22. Mendoza TR, Wang XS, Cleeland CS, *et al.* The rapid assessment of fatigue severity in cancer patients. *Cancer* 1999;**85:**1186–96.

23. Ringash J, Bezjak A. A structured review of quality of life instruments for head and neck cancer patients. *Head Neck* 2001;**23:**201–13.

24. Fung K, Terell JE. Outcomes research in head and neck cancer. *ORL* 2004;**66:**207–13.

25. Finizia C, Hammerlid E, Westin T, *et al.* Quality of life and voice in patients with laryngeal carcinoma: A post treatment comparison of laryngectomy (salvage surgery) versus radiotherapy. *Laryngoscope* 1998;**108:**1566–73.

26. Zotti P, Lugli D, Vaccher E, *et al.* The EORTC quality of life questionnaire-head and neck 35 in Italian laryngectomized patients. European organization for research and treatment of cancer. *Qual Life Res* 2000;**9:**1147–53.

27. Chen AY, Frankowski R, Bishop-Leone J, *et al.* The development and validation of a dysphagia-specific questionnaire for head and neck cancer patients: The MD Anderson Dysphagia Inventory (MDADI). *Arch Otolaryngol Head Neck Surg* 2001;**127:**870–6.

28. Sayed SI, Manikantan K, Khode S, *et al.* Perspectives on quality of life following total laryngectomy. Giornale Italiano di Medicina del Lavoro ed Ergonomia. *Supplemento B, Psicologia* 2009;**31:**3.

29. Kazi R, Singh A, De Cordova J, *et al.* Validation of a voice prosthesis questionnaire to assess valved speech and its related issues in patients following total laryngectomy. *Clin Otolaryngol* 2006;**31:**404–10.

30. Terrell JE, Ronis DL, Fowler KE, *et al.* The clinical predictors of quality of life in patients with head and neck cancer. *Arch Otolaryngol Head Neck Surg* 2004;**130:**401–8.

31. Mandrekar S, Dueck A. Future directions in QOL research. *Curr Probl Cancer* 2005;**29:**343–51.

32. Sloan JA, Loprinzi CL, Kuross SA, *et al.* Randomized comparison of four tools measuring overall quality of life in patients with advanced cancer. *J Clin Oncol* 1998;**16:**3662–73.

33. Revicki DA, Cella DF. Health status assessment for the twenty-first century: Item response theory, item banking and computer adaptive testing. *Qual Life Res* 1997;**6:**595–600.

34. Lai JS, Cella D, Chang CH, *et al.* Item banking to improve, shorten and computerize self-reported fatigue: An illustration of steps to create a core item bank from the FACIT-Fatigue Scale. *Qual Life Res* 2003;**12:**485–501.

35. Panter AT, Reeve BB. Assessing tobacco beliefs among youth using item response theory models. *Drug Alcohol Depend* 2002;**68:**S21–S39.

36. Buxton J, White M, Osoba D. Patients' experiences using a computerized program with a touch-sensitive video monitor for the assessment of health-related quality of life. *Quality Life Res* 1998;**7:**513–19.

37. Stuart GW, Laraia MT, Ornstein SM, *et al.* An interactive voice response system to enhance antidepressant medication compliance. *Top Health Info Manage* 2003;**24:**15–20.

23

TNM classification of head and neck cancer

KAPILA MANIKANTAN, RAGHAV C. DWIVEDI, ALOK PATHAK, REHAN KAZI

'A classification scheme for cancer must encompass all attributes of the tumour that define its life history', states the opening line of the manual for staging of cancer by the American Joint Committee on Cancer (AJCC) Staging. The features of a staging system should include accurate mapping of tumours to aid the physician in treatment planning, give an idea on disease prognosis, and be comparable across different centres.[1] The ability to give an accurate estimation of the prognosis is considered to be the most important attribute. To be able to do this, the staging system should divide the population into a discrete number of groups that are internally homogenous, and are yet externally dissimilar in relation to a defined outcome event.[2]

Tumour Node Metastasis (TNM) system

Halstead first proposed the concept of solid tumours spreading in a staged, stepwise fashion from the primary site of origin to regional lymphatics and subsequently to distant organs. The observation that the prognosis worsened with this pattern of spread of the tumour formed the basis of Halstead's theory.[3] Steinthal in 1905 and Paterson in 1940 used these observations for creating a staging system for breast cancer. The 'TNM system' was developed by Pierre Denoix between 1943 and 1952 at the Institut Gustave-Roussy.[3] His assessment of tumour burden was based on the size of the primary tumour (T) and presence of local/distant spread (node [N] and metastasis [M]). His proposal was formally accepted by the Union Internationale Contre le Cancer (UICC) in 1953 for staging of solid tumours as the TNM staging system. Subsequently, the UICC published 9 brochures between 1960 and 1967 with proposals for classification of tumours at 23 different anatomical body sites.[3] In 1968, these site-specific brochures were combined by the UICC working committee to develop the first edition of the TNM staging system. However, this TNM staging system was not accepted globally. In parallel, the AJCC had developed its own staging system. Finally, at the 13th International Cancer Congress in 1982, the AJCC and the UICC united to agree to a single TNM staging system. This joint effort, known as the fourth edition of the TNM, was published in 1987.[4]

Retrospective or prospective studies on patients allow the classification of different TNM categories into stage groups, such that each group is homogeneous with respect to survival, and that the survival rates for different stage groups are distinctive. There have been 7 editions of both the UICC and AJCC staging systems with the 7th edition published in 2009 and in use for patients diagnosed after 1 January 2010.[5] At present, seven distinct stages have been developed for head and neck cancer (HNC) of mucosal origin (0, I, II, III, IVa, IVb, IVc). The TNM system is widely considered to be a simple and effective tool for mapping the size of the tumour. Mutually exclusive partitions are created into which new patients with certain common characteristics are grouped, with the prognosis being based on the mean statistics of patients in that partition.[3] Any neck metastasis classifies the disease as advanced, except in select nasopharynx and thyroid cancers.

Controversies in the TNM staging

The current TNM staging system uses only three factors to

gauge tumour burden and prognosis. This over-simplicity and high dependence on anatomical/morphological characteristics, with no importance attached to other tumour- and patient-related factors, has been its major criticism. The TNM system has failed to incorporate these diverse influences whilst striving to maintain its simplicity and effectiveness. A detailed and complex system that will accurately determine prognosis will, by definition, be limited in its utility and user-friendliness. Such an effort may end up with numerous patient groupings and, therefore, making meaningful assessments of therapeutic options and prognosis rather tedious and difficult. Conversely, a very simple staging system would have a high compliance rate but would suffer from poor prognostic ability.

As more and more data from various clinical trials become available, future revisions should include the various clinical factors which have a prognostic impact on the patient. It is widely believed that host factors, patient co-morbidity and additional tumour factors, and biological and immunological markers should be incorporated to add further prognostic capabilities in the TNM system.[5]

Other staging systems

In order to address some of the perceived flaws/inadequacies of the TNM system, several researchers have tried their hand at alternate staging systems. Generally, these modifications involve either altering or adding certain tumour-related variables/characteristics, changing the existing TNM stage groupings, or developing a completely different staging system.[2]

The STNMP system for intraoral carcinoma developed by Rapidis et al. added site (S) and pathology (P) to the conventional TNM.[6] By adding scores to each of the factors they arrived at a scale of 0–155. In a comparative analysis with the conventional TNM staging in 136 patients, the STNMP was appreciably better in predicting the 5-year survival at presentation. The predictive value of the velocity of growth of the tumour (V) was also assessed in a cohort of 170 patients. The variable V was arrived at by dividing the area of the lesion by the duration of symptoms. It was seen that V was more significant when compared with the area of the tumour, or the delay in the symptoms alone. The system, however, needs to be applied to a large prospective study.[7]

Pugliano et al. developed a clinical-severity staging system for larynx cancer, which was expanded for use in the oral cavity.[2] Using multivariate techniques, they validated the prognostic importance of clinical factors in oral cavity cancer. The co-morbidity was classified using the Kaplan-Feinstein index,[8] which classifies it into three categories (mild, moderate and severe). Multivariate analysis was performed using a logistic regression model for categorical data. Several quantitative techniques were used to compare the composite staging system with the TNM system. A functional-severity staging system was developed as the symptoms and the co-morbidity describe the patient's functional status. The clinical-severity system was created by combining the functional-severity system with the TNM system. Pugliano et al.[2] showed that with the incorporation of suitable symptom severity and co-morbidity, the survival estimates can be improved. They also concluded that the composite clinical-severity staging system is a more prognostically precise system.

Alternative staging systems, which have been proposed on the basis of the TNM are the TANIS system (Tumour and Node Integer Score) and systems developed by Hall et al.[9] and Berg[10] and Kiricuta.[11] The TANIS system, in which the integers of T and N are combined to give a score was developed by Jones et al.[12] It is based on the empirical and false notion of equivalence in survival prediction between T and N. The Hall,[9] Hart[13] and Berg[10] systems were developed using statistical analysis of their specific data sets. Kiricuta's system was based on an empirical modification of Hart's system.

Cutaneous squamous cell carcinoma of the head and neck has the potential to spread to the nodes of the neck and parotid. The present TNM staging is simple in defining regional metastatic disease. To study a new staging system a retrospective study was carried out using clinical and pathopatients.[14] Patients were allocated P and N stages (parotid nodes and neck nodes, respectively) as per the staging system. On multivariate analysis clinical P3 (metastatic node >6 cm in diameter or disease involving skull base or facial nerve) parotid stage (p=0.033) and pathological N1, N2 (metastatic neck disease) neck stages (p=0.005) had independent effects on survival. The authors concluded that the addition of the P and N stages added valuable prognostic information but the value of sub groupings was uncertain.[14]

A prognostic system index for salivary gland tumours was suggested by Vander Poorten et al.[15] in a retrospective analysis of 150 patients of parotid carcinoma; pre-treatment data was incorporated in a prognostic index PS1 and the post-surgical specimen data in a post-treatment prognostic index PS2. The index was shown to give a probability of recurrence.

As yet, none of the many alternate staging systems has been widely accepted. Invariably, most systems suffer from undue complexities and impracticalities that preclude their clinical use. Therefore, caution should be exercised, and revisions to existing TNM staging systems would have to be a compromise between the ideal and the practical.[3,16]

References

1. Lydiatt WM, Schantz SP. Biological staging of head and neck cancer and its role in developing effective treatment strategies. *Cancer and Metastasis Reviews* 1996;**15**:11–26.

2. Pugliano FA, Piccirillo JF, Zequira MR, *et al.* Clinical-severity staging system for oral cavity cancer: Five-year survival rates. *Otolaryngol Head Neck Surg* 1999;**120**:38–45.

cancer syndromes. I
inherit a germline
Consequently, this a
body. It is, therefore
body will suffer con
one copy has to be r
As a result, heredit
multiple cancers at a

The hallmarks
targeted drugs

Hanahan and Wei
that occur in cance
driving their malign
represents a useful v
cancer can be target
that some of these p
others. In the follow
will be discussed an
intervention in HNC

Targeting grow

The function of gr
ligands in promotin
depicted in Fig. 2. I
to the specific ligar

3. Patel SG, Lydiatt WM. Staging of head and neck cancers: Is it time to change the balance between the ideal and the practical? *J Surg Oncol* 2008;**97**:653–7.

4. van der Schroeff MP, Baatenburg de Jong RJ. Staging and prognosis in head and neck cancer. *Oral Oncol* 2009;**45**:356–60.

5. Manikantan K, Sayed SI, Syrigos KN, *et al.* Challenges for the future modifications of the TNM staging system for head and neck cancer: Case for a new computational model? *Cancer Treat Rev* 2009;**39**:635–44.

6. Rapidis AD, Langdon JD, Patel MF, *et al.* STNMP a new system for the clinico-pathological classification and identification of intra-oral carcinoma. *Cancer* 1977;**39**:204–9.

7. Evans SJW, Langdon JD, Rapidis AD, *et al.* Prognostic significance of STNMP and velocity of tumor growth in oral cancer. *Cancer* 1982;**49**:773–6.

8. Kaplan MH, Feinstein AR. The importance of classifying initial comrbidity in evaluating the outcome of diabetes mellitus. *J Chronic Dis* 1974;**27**:387–404.

9. Hall SF, Groome PA, Rothwell D, *et al.* Using TNM staging to predict survival in patients with squamous cell carcinoma of head and neck. *Head Neck* 1999;**21**:30–8.

10. Berg H. Die prognostische relevanz des TNM-systems fur oropharynxkarzinome. *Tumor Diagn Ther* 1992;**13**:171–7.

11. Kiricuta IC. The Importance of correct stage grouping in oncology: Results of a nationwide study of oropharyngeal carcinoma in the netherlands. *Cancer* 1996;**77**:587–9.

12. Jones GW, Browmna G, Goodyear M, *et al.* Comparison of the addition of T and N integer score with TNM stage groups in head and neck cancer. *Head Neck* 1993;**15**:497–503.

13. Hart AAM, Mak-Kregar S, Hilgers FJM. The importance of correct stage grouping in oncology. Results of a nationwide study of oropharyngeal carcinoma in the Netherlands. *Cancer* 1996;**77**:587–90.

14. Andruchow JL, Veness MJ, Morgan GJ, *et al.* Implications for clinical staging of metastatic cutaneous carcinoma of the head and neck based on a multicenter study of treatment outcomes. *Cancer* 2006;**106**:1078–83.

15. Vander Poorten VLM, Balm AJM, Hilgers FJM, *et al.* the development of a prognostic score for patients with parotid carcinoma. *Cancer* 1999;**85**:2057–67.

16. Greene FL, Sobin LH. The staging of cancer: A retrospective and prospective appraisal. *CA Cancer J Clin* 2008;**58**:180–90.

Fig. 2. Growth factor i
apoptosis, angiogenesi
domain of the receptor

24

Nove
head

KEVIN J. H

Introducti

In the past 10 y
neck cancer (H
These include:
that can be en
toxicity and po
proof of the su
over radiother
treatment setti
molecular biol
and behaviour
novel targeted

Our unde
has fundamen
therapies are
occurs when t
corrupted or d
gene expression
in normal pro
changes that c
Enhancing the
survival and sp
that repress th
cancer cells acq
uncontrolled fa
a dedicated blc
and develop res

This review
that are disturb
a discussion o
opportunities in

disease control rate (complete response, partial response, stable disease) of 36%. Thirty-four per cent of patients experienced a symptomatic improvement. The median time to progression and survival was 2.6 and 4.3 months, respectively. Acneiform folliculitis was the most frequently observed manifestation of toxicity (76%), but the majority of cases were grade 1 or 2. Only 4 patients experienced grade 3 toxicity of any type (all cases of folliculitis).

Lapatinib is an oral dual TK inhibitor with action against both EGFR (c-erbB1, HER-1) and c-erbB2 (HER-2).[58,59] It has activity both *in vitro* and *in vivo*, as well as showing tolerability in phase I clinical trials.[59] A placebo-controlled randomized phase 0 biomarker study has been performed with this agent in patients with advanced HNC.[60] A single agent response rate of 17% was reported, with biomarker evidence of significantly reduced proliferation and receptor phosphorylation in the lapatinib-treated group.[60] A phase I dose escalation study of lapatinib administered during radical chemoradiotherapy in patients with stages III and IV HNC has been performed.[61] Patients were enrolled in cohorts of escalating lapatinib doses of 500 mg/day, 1000 mg/day and 1500 mg/day. Patients received 1 week of lapatinib alone, followed by 6.5–7 weeks of the same dose of lapatinib plus radiotherapy with 66–70 Gy, and cisplatin 100 mg/m^2 on days 1, 22 and 43 of radiotherapy. Endpoints included safety/tolerability and clinical activity. Thirty-one patients were enrolled (7 in each of the 500 mg and 1000 mg cohorts, 17 in the 1500 mg cohort [14 in a safety cohort]). Dose-limiting toxicities (DLT) observed were a perforated ulcer in 1 patient in the 500 mg cohort, and transient elevation of liver enzymes in 1 patient in the 1000 mg cohort. No DLTs were observed in the 1500 mg cohort. The recommended phase II dose was lapatinib 1500 mg/day with chemoradiation. The overall response rate was 81% (65% at the recommended phase II dose). The recommended phase II dose is lapatinib 1500 mg/day with chemoradiation in patients with locally advanced HNSCC, and is associated with an acceptable tolerability profile. On the basis of these findings, randomized phase II and III studies of lapatinib plus chemoradiation have been initiated.

Targeting insensitivity to anti-growth signals

A number of normal anti-growth signals counteract the positively-acting growth signals described above. Anti-growth signals work either by forcing cells into quiescence (G0 stage of the cell cycle) or by inducing their terminal differentiation such that they are permanently unable to re-enter the cell cycle. Anti-growth signalling is mediated by ligands (e.g. TGF beta [TGFβ] that act on cellular receptors (e.g. TGFβ receptor) and send signals to the nucleus via second messengers. These pathways are mainly involved in controlling the cell cycle clock and mediate their effects through proteins that include retinoblastoma protein (Rb), cyclins, cyclin-dependent

kinases (CDK) and their inhibitors (CDKi). Abnormalities in anti-growth signalling pathways are extremely common in cancer and play a role in helping cancer cells to progress through the cell cycle. Therefore, loss of Rb and members of the CDKi family and over-expression of certain cyclins and CDK have been shown to occur in a large number of tumour types.

Clinical attempts to target proliferation through cell cycle control are in their very early stages. The CDKi, Seliciclib (CYC202; R-roscovitine), has been shown to enhance apoptosis in HNC cells in preclinical studies.[62] It is the first selective, orally bioavailable inhibitor of CDK 1, 2, 7 and 9 to enter the clinic, and in a phase I trial in 21 patients at doses of 100, 200 and 800 twice daily, it caused dose-limiting toxicities at the 800 mg dose.[63] No objective tumour responses were noted, but disease stabilization was recorded in 8 patients. Other similar agents are in development and will enter clinical trials in patients with a range of malignancies, including HNC, in the near future.

Targeting the apoptotic pathway

Normal cells conduct a continual audit of their viability by assessing the balance of incoming survival (anti-apoptotic) and death (pro-apoptotic) signals. In normal cells, DNA damage leads to a block in proliferation (cell cycle arrest) while the potential for repair is assessed. If the level of damage exceeds the capacity for repair, the balance of anti- and pro-apoptotic signals tips and the cell undergoes programmed cell death (apoptosis). This prevents maintenance of DNA damage and avoids the risk that mutations will be passed to the progeny of cell division. As such, this mechanism represents a powerful barrier to the development of cancer.

Loss of normal apoptotic pathway signalling is an extremely common event in cancer. Indeed, two of the best known cancer-associated genes (p53 [TSG] and bcl-2 [oncogene]) are intimately involved in apoptosis. The two main mechanisms of apoptotic signalling (intrinsic and extrinsic pathways) are illustrated in a simplified form in Fig. 3. Cancer cells evade apoptosis through an ability to ignore signals sent through the extrinsic pathway or by re-setting the balance of intracellular pro- and anti-apoptotic molecules in favour of inhibition of apoptosis. By circumventing apoptosis, cancer cells can sustain DNA damage without it causing cell death (unless the damage is to a gene that is absolutely necessary for cell survival). Therefore, cancer cells that have switched off their apoptotic pathway are more likely to be intrinsically resistant to anti-cancer treatments. In fact, the use of these treatments may promote the accumulation of other mutations that may have a negative influence on the biology of the disease.

Therefore, targeting the apoptotic machinery represents a potentially attractive new therapeutic option in a range of

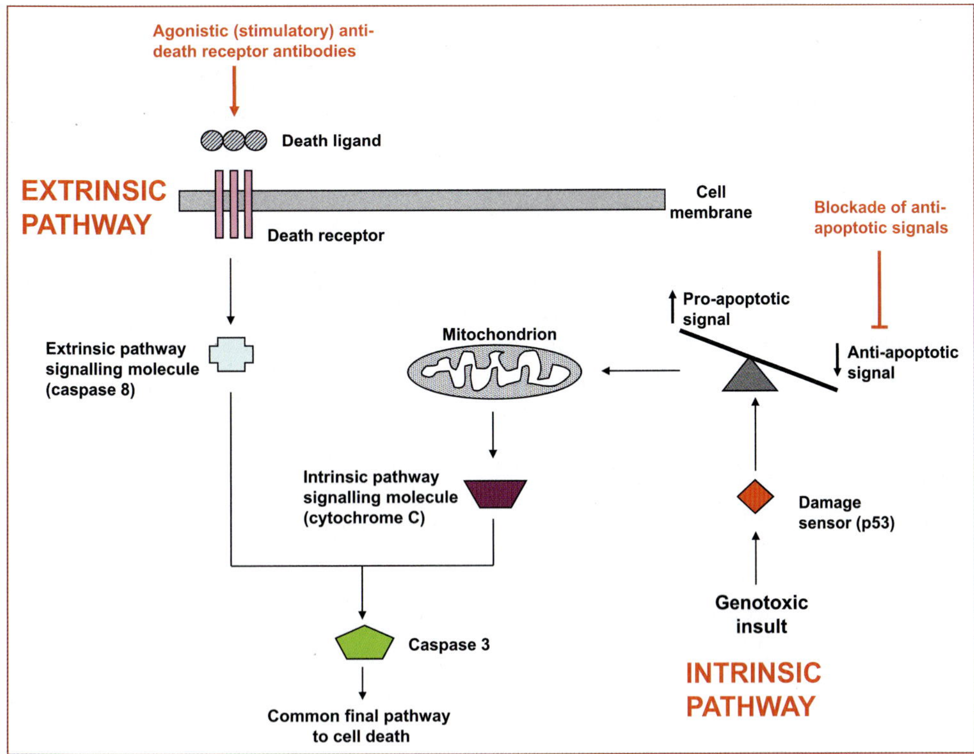

Fig. 3. Normal apoptotic signalling pathways. Cells can undergo programmed cell death in response to activation of either the intrinsic or extrinsic apoptotic pathway. Cancers frequently subvert these pathways to allow them to survive signals that would lead to the death of normal cells. The extrinsic pathway can be activated by agonistic monoclonal antibodies that can stimulate the DR4 and DR5 death receptors. Alternatively, the intrinsic pathway can be activated by inhibiting anti-apoptotic signalling (e.g. blockade of Bcl-2 or XIAP).

cancers, including those of the head and neck. In general terms, two specific strategies are under investigation: (i) Enhancing pro-apoptotic signalling by stimulating the extrinsic pathway, and (ii) blocking the anti-apoptotic regulators of the intrinsic pathway (Fig. 3).

The first of these approaches has been assessed pre-clinically and in early phase clinical trials using both recombinant pro-apoptotic receptor ligands (recombinant human apoptotic ligand 2/tumour necrosis factor-related apoptosis inducing ligand [rhApo2L/TRAIL])[64] and monoclonal antibodies that can stimulate the DR4 and DR5 death receptors.[65] Agonistic humanized or human monoclonal antibodies against DR4 and DR5 have been tested in phase I and II trials in patients with advanced cancer (other than HNC).[65] These trials have shown that these antibodies are well tolerated and are capable of producing prolonged, stable disease. Clinical studies in which TRAIL-receptor antibodies are being investigated in combination treatment regimens in patients with advanced cancer are ongoing. It is anticipated that the results from a broad spectrum of cancer therapy clinical trials will identify the activity and toxicity profiles of TRAIL death-receptor antibodies as single agents, or in combination with chemotherapy agents or radiotherapy. Studies in patients with HNC are ongoing.

The second approach to enhancing apoptosis is targeted blockade of anti-apoptotic signalling pathways. This strategy has largely relied on the approach of using anti-sense oligonucleotides to reduce the expression of proteins, such as Bcl-2. *In vitro* and *in vivo* studies in murine models have suggested that targeted reduction of Bcl-2 expression can enhance the therapeutic efficacy of chemotherapy or radiotherapy in HNC.[66,67] However, this has not yet been tested in patients with HNC in the clinic. In recent years, another means of blocking anti-apoptotic regulators of the intrinsic pathway has received considerable research attention. This approach is based on blocking the actions of inhibitors of apoptosis proteins (IAPs).[68] A prime example of this group of proteins is provided by the X-linked IAP (XIAP), which is a component of the final common pathway that inhibits caspases and suppresses apoptosis. XIAP is over-expressed in many cancer cell lines and cancer tissues, and its expression has been correlated with resistance to chemotherapy and radiotherapy, and to poor clinical outcome. Inhibition of XIAP can be achieved with either antisense oligonucleotides or small molecule inhibitors. *In vitro*, XIAP antagonists produce XIAP knockdown and apoptosis which is associated with sensitization of tumour cells to radiotherapy and cytotoxic drugs.[68] *In vivo*, XIAP antagonists have anti-tumour effects and sensitize tumours to the effects of chemotherapy. This group of agents is currently undergoing phase I evaluation and may have potential in solid cancers, such as those of the head and neck.

Targeting cellular immortalization

Normal somatic cells can only undergo a finite number of cell divisions (Hayflick limit) before they enter a period of permanent growth arrest known as replicative senescence. This process occurs as a result of the cells' inability to replicate the ends of their chromosomes (the telomeres) fully at each division. Therefore, over time the telomeres get progressively shorter, effectively acting as molecular clocks that count down the cells' lifespan. In contrast, stem cells and malignant cells have acquired immortality by maintaining the length of their telomeres. In most tumours, this occurs through upregulation of the enzyme telomerase, but in 10%–15% of cases a different mechanism, called alternative lengthening of the telomeres, is responsible. Telomerase enzymatic activity involves a large number of proteins, but its two main components are an RNA template (hTR) and a reverse transcriptase enzyme (hTERT); the reverse transcriptase uses the hTR RNA template as a guide in the resynthesis of the DNA sequence of the telomere. Therefore, tumours that have reactivated the expression of telomerase are able to re-build the parts of their telomeres that they lose with each round of cell division and are thus able to avoid being sidelined into replicative senescence.

At present, efforts to target the immortalized, stem cell compartment within tumours remains in its infancy. Nonetheless, recognition of the importance of these cells to the overall behaviour of the tumour—in terms of its ability to self-propagate, spread and resist therapeutic intervention—means that active efforts will be made to devise specific targeted therapies against this compartment. Such developments are likely to result in novel approaches to the treatment of a range of tumour types, including those of HNC.

Targeting sustained angiogenesis

In normal tissues, the growth of new blood vessels (angiogenesis) is held very tightly in check by a balance between positive (pro-angiogenic) and negative (anti-angiogenic) signals (Table 1). The growth of cancer deposits is intimately related to their ability to secure a blood supply. A small cluster of cancer cells can grow to 60–100 μm by deriving a supply of oxygen and nutrients by direct diffusion, but beyond this size the fledgling tumour must acquire a dedicated blood supply. Cancers acquire their new blood supply by subverting the balance between pro- and anti-angiogenic factors.[69,70] Essentially, cancers switch to an 'angiogenic phenotype' by upregulating production of pro-angiogenic proteins, such as vascular endothelial growth factor (VEGF), basic fibroblast growth factor and platelet-derived growth factor, and/or by downregulating production of anti-angiogenic proteins, such as thrombospondin-1, angiostatin and endostatin. Cancer-associated endothelial cells have receptors for both growth promoting and inhibitory factors (Fig. 4). Binding

Table 1. Pro- and anti-angiogenic factors

Pro-angiogenic
• Vascular endothelial growth factor (VEGF)
• Basic fibroblast growth factor (bFGF)
• Acidic fibroblast growth factor (aFGF)
• Transforming growth factors alpha and beta (TGF-α, TGF-β)
• Platelet derived growth factor (PDGF)
• Tumour necrosis factor alpha (TNF-α)

Anti-angiogenic
• Angiostatin
• Endostatin
• Thrombospondin-1 and -2 (TSP-1, TSP-2)
• Interleukins (IL-1β, IL-12, IL-18)
• Anti-thrombin III

of cognate ligand to a VEGF receptor on the endothelial cell causes receptor TK activation and downstream signalling to stimulate endothelial cell proliferation, vessel permeability and migration. The net result is formation of new blood vessels. VEGF production in tumour cells is frequently under the control of hypoxia inducible factor-1α, which is a transcription factor that is activated by low cellular oxygen tension.

Drugs that target angiogenesis can be classified into two main groups: (i) Vascular disrupting agents; and (ii) anti-angiogenic agents.[71] Vascular disrupting agents cause rapid and selective dysfunction of existing tumour vasculature leading to tumour death. Tubulin-destabilizing agents, such as combretastatin A4 phosphate and ZD6126, are two such agents.[71–73] The attraction of these agents is their potential ability to deprive large areas of tumour of a blood supply, with resulting widespread tumour cell death. As such, they are likely to lead to tumour regressions. However, their ability to cause vascular shutdown may also theoretically increase the presence of tumour hypoxia—a factor that is known to be correlated with resistance to standard therapeutics. Anti-angiogenic agents work in a completely different fashion by inhibiting new blood vessel formation, without having an effect on established tumour vasculature. This is achieved by either binding VEGF or inhibiting VEGF-R activation.[70] Bevacizumab (AvastinTM) is a humanized monoclonal antibody to the VEGF-R ligand VEGF-A. VEGF-R TKIs also have anti-angiogenic properties through their ability to inhibit phosphorylation of the tyrosine residues in the cytoplasmic domain of the receptor. A number of small molecule TKIs (SU6668, SU5416 [semaxanib], SU11248 [sunitinib], SU11657, PTK787/ZK222584 [vatalanib] and ZD6474) have shown promise in tumour types other than HNC.[70] It is highly likely that these agents will be assessed in HNC in combination with chemotherapy and/or radiotherapy in the near future.

As regards the combination of vascular disrupting or anti-angiogenic agents with standard therapeutic agents (radiotherapy, chemotherapy), there are theoretical

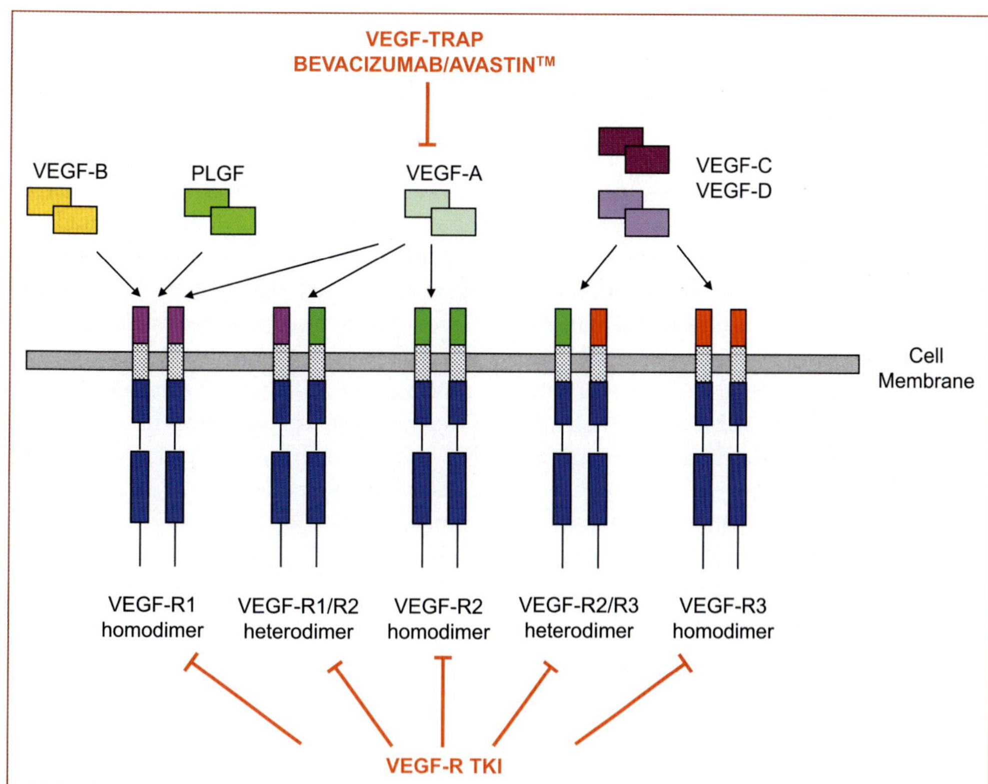

Fig. 4. Vascular endothelial growth factor receptor signalling. VEGF-R can form homo- or heterodimeric complexes that are capable of binding different activating ligands. VEGF-A is the dominant ligand involved in signalling through VEGF-R2 to mediate new blood vessel formation in tumours. Activation of this receptor can be inhibited by binding of the ligand by an anti-VEGF-A antibody (Bevacizumab) or by small molecule VEGF-receptor TK inhibitors (VEGF-R TKI).

considerations that suggest that this approach could be detrimental. For example, depriving a tumour of its blood supply (either acutely by vascular disruption or chronically by reducing angiogenesis) is likely to increase tumour hypoxia. However, for the anti-angiogenic agents, Fukumura and Jain have suggested that treatment can lead to normalization of the tumour vasculature—if the dose and duration of treatment lies within certain parameters.[74,75] The existence of this so-called 'vascular normalization window' is supported by experimental data, but not yet by clinical trial findings. In addition, for the vascular disrupting drugs, it is possible that they can be used to trap radiosensitizing compounds or cytotoxic drugs within tumour tissue by collapsing the vascular networks that will serve to wash the drug out of the tissue. In view of both of these rationalizations, there is enormous interest in combining anti-VEGF monoclonal antibodies, VEGF-R TKIs and vascular disrupting agents with radiation and/or chemotherapy in HNC.

Targeting invasion and metastasis

Distant metastases cause 90% of cancer deaths. Invasion and metastasis involves careful orchestration of a series of complex biological processes: (i) Detachment from immediate neighbours and stroma at the local site; (ii) enzymatic digestion of the extracellular matrix followed by specific directional motility; (iii) penetration (intravasation) of blood or lymphatic vessels and tumour embolization; (iv) survival in the circulation until arrival at the metastatic site that may be chosen on the basis of provision of a favourable supply of appropriate growth factors; (v) adhering to the endothelium of blood vessels at its destination and extravasating from the vessel; and (vi) beginning to proliferate and invade its new location and set about recruiting a new blood supply.

The development of metastatic disease in loco-regional cervical lymph nodes is a hallmark of HNSCC. Such is the predilection of this disease for lymphatic metastasis that patients may present with pathologically involved cervical nodes at any time during the natural history of the disease.[76] The phenomenon of cervical nodal metastasis from an occult primary mucosal site in the head and neck is well recognized.[77] In addition, involved cervical nodes can present synchronously with the primary tumour or metachronously as the first sign of disease relapse. The presence or absence of lymphatic metastasis is the most important prognostic factor for patients with HNSCC.[78] On the basis of this fact, most patients who are diagnosed with HNSCC will have radiological investigations, such as computed tomography (CT) or magnetic resonance imaging (MRI) in an attempt to identify nodal metastases. Even if these tests suggest that the neck is not involved (clinically node negative, or cN0, disease), patients frequently undergo prophylactic treatment of the neck, either by elective neck dissection or radiotherapy, in an attempt to ablate occult micrometastases. Such additional treatment carries a significant morbidity for the patient. For those patients who present with N+ disease, the risk of systemic metastasis is greater; the metastasis increases with increasing N stage and involvement of nodes lower in the neck (e.g. level IV compared with level I). Identification of a panel of biomarkers that could predict the likelihood of nodal metastases would represent a useful tool for patient selection for elective or adjuvant treatment of the neck. Alternatively, novel therapies that could reduce the risk of local or systemic metastasis would represent a significant advance in the treatment of HNC.

Evolving evidence suggests that the patterns of metastasis of different cancers to specific organs (e.g. HNC to cervical lymph nodes; breast cancer to liver, bone and brain; lung cancer to brain and adrenal gland) are not random, but appear to be driven by expression of chemokine receptors by tumour cells that allow them to 'seek' a suitable environment in which to establish a colony. Chemokines are small, secreted proteins with characteristic cysteine motifs in their amino acid sequences.[79] Chemokines interact with their cognate receptors, which are G-protein coupled, seven-transmembrane receptors.[80] Chemokines were initially shown to be involved in controlling the targeted migration of haematopoietic cells, but more recently they have been implicated in a diverse range of physiological and pathological functions, including wound healing, the control of angiogenesis and the development of tumour metastases.[79] Indeed, there has been an evolving interest in the role of chemokines and their receptors in the process of tumour metastasis in recent years. A landmark study clearly demonstrated that breast cancer cells that expressed the chemokine receptors, CXCR4 and CCR7, were capable of preferentially homing to particular tissues.[81]

CCR7 is known to be the functional receptor for SLC (secondary lymphoid organ chemokine). It acts by influencing the migration of activated dendritic cells to regional lymph nodes. In a recent study, a strong association was reported between CCR7 expression and synchronous nodal metastasis in patients with tonsillar cancer.[82] Blockade of CCR7 signalling has been shown to increase the therapeutic efficacy of cisplatin and anti-EGFR therapy in murine models of HNC.[83] Clearly, this is an interesting area for future clinical development, although clinical trials of targeted anti-chemokine therapeutics have not yet been initiated.

Conclusion

Despite significant improvements in treatment outcome in patients with HNSCC, which have resulted from technological advances in radiation delivery and the use of cytotoxic chemotherapy, there is an urgent need for novel therapies. The molecular biology revolution has provided us with a new framework for developing specific targeted therapies. The first major success of this approach was the anti-EGFR monoclonal antibody, cetuximab, which has been shown to increase control rates in newly diagnosed disease (in combination with radiotherapy) and to prolong survival in relapsed disease (in combination with chemotherapy). This agent is likely to be the first of a series of new agents that will target specific molecular defects in HNC. It is likely that the next wave of developments will include active small molecule inhibitors of EGFR (and other members of the c-erbB family of receptors), anti-angiogenic agents and drugs that can increase pro-apoptotic signalling in cancer cells. As with cetuximab, it is most likely that these new agents will first find a niche in the context of combination regimens with standard anti-cancer therapeutics.

References

1. Nutting C. Intensity-modulated radiotherapy (IMRT): The most important advance in radiotherapy since the linear accelerator? *Br J Radiol* 2003;**76**:673.

2. Lee NY, Le QT. New developments in radiation therapy for head and neck cancer: Intensity-modulated radiation therapy and hypoxia targeting. *Semin Oncol* 2008;**35**:236–50.

3. Guerrero UT, Clark CH, Hansen VN, *et al.* A phase I study of dose-escalated chemoradiation with accelerated intensity modulated radiotherapy in locally advanced head and neck cancer. *Radiother Oncol* 2007;**85**:36–41.

4. Bhide S, Clark C, Harrington K, *et al.* Intensity modulated radiotherapy improves target coverage and parotid gland sparing when delivering total mucosal irradiation in patients with squamous cell carcinoma of head and neck of unknown primary site. *Med Dosim* 2007;**32**:188–95.

5. Miles EA, Clark CH, Urbano MT, *et al.* The impact of introducing intensity modulated radiotherapy into routine clinical practice. *Radiother Oncol* 2005;**77**: 241–6.

6. Pignon JP, Bourhis J, Domenge C, *et al.* Chemotherapy added to locoregional treatment for head and neck squamous-cell carcinoma: Three meta-analyses of updated individual data. MACH-NC Collaborative Group. Meta-Analysis of Chemotherapy on Head and Neck Cancer. *Lancet* 2000;**355**:949–55.

7. Bernier J, Domenge C, Ozsahin M, *et al.* European organization for research and treatment of cancer trial 22931. Postoperative irradiation with or without concomitant chemotherapy for locally advanced head and neck cancer. *N Engl J Med* 2004;**350**:1945–52.

8. Cooper JS, Pajak TF, Forastiere AA, *et al.* Radiation therapy oncology group 9501/Intergroup. Postoperative concurrent radiotherapy and chemotherapy for high-risk squamous-cell carcinoma of the head and neck. *N Engl J Med* 2004;**350**:1937–44.

9. Singh B. Molecular pathogenesis of head and neck cancers. *J Surg Oncol* 2008;**97**:634–9.

10. Harrington KJ. Biology of cancer. *Medicine* 2008;**36**:1–5.

11. Hanahan D, Weinberg RA. The hallmarks of cancer. *Cell* 2000;**100**: 57–70.

12. Rogers SJ, Harrington KJ, Rhys-Evans P, *et al.* Biological significance of c-erbB family oncogenes in head and neck cancer. *Cancer Metastasis Rev* 2005;**24**:47–69.

13. Khademi B, Shirazi FM, Vasei M, *et al*. The expression of p53, c-erbB-1 and c-erbB-2 molecules and their correlation with prognostic markers in patients with head and neck tumors. *Cancer Lett* 2002;**184**:223–30.

14. Dassonville O, Formento JL, Francoual M, *et al*. Expression of epidermal growth factor receptor and survival in upper aerodigestive tract cancer. *J Clin Oncol* 1993;**11**: 1873–8.

15. Kusukawa J, Harada H, Shima I, *et al*. The significance of epidermal growth factor receptor and matrix metalloproteinase 3 in squamous cell carcinoma of the oral cavity. *Oral Oncol* 1996;**32**:217–21.

16. O-charoenrat P, Rhys-Evans P, Modjtahedi H, *et al*. The role of cerbB receptors and ligands in head and neck squamous cell carcinoma. *Oral Oncol* 2002;**38**:627–50.

17. Downward J, Yarden Y, Mayes E, *et al*. Close similarity of epidermal growth factor receptor and v-erb-B oncogene protein sequences. *Nature* 1984;**307**:521–7.

18. Grandis JR, Tweardy DJ. Elevated levels of transforming growth factor alpha and epidermal growth factor receptor messenger RNA are early markers of carcinogenesis in head and neck cancer. *Cancer Res* 1993;**53**:3579–84.

19. Shin DM, Ro JY, Hong WK, *et al*. Dysregulation of epidermal growth factor receptor expression in premalignant lesions during head and neck tumorigenesis. *Cancer Res* 1994;**54**:3153–9.

20. Grandis JR, Tweardy DJ, Melhem MF. Asynchronous modulation of transforming growth factor alpha and epidermal growth factor receptor protein expression in progression of premalignant lesions to head and neck squamous cell carcinoma. *Clin Cancer Res* 1998;**4**:13–20.

21. Ibrahim SO, Vasstrand EN, Liavaag PG, *et al*. Expression of c-erbB proto-oncogene family members in squamous cell carcinoma of head and neck. *Anticancer Res* 1997;**17**:4539–46.

22. Werkmeister R, Brandt B, Joos U. Clinical relevance of erbB-1 and –2 oncogenes in oral carcinomas. *Oral Oncol* 2000;**36**:100–105.

23. Wilkman TS, Heitanen JH, Malstrom MJ, *et al*. Immunohistochemical analysis of the oncoprotein c-erbB-2 expression in oral benign and malignant lesions. *Int J Oral Maxillofac Surg* 1998;**27**:209–12.

24. Chen Z, Zhang K, Zhang X, *et al*. Comparison of gene expression between metastatic derivatives and their poorly metastatic parental cells implicates crucial tumor-environment interaction in metastasis of head and neck squamous cell carcinoma. *Clin Exp Metastasis* 2003;**20**:335–42.

25. Sok JC, Coppelli FM, Thomas SM, *et al*. Mutant epidermal growth factor receptor (EGFRvIII) contributes to head and neck cancer growth and resistance to EGFR targeting. *Clin Cancer Res* 2006;**12**:5064–73.

26. Hellyer NJ, Kim MS, Koland JG. Heregulin-dependent activation of phosphoinositide 3-kinase and Akt via the ErbB2/ErbB3 co-receptor. *J Biol Chem* 2001;**276**:42153–61.

27. Hou L, Shi D, Tu SM, *et al*. Oral cancer progression and c-erbB-2/neu proto-oncogene expression. *Cancer Lett* 1992;**65**:215–20.

28. Bei R, Pompa G, Vitolo D, *et al*. Co-localization of multiple ErbB receptors in stratified epithelium of oral squamous cell carcinoma. *J Pathol* 2001;**195**:343–8.

29. Xia W, Lau Y-K, Zhang H-Z, *et al*. Combination of EGFR, HER-2/neu and -3 is a stronger predictor for the outcome of oral squamous cell carcinoma than any individual family members. *Clin Cancer Res* 1999;**5**:4164–74.

30. Barnes CJ, Kumar R. Epidermal growth factor receptor family tyrosine kinases as signal integrators and therapeutic targets. *Cancer Met Rev* 2003;**22**:301–7.

31. Huang SM, Harari PM. Modulation of radiation response after epidermal growth factor receptor blockade in squamous cell carcinomas: Inhibition of damage repair, cell cycle kinetics, and tumor angiogenesis. *Clin Cancer Res* 2000;**6**:2166–74.

32. Harari PM, Huang SM. Head and neck cancer as a clinical model for molecular targeting of therapy: Combining EGFR blockade with radiation. *Int J Radiat Oncol Biol Phys* 2001;**49**:427–33.

33. Herbst RS, Kim ES, Harari PM. IMC-C225, an anti-epidermal growth factor receptor monoclonal antibody, for treatment of head and neck cancer. *Expert Opin Biol Ther* 2001;**1**:719–32.

34. Huang SM, Li J, Harari PM. Molecular inhibition of angiogenesis and metastatic potential in human squamous cell carcinomas after epidermal growth factor receptor blockade. *Mol Cancer Ther* 2002;**1**:507–14.

35. Baselga J, Pfister D, Cooper MR, *et al*. Phase I studies of anti-epidermal growth factor receptor chimeric antibody C225 alone and in combination with cisplatin. J Clin Oncol 2000;**18**:904–14.

36. Shin DM, Donato NJ, Perez-Soler R, *et al*. Epidermal growth factor receptor-targeted therapy with C225 and cisplatin in patients with head and neck cancer. *Clin Cancer Res* 2001;**7**:1204–13.

37. Robert F, Ezekiel MP, Spencer SA, *et al*. Phase I study of anti-epidermal growth factor receptor antibody cetuximab in combination with radiation therapy in patients with advanced head and neck cancer. *J Clin Oncol* 2001;**19**:3234–43.

38. Herbst RS, Arquette M, Shin DM, *et al*. Phase II multicenter study of the epidermal growth factor receptor antibody cetuximab and cisplatin for recurrent and refractory squamous cell carcinoma of the head and neck. *J Clin Oncol* 2005;**23**:5578–87.

39. Baselga J, Trigo JM, Bourhis J, *et al*. Phase II multicenter study of the antiepidermal growth factor receptor monoclonal antibody cetuximab in combination with platinum-based chemotherapy in patients with platinum-refractory metastatic and/or recurrent squamous cell carcinoma of the head and neck. *J Clin Oncol* 2005;**23**:5568–77.

40. Bonner JA, Harari PM, Giralt J, *et al*. Radiotherapy plus cetuximab for squamous-cell carcinoma of the head and neck. *N Engl J Med* 2006;**354**:567–78.

41. Bonner JA, Harari PM, Giralt J, *et al*. Radiotherapy plus cetuximab for locoregionally advanced head and neck cancer: 5 year survival data from a phase 3 randomised trial, and relation between cetuximab-induced rash and survival. *Lancet Oncol* 2010; (in press).

42. Harrington KJ. Rash conclusions from a phase 3 study of cetuximab? *Lancet Oncol* 2010; (in press).

43. Vermorken JB, Mesia R, Rivera F, *et al*. Platinum-based chemotherapy plus cetuximab in head and neck cancer. *N Engl J Med* 2008;**359**:1116–27.

44. Heymach JV, Nilsson M, Blumenschein G, *et al*. Epidermal growth factor receptor inhibitors in development for the treatment of non-small cell lung cancer. *Clin Cancer Res* 2006;**12**:4441s–4445s.

45. Wu M, Rivkin A, Pham T. Panitumumab: Human monoclonal antibody against epidermal growth factor receptors for the treatment of metastatic colorectal cancer. *Clin Ther* 2008;**30**:14–30.

46. Kruser TJ, Armstrong EA, Ghia AJ, *et al*. Augmentation of radiation response by panitumumab in models of upper aerodigestive tract cancer. *Int J Radiat Oncol Biol Phys* 2008;**72**:534–42.

47. Baselga J, Averbuch SD. ZD1839 ('Iressa') as an anticancer agent. *Drugs* 2000;**60** (Suppl 1):33–40

48. Sirotnak FM, Zakowski MF, Miller VA, *et al*. Efficacy of cytotoxic agents against human tumor xenografts is markedly enhanced by coadministration of ZD1839 (Iressa), an inhibitor of EGFR tyrosine kinase. *Clin Cancer Res* 2000;**6**:4885–92.

49. Norman P. ZD-1839 (AstraZeneca). *Curr Opin Investig Drugs* 2001;**2**:428–34.

50. Baselga J, Rischin D, Ranson M, *et al*. Phase I safety, pharmacokinetic, and pharmacodynamic trial of ZD1839, a selective oral epidermal growth factor receptor tyrosine kinase inhibitor, in patients with five selected solid tumor types. *J Clin Oncol* 2002;**20**:4292–302.

51. Ranson M, Hammond LA, Ferry D, *et al.* ZD1839, a selective oral epidermal growth factor receptor-tyrosine kinase inhibitor, is well tolerated and active in patients with solid, malignant tumors: Results of a phase I trial. *J Clin Oncol* 2002;**20**:2240–50.

52. Herbst RS, Maddox AM, Rothenberg ML, *et al.* Selective oral epidermal growth factor receptor tyrosine kinase inhibitor ZD1839 is generally well-tolerated and has activity in non-small-cell lung cancer and other solid tumors: Results of a phase I trial. *J Clin Oncol* 2002;**20**:3815–25.

53. Nakagawa K, Tamura T, Negoro S, *et al.* Phase I pharmacokinetic trial of the selective oral epidermal growth factor receptor tyrosine kinase inhibitor gefitinib ('Iressa', ZD1839) in Japanese patients with solid malignant tumors. *Ann Oncol* 2003;**14**:922–30.

54. LoRusso PM, Herbst RS, Rischin D, *et al.* Improvements in quality of life and disease-related symptoms in phase I trials of the selective oral epidermal growth factor receptor tyrosine kinase inhibitor ZD1839 in non-small cell lung cancer and other solid tumors. *Clin Cancer Res* 2003;**9**:2040–8.

55. Cohen EE, Rosen F, Stadler WM, *et al.* Phase II trial of ZD1839 in recurrent or metastatic squamous cell carcinoma of the head and neck. *J Clin Oncol* 2003;**21**:1980–7.

56. Cohen EE, Kane MA, List MA, *et al.* Phase II trial of gefitinib 250 mg daily in patients with recurrent and/or metastatic squamous cell carcinoma of the head and neck. *Clin Cancer Res* 2005;**11**:8418–24.

57. Kirby AM, A'Hern RP, D'Ambrosio C, *et al.* Gefitinib (ZD1839, Iressa) as palliative treatment in recurrent or metastatic head and neck cancer. *Br J Cancer* 2006;**94**:631–6.

58. Xia W, Mullin RJ, Keith BR, *et al.* Anti-tumor activity of GW572016: A dual tyrosine kinase inhibitor blocks EGF activation of EGFR/erbB2 and downstream Erk1/2 and AKT pathways. *Oncogene* 2002;**21**:6255–63.

59. Burris HA III, Hurwitz HI, Dees EC, *et al.* Phase I safety, pharmacokinetics, and clinical activity study of lapatinib (GW572016), a reversible dual inhibitor of epidermal growth factor receptor tyrosine kinases in heavily pretreated patients with metastatic carcinomas. *J Clin Oncol* 2005;**23**:5305–13.

60. Del Campo JM, Sebastian P, Hitt R, *et al.* Effect of lapatinib on apoptosis and proliferation: Results of a phase II randomised study in patients with locally advanced squamous cell carcinoma of the head and neck (SCCHN). *Ann Oncol* 2008;**19** (supplement 8):viii217 (abstract 688O).

61. Harrington KJ, El-Hariry IA, Holford CS, *et al.* A phase I study to establish the recommended phase II dose of lapatinib in combination with chemoradiation in patients with locally advanced squamous cell carcinoma of the head and neck. *J Clin Oncol* (in press).

62. Mihara M, Shintani S, Kiyota A, *et al.* Cyclin-dependent kinase inhibitor (roscovitine) suppresses growth and induces apoptosis by regulating Bcl-x in head and neck squamous cell carcinoma cells. *Int J Oncol* 2002;**21**:95–101.

63. Benson C, White J, De Bono J, *et al.* A phase I trial of the selective oral cyclin-dependent kinase inhibitor seliciclib (CYC202; R-Roscovitine) administered twice daily for 7 days every 21 days. *Br J Cancer* 2007;**96**:29–37.

64. Ashkenazi A, Holland P, Eckhardt SG. Ligand-based targeting of apoptosis in cancer: The potential of recombinant human apoptosis ligand 2/Tumor necrosis factor-related apoptosis-inducing ligand (rhApo2L/TRAIL). *J Clin Oncol* 2008;**26**:3621–30.

65. Buchsbaum DJ, Forero-Torres A, LoBuglio AF. TRAIL-receptor antibodies as a potential cancer treatment. *Future Oncol* 2007;**3**:405–9.

66. Yip KW, Mocanu JD, Au PY, *et al.* Combination bcl-2 antisense and radiation therapy for nasopharyngeal cancer. *Clin Cancer Res* 2005;**11**:8131–44.

67. Lacy J, Loomis R, Grill S, *et al.* Systemic Bcl-2 antisense oligodeoxynucleotide in combination with cisplatin cures EBV+ nasopharyngeal carcinoma xenografts in SCID mice. *Int J Cancer* 2006;**119**:309–16.

68. Danson S, Dean E, Dive C, *et al.* IAPs as a target for anticancer therapy. *Curr Cancer Drug Targets* 2007;**7**:785–94.

69. Folkman J. Angiogenesis. *Annu Rev Med* 2006;**57**:1–18.

70. Seiwert TY, Cohen EE. Targeting angiogenesis in head and neck cancer. *Semin Oncol* 2008;**35**:274–85.

71. Lippert JW 3rd. Vascular disrupting agents. *Bioorg Med Chem* 2007;**15**:605–15.

72. el-Zayat AA, Degen D, Drabek S, *et al. In vitro* evaluation of the antineoplastic activity of combretastatin A-4, a natural product from Combretum caffrum (arid shrub). *Anticancer Drugs* 1993;**4**:19–25.

73. Chaplin DJ, Pettit GR, Parkins CS, *et al.* Antivascular approaches to solid tumour therapy: Evaluation of tubulin binding agents. *Br J Cancer Suppl* 1996;**27**:S86–8.

74. Jain RK. Normalization of tumor vasculature: An emerging concept in antiangiogenic therapy. *Science* 2005;**307**:58–62.

75. Fukumura D, Jain RK. Tumor microvasculature and microenvironment: Targets for anti-angiogenesis and normalization. *Microvasc Res* 2007;**74**:72–84.

76. Munro AJ, MacDougall RH, Stafford ND. Head and Neck Chapter in Treatment of Cancer. In: Price P, Sikora K.(ed). *Treatment of Cancer.* London, UK: Chapman and Hall Medical; 2002:313–90.

77. De Braud F, al-Sarraf M. Diagnosis and management of squamous cell carcinoma of unknown primary tumor site of the neck. *Semin Oncol* 1993;**20**:273–8.

78. Layland MK, Sessions DG, Lenox J. The influence of lymph node metastasis in the treatment of squamous cell carcinoma of the oral cavity, oropharynx, larynx and hypopharynx: N0 versus N+. *Laryngoscope* 2005;**115**:629–39.

79. Rossi D, Zlotnik A. The biology of chemokines and their receptors. *Ann Rev Immunol* 2000;**18**:217–42.

80. Gerard C, Rollins BJ. Chemokines and disease. *Nat Immunol* 2001;**2**:108–15.

81. Muller A, Homey B, Soto H, *et al.* Involvement of chemokine receptors in breast cancer metastasis. *Nature* 2001;**410**:50–6.

82. Pitkin L, Corbishley C, Dalton P, *et al.* Expression of CC chemokine receptor 7 in tonsillar cancer predicts cervical nodal metastasis, systemic relapse and survival. *Br J Cancer* 2007;**97**:670–77.

83. Wang J, Seethala RR, Zhang Q, *et al.* Autocrine and paracrine chemokine receptor 7 activation in head and neck cancer: Implications for therapy. *J Natl Cancer Inst* 2008;**100**:502–12.

25

Post-treatment surveillance in head and neck cancer

KAPILA MANIKANTAN, RAGHAV C. DWIVEDI, REHAN KAZI

Introduction

The definitive management of patients with head and neck cancer (HNC) involves a period of post-treatment follow up. The main aim of follow up is the early detection of loco-regional recurrence, persistent disease, metastasis, or secondary primary tumours. Early detection may allow definitive treatment with curative intent.[1] In addition, evaluation of disease control, rehabilitation of functional loss, pain management, and assessment of the impact on quality of life (QOL) can be done during follow up. Second primary tumours in the upper aerodigestive tract (UADT) occur at a rate of 10%–20%, or at approximately 5% per year as a result of risk factors related to tobacco use.[2–5] There is no consensus in the literature on the optimum frequency of follow-up visits required after treatment with curative intent.

Head and neck surgeons and oncologists across the globe are using a variety of interventions, such as clinical examinations, blood tests, measurement of serum tumour markers, imaging studies, and endoscopies to follow up patients. These investigations and interventions have to be used in an effective manner for optimal detection of residual disease, recurrences and second primaries at the earliest opportunity so that appropriate treatment can be instituted.[6] The scant data in the literature makes it difficult to compare conclusively the different surveillance schemes, and to suggest whether they should be based on patient survival, QOL or cost-adjusted parameters. The lack of accepted guidelines on follow-up practices for post-treatment HNC patients means that there are significant variations across the globe.

Follow-up visits

A number of recommendations have been documented in the literature for post-treatment follow up of HNC patients. These may be either site-specific or applicable to all sites (generic). The recommendations usually suggest 8–27 clinic visits and around 18 chest radiographs for all sites of head and neck cancer during the first 5 years post-treatment.[7–18] Published site-specific recommendations vary greatly.[6,19–26] Randomized controlled trials comparing a pre-defined follow-up strategy with no definite follow-up strategy are lacking, which makes it difficult to identify a programme that is best suited to, or more efficient in detecting recurrences, or improving the survival time, or, indeed, QOL. Fischer,[25] in his handbook, recommended an average of 23 clinic visits and five chest radiographs for all cancers except those of the lip, nasopharynx and larynx in the 5 years post-treatment. The American Head and Neck Society proposed guidelines for surveillance in HNC in1996, which recommended an average of 28 visits and five chest radiographs in the first 5 years post-treatment.[24] Additional tests varied, according to the site. Practice care guidelines published in the *European Journal of Surgical Oncology* in 2001 for clinicians participating in the management of HNC recommended a 4–6 week follow-up schedule in the first 2 years, 3 monthly follow ups for the third year, 6 monthly follow-ups in years 4 and 5, and finally annual visits thereafter.[27]

Members of the Society of Head and Neck Surgeons and American Society for Head and Neck Surgery conducted a survey to study the effect of Tumour, Node, Metastasis

(TNM) stage on follow-up strategy.[13] The results showed that 70% of the respondents follow the same strategy irrespective of the TNM stage. It was concluded that the cost of detecting a recurrence is high and that few patients benefit from detecting a recurrence.

De Visscher *et al.*[6] concluded that routine follow up or surveillance post-treatment was indispensable and the site and stage of the tumour determined the length of follow up rather than the differentiation grade of the tumour or type of initial treatment. A prospective study by Boysen *et al.*[7] showed that follow up is not indicated 3 years after completion of treatment, and should only be routine for patients who still have a treatment option left. They estimated that about one-third of the follow-up consultations could be dropped without sacrificing the number of early recurrences that are detected. For detecting second primary tumours of the respiratory and UADT, follow up after the third year should be for long periods, or even lifelong. The main implications from this study are that patients for whom a salvage treatment option exists should have a strict follow-up regimen for the first 3 years, and that in patients who have been treated by combined modality therapy, the focus should be on providing care and support rather than on detecting recurrence.

Schwartz *et al.*[28] conducted a retrospective study on 115 patients who had received primary or postoperative radiotherapy and who were followed up at the discretion of the providers. It was reported that 86% of failures were symptomatic and were detected by patient-related complaints and only 14% of recurrences were detected on routine follow up. Of the recurrences, 90% occurred within the first year of follow up. All patients who developed recurrence had a poor overall survival, irrespective of the mechanism of its detection. The follow-up intensity was between 5–6 visits per year. Intensive follow up was associated with higher TNM staging and high-risk pathological features. The authors concluded that there was an inconsistent follow-up strategy among centres worldwide, divergent secondary costs, recurrence was better detected by symptoms rather than routine testing, and that post-recurrence survival rates were poor.[28]

A study by Cooney *et al.*[29] to evaluate the efficacy of routine follow up in conferring an advantage in long-term survival of patients receiving combined modality treatment for advanced HNC showed that routine follow up was important for emotional support and evaluation of treatment results, rather than for improving patient survival. Patients included in the study had stages III and IV cancers of the oral cavity, oropharynx and larynx, which were treated with curative intent by surgery and radiotherapy. The follow-up regimen used was history taking and examination at monthly intervals for 3 months initially, then every 2–3 months for 2 years, and finally every 4–6 months for 5 years. A chest X-ray was performed annually and other investigations were done as per indication. Of the 302 patients included in the study,

52% were disease-free at 5 years. Relapses occurred in 119 patients, with 50% of these being detected within 1 year, and 89% being detected within 3 years. Of the 49 patients in whom salvage treatment was attempted with varying combinations of surgery, radiotherapy and chemotherapy, only 2 survived to 5 years after relapse, and both patients had been symptomatic at the time of detection of the relapse.

Studies on patient awareness of recurrent disease have quoted a wide range from 22% to 86%.[6,28] Schwartz *et al.* quoted a salvage cure rate in recurrent squamous cell carcinoma of the oral cavity of around 21%, and found that patients who were most likely to benefit were those in whom the primary disease was stage I or II; recurrence occurred after 6 months and was amenable to surgical excision.[28] In a series of 100 patients with recurrent HNC, Pearlmann found 30% amenable to further surgery and 45%, who were initially node negative, were amenable to neck surgery.[30]

Imaging studies

Imaging is crucial for the detection of recurrences, especially for patients in whom only the primary tumour has been treated, or in whom the neck has been treated just by radiotherapy, chemoradiation, or limited surgery. Computed tomography (CT), magnetic resonance imaging (MRI) and ultrasound (US) have poor specificity in differentiating postoperative oedema from recurrence.[31,32] Various authors have shown the efficacy of US and US-guided fine needle aspiration cytology (US-FNAC) in the follow up of the treated neck; Westhofen reported that US-FNAC is superior to CT in detecting recurrences.[33]

Chest radiography is done as part of a routine follow up of HNC to detect lung metastasis and second primaries in the lung. However, in the study by O'Meara *et al.* it was seen that <5% of the patients with abnormal chest X-rays had second primary tumours and that the abnormality was due to metastasis.[34]

De Visscher *et al.* concluded that routine chest radiography is of value only in patients with index tumours of the larynx.[6] Engelen *et al.* retrospectively studied the incidence and prognosis of lung malignancies in 556 laryngeal cancer patients by yearly chest radiography.[22] Supraglottic cancer showed a higher incidence of second primaries and metastatic tumours in comparison to glottic cancers. Routine chest radiography detected lung malignancies in 68% of patients without symptoms, and this gave a significantly higher survival benefit compared with symptomatic patients of 10 and 4 months, respectively. However, *in lieu* of the lead time bias the authors concluded that the observed survival benefit of yearly chest radiography was nil.[22] O'Meara *et al.* concluded from their study that chest radiography, as part of a routine follow up, was not imperative unless the patients' clinical situation required aggressive treatment of lung disease.[34] In a retrospective study of 26 patients undergoing treatment for

HNC who were screened by both chest radiography and chest CT, 4 patients were seen to have a normal chest radiograph but abnormal chest CT. The authors concluded that chest CT should be used instead of chest radiograph as a screening tool in patients of advanced head and neck squamous cell carcinoma.[35] Hsu *et al.* studied 192 patients with head and neck squamous cell carcinoma to determine the role of chest CT.[36] They found that the rate of abnormal scans was significantly higher in patients on follow up (44.2%) than in new cases (14.2%). The authors concluded that chest CT was necessary for the follow-up of high-risk patients. A study of 168 scans performed on 93 patients to establish the number of malignancies detected by chest CT in HNC patients showed that CT detected malignancy in 9 of 57 patients during diagnosis of neck disease, 9 of 43 during follow up, and 6 of 18 patients with local or loco-regional recurrence.[37]

A prospective study on 127 patients who had undergone treatment for HNC evaluated the efficacy of sonography and palpation in follow-up.[38] The authors concluded that ultrasound was well suited to detect enlarged lymph nodes, with an accuracy of 97.5%. In another prospective randomized study conducted on 43 patients treated for HNC, the mean follow-up period was 28 months. In addition to clinical and colour-duplex echography (CDS) examinations, CT and positron emission tomography (PET) were performed.[39] The sensitivity and specificity of CDS in detecting recurrences was 80% and 78.6%, respectively. The authors concluded that CDS could contribute to the successful treatment of recurrences in HNC.

Information obtained from cross-sectional imaging is important in the post-treatment follow up of HNC. Residual and recurrent tumours are difficult to detect in the post-irradiation neck because of oedema and fibrosis.[31] Accurate interpretation of CT images is necessary to differentiate between post-irradiation and residual or recurrent disease. A baseline CT or MRI done 3–6 months after treatment of high-risk HNC by surgery, radiation, or combined treatment can be compared with subsequent images for earlier detection of abnormalities.[28,40] A study using post-irradiation CT scans performed 6 months after radiotherapy in patients with laryngeal cancer found that those with a focal laryngeal mass of ≤1 cm or a tumour volume reduction of < 50% have a high chance of recurrence.[32] Hermans *et al.* studied 66 patients who underwent radiotherapy for laryngeal cancer who were followed up with CT scans 1–6 months after therapy.[40] The scans were done as part of a routine follow up, or in patients with symptoms suggestive of local failure. Whereas 56% patients were seen to be free of disease, 44% developed a local failure. In 12 of the 29 patients with local failure, CT findings were apparent before clinical examination and were confirmed on biopsy or after total laryngectomy. In the study, the sensitivity was 83%, specificity 95%, accuracy 89%, negative predictive value 88% and positive predictive value 92%. The authors concluded that close clinical and imaging follow up

was necessary to detect progressive soft tissue changes, and recommended an interval of 3–4 months between studies, for a duration of 2 years after radiation therapy. Misiti *et al.* studied 72 laryngeal cancer cases treated by surgery and followed up by CT. It was confirmed that CT scan was essential to assess correctly the extent of relapse and recurrence.[41] The criteria for a recurrent tumour on MRI is an enlarging, enhancing and infiltrating mass that is of intermediate to high signal intensity on T_2-weighted imaging. The ability of MRI to detect recurrence is dependent on the individual interpreting the study. MRI is preferred in patients with sino-nasal, skull base, and nasopharyngeal tumours, and in whom there is evidence of early perineural or intracranial spread.

Tissues can exhibit changes in physiological and metabolic functions before any structural changes are visible. Hence, anatomical imaging techniques can struggle to identify residual tumour cells, particularly when the tumour cells are replaced by fibroblasts without significant changes in the tumour volume.[42] PET with the glucose analogue18 F-fluoro-deoxyglucose (FDG), adapted for clinical use in the late 1980s, has found widespread acceptance in the initial staging, restaging and detection of second primary tumours in head and neck squamous cell cancer. However, PET has been shown to produce a high ratio of false-positive results in patients with suspected recurrent HNC.

The introduction of FDG-PET in combination with CT, known as PET-CT, helps in accurate anatomical localization of the functional information given by the FDG-PET scans and, to some extent, may reduce the false-positive results of stand-alone PET.[43] PET-CT is a whole body study from the vertex to the mid-thighs and this may help in detecting distant lesions that are not normally detectable by the traditional imaging techniques of chest radiography and chest CT. PET-CT is reported to have a sensitivity of 92% for the detection of recurrent cancer of the larynx.[44] The accuracy of diagnosis of PET-CT for distant metastasis in patients with laryngeal cancer is in the region of 100%, probably due to the absence of treatment-related changes in the region outside the neck.[44] Ong *et al.* studied 65 patients undergoing chemo-radiotherapy for HNC by FDG-PET-CT scan done no later than 6 months post-therapy, and showed it had a negative predictive value (NPV) of 98% for excluding viable cancer in neck nodes.[45] The combination of PET with CT reduced the false-positive rates by >50% compared with CT alone. The authors felt that planned neck dissection could be withheld in the event of negative PET and no residual lymphadenopathy in CT. They also found that in the event of lymphadenopathy of >1 cm and normal PET findings, the NPV remained high at >90%, but nonetheless felt that large prospective studies were required before the debate on planned neck dissections in such a scenario could be put to rest. In a meta-analysis to study the effectiveness of PET scan in detecting recurrence or relapse after HNC treatment by radiotherapy and chemoradiotherapy,[46] it was seen that in the 27 studies included, the pooled sensitivity and specificity were 94% (95% confidence interval [CI] 87%–97%) and 82% (95% CI 76%–86%), respectively. The positive predictive value was 75% (95% CI 68%–82%), negative predictive value 95% (95% CI 92%–97%), and the sensitivity was greater for scans performed after 10 weeks of treatment. Abgral *et al.* prospectively studied the role of hybrid FDG-PET-CT in detecting subclinical loco-regional recurrence of head and neck squamous cell carcinoma and distant metastasis in 91 patients without evidence of recurrence[47] on the basis of 12 months of conventional follow up. The gold standard was 6 months of imaging or histopathology. The examination had negative results in 52 patients and positive results in 39 patients. Of the 39 patient with positive scans, 9 had false-positive results and 30 had proven recurrence. In this study the sensitivity of FDG-PET-CT was 100%, specificity 85%, positive predictive value was 77% and NPV was 100%, with an overall accuracy of 90%. The authors concluded that FDG-PET-CT was more accurate than conventional follow-up alone for assessment of recurrent HNC and recommended that it be done after 12 months of follow up.

Endoscopy

Pan-endoscopy is usually included as part of an initial work-up of HNC patients to rule out second primary tumours, although a majority of these occur more than 6 months after treatment, i.e. metachronously. In a meta-analysis of second primary tumours of the head and neck, it was found that overall prevalence of second primary tumours was 14.2% in 40,287 patients.[48] A significantly higher detection rate was seen for prospective pan-endoscopy studies. The authors recommended routine endoscopic evaluation within 2 years of completion of treatment and clinical surveillance beyond 5 years to detect second primary tumours. Pan-endoscopy is unpleasant and a significant cost burden on both the healthcare system and the patient. Rachamat *et al.* studied 170 patients with laryngeal cancer who were followed up by twice yearly bronchoscopy with sputum cytology.[49] Five second primary tumours and six metastases in the lung were detected. The patients found the procedure to be unpleasant, an emotional burden and time consuming. The authors concluded that the procedure was not useful or justifiable. Chao *et al.* prospectively studied 57 patients treated for nasopharyngeal cancer by irradiation to evaluate the efficacy of different modalities in detecting disease in the early post-treatment period.[50] The patients were studied by CT scan, post-nasal space (PNS) biopsy and an endoscopic examination 4 months after treatment. PNS biopsy is taken as the gold standard for disease detection in nasopharyngeal carcinoma. Endoscopic studies revealed a sensitivity of 75%, specificity of 94.3%, positive predictive value of 50% and negative predictive value of 98%. For CT scan studies, the sensitivity

was 50%, specificity 49.1%, positive predictive value of 6.9% and negative predictive value of 92.9%. The authors felt that routine PNS biopsies were not necessary in the presence of normal endoscopic findings. Guardiola *et al.* studied 487 HNC patients by triple endoscopy during the initial work-up of the primary cancer.[51] It was seen that a synchronous tumour was detected in the lung in 1% of patients and in the oesophagus in 2% of patients. Oesophageal carcinoma was detected in 1.3% of patients with oropharyngeal tumours, in 2% of patients with a laryngeal tumour, and in 9.2% of patients with a hypopharyngeal tumour. The reported incidence of a second primary in the oesophagus after treatment of the primary in the head and neck is around 0%–3.2% over a follow-up period of 2–10 years. All the authors of the studies cited were of the opinion that a systematic search for a second primary during routine surveillance is not warranted.

Tumour markers

Various tumour markers have been studied for their role in the diagnosis, prognosis and treatment monitoring in HNC. These markers, however, lack sensitivity for use in HNC. Söderholm *et al.* studied 63 patients with oral cancer monitored by liver function tests, tumour markers and radiological examination.[20] It was seen that carcino-embryonic antigen (CEA) was not sensitive enough as a marker and radiological examination did not detect any recurrences or metastasis. The authors concluded that the cost–benefit of these examinations was low.

Thyroid function tests

External beam irradiation is an integral part of HNC treatment, and part or whole of the thyroid gland is often included in the target volume of tissue that is irradiated. The reported incidence of hypothyroidism after radiation to the thyroid gland is between 3% and 44%.[52] Most patients with hypothyroidism are asymptomatic at follow up. With this incidence of hypothyroidism in all patients receiving irradiation for the head and neck it seems necessary that these patients undergo regular follow up with thyroid function tests.[34] In a study of 378 patients receiving radiotherapy for HNC, it was seen that hypothyroidism affected only patients treated by surgery and radiotherapy.[53] The authors concluded that thyroid function tests should be done in these patients prior to and 3–6 months after completion of therapy. Garcia-Serra *et al.* retrospectively studied 504 patients with HNC in whom the radiation fields included the thyroid gland.[54] Hypothyroidism was defined as thyroid stimulating hormone (TSH) ≥4.5 mIU/L. Of the 504 subjects, 206 had post-treatment documented TSH values, and the actuarial freedom from hypothyroidism was 58% at 5 years and 26% at 10 years. Not surprisingly, patients who had undergone surgery involving partial removal of the thyroid

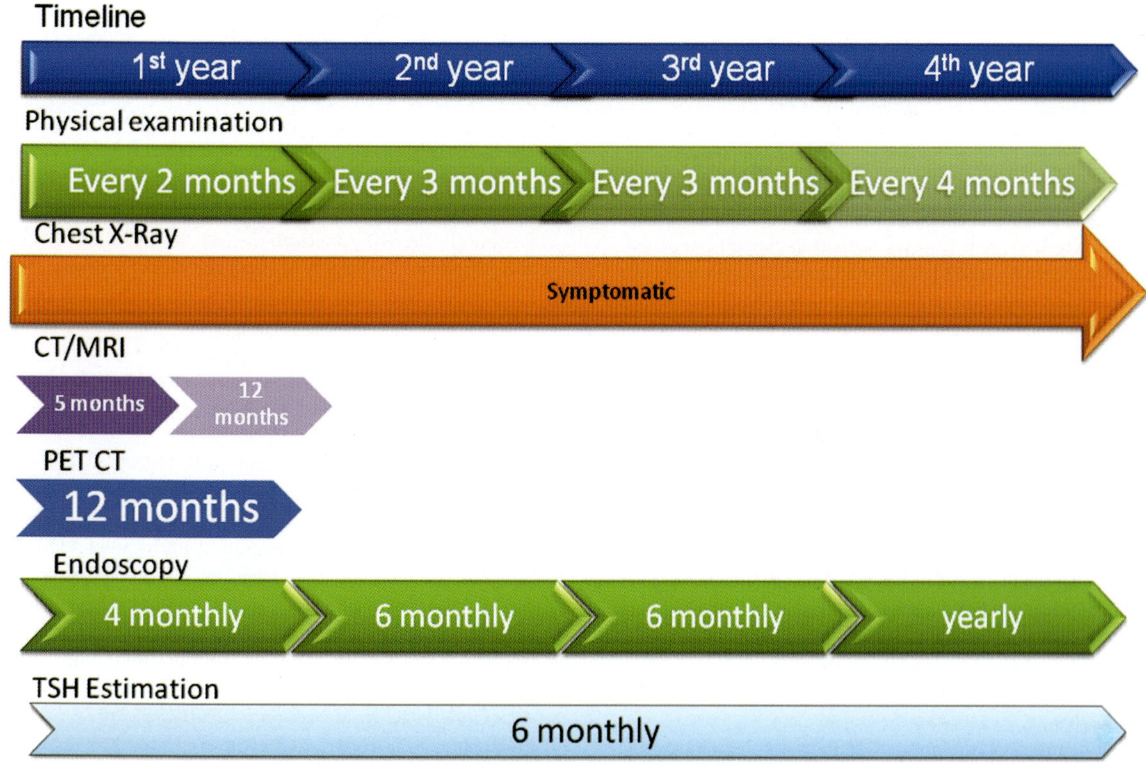

- Chest X –ray can be done in symptomatic patients
- USG-FNAC in patients who were N0 on primary diagnosis
- Serum investigations other than TSH is to be done in patients who are symptomatic
- Chest CT can be done instead of chest-x ray in patients who can be actively treated if chest metastases is found
- If CT/MRI is inconclusive at 6 months PET or PET/CT can be done
- Further follow-up with imaging studies can be done as per the merits of the case

Fig. 1. Time-tagged visual flow chart for surveillance in the post-treatment period of head and neck cancer patients

gland had a higher chance of developing hypothyroidism. The authors concluded that serum TSH should be checked 6 monthly for the first 5 years and yearly thereafter in patients receiving radiotherapy to the low-neck region. They also felt that thyroid hormone replacement therapy should be initiated if the TSH value was >4.5 mIU/L.

Cost–benefit analysis

Most analyses of follow-up strategies lack precise information on cost or charge data. The cost of the follow up is often very difficult to calculate accurately as any true estimate would have to include the cost of each visit to the medical practitioner, the cost of travel, the cost of routine and other investigations ordered as a result of follow up, the cost of treatment (including complications) if recurrent disease was found, and the cost borne by the community resulting from loss of productivity of the patient. In a study analysing 31 different strategies for follow up, the cost of each strategy was analysed for one patient for 5 years and compared.[55] Of the

strategies, the one by Jones[12] was seen to be the most intense, with 27 office visits, 8 complete blood counts (CBCs), 8 liver function tests, 8 serum electrolyte level measurements and 8 chest radiographs. On the other hand, the strategy by Byers[17] was the least intense, with 8 office visits, 6 CBCs and 6 chest radiographs. No data were available to demonstrate greater efficiency for higher cost strategies. There was a 9- to 12-fold difference between the least and most expensive strategy. The authors recommended a minimalist approach towards follow up. They, however, also pointed out that their analysis was not performed on actual patients and was done prospectively.

Randomized controlled trials on the benefit of routine surveillance in HNC are singularly lacking. All recommendations are from retrospective data. From the observation that recurrences found by routine follow up resulted in better post-recurrence survival compared with disease found by symptoms, De Visscher and Manni concluded that routine follow up is indispensable.[6] Time-tagged visual flow-chart for surveillance in post-treatment head and neck cancer patients.(Fig. 1)

References

1. Ridge JA. Squamous cancer of the head and neck: Surgical treatment of local and regional recurrence. *Semin Oncol* 1993;**20**:419–29.

2. Schwartz L, Ozsahin M, Zhang G, *et al.* Synchronous and metachronous head and neck carcinomas. *Cancer* 1994;**74**:1933–8.

3. Sturgis E, Miller R. Second primary malignancies in the head and neck cancer patient. *Ann Otol Rhinol Laryngol* 1995;**104**:946–54.

4. Vikram B, Strong EW, Shah JP, *et al.* Second malignant neoplasms in patients successfully treated with multimodality treatment for advanced head and neck cancer. *Head Neck Surg* 1984;**6**:734–7.

5. Tepperman BS, Fitzpatrick PJ. Second respiratory and upper digestive tract cancer after oral cancer. *Lancet* 1981;**62**:547–9.

6. DeVisscher AVM, Manni JJ. Routine long-term follow-up in patients treated with curative intent for squamous cell carcinoma of the larynx, pharynx, and oral cavity. *Arch Otolaryngol Head Neck Surg* 1994;**120**:934–9.

7. Boysen M, Lövdal O, Tausjö J, *et al.* The value of follow-up in patients treated for squamous cell carcinoma of the head and neck. *Eur J Cancer* 1992;**28**:426–30.

8. Schantz SP, Andersen PE. Head and neck carcinoma. In: Johnson FE, Virgo KS (eds). *Cancer patient follow-up.* St Louis, Mo: Mosby–Year Book; 1997:57–64.

9. Boysen M. Value of follow-up in patients treated for squamous cell carcinomas of the oral cavity and oropharynx. *Recent Results Cancer Res* 1994;**134**:205–14.

10. Loree TR. Head and neck carcinoma: Counterpoint. In: Johnson FE, Virgo KS (eds). *Cancer Patient Follow-up.* St Louis, Mo: Mosby–Year Book; 1997:72.13.

11. Weymuller EA Jr. Head and neck carcinoma: Counterpoint. In: Johnson FE, Virgo KS (eds). *Cancer Patient Follow-up.* St Louis, Mo: Mosby–Year Book; 1997:72–5.

12. Jones AS. Head and neck carcinoma: Counterpoint. In: Johnson FE, Virgo KS (eds). *Cancer Patient Follow-up.* St Louis, Mo: Mosby–Year Book; 1997:65–71.

13. Johnson FE, Johnson MH, Virgo KS. Current follow-up strategies after potentially curative resection of upper aerodigestive tract epidermoid carcinoma: Results of a survey of members of the Society of Head and Neck Surgeons. *Int J Oncol* 1997;**10**:927–31.

14. Marchant FE, Lowry LD, Moffitt JJ, *et al.* Current national trends in the post-treatment follow-up of patients with squamous cell carcinoma of the head and neck. *Am J Otolaryngol* 1993;**14**:88–93.

15. Boysen M, Natvig K, Winther FÖ, *et al.* Value of routine follow-up in patients treated for squamous cell carcinoma of the head and neck. *J Otolaryngol* 1985;**14**:211–14.

16. Austin JR. Carcinoma of the head and neck. In: Berger DH, Feig BW, Fuhrman GM (eds). *The M.D. Anderson surgical oncology handbook.* Boston, Mass: Little Brown; 1995.

17. Byers RM. Head and neck cancer. In: Eiseman B, Robinson WA, Steele G Jr (eds). *Follow-up of the cancer patient.* New York, NY: Thieme-Stratton; 1982:36–40.

18. Coniglio JU, Netterville JL. Guidelines for patient management. In: Bailey BJ, Johnson JT, Pillsbury HC, *et al.* (eds). *Head and neck surgery otolaryngology.* Philadelphia, Pa: JB Lippincott; 1993:1021–8.

19. Nakashima T. Head and neck carcinoma: Counterpoint. In: Johnson FE, Virgo KS (eds). *Cancer patient follow-up.* St Louis, Mo: Mosby–Year Book; 1997:64–5.

20. Söderholm AL, Lindqvist C, Haglund C. Tumour markers and radiological examinations in the follow-up of patients with oral cancer. *J Craniomaxillofac Surg* 1992;**20**:211–15.

21. Lara PC, Cuyás JM. The role of squamous cell carcinoma antigen in the management of laryngeal and hypopharyngeal cancer. *Cancer* 1995;**76**:758–64.

22. Engelen AM, Stalpers LJ, Manni JJ, *et al.* Yearly chest radiography in the early detection of lung cancer following laryngeal cancer. *Eur Arch Otorhinolaryngol* 1992;**249**:364–9.

23. Stalpers LJ, van Vierzen PB, Brouns JJ, *et al.* The role of yearly chest radiography in the early detection of lung cancer following oral cancer. *Int J Oral Maxillofac Surg* 1989;**18**:99–103.

24. Clinical Practice Guidelines Task Force. Clinical practice guidelines for the diagnosis and management of cancer of the head and neck. Pittsburgh, Pa: The American Society for Head and Neck Surgery, and Arlington, Va: Society of Head and Neck Surgeons; 1996.

25. Fischer DS. Head and neck cancers. In: Fischer DS (ed). *Follow-up of cancer: A handbook for physicians.* 4th ed. Philadelphia, Pa: Lippincott Williams & Wilkins; 1995:8–25.

26. Yuen AP, Wei WI, Wong SH, *et al.* Comprehensive analysis of nodal recurrence of advanced laryngeal carcinoma following surgery. *Eur J Surg Oncol* 1996;**22**:350–3.

27. British Association of Head and Neck Oncologists. Practice care guidance for clinicians participating in the management of head and neck cancer patients in the UK. Drawn up by a Consensus Group of Practising Clinicians. *Eur J Surg Oncol* 2001;(Suppl A):S1–S17.

28. Schwartz DL, Barker J Jr, Chansky K, *et al.* Post-radiotherapy surveillance practice for head and neck squamous cell carcinoma – too much or too little? *Head Neck* 2003;**25**:990–9.

29. Cooney TR, Poulsen MG. Is routine follow-up useful after combined-modality therapy for advanced head and neck cancer? *Arch Otolaryngol Head Neck Surg* 1999;**125**:379–82.

30. Pearlmann NW. Treatment outcome in recurrent head and neck cancer. *Arch Surg* 1979;**114**:39–42.

31. Mukherji SK, Mancuso AA, Kotzur IM, *et al.* Radiologic appearance of the irradiated larynx. Part II. Primary site response. *Radiology* 1994;**193**:149–54.

32. Pameijer FA, Hermans R, Mancuso AA, *et al.* Pre- and post-radiotherapy computed tomography in laryngeal cancer: Imaging-based prediction of local failure. *Int J Radiat Oncol Biol Phys* 1999;**45**:359–66.

33. Westhofen M. Ultrasound B-scans in the follow-up of head and neck tumors. *Head Neck Surg* 1987;**9**:272–8.

34. O'Meara WP, Thiringer JK, Johnstone PA. Follow-up of head and neck cancer patients post-radiotherapy. *Radiother Oncol* 2003;**66**:323–6.

35. Warner GC, Cox GJ. Evaluation of chest radiography versus chest computed tomography in screening for pulmonary malignancy in advanced head and neck cancer. *J Otolaryngol* 2003;**32**:107–9.

36. Hsu YB, Chu PY, Liu JC, *et al.* Role of chest computed tomography in head and neck cancer. *Arch Otolaryngol Head Neck Surg* 2008;**134**:1050–4.

37. Mercader VP, Gatenby RA, Mohr RM, *et al.* CT surveillance of the thorax in patients with squamous cell carcinoma of the head and neck: A preliminary experience. *J Comput Assist Tomogr* 1997;**21**:412–17.

38. Steinkamp HJ, Knöbber D, Schedel H, *et al.* Palpation and sonography in after-care of head-neck tumor patients: Comparison of ultrasound tumor entity parameters. *Laryngorhinootologie* 1993;**72**:431–8.

39. Di Martino E, Hausmann R, Krombach GA, *et al.* Relevance of colour-duplex echography for detection and therapy of recurrences in the follow-up of head and neck cancer. *Laryngorhinootologie* 2002;**81**:866–74.

40. Hermans R, Pameijer FA, Mancuso AA, *et al.* Laryngeal or hypopharyngeal squamous cell carcinoma: Can follow-up CT after definitive radiotherapy be used to detect local failure earlier than clinical examination alone? *Radiology* 2000;**214**:683–7.

41. Misiti A, Macori F, Caimi M, *et al.* Computerized tomography in the evaluation of the larynx after surgical treatment and irradiation. *Radiol Med* 1997;**94**:600–6.

42. Kostakoglu L, Goldsmith SJ. PET in the assessment of therapy

response in patients with carcinoma of the head and neck and of the esophagus. *J Nucl Med* 2004;**45**:56–68.

43. Schoder H, Yeung HWD, Gonen M, *et al.* Head and neck cancer: Clinical usefulness and accuracy of PET/CT image fusion. *Radiology* 2004;**231**:65–72.

44. Gordin A, Daitzchman M, Doweck I, *et al.* Fluorodeoxyglucose-positron emission tomography/computed tomography imaging in patients with carcinoma of the larynx: Diagnostic accuracy and impact on clinical management. *Laryngoscope* 2006;**116**:273–8.

45. Ong SC, Schöder H, Lee NY, *et al.* Clinical utility of 18F-FDG PET/CT in assessing the neck after concurrent chemoradiotherapy for loco-regional advanced head and neck cancer. *J Nucl Med* 2008;**49**:532–40.

46. Isles MG, McConkey C, Mehanna HM. A systematic review and meta-analysis of the role of positron emission tomography in the follow-up of head and neck squamous cell carcinoma following radiotherapy or chemoradiotherapy. *Clin Otolaryngol* 2008;**33**:210–22.

47. Abgral R, Querellou S, Potard G, *et al.* Does 18F-FDG PET/CT improve the detection of post-treatment recurrence of head and neck squamous cell carcinoma in patients negative for disease on clinical follow-up? *J Nucl Med* 2009;**50**:24–9.

48. Haughey BH, Gates GA, Arfken CL, *et al.* Meta-analysis of second malignant tumors in head and neck cancer: The case for an endoscopic screening protocol. *Ann Otol Rhinol Laryngol* 1992;**101**:105–12.

49. Rachmat L, Vreeburg GC, de Vries N, *et al.* The value of twice yearly bronchoscopy in the work-up and follow-up of patients with laryngeal cancer. *Eur J Cancer* 1993;**29A**:1096–9.

50. Chao SS, Loh KS, Tan LKS. Modalities of surveillance in treated nasopharyngeal cancer. *Otolaryngol Head Neck Surg* 2003;**129**:61–4.

51. Guardiola E, Pivot X, Dassonville O, *et al.* Is routine triple endoscopy for head and neck carcinoma patients necessary in light of a negative chest computed tomography scan? *Cancer* 2004;**101**:2028–33.

52. Zohar Y, Tovim RB, Laurian N, *et al.* Thyroid function following radiation and surgical therapy in head and neck malignancy. *Head Neck* 1984;**6**:948–52.

53. Cetinayak O, Akman F, Kentli S, *et al.* Assessment of treatment-related thyroid dysfunction in patients with head and neck cancer. *Tumori* 2008;**94**:19–23.

54. Garcia-Serra A, Amdur RJ, Morris CG, *et al.* Thyroid function should be monitored following radiotherapy to the low neck. *Am J Clin Oncol* 2005;**28**:255–8.

55. Virgo KS, Paniello RC, Johnson FE. Costs of post-treatment surveillance for patients with upper aerodigestive tract cancer. *Arch Otolaryngol Head Neck Surg* 1998;**124**:564–72.

Index*

American Joint Committee on Cancer (AJCC)   24, 105–8, 145, 157, 168, 189, 253–4

Basal cell carcinoma (BCC) of the head and neck   215–16
  cicatricial (morphoeic) type   215
  clinical presentation   215–16
  cystic type   215
  histology   216
  management   216
  nodulo ulcerative type   215
  pigmented type   216
  superficial (multicentric) type   215
Biofilms on voice prostheses   240; *see also* Voice restoration
Bone tumours of the jaws and skull   40–2

Caldwell–Luc approach   156
Ceruminoma of the head and neck   218
Cervical lymphatics   94, 95t
Cervical metastases
  en bloc/radical neck dissection   93
  management of the N0 neck   96–8
  neck dissection
    factors affecting choice of   95
    modified (MND)   93–5
    morbidity   95
    radical (RND)   94
    selective (SND)   94, 97, 97t
  surgical treatment   93
Chemoradiation/chemotherapy, postoperative   69–70, 70t
  criteria for selecting patients   70t
  palliative   70–71
  role in HNC   67, 67t
  and radiation interaction   67–8
  and radiotherapy   68–9, 69t
Craniofacial resection, nose and paranasal sinuses   162–3

Dysphagia following laryngeal surgery   228
Dysphagia following surgery for HNC   226; *see also* Swallowing rehabilitation

Ear
  cylindroma   43
  embryonal rhabdomyosarcoma   43
  external, tumour of the   218–19
  extostosis   43
  middle, tumour of the   219
  tumours of the angiolymphoid hyperplasia with eosinophilia   43
  tumours of the   42, 217–23
  WHO classification, tumours of the   217–18
Ear and temporal bone
  lateral temporal bone resection   222
  prognosis and outcomes following treatment   223–4
  radiotherapy   223
  reconstruction   223
  rehabilitation   24
  sleeve resection of tumours   222
  spread and natural history of tumours   220–1
  staging   221
  subtotal temporal bone resection   222
  total temporal bone resection   223
  treatment   221–2
Electrolarynx   240–1
  intraoral placement devices   241
  neck placement devices   241
Endoscopic laser surgery of the larynx   228

Flap   *see also* Skin Flap
  deltopectoral   76–8
  forehead   75–6
  latissimus dorsi   81
  myocutaneous   78–81
  nasolabial   74–5
  pectoralis major myocutaneous (PMMC)   78–81
  platysma   82–3
  sternomastoid island myocutaneous   84
  submental artery island   84–6
  trapezius myocutaneous   82
Free flap, common   89, 90, 91; *see also* Flap
  and conventional flaps   86–8

---

*In this index, HNC stands for head and neck cancer and the letter 't' after a page number represents a table and 'f' represents a figure.

Free skin graft　72–3
Free tissue transfer　86–8, 119–20

Hands-free speech　240; *see* Voice restoration
Head and neck malignancies, role of imaging in　47–55
HNC
　　acantholytic SCC　35
　　advanced stage　28
　　aetiology　8–11, 9t
　　apoptotic pathway　260
　　basaloid SCC　35
　　carcinoma *in situ*　34
　　chemotherapy　28, 67–71
　　classification　24–6, 25t
　　dietary factors　10
　　distant spread　14–15
　　dysphagia following surgery for　226
　　early stage　28
　　epidemiology　2–8
　　epithelial premalignant lesions　34
　　epithelial tumours　33–7
　　evaluation　19–22
　　familial and genetic factors　11
　　fibreoptic examination　22
　　focal epithelial hyperplasia　34
　　follow up and rehabilitation　28–9
　　functional outcomes and QOL　29, 247–51
　　germ cell tumours　38
　　glandular lesions　36
　　historical perspective　1–2
　　history-taking　19–20
　　immature teratomas　38
　　invasive SCC　34–5
　　investigations　22–4, 61
　　keratoacanthoma　34
　　lymphatic spread　13–14
　　management　22–9
　　mature teratoma　39
　　metastatic work-up　22
　　microscopy of chondrosarcomas　41
　　molecular biology　256
　　multidisciplinary team (MDT) approach　19
　　multiple primaries　15
　　N-stage classification　26t
　　neck node levels　20, 21t
　　newer agents　28
　　nutritional assessment　22
　　oral submucous fibrosis　34
　　outcomes　29
　　papillary squamous hyperplasia　34
　　papilloma of the sinonasal tract　33
　　paraganglioma　42
　　pathogenesis and natural history　11–15
　　pathology of　33–46
　　physical examination　20–2
　　post-treatment surveillance　267–71
　　primary lesion　12–13
　　psychosocial assessment　22
　　quality of life　29
　　radiology of　47–55

HNC (*continued*)
　　radiotherapy　28, 57–65
　　reconstruction in　72–92
　　rehabilitation in　28
　　sensory-motor examination　22
　　sinonasal terato carcinosarcoma　39
　　sites of　2, 4f
　　spindle cell carcinoma　35
　　squamous papillomas　33
　　staging of　26, 26t
　　surgery for　27–8
　　survival, influencing factors　29
　　swallowing rehabilitation following　225–34
　　targeted drugs　257
　　therapeutic approaches　256–64
　　TNM classification　24–5
　　treatment　26–7, 27t
　　upper aerodigestive tract (UADT)　20
　　variants of SCC　35
　　verrucous carcinoma　35
　　and swallowing　226
Human immunodeficiency virus (HIV)　10, 111
Human papillomavirus (HPV)　10, 104, 110
Hypopharynx, cancer of the　51, 143, 144
　　locally advanced　146
　　management　145–8
　　radiation in　49, 65
　　surgery after radiotherapy failure　148
　　TNM staging　25, 145
　　voice rehabilitation after surgery　148

Induction chemotherapy　68, 68t
　　followed by concurrent chemoradiation therapy　69
　　role of taxanes in　68, 69t
Intensity-modulated radiation therapy (IMRT) in cancer of the
　　oropharynx　120

Jaws and skull, bone tumours of　40–2

Kadish staging system　154

Laryngeal malignancies　124t
Laryngectomy
　　near total　138
　　total　138–9
Larynx, cancer of the　25, 49, 50–1
　　early stage　123–34
　　　　anatomical considerations　123–4, 124f
　　　　conservative salvage surgery after failed RT　128–9
　　　　conservative surgical strategies after failure of RT　129–3
　　　　horizontal laryngectomies　126–8, 127t
　　　　management principles　125–6
　　　　open partial laryngectomy (OPL)　133
　　　　pattern of tumour spread　124, 125, 125f
　　　　radiation in　65
　　　　staging of laryngeal carcinoma　129
　　　　supracricoid laryngectomy (SCL) after failure of RT　130–3
　　　　transoral laser surgery after failure of RT　130
　　　　treating neck lymph node metastases　133

Larynx, cancer of the (*continued*)
    advanced stage   136–41
        anatomy   136
        chemoradiation   137–8
        diagnosis and evaluation   137
        management   137–41
Lip and oral cavity, cancer of   103–12; *see also* Oral cancers

Malignant melanoma   213–14
    desmoplastic melanomas (DMs)   213
    histology   213
    lentigo maligna (LM) melanoma   213
    management   214
    microstaging   213–14
    mucosal melanomas   213
    nodular melanoma   213
    superficial spreading melanoma   213
Malignant tumours of the ceruminous glands   218
Malignant tumours of the parotid   188–9, *see* Parotid
Merkel cell carcinoma of the head and neck   217
Metastatic tumours in the head and neck   42
    metastasis to craniofacial bones and sinuses   42
    metastasis to lymph nodes   42
Microvascular free tissue transfer   86–92; *see also* Flap
Middle ear
    acoustic neuroma   43
    benign tumours   219
    endolymphatic sac tumour   43
    Langerhans cell histocytosis   143
    malignant tumours   219
    papillary adenocarcinoma   43
    Schneiderian papilloma and inverted papilloma   43
    tumours of the   43, 219–20
Molecular biology of HNC   256–7
Molecularly targeted drugs for HNC   257, 257f
Mucosal melanoma of the head and neck   214–15
    investigations   214–15
    prognosis   215
    staging   214
    treatment   215
Multinodular goitre   179–80

N0 neck   96–7
N+ neck   98
    adjuvant radiation therapy/chemotherapy   100
    adverse histological features   99
    bilateral nodes and the second jugular vein   99
    carotid artery   99
    contralateral N0 neck   99
    cystic cervical metastases   99
    dissection after chemoradiation   100
    fixed nodes   99–100
    palliative treatment   100
    primary unknown 100
    retropharyngeal nodes   100
    salvage neck dissection   100
    specificity of clinical staging   98
    type of dissection   98
Nasal airflow inducing manoeuvre (NAIM)   244; *see also* Olfactory
    rehabilitation

Nasopharynx   167
    anatomy   168, 169t
    angiofibroma   38
    brachytherapy   172
    cancer of the   38, 49–50, 156, 167–71
    concurrent chemoradiation followed by adjuvant chemotherapy   172
    diagnostic and staging work-up   170–1
    induction chemotherapy followed by RT   172
    laboratory studies   170
    local extension   168–9
    otological assessment   170
    radiological investigations   49, 170
    recurrent carcinoma   172
    re-irradation   173
    role of palliative radiation   172
    surgery   172
    treatment   171–3
    TNM staging   25, 168
    WHO classification   167
Neck dissection, nose and paranasal sinuses, cancer of the   165
Neuroectodermal tumours   38
    Ewing sarcoma/primitive neuroectodermal tumour (EWS/PNET)   38
    of infancy   38
    olfactory neuroblastoma   38
    mucosal malignant melanoma   38
    nasal glioma   38
Neuroendocrine tumours   37–8
Nose and paranasal sinuses, cancer of the
    adenocarcinoma   154
    adenoid cystic carcinoma   154–5
    aetiology   151–2
    benign epithelial tumours   152–3
    benign non-epithelial tumours   152
    chondrosarcoma   153
    classification of cancer by site   156
    clinical features   155
    extramedullary plasmacytoma   154
    haemangiopericytoma   153
    lateral rhinotomy with medial maxillectomy   158–60
    lymphoma   154
    malignant epithelial tumours   154
    malignant non-epithelial tumours   153
    management of the orbit   162
    melanoma   154
    metastatic tumours   155
    midfacial degloving approach   160
    neurogenic sarcomas   153
    olfactory neuroblastoma   154
    osteosarcoma   153
    pathology   152–5, 152t
    rhabdomyosarcoma   153
    sinonasal undifferentiated carcinoma   155
    squamous cell carcinoma   155
    surgical anatomy   150–1
    surgical treatment   158–62
    treatment rationale   157–8
    TNM classification   157

Odontogenic tumours   39
    ameloblastic adenomatoid tumour   39

Odontogenic tumours (*continued*)
  ameloblastoma 39
  calcifying epithelial odontogenic tumours (Pindborg tumours) 39
  myxoma (fibromyxoma) 40
  soft mixed odontoma 39–40
Oesophageal speech 241–2
  inhalation method 242
  injection method 241
Olfactory rehabilitation after total laryngectomy 242–3
  anatomical and physiological changes 242–3
  different manoeuvres 243–4
  nasal airflow inducing manoeuvre (NAIM) 244
  prosthetic device to improve the olfaction 243
  techniques 243–4
Oral cancer and mandible 111
  invasion of OSCCs 111–12
  surgical significance of 112
Oral cancer in young adults 110–11
Oral cancers/malignancies 47–9, 103–5
  advanced oral cancers 109
  alcohol 104
  anatomy 103
  carcinogenesis 104
  chronic carcinogen exposure 104
  classification 25, 105
  clinical features 105
  differential diagnosis 105
  endoscopic examination 105
  epidemiology 103
  gene therapy 110
  histopathological tissue diagnosis 105
  history and physical examination 105
  human papillomavirus (HPV) 104
  imaging 105
  locally advanced inoperable and metastatic disease 110
  locally advanced operable lesions 110
  lymphatic drainage 103
  postoperative radiotherapy 109
  preoperative chemotherapy 109
  surgery for primary disease 109, 109t
  survival 110
  TNM staging 105–8
  tobacco and betel quid 104
  treatment 108–9
Oropharynx, cancer of the 114, 115
  evaluation and staging 116
  multidisciplinary management team 114
  pattern of tumour spread 115-16
  photodynamic therapy 120
  principles of treatment 117
  radiotherapy and chemo-radiotherapy, chemotherapy 120–1
  radiation in 64–5
  rehabilitation 121
  reconstruction 119
  surgery 118–19
  treatment options 117–18
  TNM staging 25
Osteoid-producing tumours 40
  chondroid tumours 41
  chordoma 41

Osteoid-producing tumours (*continued*)
  fibrous dysplasia 41-2
  osteoma of the skull 40
  osteosarcoma 40–1
Osteomas and exostosis 218–19

Paranasal sinuses
  carcinoma of the 156
  ethmoid sinuses, carcinoma of the 156–7
Parathyroid glands 177–8
Parotid tumour, treatment 189–92
  anatomy 185–6
  benign tumours of the parotid 187–8
    oncocytoma 188
    pleomorphic adenoma 187
    Warthin tumour 187–8
  vasculature of the 186–7
Pedicled flap, reconstruction of the oropharynx 119
Pemberton manoeuvre 179
Pharynx *see* Nasopharynx
Photodynamic therapy (PDT) 120; *see also* Oropharynx
Pindborg tumours 39
Post-laryngectomy voice restoration with TEP 240; *see also* Voice restoration
Post-treatment surveillance in HNC 267
  cost–benefit analysis 271
  endoscopy 270
  follow-up visits 267–8
  imaging studies 268–70
  thyroid function tests 270
  tumour markers 270
Pulmonary rehabilitation after total laryngectomy 242; *see also* Olfactory rehabilitation

Quality of life (QOL) 29, 141, 247–51
  outcome measures 248–9, 249f, 250t
  outcomes in HNC 247–8, 248f
  outcomes, limitations of research in HNC 249–51, 250t
  issues in cancer of the larynx, advanced stage 141

Radiation oncology 58–9
Radiobiology 58
Radiotherapy 57–62, 120, 190
  combined with chemotherapy 61
  combined with surgery 61
  delivery techniques 58–63
  fractionation 59
  oral cavity 63–4
  postoperative indications for 62
  side-effects 60
  and dental care 63
Reconstruction in HNC, *see also* Skin graft, Flap
Reconstruction, nose and paranasal sinuses 164–5, 165t

Salivary glands, cancer of the; *see also* Parotid tumour
  acinic cell carcinoma 36
  adenoid cystic carcinoma 36–7
  basal cell adenoma 36
  canalicular adenoma 36
  carcinoma ex-pleomorphic adenoma 37

Salivary glands, cancer of the (*continued*)
    cystadenoma   36
    epithelial–myoepithelial carcinoma   37
    mucoepidermoid carcinoma   36
    myoepithelial carcinoma   37
    myoepithelioma   36
    occurrence of cancer   185, 185f
    oncocytoma   36
    pleomorphic adenoma   36
    polymorphous low-grade adenocarcinoma   37
    radiation in   65
    salivary duct carcinoma   37
    staging of primary   189
    Warthin tumour   36
Secondary speech restoration   239; *see* Speech restoration, Voice
        restoration
Sinonasal neoplasms   51, 51t
    adenoid cystic carcinomas   52, 53f
    challenges in imaging   51
    lymphomas   52–3
    olfactory neuroblastomas   53, 53f
    undifferentiated carcinoma   38
Skin flap for local reconstruction   73–4; *see* Flap
Skin graft   73; *see also* Free skin graft
    composite graft (full thickness skin and cartilage)   73
    full thickness skin graft   73
    oropharynx, reconstruction of   119
    split thickness skin graft   73
Skin tumours   212–17, 212t
Skull base, cancer of the
    imaging   198–200
    cerebral blood flow evaluation   199–200
    rare tumours   196–8
    surgical anatomy   193–5
    tumour spread   195–6
Skull base surgery   200
    approaches to the anterior skull base   201
        basal sub-frontal approach   203–4
        craniofacial approach   201
        craniotomy   201–2
        facial approach   201
        reconstruction   202–3
        technique of craniofacial approach   201
    approaches to the middle skull base   205–9
        facial translocation approach   206–7
        infratemporal approaches of Fisch types A, B and C   207–8
        petrosectomy   208–9
        preauricular approach   205–6
    approaches to the posterior skull base   209
        transtemporal approaches   209
    complications   209–10
    preoperative embolization   200
Speech rehabilitation after total laryngectomy   237–8; *see also* Voice
        restoration
Speech restoration after laryngectomy, non-surgical   240–2
    primary   238–9
        insertion of voice prostheses   238–9
        selection of patients   238
    secondary   239–40
        common problems   239–40

Speech restoration after laryngectomy, non-surgical (*continued*)
    Secondary
        indwelling versus non-indwelling voice prostheses   240
        leakage around the prostheses   239–40
        leakage through the prostheses   239
Squamous cell carcinoma (SCC)
    of the external meatus   218
    of the head and neck   216–17, 219
Surgical restoration of alaryngeal speech   237–8
    neoglottic reconstruction   237
    shunt techniques   237–8
Swallowing mechanism   225–6, 225f
    oesophageal phase   226
    oral preparatory phase   226
    pharyngeal phase   226
Swallowing rehabilitation   232–4
    chemotherapy   231
    dysphagia and aspiration   225
    hypopharyngeal surgery   229–30
    near total laryngectomy   229
    oral and oropharyngeal surgery   226–8
    partial laryngectomy   228
    radiotherapy   230
    skull base surgery   230–1
    supracricoid laryngectomy   229
    supraglottic laryngectomy   228–9
    total laryngectomy   229
    tracheostomy   228

Targeting cellular immortalization   262
Targeting growth factor independence   257–60, 257f
Targeting insensitivity to anti-growth signals   260
Targeting invasion and metastasis   263–4
Targeting sustained angiogenesis   262, 262t, 263f
    anti-angiogenic agents   262
    vascular disrupting agents   262
Targeting the apoptotic pathway   260–1, 261f
Therapeutic approaches to HNC   256–64
Thyroid, cancer of the
    aetiology and pathophysiology   178
    clinical features   178–9
    follicular neoplasm   44
    lymphatic drainage of the   178
    malignancies of   180
    malignant lymphoma   45
    medullary thyroid carcinoma (MTC)   44
    papillary carcinoma and variants   43–4
    paraganglioma   45
    poorly differentiated carcinoma (insular carcinoma)   44–5, 45t
    primary squamous cell carcinomas   45
    sarcomas of the thyroid   45
    secondary tumours   45
    surgical pathology   178
    TNM staging   25
    undifferentiated (anaplastic) carcinoma   45
Thyroid and parathyroid glands, surgical anatomy   175–6
Thyroid malignancies, imaging   53–5
Thyroid nodule   181–2, 182t
    managing the upper pole   184
    subcapular dissection   183

Thyroid nodule (*continued*)
    surgical pearls 183–4
    treatment policy
        benign thyroid swellings 182
        malignant thyroid lesions 182
        management of neck nodes in well differentiated thyroid
            carcinoma 182–3
        total versus partial thyroidectomies (essential
            lobectomy) 183
TNM (Tumour Node Metastasis) classification in HNC 25–6, 253–5
    hypopharynx 145
    nose and paranasal sinuses 157
    nasopharynx 168
    controversies in TNM staging 253–4
    lip and oral cavity 105–8

TNM (Tumour Node Metastasis) classification in HNC (*continued*)
    other staging systems 254
    salivary grands 189
Tracheo-oesophageal (TE) voice using prostheses 238

UCLA (University of California, Los Angeles) staging system 154
University of Pittsbergh staging system 218

Voice restoration after total laryngectomy 139–41, 237
Voice rehabilitation after surgery for hypopharyngeal cancer 148

Well differentiated carcinoma, pathology of 180–8
WHO classification
    ear, tumour of the 217
    nasopharynx, tumour of the 167